Textbook of
Biotechnology
(Fundamentals of Molecular Biology)

Textbook of Biotechnology
(Fundamentals of Molecular Biology)

S.K. Jain
M.Sc., Ph.D.
Professor of Biotechnology,
Head, Centre for Biotechnology, &
Dean, Faculty of Science
Hamdard University, New Delhi

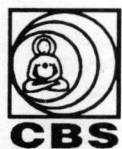

CBS

CBS Publishers & Distributors Pvt. Ltd.

New Delhi • Bengaluru • Chennai • Kochi • Kolkata • Mumbai
Hyderabad • Uttarakhand • Nagpur • Patna • Pune • Jharkhand

ISBN: 81-239-0699-4

First Edition: 2000
Reprint: 2002, 2003, 2004, 2006, 2008, 2011, 2018

Published by **Satish Kumar Jain** and produced by **Varun Jain** for
CBS Publishers & Distributors Pvt. Ltd.,
4819/XI Prahlad Street, 24 Ansari Road, Daryaganj, New Delhi - 110002
delhi@cbspd.com, cbspubs@airtelmail.in • www.cbspd.com
Ph.: 23289259, 23266861, 23266867 • Fax: 011-23243014

Corporate Office: 204 FIE, Industrial Area, Patparganj, Delhi - 110 092
Ph: 49344934 • Fax: 011-49344935
E-mail: publishing@cbspd.com • publicity@cbspd.com

Branches:
• *Bengaluru:* 2975, 17th Cross, K.R. Road, Bansankari 2nd Stage,
  Bengaluru - 70 • Ph: +91-80-26771678/79 • Fax: +91-80-26771680
  E-mail: cbsbng@gmail.com, bangalore@cbspd.com
• *Chennai:* No. 7, Subbaraya Street, Shenoy Nagar, Chennai - 600030
  Ph: +91-44-26681266, 26680620 • Fax: +91-44-42032115
  E-mail: chennai@cbspd.com
• *Kochi:* Ashana House, 39/1904, A.M. Thomas Road, Valanjambalam,
  Ernakulum, Kochi • Ph: +91-484-4059061-65
  Fax: +91-484-4059065 • E-mail: cochin@cbspd.com
• *Kolkata:* 6-B, Ground Floor, Rameshwar Shaw Road, Kolkata - 700014
  Ph: +91-33-22891126/7/8 • E-mail: kolkata@cbspd.com
• *Mumbai:* 83-C, Dr. E. Moses Road, Worli, Mumbai - 400018
  Ph: +91-9833017933, 022-24902340/41 • E-mail: mumbai@cbspd.com

Representatives:

• Hyderabad: 0-9885175004   • Nagpur: 0-9021734563
• Patna: 0-9334159340   • Pune: 0-9623451994
• Jharkhand: 0-9811541605   • Uttarakhand: 0-9716462459

Printed at:
J.S. Offset Printers, Delhi (India)

Preface

Biotechnology is an ancient science as old as the civilization itself. It began with the domestication of useful plants and animals. The use of yeast to make bread and wines dates back to more than 5000 years. With the advent of scientific approach, various new techniques were developed and used for the welfare of mankind. However, last 50 years have seen fast changes in the field of biotechnology.

Modern biotechnology started with the discovery of double helical structure of DNA. Subsequent investigations that helped in unravelling the processes of inheritance pattern provided further impetus to biotechnological research. The elaborate information on gene structure, function and regulation laid the foundation of biotechnology on a firm footing. Synthesis of artificial genes that could function in vitro and the process of reverse transcription discovered in certain organisms paved the way for a new field of science, namely genetic engineering and the comprehensive utilization of the technique in biotechnology.

Recombinant DNA technology has opened new vistas in promoting human welfare. The feasibility of the technique has been established and it has many practical applications in the production of various biochemicals including the enzymes and drugs as well as other industrial chemicals by commercially viable methods. The technique also has applications in creation of novel nucleic acid and protein molecules and in obtaining these in abundant amounts. Use of biotechnology is gaining importance in generation of improved varieties of economically important plants with desired traits such as disease resistance, requirement of lesser amounts of fertilizer etc., thus making large savings on fertilizers, insecticides, herbicides and pesticides etc. The isolation and characterization of desired genes have been accomplished and used fruitfully. Another approach of genetic engineering that can be successfully used is in creation of genetically designed organisms with economically important features.

In order to develop an expertise in genetic engineering and biotechnology it is essential that the fundamental principles of molecular biology are well understood. The life itself is an organized interaction of various biomolecules. Any interference in correct organization of these molecules leads to pathological state, disease and even death. Here I would like to quote a couplet written by an Urdu poet, Shri Chakbast Lucknawi, which explains the importance of molecular components in life. The couplet is:

Zindgi kya hai, ansair mein zahur-e-tarteeb.
Maut kya hai, inhin ajza ka pareeshan hona.

This can be translated as following:

> What is life? It is a systematic arrangement of components (biomolecules).
>
> What is death? It is the disorganization of the same components.

It is almost impossible to understand the biological science without the fundamental knowledge of molecular biology. Though molecular biology has also evolved along with other sciences, it has made very rapid strides during the last 25 years. Earlier as a student and then as a teacher of molecular biology I had felt the need for clear and concise books in this field. Most of the currently available books are by foreign authors and are often difficult to understand by an average Indian student who is beginning his venture in the field of molecular biology.

The present book is aimed at filling this gap. The book covers the entire gamut of molecule biology; from structure of DNA to gene structure; regulation of its expression and principles of genetic engineering in detail in a simple and easy to understand language. The book covers the syllabus of Indian Universities and shall fulfill the requirement of students of Biology, Biochemistry, Biotechnology and other biological sciences at both the undergraduate and postgraduate level.

It has not been an easy job to write this book. A number of my colleagues and students have directly or indirectly contributed in preparation of the manuscript and I express my gratitude to them all. The understanding and encouragement I received from my family motivated me to finish the task in time. Feedbacks and suggestions from my son, Pankaj, have been very useful. I would like to express my appreciation for Sri Satish Jain, Sri Vinod Jain and a number of staff members of CBS Publishers & Distributors, New Delhi, for their help in timely publication of the book.

January, 2000   S.K. Jain
Hamdard University, New Delhi - 110 062

Contents

Rho independent termination). Eukaryotic transcription. Post-transcriptinal modifacations. Splicing of pre-mRNA. Nuclear splicing: lariat formation. Role of SnRNPs: the splisomes. Autosplicing. Splicing of tRNAs. Production of multiple mRNA from one gene: the alternate splicing. Self-cleavage of viroids and virusoids. RNA processing. Cap formation and polyadenylation. Replication of genome of RNA viruses (By reverse transcriptase; By RNA dependent RNA polymerase).

Messenger RNA. Essential features of mRNA structure. Abundance of mRNAs. Genetic code. Genetic code is universal. Degeneraticity of genetic code. Exception to universal code. Anticodons. Machinery for translation. Ribosomes. Transfer RNA. Wobble theory. Aminoacyl tRNA synthetase. Prokaryotic and eukaryotic translation factors. Events in protein synthesis. Role of SD sequences. Kozak's scanning model for initiation of eukaryotic translation. Activation of aminoacids and aminoacyl tRNA formation. Initiation. Elongation. Termination of translation. Fidility of protein synthesis. Role of tRNA synthetase. Proof reading function of ribosomes. GTPase timer. Post-translational modifications. Modification of N-terminal ends. Formation of disulphide bond. Oligomerization. Proteolytic cleavage. Cleavage of signal peptide. Addition of prosthetic group. Protein phosphorylation. Glycosylation. O-liked glycosylation. N-linked glycosylation. Dolichol. High mannose carbohydrate addition. Processing of carbohydrate moity. The events in Golgi and ER. Other modifications.

Gene expression is related to metabolic state of the cell. Constitutive expression. Regulated expression. Role of transcription factors. DNA binding. Motifs. Helix-turn-helix motif. Zinc finger motif. Leucine zippers. Helix-loop-helix motif. Catabolic repression. Operon theory. Lac operon. Trp operon. Gal operon. Ara operon. Attenuation: role of alternate RNA structure. Gene regulation in lambda phage: lytic and lysogenic cascade. Regulation of gene expression by genetic recombination. Regulation of gene expression in yeast cell specificity. Regulation of yeast mating types. Regualtion of gene expression in drosophila. Alternate splicing plays regulatory role. Factors affecting gene expression. Role of Sigma factors. Heat shock genes. Regulation by heavy metals. Other stress genes. Hormone dependent genes. Cell surface receptor-ligand interaction. Regulation of proto-oncogenes. Other mechanisms. Cytoplasmic control of gene expression. Poly (A) tail. Sequences at the 3'-untranslated region of mRNA. Autoregulation. Hormonal regulation. Concentration of micronutrients. Other factors affecting rate of translation.

Free and membrane bound polysomes. Membrane bound proteins. Signal peptide and signal recognition particles. The signal hypothesis. Transport vesicles. Clathrin containing and non-clathrin vesicles. Direction of protein transport. Translocation of proteins to organelles.

1

Pathway for the Transfer of Genetic Information
The Central Dogma of Molecular Biology

A cell is the basic unit of life. The living cells are seemingly very complex entities with a number of intracellular compartments and cell organelles. However, critical analysis of entire cell content reveals that it is composed of a number of chemical substances which are similar to other chemicals in their nature and follow the basic principles of physics, chemistry and thermodynamics. How does the living cell, then differ from a test tube with all these chemicals? In the cell these compounds are present in a well defined and organized manner. Some of these cell constituents are simple chemicals such as NaCl, glucose, ATP etc. while others are very complex compounds of large molecular weight. Many of the complex substances, referred as bio-macromolecules, are found only in living cells. The numerous compounds of different size, shape and chemical composition as well as having different properties interact with each other and many chemical reactions are continuously and simultaneously taking place in the cell at any given moment. Again these reactions take place in a highly ordered manner and are very precisely regulated. The proper organization of the complex chemicals and the precise regulation of the biochemical reactions is the basis of life. Any distortion or impairment of these events results in pathological conditions and may even lead to cell death.

The principal bio-macromolecules can be divided into four major classes namely, proteins, lipids, carbohydrates and nucleic acids. Each of these has diverified but well defined roles. The carbohydrates and lipids are the main source of energy in the body. Besides being the source of energy, the lipids have certain other roles also, such as these are the essential part of the membrane structure. Majority of the cellular functions are mediated through enzymes, which are mostly protein in nature. Proteins also serve as important structural constituent of the cell. Besides, a number of protein factors serve as the regulator of various metabolic pathways. Nucleic acids on the other hand, are involved in storage and transfer of genetic information and provide the biological diversity and specific characters to different organism and also to cells.

Nucleic acids are complex molecules, synthesized by polymerization of small building blocks, the nucleotides. Two types of structurally related but functionally distinct nucleic acids, the ribonucleic acid (RNA) and deoxy-ribonucleic acid (DNA), are found in the cell. DNA is the basic genetic material in almost all the organisms. Further, it is the only molecule which has the capability to produce its own copies by a process known as replication. The only known exceptions to these fundamental rules are certain viruses (retroviruses and the reoviruses), which have RNA as their genetic material. In retroviruses, the replication of genomic RNA requires an obligatory synthesis of DNA as an intermediate in the process However, the RNA genome of reoviruses replicates without any asistance or involvement of DNA. The DNA is arranged in a highly ordered manner to form long thread like structures, the chromosomes. A number of proteins participate in the organization of chromosomal structure. The chromosomes are highly condensed structure and accomodate large amounts of DNA in relatively small space. There are usually more than one chromosomes in a cell, the number of chromosomes depends upon the evolutionary complexity of the organism. The amount of DNA, its organization and the number of chromosomes are the characteristic properties of any species. These properties do not vary from cell to cell or individual to individual within the same species. However, these vary from species to species. The chromosomes are present in the nucleus of eukaryotes. Prokaryotes donot have defined nucleus. However, the DNA in prokaryotes is also arranged in form of a chromosome. The bacterial chromosomes are present in a relatively dense region of the cytoplasm, referred as nucleoid. While DNA stores and transfers the genetic information from one generation to another, most of the cellular functions are mediated through proteins. This information is finally expressed in the form of a protein by a series of intermediary processes. The first step in the expression of genetic information involves the transfer of the information present in DNA to RNA. The DNA and RNA, both have similar basic structure and are made with four different types of nucleotides (the A,T,C and G in DNA and A,U,C and G in RNA) which are their building blocks. Different informations are stored in coded form by different sequence of these four nucleotides. This process of transfer of information from DNA to RNA is known as the transcription. Transcription is primarily carried out by the enzyme RNA poly-merase, though a number of other enzymes and trans acting factors assist in this process. In the retroviruses (which have RNA as their genetic material but replicate through DNA) first a true copy of the genome in the form of DNA which is complementary to RNA, is synthesized by a process which is the reversal of transcription. This process is mediated by reverse transcriptase, an enzyme present only in retro-viruses and not in any other organism. The DNA is then replicated and transcribed by normal pro-cesses to produce multiple copies of genomic RNA. The genomic RNA of reoviruses, on the other hand, is self replicated through a specialized enzyme, the RNA dependent RNA polymerase or the RNA replicase. The RNA is then transported to cytoplasm where the information carried by it is decoded and transferred to a structurally unrelated form, the proteins. This process is probably the most complex cellular process and is referred as the translation. The ribosomes serve as the site of protein synthesis and a number of enzymes and other trans acting factors participate in this process. As will be discussed later, the proteins are madeup of totally unrelated building blocks, the aminoacids. There are twenty different aminoacids which participate in the synthesis of proteins. Thus an information written in a language of only four letters is finally translated to a entirely different language with a complex alphabet of twenty aminoacids. This general pathway for the transfer of genetic information from DNA to proteins constitutes the central dogma of molecular biology. It has been diagrammatically illustrated in Fig. 1.1.

It is thus clear that the transfer of information between two types of nucleic acids is reversible and it is possible to interchange it from one form to another. However, once the information has been transfered to the proteins, the transfer is irreversible and it can not revert back to nucleic acid.

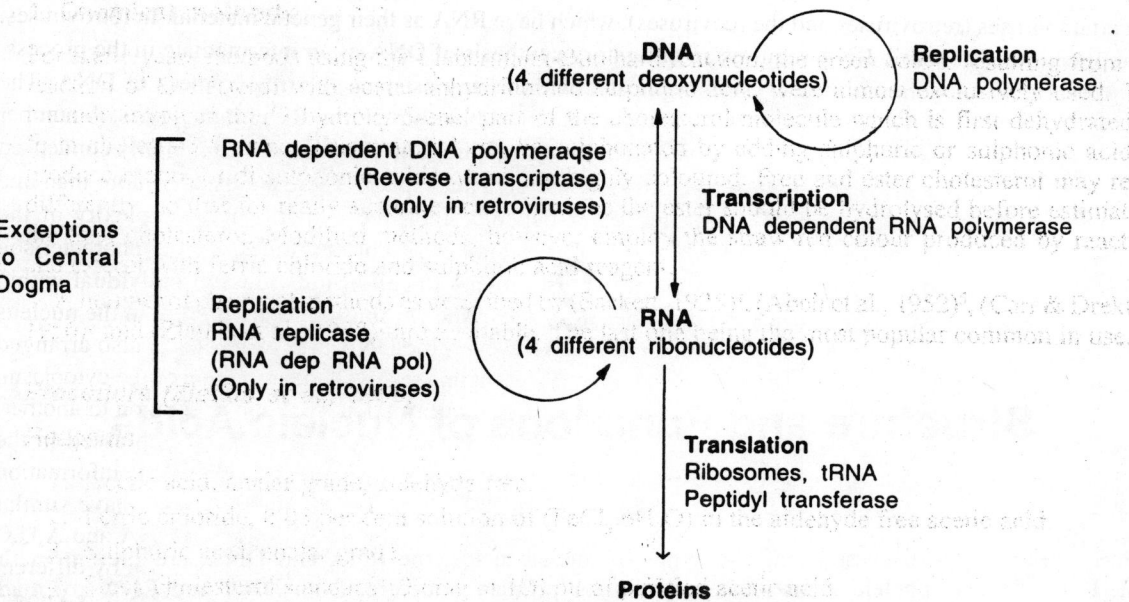

DNA
(4 different deoxynucleotides)

Replication
DNA polymerase

Exceptions to Central Dogma

RNA dependent DNA polymeraqse
(Reverse transcriptase)
(only in retroviruses)

Transcription
DNA dependent RNA polymerase

Replication
RNA replicase
(RNA dep RNA pol)
(Only in retroviruses)

RNA
(4 different ribonucleotides)

Translation
Ribosomes, tRNA
Peptidyl transferase

Proteins
(20 different Aminoacids)

Fig. 1.1. Central dogma of molecular biology.

2

Structure and Functions of Nucleic Acids

It has already been discussed that two types of nucleic acids, the RNA and DNA, are present in the cell. Both of these nucleic acids have very similar primary structure. Both DNA and RNA are made of three basic components, a nitrogeneous base, the sugar and the phosphate groups. The bases are of two types, the purines and the pyrimidines. Two purines, adenine and guanine and two pyrimidines, thymine and cytosine are present in DNA. In RNA thymine is not present but another pyrimidine, the uracil, is present in its place. The sugar moiety is always a pentose. The sugar in RNA is β–D–ribose, while DNA has β–D–2–deoxy ribose (d–ribose). The sugar is always present in its β–furanose configuration. The nitrogen at position 9 of purines and at position 1 of pyrimidines is attached to 1st carbon atom of the sugar through a N–glycosidic bond. The base and sugar together are called as the nucleoside. To differentiate between the positions of carbon and nitrogen atoms constituting the ring of purine and pyrimidine bases from the positions of carbon atoms present in the sugar moiety, the carbons and nitrogens in the base are numbered 1–9 in purines and 1–6 in pyrimidines while the carbon atoms of sugar are numbered as 1'–5'. The 5'–carbon of the sugar is attached to the phosphate group(s) by an ester bond. A maximum of three phosphate groups can be associated with a nucleoside. The phosphorylated form of nucleoside is known as the nucleotide. When more than one phosphate groups are attached, these are present in a linear manner in a nucleotide. The phosphates are numbered as α (the first phosphate attached to the sugar), β (the second) and γ (the third), respectively. Depending on the number of phosphate groups, the nucleotide is a nucleoside monophosphate (NMP), nucleoside diphosphate (NDP) or nucleoside triphosphate (NTP). A nucleotide triphosphate (rNTP in RNA and dNTP in DNA) is the basic building block of nucleic acid. Depending on the base, it is adenosine triphosphate (ATP), cytidine triphosphate (CTP), thymidine triphosphate (TTP, present only in DNA) or uridine triphosphate (UTP, present only in RNA) and guanosine triphosphate (GTP). Usually the bases as well as the nucleotides are written with a single letter as A, T, G, C and U. While talking of DNA, it is understood that nucleotides are deoxy–nucleotides while in RNA these are ribonucleotides. The basic structures of purine and pyrimidine rings, the bases, sugars, nucleosides, and nucleotides and their relationship has been summarised in Fig. 2.1.

Polymerization of nucleotides to form nucleic acids

Nucleotides are polymerised in a linear fashion through enzymatic condensation to form long polymers. The sugar moieties of two adjacent nucleotides are joined together through a bond mediated by the phosphate

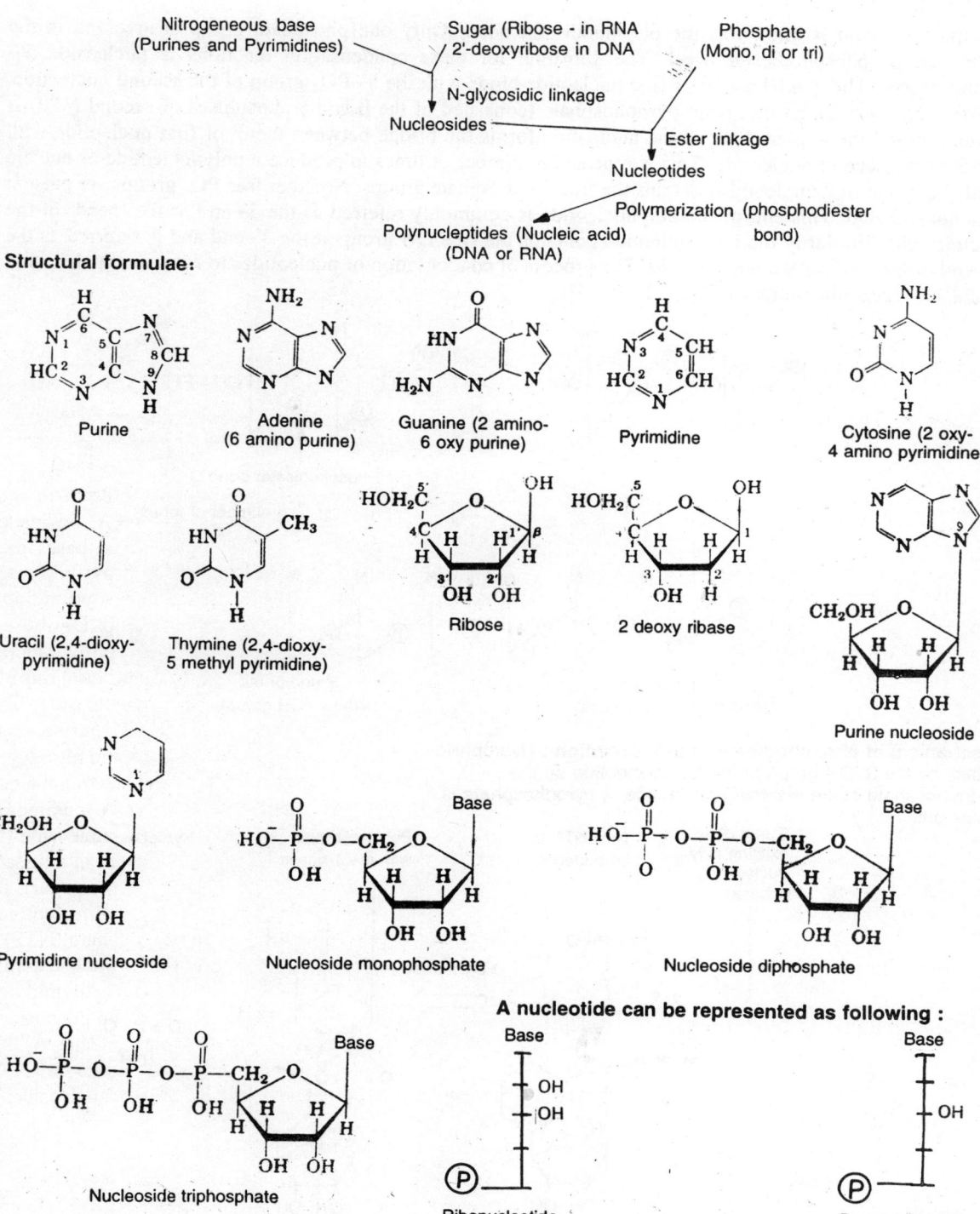

Fig. 2.1. Basic units of nucleic acids.

group. This bond is known as the phosphodiester bond. Only one phosphate group is involved in the formation of phosphodiester bond. The substrate for these condensation reactions is nucleoside 5'–triphosphates. The 3'–OH group of first nucleotide binds with the 5'–PO_4 group of the second nucleotide. During this process, an inorganic pyrophosphate (consisted of the β and γ phosphates of second NTP) is given out and the α phosphate of the nucleotide forms the bridge between the 3' of first nucleotide with the 5' of the second nucleotide. This repeated n number of times to produce a polynucleotide or nucleic acid. Thus, the first nucleotide contains the free 5'–phosphate groups. No other free PO_4 groups are present in a nucleic acid. This end of the polynucleotide is commonly referred as the 5'–end or the 'head' of the nucleic acid. Similarly the last nucleotide contains the free OH group at the 3'–end and is referred as the 3'–end or the 'tail' of the nucleic acid. The process of condensation of nucleotides to form the nucleic acid chain has been illustrated in **Fig. 2.2.**

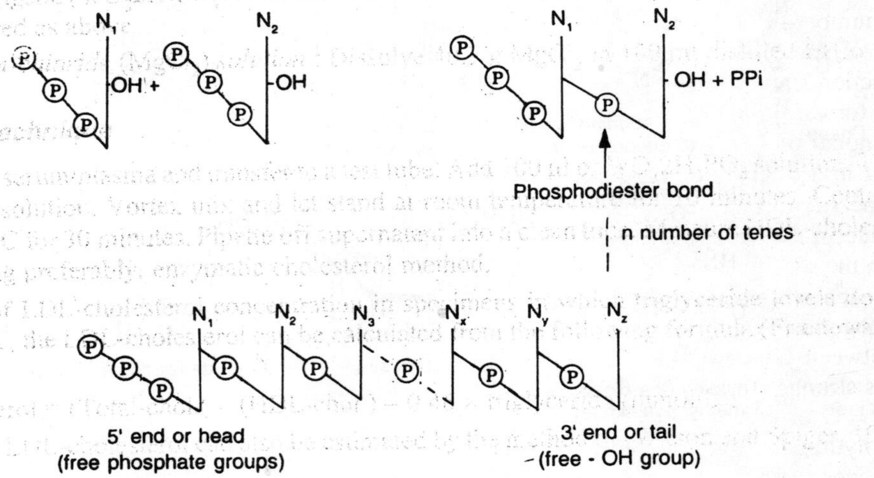

Mechanism of phosphodiester bond formation : Hydrophilic attack by the 3'-OH group of the last nucleotide on the 5'-triphosphate of the incoming nucleotide, a pyrophosphate is given out.

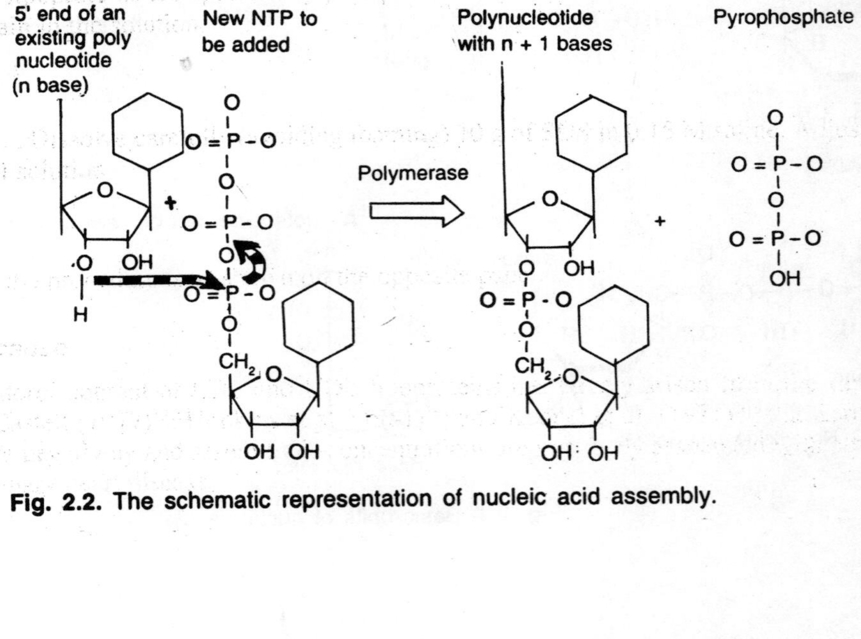

Fig. 2.2. The schematic representation of nucleic acid assembly.

Structure of DNA

The presence of DNA in living cells was established long time back. In 1868, Friedrich Miescher while studying the nucleus of animal cells, found a phosphorus containing material in it. He called it as nuclein. He later isolated nuclein from the nucleus of pus cells obtained from the used surgical bandages. Later it was fractionated into two parts, an acidic material and a basic portion. The acidic part was later called nucleic acid and the basic part consisted of the proteins.

The analysis of DNA from a number of organisms (selected at different positions on the evolutionary ladder) revealed that the base composition of DNA from different organism vary and is unique for a given organism. However, its composition was constant within a particular species and did not vary from individual to individual or from cell to cell within the same individual. Further analysis of the DNA revealed a very interesting observation. It was found that the number of purine nucleotides always equals to pyrimidine nucleotides (A + G = C + T). Further, the number of A residues always equals to the number of T residues and the number of G residues always equals to the number of C residues. This observation suggested the presence of some type of co–relation between the A and T and between the G and C residues. The X–ray defraction studies further depicted these relationships and a number of models for the structure of DNA were put forward. Finally, Watson and Crick analysed these structures in detail and in 1952 proposed their famous model of DNA structure which is now universally accepted. According to this model, the DNA is present in a double stranded from. The two strands are running antiparallel to each other and the 5'–end of one strand faces the 3'–end of the other strand. Further, an A residue in one strand always faces a T residue in the second strand and vice–versa. Similarily a C residue in one strand is paired with a G residue in the second strand and vice–versa. The A and T and the C and G are known as the complementary bases to each other and the two strands of a DNA molecule are complementary strands. The two strands are held together by hydrogen bonds between the complementary bases. There are three possible hydrogen bonds between G and C while only two hydrogen bonds can be formed between A and T. Thus a G : C bond is stronger than the A : T bond. The hydrogen bonds are formed between the $-NH_2$ group of one base and = O of complementary base or between = NH of one and $-N$ of other base. For the formation of stable hydrogen bonds, the N–N distance is 0.30 nm and O–N distance is 0.28–0.29 nm. The positions and distances of these bonds has been shown in Fig. 2.3.

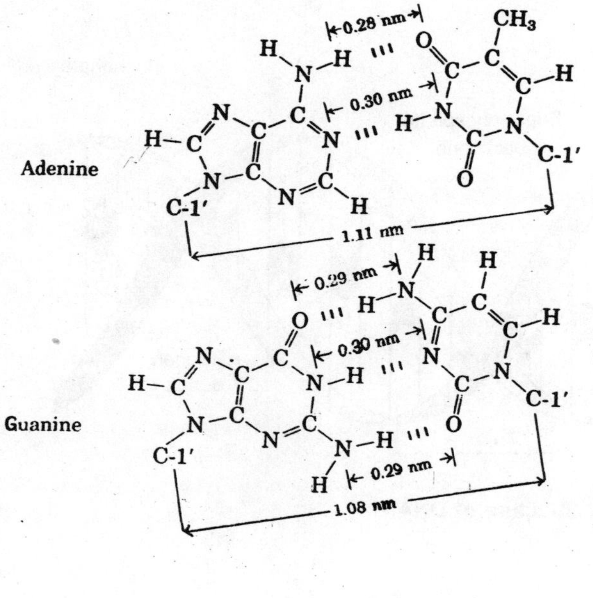

Fig. 2.3. The hydrogen bonds between complementary nucleotides.

It has been found that the two strands of DNA molecule are not present as a linear structure but are coiled in a spring like manner around a common axis. This coiled structure, known as the double helical structure, is highly organised. It is present as a right handed helix having ten bases in a turn. Each base is thus at an angle of 36° to the adjoining base. The linear distance of one complete turn is 34 Å and therefore each base is 3.4 Å away from the adjoining base. The diameter of the helix is 20 Å. The sugars and the phosphates together form the backbone of the helix. In its double helical form, the bases are perpendicular to the axis of the helix and face each other. The position of the sugar–phosphate backbone is towards the outside of the helix at a 90° to the bases. The three dimensional structure of DNA has been shown in Fig. 2.4. As represented in the diagram, the three dimensional structure creates two grooves of different sizes in each turn of the DNA molecule. One of these is large and is known as the major groove while the other is relatively smaller and is known as the minor groove.

SUGAR PHOSPHATE BACKBONE OF DNA

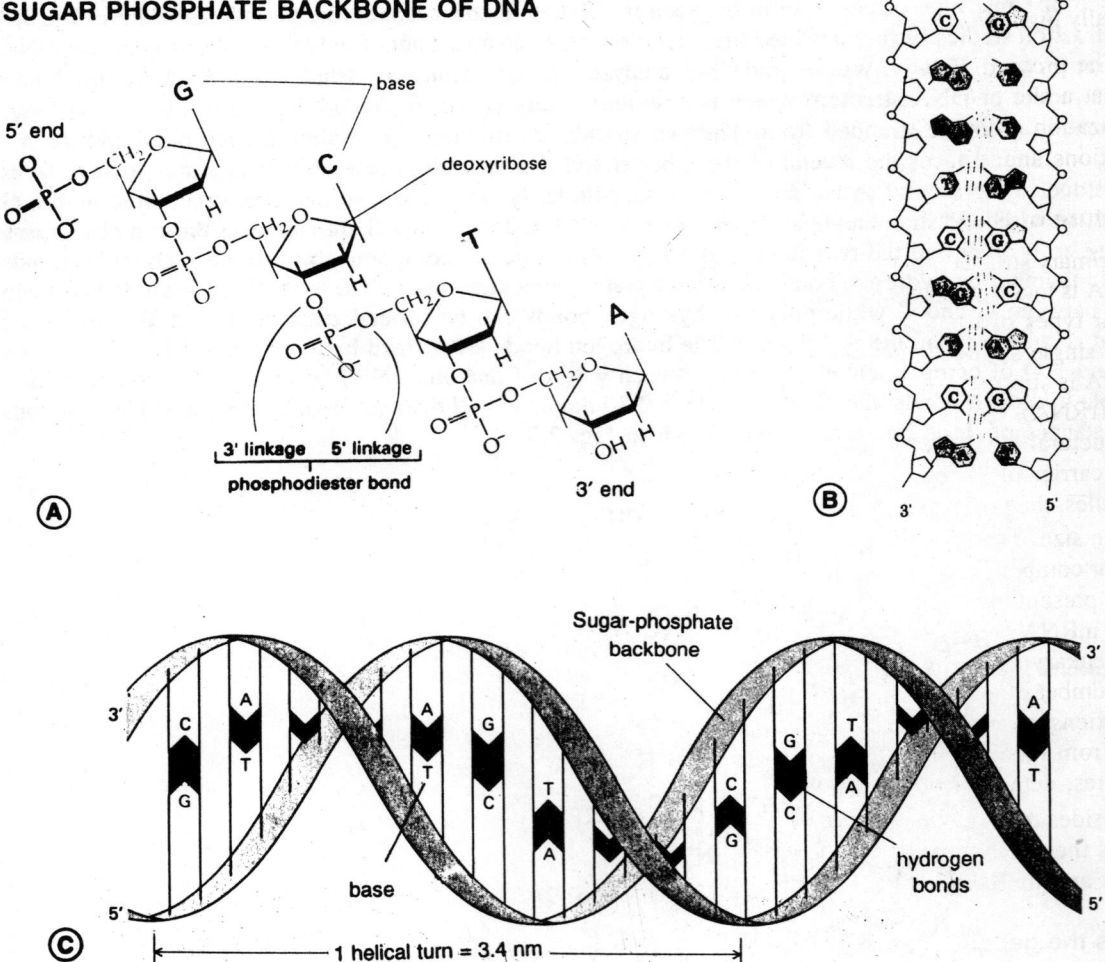

Fig. 2.4. Structure of DNA.

Various Forms of DNA

Majority of DNA of the cell has the three dimensional structure as represented by the Watson–Crick's model described earlier. This form of DNA is known as the 'B–DNA'. However, small amounts of the DNA having alternate molecular structure with certain differences from the B–DNA, are also present. These represent only very minor species. The first alternate structure is that of the A form of DNA which varies from B–DNA in having 11 bases/turn and is more compact than the B–DNA. The presence of A–DNA has been demonstrated in vitro in relatively less hydrous environment and with higher Na+ and K+ concentration. In its three dimensional structure, A form of DNA has close resemblance with the double stranded RNA. Z–DNA, yet another alternate form of DNA, has left handed helix. It contains about 12 bases/turn and the phosphodiester backbone is present in a zig zag manner along the molecule. Defined major and minor grooves are thus not present in Z–DNA. In experimental conditions the existance of Z–DNA had been shown in presence of either high salt conditions or in presence of specific cations such as spermine and spermidine. It has high degree of negative supercoiling and has certain specific proteins attached to it. Besides, there is usually high degree of methylation of C residues at the C5 positions in the Z–DNA.

The precise role of the alternate forms of DNAs is not very clear. These may play certain regulatory roles at a site near to them as well as at the distal sites also. Besides, they may also play some role in stabilization of DNA structure. The possibility that some of these may be the artefacts of experimental conditions and are not present under in vivo conditions may not be completely ruled out.

Structure of RNA

The primary structure of RNA is very similar to the structure of DNA. Though the three dimentional structure of RNA is totally different than the DNA. Similar to DNA, the RNA is also synthesized by the polymerization of four types of ribonucleotides, joined together by a phosphodiester bond. Majority of the RNA in the cell is single stranded. However, some double stranded RNA is also present in the cell. The structure of ds RNA is similar to A–DNA. Three major classes of RNA are present in the cell. These are (a) ribosomal RNA (rRNA), (b) transfer RNA (tRNA) and (c) messenger RNA (mRNA). The rRNA and the tRNA are the structural molecules which play an important role in protein synthesis. The mRNA, on the other hand, is the carrier of genetic information and transfers this information from DNA to the ultimate functional molecules, the proteins. Ribosomal RNAs are the most predominant class of cellular RNA and are relaively large in size. The main rRNAs are 28S and 18S in eukaryotes and 23S and 16S in prokaryotes along with a minor component of 5S present in both eukaryotes and prokaryotes. Besides, another small RNA of 5.8S is also present in eukaryotic ribosomes. The tRNA is relatively small (4S, 75–100 nucleotide) in size. The size of mRNA on the other hand is very heterogeneous, varying from less than 5S to more than 30S. Majority of the eukaryotic mRNA has a size range of 7–15S. Each class of RNA has certain special features. There are a number of modified bases in tRNAs, both tRNA and rRNAs have a highly compact secondary structure with extensive regions of intramolecular double strands and the eukaryotic mRNA has a special structure made from modified bases, the cap, at the 5'–end and a poly(A) tail at the 3'–end. These are specialized structures, details of which will be discussed later.

Besides the three major classes of RNA, a number of small RNA molecules of various size and shape, such as the SnRNA, ScRNA are also present in the cells. These RNAs together form only a very minor species and the details of these will be discussed elsewhere when their role is discussed.

DNA is the genetic material

Even though the DNA was discovered long time back, its role as the carrier of genetic information was established only in 1943. Previously it was believed that the genetic information is transferred through the proteins. Though many biologists had been suspecting that DNA ought to be playing some role in the cell inheritance. For a molecule to carry genetic information from one generation to another generation, it was necessary that the compound should on one hand, be relatively stable and should also be able to replicate itself with a high degree of fidelity, so that it can be transmitted from one generation to another generation countless time without any loss or alteration. On the other hand, it should have enough flexibility so that it can get altered and can account for the evolution. DNA fulfills both these requirements. Way back in 1928, Frederick Griffith did an experiment in which he injected a encapsulated virulent strain of Streptococcus pneumoniae to a mouse and found that mouse developed pneumonia and died. The injection of a non–virulent strain didnot result in either manifestation of the disease or in the death of the animal. He later heat killed the virulent strain and injected these dead bacteria to mouse. These were non–pathogenic and the mouse remained healthy. However, when he injected a mixture of heat killed organisms of the virulent strain along with the living organisms of the non–virulent strain (both of which are non–pathogenic separately), the mouse became sick and died. It suggested that a heat resistant factor was present in the virulent strain which was able to transform the organisms of the non–virulent strain into virulent form (Fig. 2.5). Later, Oswald Avery, Colin MacLeod and Maclyn McCarty in 1943 extracted the material from virulent Pneumococcus which was responsible for the transformation of non–virulent strain. The extracted material was later identified to be DNA by the fact that it had the physical characteristics and elemental analysis of DNA molecule. The transforming property was not lost upon the extraction of lipids and polysaccharides from this material. Further, its transforming property was not lost by its complete enzymatic digestion with proteases. Similarly, upon treatment with RNases, the transforming activity was not lost but treatment with DNase resulted in the loss of this transformation property. These experiments established the identity of the transformationally active material to be DNA. They also found that addition of this DNA to non–virulent strain resulted in its permanent transformation into the virulent form. These experiments clearly showed that DNA was responsible for the transformation of non–virulent strain. However, some scientists still expressed doubts and believed that the transformation of non–virulent strain as seen by Avery et al, was due to small amounts of proteins which might have co–purified with DNA during the isolation procedure and may have been present as the contaminant in their DNA preparation.

Live Virulent strain of S. pneumoniae	injected to ———→ mouse	Mouse died
Heat killed virulent Bacteria	injected to ———→ mouse	Mouse remained alive
Live Non-virulent strain of bacteria	injected to ———→ mouse	Mouse remained alive
Heat killed virulent Strain + live non- virulent strain together	injected to ———→ mouse	Mouse died

Inference : A heat stable factor from killed bacterial of virulent
strain can transform the bacteria of non-virulent strain

Fig. 2.5. The Avory-MacLeod-McCorty experiment.

Later a direct double labelling experiment was carried out by Alfred Hershey and Martha Chase in 1952. They incorporated two separate radioactive precursors into the bacteriophage T$_2$; using the radiolabelled nucleotides, the phage DNA was labelled with ^{32}P and using radiolabelled methionine, the proteins were labelled with ^{35}S. This doubly-labelled phage was used to infect the *E. coli* and the fate of radioactivity was followed. It was found that the ^{32}P has entered inside the host cells and can be recovered from there. The ^{35}S, on the other hand, did not enter the host cell and could be isolated from the cell supernatant (Fig. 2.6). This experiment unambiguously proved that the genetic information is transferred through DNA. We now know it very well that the DNA is the carrier of the genetic information.

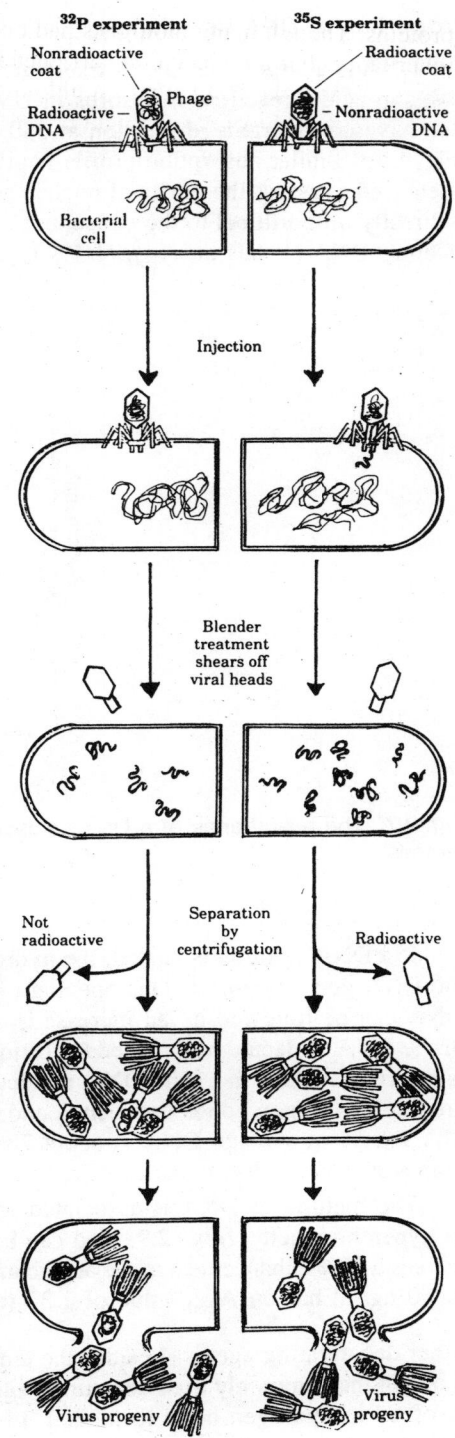

Fig. 2.6. The Hershey-Chase experiment of isotopically-labelled bacteriophage particles were prepared. One was labelled with ^{32}P in the phosphate groups of the DNA and the other with ^{35}S in the sulfur-containing amino acids of the protein coats (capsids). (Note that DNA contains no sulfur, and viral protein no phosphorus.) The two batches of labelled phage were then added to separate suspensions of unlabelled bacteria. Each suspension of phage-infected cells was agitated in a blender to shear the viral capsids from the bacteria. The bacteria and empty viral coats (ghosts) were then separated by centrifugation. The cells infected with the ^{32}P-labelled phage were found to contain ^{32}P, indicating that the labelled viral DNA had entered the cells, and the viral ghosts contained no radioactivity. The cells infected with ^{35}S-labelled phage were found to have no radioactivity after blender treatment, but the viral ghosts contained ^{35}S. Progeny virus particles were produced in both batches of bacteria some time after the viral coats were removed, thus the genetic message for their replication had been introduced by viral DNA, not by viral protein.

Properties of DNA in solution

The DNA is a large molecule. It freely dissolves in water and in many other solvents. In solution the DNA gives an acidic reaction. It absorbs in UV range and has an absorption maxima at 260 nm. However, it also have considerable absorption at 280 nm and the A_{260}/A_{280} ratio of pure DNA is approximately 2.0 (Fig. 2.7). Similar absorption profile is given by single stranded DNA and also by RNA. This property is often used to assess the purity of nucleic acids. The absorbance at 260 nm follows the Beer's law and A_{260} is directly proportional to the concentration of nucleic acid. A solution of ds DNA having a concentration of 50ug DNA/ml has an A_{260} of 1.0 in 1.0 cm light path.

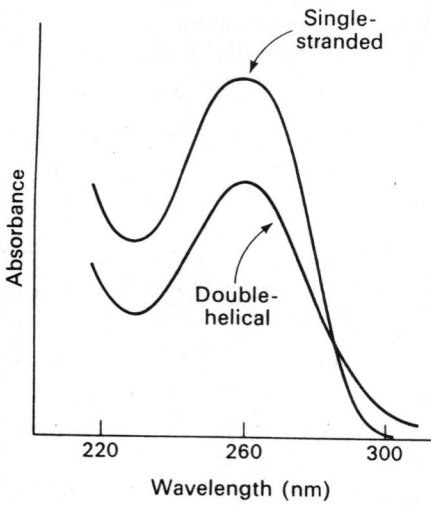

Fig. 2.7. The absorbance of a DNA solution at 260 nm increases when the double helix is melted into single strands.

If a DNA solution is heated, the hydrogen bonds between the complementary bases start breaking and the DNA gets denatured. This opening of two strands is referred as the melting of DNA. The melting of DNA can be followed by an increase in absorbance (see later) at 260nm. The temperature at which half of the DNA molecule has opened (as estimated by the rise in absorbance, see later) has been half achieved, is referred as the Tm of the DNA molecule. The Tm depends on the G:C content of the DNA. As there are three hydrogen bonds between G and C, the breakage of bonds requires higher temperature (Fig. 2.8). The Tm of an average DNA is about 78°. The Tm can be altered if salts are added to DNA solution, a high salt solution has enhanced Tm.

The melting of DNA is associated with an increase in absorbance at 260 nm. This effect is known as hyperchromacity (Fig. 2.9) and can be used to estimate the amount of denatured DNA. For example, there is a 37% enhancement in the absorbance of DNA when it is fully denatured. A ss DNA at a concentration of 50 ug/ml has an A_{260} value of 1.37 (compared to 1.0 for the ds DNA).

Other denaturating agents: Besides the temperature, a number of chemicals can denature the DNA. Alkali is one of the commonly used denaturing agent. The alkali acts by changing the ionic properties of the groups involved in hydrogen bond formation. In a solution of pH higher than 11.5, all the hydrogen bonds are broken and the DNA is present in ss form. Similarly denaturing agents such as urea or formamide can be

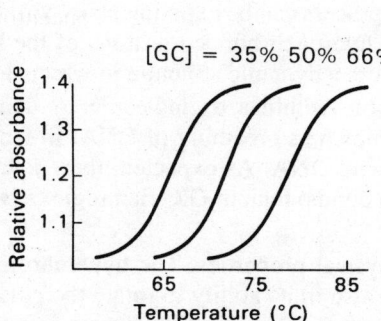

Fig. 2.8A. DNA melting curves. The absorbance (at 260 nm) relative to that at 25°C is plotted against temperature.

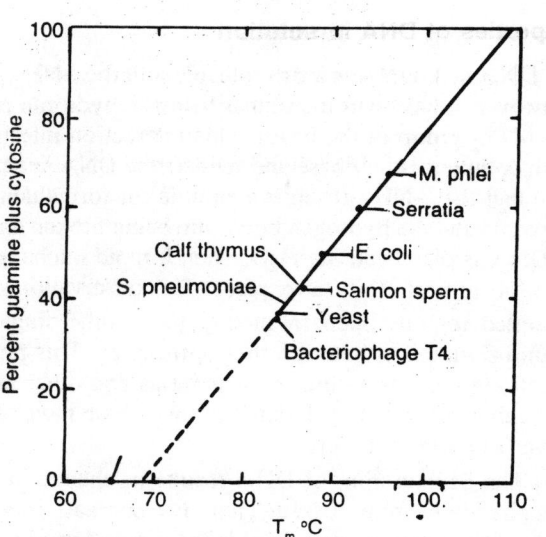

Fig. 2.8B. Relationship between DNA melting temperature and GC content. AT-DNA refers to synthetic DNA composed exclusively of A and T (GC content = 0).

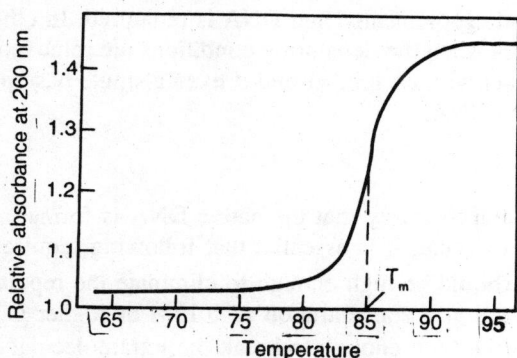

Fig. 2.9. Melting curve of *Streptococcus pneumoniae* DNA. The DNA was heated, and its melting was measured by the increase in absorbance at 260 nm. The point at which the melting is half complete is the melting temperature, or T_m. The T_m for this DNA under these conditions is about 85°C.

used to denature the DNA. The Tm of DNA is decreased by 1/2° for each 1% of formamide added to DNA solution. Thus in presence of 90% formamide the Tm of DNA will be about 33°.

In biological systems, a number of helix destabilizing proteins are present which can unwind a DNA helix. Many of these proteins open the DNA by binding to individual strands and breaking the hydrogen bonds. Such unwinding may be essential for many of the biological activies of the DNA. The DNA replication and transcription are some of the processes where DNA melts for carrying out the biological function.

Breathing in DNA structure

As discussed, DNA is a ds molecule and the $-NH_2$ groups of the bases are involved in hydrogen bonding. However, it has been found that formaldehyde can react with DNA, the interaction being taking place with the $-NH_2$ group of the bases. This interaction interferes with the ability of $-NH_2$ group to hydrogen bond with complementary base and renders the DNA denatured. This denaturing of DNA is slow and irreversible. The fact that $-NH_2$ group is available for formaldehyde to react means that the bases are being paired and unpaired and the hydrogen bonds are being broken and formed. The process can be experimentally visualized if DNA is dissolved in ^3H_2O when a rapid exchange between the hydrogen bonded protons of the bases and $^3H^+$ ions of ^3H_2O takes place. This observation shows that DNA is a dynamic structure in which double stranded regions open frequently to become single stranded bubble within a ds molecule. A dynamic equilibrium exists between these processes. This phenomenon is known as breathing of DNA. In fact this breathing permits a number of proteins and other factors to react with DNA. As expected, there is higher breathing within the A:T rich regions (which have only 2 hydrogen bonds) than in G:C rich regions (which have 3 hydrogen bonds).

The denaturation of DNA results in change in some of its physical properties. The hyperchromacity has already been discussed. There is a decrease in its viscosity and also in its ability to rotate the polarized light. This indicates that there is the disruption of the helical structure of DNA. The DNA strands are very large and previously it was thought that complete opening of the strands may not be possible. However, direct experiments using one ^{15}N–labelled strand in a ds DNA have confirmed that the two strands are separated in during denaturation.

It has been observed that DNA can be denatured by heat treatment. However, if a DNA solution is heated to a temperature where most but not all of the hydrogen bonds are broken and is subsequently cooled to room temperature, the strands get annealed and DNA is renatured. In other words, if strand separation is incomplete, the DNA rewinds when the denaturing conditions are removed. When two DNA strands are allowed to come in close contact with each other and if even a single base pair is formed, the two strands can anneal together to form ds DNA.

Renaturation of DNA

If denatured DNA is treated in such a way that the native DNA is formed, the process is referred as the renaturation. For renaturation to occur, it is essential that following requirements are met.

1. The salt concentration should be high enough to eliminate the repulsiveness of the PO_4 groups in two strands, usually NaCl at a concentration of 0.15M or higher is used for this purpose.
2. The temperature should be high enough to break the intramolecular hydrogen bonds. However, it should not be too high otherwise interstrand base pairing will not take place. Usually the temperature of $20-25°$ below the Tm is optimal for renaturation.

The renaturation of DNA is a relatively slow process. The actual winding of the strands is not the rate limiting step but the precise collision between complementary strands is responsible for this slow renaturation. The collision of strands is the result of a random motion and is concentration dependent (see later). Under most of the experimental conditions, it takes several hours for a sample of denatured DNA to fully renature.

The molecular mechanism of renturation can be explained by taking the example of a hypothetical molecule with a number of repeats of the sequence. Each of the two strands are long molecules, say 100,000 bases and the base sequences of the two strands are complementry to each other. Should there be a collision of two strands in such a way that A_1 hits the B_1, two strands will be in correct position and will form a ds DNA. However, collision of A_1 with B_2 will be ineffective as the two regions are not complementary.

On the other hand, by virtue of the internal homology between the regions A_1, A_2 and A_4 in the sequence, it is possible that base pairing between A_1 and B_4 can take place. However, this base pairing will be short lived as the bases sorrounding this short region of complementarity are not complementary and cannot base pair. Only when the regions such as A_1 and B_1 pair, the sorrounding bases also pair and renaturation takes place.

Now let us take another case where multiple molecules of DNA are present. Each has been denatured and there are many single stranded DNAs. Each strand will have equal chance to hit any other strand and will join at random, whenever it finds a complementary strand. This molecular mixing is known as the hybridization. The molecular hybridization is a strong tool to identify the related sequences in a pool of nucleic acid and is extensively used in rDNA technology.

The renaturation is concentration dependent

As the initial event during the renaturation is the collision between complementary bases, the rate of renaturation has to be dependent on the concentration of the DNA. Based on the concentration dependence, some striking behaviour of both eukaryotic and prokaryotic DNAs has been observed.

If the mixture of equal amounts of two DNAs of different size are mixed together, their molar ratio will depend on their sizes. Let us take the case of DNAs of two phages, the T_7 (MW 2.5×10^7) and T_4 (MW 1.1×10^8). If the concentration of two DNAs is same, the molar ratio of T_7 DNA will be 4.4 times of the T_7 DNA. If there is no sequence homology between the two DNAs, the renaturation curve shows that half of the DNA renatures faster than the other half. As the molar ratio of T_7 DNA is higher, the faster renaturating species has to be the T_7 DNA. However, if the DNA of both types are broken into many pieces, the renaturation kinetics will change. But the two basic parameters, namely that the DNA will renature as two independent components which will take different time for renaturation will remain the same.

This introduces a new parameter to the renaturation, the complexity of the sequences. Let us assume a situation where a long molecule of DNA has a repeating base sequence within itself. This sequence accounts for 2% the total DNA and let us assume that 6 copies of this repeat are present in the genome. Now if the DNA is fragmented into very small fragments, the weight of the repeated fragments will be 12% of total fragments (2% × 6 repeats) but its molar ratio will be 6 times higher than that of other regions (which are not repeated i.e. present in single copy). Thus 12% of the total DNA will renature much faster than the rest of DNA. The kinetics of renaturation will be dependent on complexity of the repeats and can be determined from the curve.

The cot curve

If initial DNA concentration is Co (expressed as moles of bases/litre), concentration of DNA which remains unrenatured at time t is C and k is a rate constant (which will depend on temperature and the size of DNA fragment), then

$$C/Co = 1/(1 + k \, Cot).$$

If, $\quad C/Co = 1/2$

then $Cot_{1/2} = 1/k$

As k is inversely proportional to N (the number of bases in the DNA fragment), the $Cot_{1/2}$ (the time at which half of the DNA is present in renatured form) is directly proportional to N or the complexity of DNA. If there are no repeats in the DNA, N represents the size of the total DNA molecule.

Thus by following the denaturation–renaturation kinetics of a DNA molecule, it is possible to estimate the repeats, if any, and size of these repeats as well as the complexity of the DNA. The Cot curve of eukaryotic DNA has been shown in Fig. 2.10.

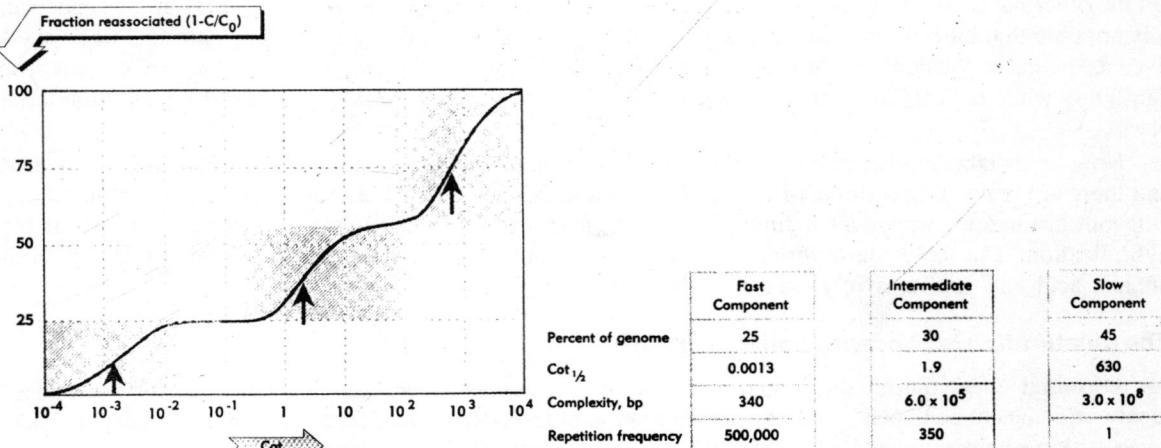

	Fast Component	Intermediate Component	Slow Component
Percent of genome	25	30	45
$Cot_{1/2}$	0.0013	1.9	630
Complexity, bp	340	6.0×10^5	3.0×10^8
Repetition frequency	500,000	350	1

Fig. 2.10. The reassociation kinetics of eukaryotic DNA show three types of component (indicated by the shaded areas). The arrows identify the $Cot_{1/2}$ values for each component.

The behaviour of repeatitive sequences has been shown in Fig. 2.11.

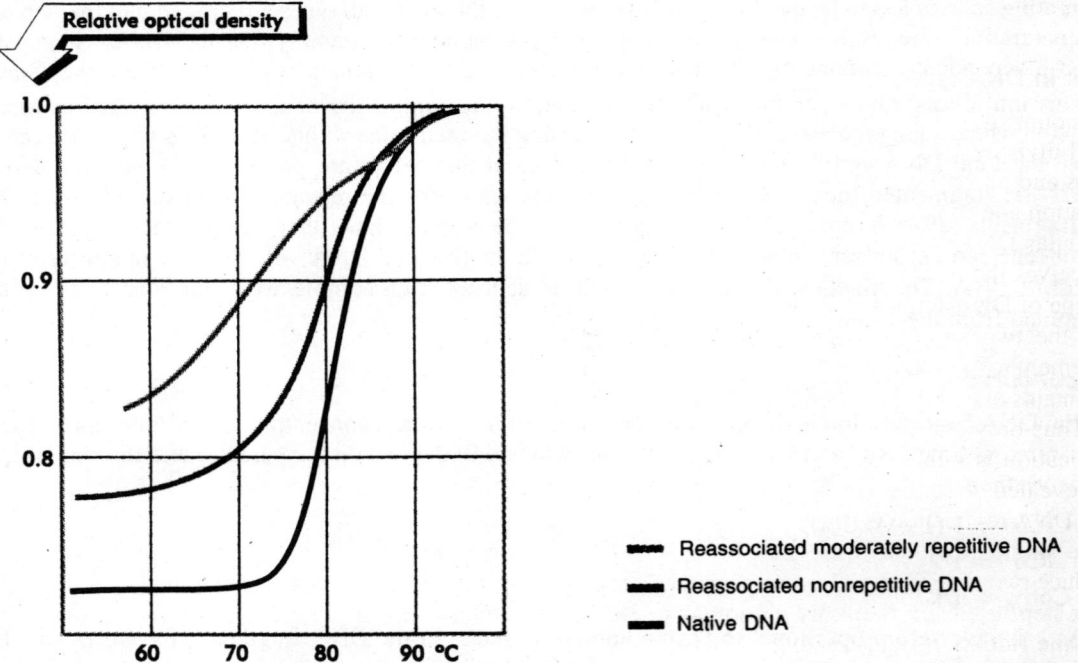

━━ Reassociated moderately repetitive DNA

━━ Reassociated nonrepetitive DNA

━━ Native DNA

Fig. 2.11. The denaturation of reassociated nonrepetitive DNA takes place over a narrow temperature range close to that of native DNA, but reassociated repetitive DNA melts over a wide temperature range.

3

DNA Replication

As discussed earlier, DNA is the genetic material of the cell. It stores all the information necessary for normal functioning of the cell. It is, therefore, necessary that during the cell division, each of the daughter cells receives a true copy of the genome of the parent cell. The DNA has to multiply and the fidelity of the primary structure has to be maintained during this duplication of DNA, so that the composition of DNA in daughter cells is precisely the same as that of the parent cell. This fidelity of DNA structure is maintained by the complimentarity between the bases, A and T and the bases C and G, which always pair with each other.

Events in DNA replication

The amount of DNA in a cell remains constant. Therefore, the DNA replication is always coupled with the cell division. During the S phase of cell cycle, immediately prior to cell division the DNA of the cell doubles and one copy of the genome is transferred to each of the daughter cells. Thus the process of DNA duplication and its distribution in two daughter cells presents two possible scenerios, first possibility is that the cellular DNA is duplicated and one cell receives the pre-existing (the original) DNA while the other cell receives the newly synthesized DNA. In other words, the integrity of pre-existing DNA is conserved. This type of DNA replication will be called as the *conservative mode of DNA repilcation*. Other possibility is that the two strands of the original DNA are separated, each is duplicated by the synthesis of the complementary strand, thus producing two exact replica of the parent DNA. Each of the two molecules thus contains one original strand and one newly synthesized strand, which are then distributed to two daughter cells. Thus only one of the two strands of the original DNA is conserved in each of the cells. This mode of replication is known as *semiconservative mode of replication*. The studies with isotope incorporation have revealed that the DNA replication takes place by semiconservative mode (Fig. 3.1). The first step in DNA replication is, therefore, the opening of DNA chain and conversion of a double stranded DNA into the single stranded form. Each of these strands are then duplicated by a series of enzymatic events to produce two replica copies of the original DNA. The cell constantly applies a number of different checks at each step to ensure that only a complementary base is incorporaed for each base of the parent strand so that the fidelity in the structure of DNA is maintained. We will discuss the details of these events one by one.

Enzymes involved in DNA replication

A number of enzymes participate in DNA replication. The details of these enzymes have been discussed below.

The Meselson-Stahl experiment using light (^{14}N) and heavy (^{15}N) nitrogen showed that first generation DNA is hybrid.

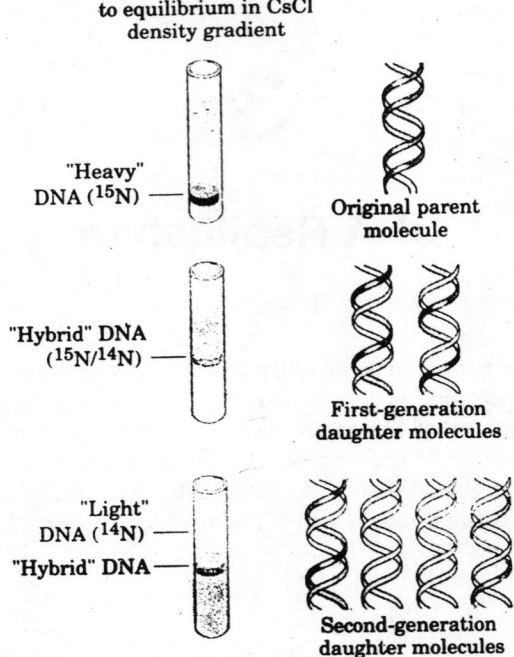

Fig. 3.1. DNA replication is semi conservative.

DNA polymerase

The primary enzyme which carries out the condensation of nucleotides to form a polynucleotide chain is the DNA polymerase. DNA polymerase was originally isolated from E. coli by Arther Kornburg and is also referred as Kornberg's enzyme. It is a single polypeptide with a molecular weight of 109KD. It catalyses the synthesis of the DNA from 5' to 3' direction i.e. starts copying the template DNA from its 3'-end. It can not act in the opposite direction. Even though a single protein, it has three distinct catalytic properties.

(i) A 5'→3' polymerase activity which is the predominant function of the enzyme and is responsible for the esterification of nucleotides to form the DNA chain. It causes the addition of a new nucleotide at the 3'-OH group of an existing oligonucleotide. For its activity it requires a single stranded DNA which is copied by it. This DNA strand which is to be copied, is known as the template. The enzyme thus depends on a template DNA and is referred as the DNA-dependent DNA polymerase. While copying a template, it cannot initiate the synthesis of a new DNA chain. However, it can add more nucleotides to an existing molecule and can extend it. This pre-existing nucleic acid molecule is known as the primer. Either a DNA or an RNA can act as primer for DNA polymerase. The DNA polymerase has an obligatory requirement for the primer and can not act in its absence. The reaction can be written in following form.

$$\text{(Polynucleotide)n} + \text{dNTP} \longrightarrow \text{(Polynucleotide)n+1} + \text{PPi}$$

In fact the enzyme actually transfers a nucleotide to an existing nucleic acid molecule. It is, therefore, a transferase in true sense. The E.C. name of the enzyme is DNA-nucleotidyl transferase (E.C. 2.7.7.7.). Deoxynucleotide triphosphates (dNTPs) serve as the substrate for this polymerization reaction. The enzyme can not use either dNDPs or dNMPs as the substrate. Besides, these requirements, it also has an obligatory requirement for Mg^{++} ions.

(ii) A 5'→3' exonuclease activity which is responsible for the removal of nucleotides from the 5' end of the DNA chain. This activity is primarily responsible for the removal of the RNA primer from the 5' end of the newly synthesized chain (see later).

(iii) A 3'→5' exonuclease activity which catalyses the removal of nucleotides from the 3'-end of the DNA chain. This reaction is just opposite to the polymerase function. However, the polymerase activity is several fold higher than the exonuclease activity. Thus for all practical purposes the enzyme acts as the polymerase and not nuclease in presence of the four dNTPs, the template, the primer and all other requirements. The function of 3'→5' exonuclease activity is in proof reading which helps in removing any mismatched nucleotide and is essential for maintaining the accuracy of replication and will be discussed later.

By tryptic digestion, the DNA polymerase can be cleaved in two bioactive molecules, a large fragment or the Klenow polymerase (named after the scientist who discovered it) of 75KD which has the polymerase and the 3'→5' exonuclease activities and a small fragment of 38KD which has the 5'→3' exonuclease activity.

The DNA polymerse discussed above, at the time of its discovery by Kornberg, was thought to be the only DNA polymerase present in the cells. However, later a number of other enzymes with similar activities were discovered and the original Kornberg's enzymes is often designated as DNA polymerase I (Pol I). We now know that Pol I is not the primary enzyme involved in DNA synthesis and it does not play very important role during the replication of DNA. However, its basic responsibility is in the proof reading and DNA repair. Another enzyme, Pol II with a molecular weight of 120KD has been isolated whose in vivo function is not very well understood. It is probably a very specialised enzyme involved in DNA repair. The third enzyme Pol III, a hetero–multimeric enzyme with a molecular weight of >250KD is the main enzyme which is responsible for the DNA replication.

DNA Polymerase III

DNA polymerase III (Pol III) is a hetro-multimer of several subunits. In. E. coli, the 160 KD catalytic core of Pol III is made of one α-subunit (MW 130 KD, product of the gene, polC) which is responsible for DNA synthesis, one ε subunit (25 KD, product of the gene, dnaQ) and a 10 KD θ subunit. The ε and θ subunits help in the assembly for proof reading along with the help of PolI. Two molecules of core enzyme condense together with the help of two τ subunits (71 KD, product of the gene, dnaX). The presence of τ subunits is essential for the dimer formation. This dimer, referred Pol III* (molecular mass, 470 KD), has increased processivity. To one of the α-subunits in Pol III*, two γ-subunits (52 KD each) and two δ-subunits (32 KD each), get associated. This results in the formation of a 750KD asymmetrical complex (pol III'), which can bind to template DNA. However, a number of other subunits, especially the β subunit (product of the gene, dnaN) binds to the Pol III' molecule and assemble the holoenzyme (900 KD) which is the complete Pol III and can carry out all the functions of the enzyme. The characteristics of various subunits are summarized in Table 3.1 and the structure of Pol III, which is an asymetrical dimer, is shown in Fig. 3.2.

Table 3.1. The subunits of DNA polymerase III

Subunit	Gene	Mol. wt. KD	No. of subunits/ mol. of enzyme	Function
α	polC (dnaE)	130	2	DNA synthesis (dnaE), part of the core enzyme
β	dnaN	37	4	Template association?
γ	dnaX	52	2	Template binding, increased processivity
δ	holA	32	2	Increased processivity
ε	dnaQ (mutD)	25	2	Proof reading (mutD), core subunit
θ	holE	10	2	Assembly?
τ	dnaX*	71	2	Stable template binding dimer formation

Other subunits with unknown function which may be part of polIII

δ'	holB	33		
χ	holC	15		
ψ	holD	12		

* The gene dnaX codes for the τ subunit and also for the γ subunit of polymerase III. The 80% of the N terminal of τ subunit has same sequence as the γ subunit. However, a frame shifting mechanism results in the premature termination and formation of γ subunit.

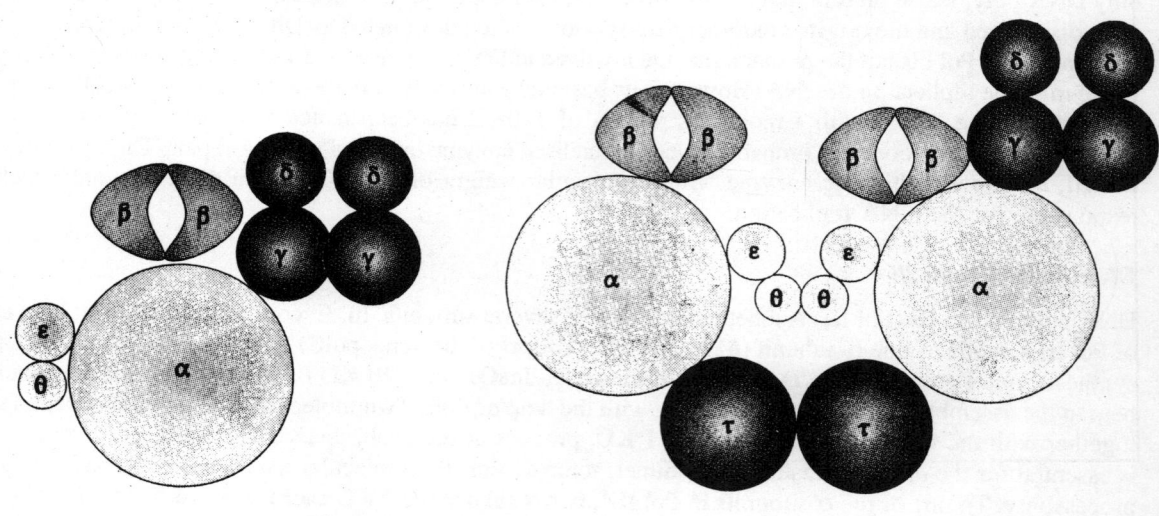

A. The core enzyme

B. The holoenzyme

Fig. 3.2. Structure of DNA polymerase III.

The assembly of Pol III takes place in a systematic and stage wise manner. The early events during the assembly are energy dependent and require the hydrolysis of ATP. The assembly of prokaryotic Pol III has been schematically represented in Fig. 3.3.

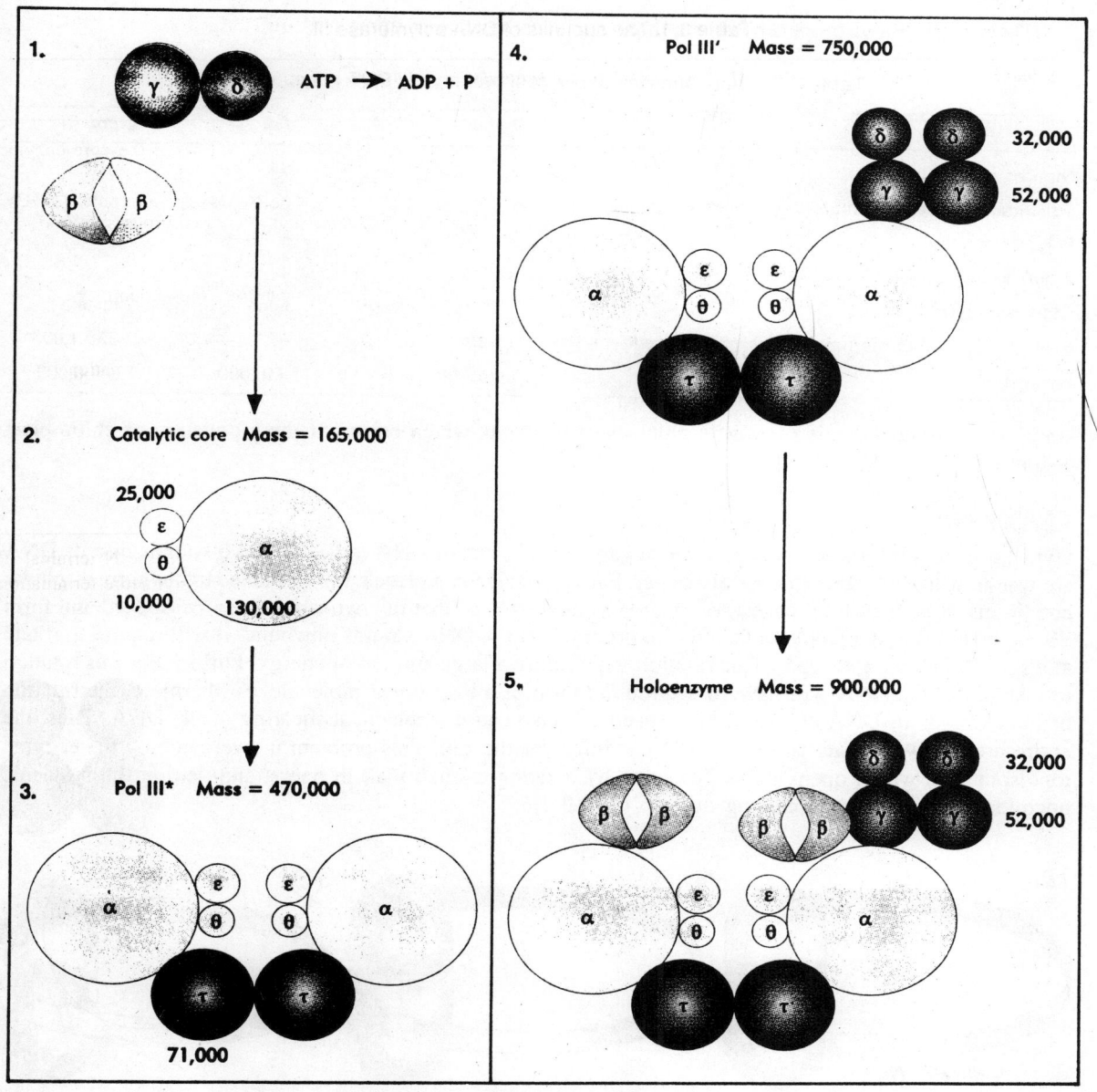

Fig. 3.3. Assembly of Polymerase III.

Similar to prokaryotes, three different DNA polymerases are present in eukaryotes also. All these enzymes are complex multimeric molecules and are referred as polymerase α, polymerase β and polymerase γ. The polymerase α is the main enzyme which is present in the nucleus of the cell. It along with another enzyme, polymerase δ, is responsible for the DNA replication. The DNA polymerase β is primarily responsible for DNA repair. It may be assisted by another enzyme, polymerase ε also. Polymerase γ, on the other hand, is the mitochondrial enzyme responsible for the replication of mitochondrial DNA. An enzyme

The structure and properties of the three enzymes have been compared in Table 3.2

Table 3.2. Characteristics of different prokaryotic DNA polymerases

	Pol I	Pol II	Pol III
Number of subunits	1	>4	>10
Structural gene for subunit with polymerase activity	polA	polB (dnaB)	polC (dnaC)
Polymerase activity	+	+	+
Proof reading function	+	+	+
Other activity(ies)	5'-3' exo-nuclease	none	none
Rate of DNA synthesis (nucleotides polymerised/sec)	15-20	~7	250-1,000
Processivity	upto 200	>10,000	>500,000

similar to polymerase γ is present in chloroplast of plants which carry out the replication of chloroplast genome.

DNA gyrase

Gyrases or the topoisomerases cause the negative supertwist in DNA molecule. Two strands of a ds DNA are wound with each other in a spiral manner. Further, the DNA molecule is supercoiled under normal cellular conditions. It is, therefore, necessary to unwind the DNA, so that the two strands can be opened and form SS regions during the DNA replication. In order to get the DNA strands unwound, it will require to rotate at a speed of about 4500 rpm. This rotation will require a large amount of energy. Further, for this rotation to take place, the DNA will have to acquire the form of a long linear molecule. Furthermore, the rotation of long strands of DNA at such a high speed can also cause mechanical shearing of the DNA. Thus, the entire process will create an undesirable condition for the cell. This problem is overcome by the enzyme topoisomerase which opens the coiled turns by creating a small nick in one strand, letting the molecule uncoiled by one turn and closing the gap (Fig. 3.4).

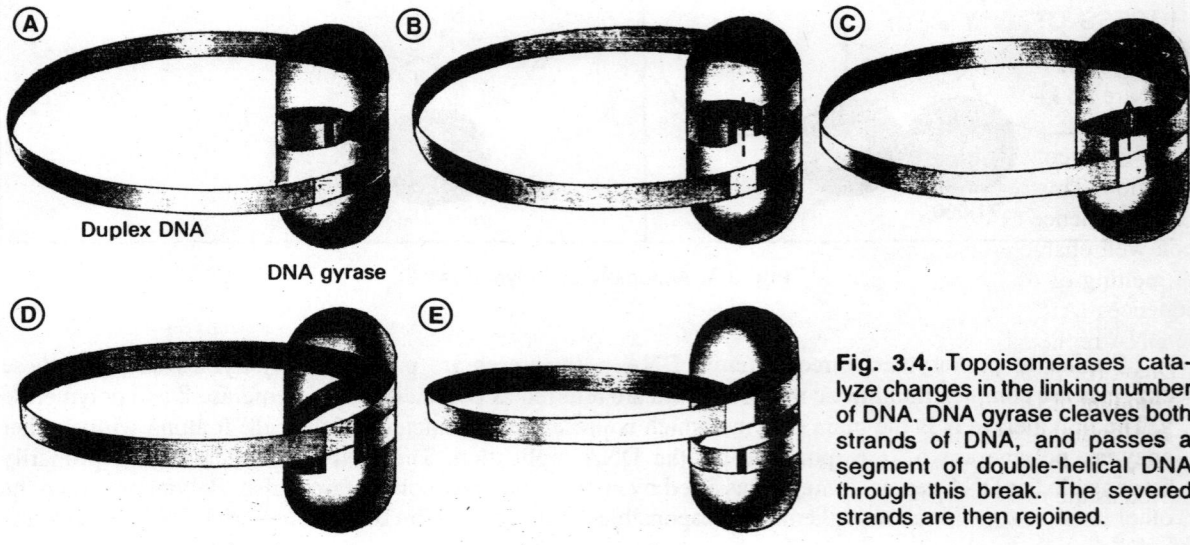

Duplex DNA

DNA gyrase

Fig. 3.4. Topoisomerases catalyze changes in the linking number of DNA. DNA gyrase cleaves both strands of DNA, and passes a segment of double-helical DNA through this break. The severed strands are then rejoined.

The DNA gyrase belongs to the general class of type II DNA topoisomerases. The topoisomerases inter–convert the DNA to diffrent topoisomers. The topoisomers are different physical forms of same DNA which differ only in their linking number. The linking number is defined as the number of times a strand winds around the other strand in the right handed manner. The type II topoisomerases, including the gyrase, cleave both the strands and require ATP for their action. Type I topoisomerases, on the other hand, cleave only one strand and do not need ATP. These are involved in relaxation of negative supercoiling of DNA.

DNA ligase

It can join two pieces of DNA by the formation of a phosphodiester bond between these molecules. For this, the two DNAs should have a free 3'-OH and a 5'-PO_4 groups, respectively. It should be noted that the DNA ligase can only close a nick but cannot incorporate any new nucleotide to fill a gap. The enzyme is used to join the polynucleotide fragments in the lagging strand during the DNA replication (see later).

Primase

It is a specific RNA polymerase which is responsible for the synthesis of a sequence specific RNA molecule which serves as the primer to initiate the DNA synthesis. This is a monomer of 66 KD and is the product of the gene dnaG. This enzyme is simpler and much smaller than the RNA polymerase involved in the transcription and is distinct from it.

Helicase

The enzyme, also referred as unwinding protein, is responsible for the melting of DNA and formation of SS DNA at the begining of the replication fork. It requires ATP for its action. The active form of helicase is the homo-hexamer of a 330 KD protein.

Other DNA binding factors

Besides the enzymes described above, a number of other protein factors also participate in DNA replication. These will be discussed as and when their role is discussed.

PROCESS OF DNA REPLICATION

The synthesis of DNA starts at a defined locus in the genome which is known as the 'origin of replication'. There are no known conserved sequences to define the origin of replication. Most of the eukaryotic DNAs have multiple origins of replication. Prokaryotes, on the other hand, generally have only one origin. The origin in E. coli genome has been well characterized. It is referred as 'OriC' and is present within a 245 bp region. This region has three repeats of a 13 bp long sequence (GATCTNTTNTTTT) and 4 repeats of a 9 bp sequence (TTATNCANA). The origin of replication in a number of plasmids and phages have also been well characterized. In general, the sequences at the origin of replication are A:T rich, which makes the melting of ds DNA easier. The origins of replication in yeast are referred as autonomous replicating sequences (ARS). However, the origins from higher organisms have not been well identified. To initiate the DNA replication a protein factor, DnaA, recognizes and binds at the origin of replication. The binding of DnaA (or priA in phages) is with the repeat regions of OriC. DnaA is a monomer of a 82 KD protein. The binding of DnaA may be preceded by the binding of a pre-priming factor DnaT (66 KD). This is followed by the binding of helicase which causes the melting of a small stretch of DNA. This region of the DNA opens up to form a single stranded region and the separation of two strands takes place. This structure is referred as the replication fork. The single stranded character of replication fork is maintained by the binding of single strand specific DNA binding proteins referred as SSB proteins. The association of these proteins prevent the reformation of ds DNA. The SSBs are the tetramer of a 74 KD protein, the DnaB. Another ancillary protein causes the activation of primase which synthesizes the RNA primer. The primer is complementary to 3'-end of the template. The activity of DnaB is facilitated by the binding of another protein, DnaC to DnaB. DnaB is present in form of a hexamer. There are six molecules of DnaC for each DnaB molecule. One monomer of DnaC binds to each of the subunits of the DnaB hexamer. Once the primer has initiated the DNA synthesis, DNA polymerase takes over and adds more nucleotides, one at a time, to the primer and continues to extend the DNA chain. Thus a number of factors get associated to DNA to initiate the replication. The entire complex is referred as the primosome. Once initiation has taken place, the DNA synthesis continues. The entire process has been diagrammatically represented in Fig. 3.5. Primosome formation in phage φX174 takes place at a specific site, pas (for primosome assembly site), and involves priA, priB, and priC proteins along with the DnaT, DnaB and DnaC proteins. The primosome can move along the SS DNA and priming can also occur at sites other than the pas site. DnaB is a central component in both types of events and a primase is required for initiating the replication. During the entire process the helicase keeps binding ahead of the fork so that there is a forward movement of the fork. The elongation of the chain is relatively simple process. The new nucleotide-ancillary factor complex of a growing chain is referred as the replisome.

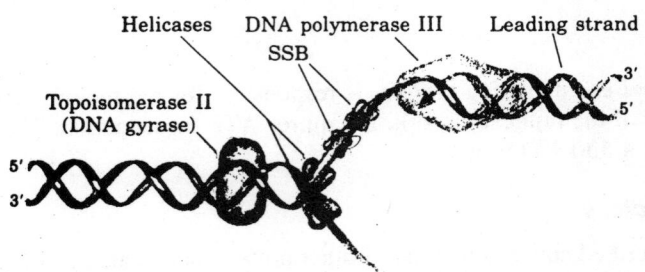

Fig. 3.5. Replication of DNA (only leading strand has been shown).

Leading and lagging strands

The mechanism of DNA replication described above very well explains the synthesis of DNA for one strand, namely 3'–5' of template which will be copied in the 5'–3' direction by the DNA polymerase. How does the synthesis of the other strand (5'–3' of template) which apparantly seems to grow in 3'–5' direction, takes place? It was a big puzzle for a long time as there is no known DNA polymerase which can carry out such an extension. The problem was solved in 1960s when Reiji Okazaki and his colleagues discovered the presence of a large number of small DNA fragments, each with an RNA primer attached to it, in the dividing cells. He analysed the importance of these DNA pieces which are called as Okazaki fragments and explained the replication of the 5'–3' template. It has been well established now that the synthesis of this strand also takes place only in the 5'–3' direction. The primase initiates the synthesis of DNA at the 3'–end of the opened region of the fork and polymerase extends this primer towards the 5' side (of template), synthesizing the new DNA in 5'–3' direction. When more bases of template DNA open up and the size of the fork is increased, a new primer is synthesized and gets annealed at the 5'– end of the fork and the entire process is repeated until the polymerase has reached to the first primer. The 5'–3' exonuclease activity of Pol I, at this stage, digests the RNA primer and the polymerase fills the gap with DNA. Thus the synthesis of this strand takes place in pieces. These pieces are then joined by DNA ligase to form a continuous

DNA strand. There are separate primases for leading and lagging strands. The process has been illustrated in Fig. 3.6. The synthesis of two strands, thus takes place in slightly different manner. One strand which is known as the leading strand is synthesized in a continuous manner while the other strand called as lagging strand is synthesized in discontinuous manner. The DNA replication is, therefore, semi-discontinous in nature. The small fragments of DNA which are synthesized in the lagging strand are known as Okazaki fragments. It should be noted that there is a single primosome formation for the leading strand while multiple primosomes are formed on the lagging strand. Each primosome results in the formation of a single Okazaki fragment.

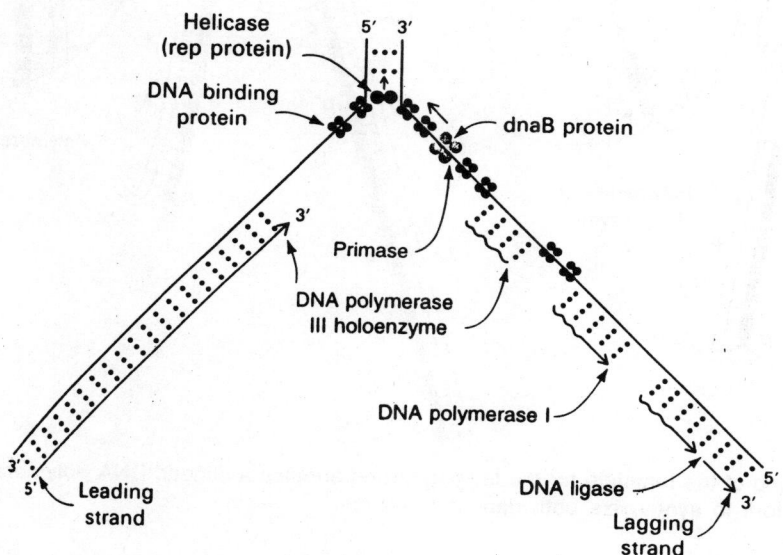

Fig. 3.6. Schematic diagram of the enzymatic events at a replication fork of *E. coli.*

According to above model the two strands are replicated in different directions. This can take place only if two separate DNA polymerase molecules are involved in the replication of the leading and the lagging strand. As discussed, the holoenzyme Pol III is made up of two catalytic cores. It was found that one of the two cores of same molecule catalyses the replication of leading strand while the other catalyses the replication of lagging strand. How does it take place? The detailed analysis revealed that at the point of polymerase action, the lagging strand folds back which changes the physical direction of the strand. Thus two strands grow in same physical direction but in different biological direction and maintain the 5'-3' orientation (Fig. 3.7).

Multiple origins of replication

The eukaryotic genome is very large. If the entire replication of DNA was to take place from one end, as has been depicted above, the time taken for the replication of DNA will be much longer than the actual time it takes. The size of human genome, for example, is 6×10^6 kb. The average rate of replication is 2.2 kb/min. It will, therefore, take about 45,000 hr for the replication of the entire genome. However, it actually takes only 9 hr to duplicate the entire human genome in a dividing cell. How can one account for this discrepancy? It has been found that there are multiple origins of replication in eukaryotic DNA. These are referred as the replicons. The average size of an replicon and the efficiency of DNA polymerase for a number

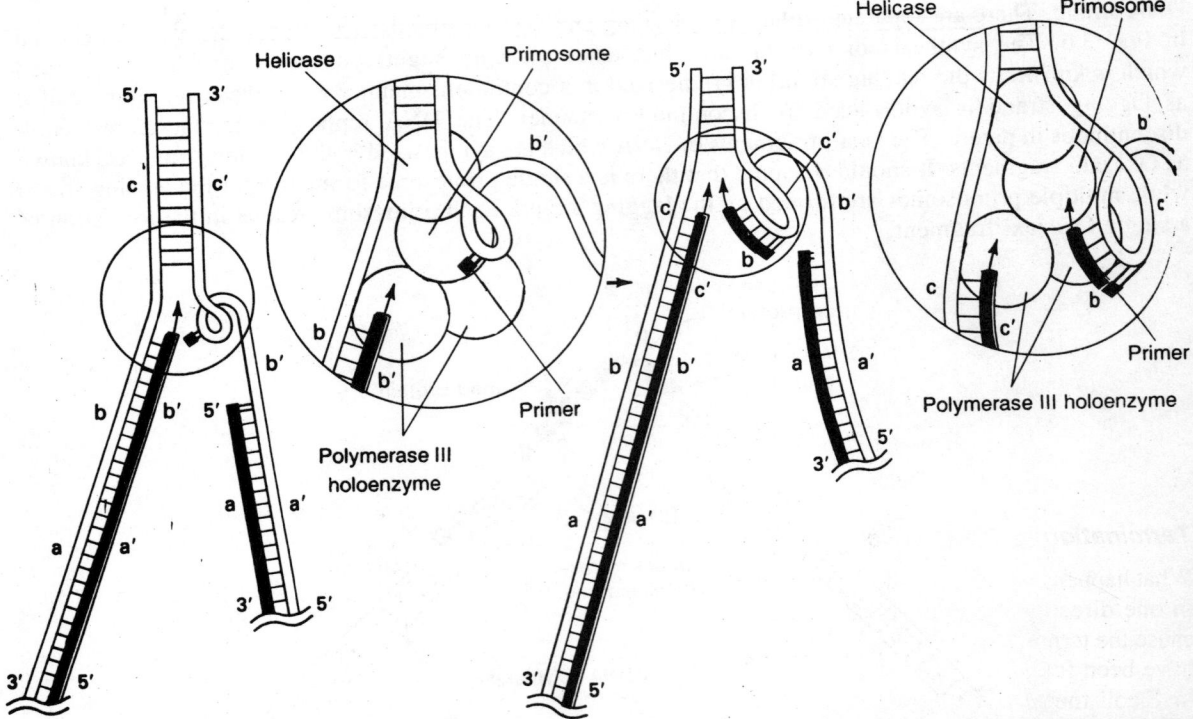

Fig. 3.7. The looping of the template for the lagging strand enables a dimeric DNA polymerase III holoenzyme at the replication fork to synthesize both daughter strands.

of organisms have been shown in Table 3.3. Entire process of replication continues from each of these origins. Further, the replication proceeds in both direction from each of the origins. Thus each strand serves as leading strand at one direction and lagging strand at the other direction. At the point where two growing chains from opposite direction meet, the DNA ligase seals the nick and a continuous DNA molecule is produced. These multiple origins of replication working simultaneously are called replication bubbles or replication eye (Fig. 3.8).

Table 3.3. Eukaryotic and prokaryotic replicons

Organism	Average genome size (Kb)	Average replicon size (Kb)	No. of replicons per genome	Rate of DNA synthesis(bp/s)
E. coli	4,200	4,200	1	800-1000
S. cerevisiae	20,000	40	500	50-60
D. melanogaster	140,000	40	3500	40-50
X. laevis	3,000,000	200	15,000	8-10
M. musculus	3,750,000	150	25,000	35-40
V. faba (Plant)	105,000,000	300	35,000	?

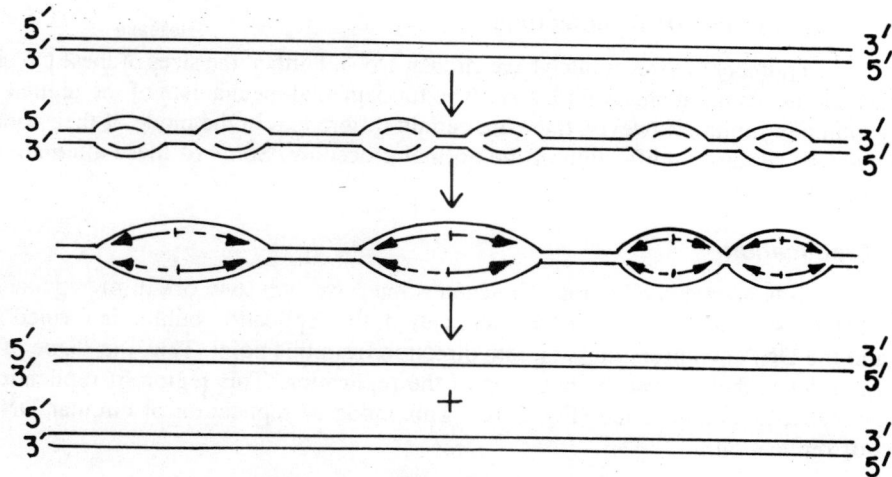

Fig. 3.8. Multiple origins of replication.

Termination of DNA replication

What happens when the replication fork (or bubble) grows on both sides? Is there a crash of one fork (growing in one direction) with the other fork growing in opposite direction? Are there specific sequences which cause the termination of replication at the point of meeting of the two forks? In E.coli certain specific features have been found which result in termination of replication at the point of meeting. It should be noted that in E.coli the DNA is circular and even though there is only a single origin of replication, the growing forks will meet each other at about the half way around the chromosome. Two termination regions, referred as terD/terA and terB/terC have been identified which are responsible for the termination of fork 1 and fork 2 respectivel, (Fig. 3.9). These are located on either side of the meeting point and are specific for the fork growing in one of the directions. The location of these points ensures that the fork has to cross the terminus specific for other fork before reaching to the meeting point. If one of the two forks is delayed, the faster fork will be terminated immediately after the meeting point. Thus it will avoid the crash of the two forks.

There is a region of 23 bp which is present at each of these ter regions. The concensus sequence is AATTAGTATGTTGTAACTAAAGT. This sequence causes the termination of DNA synthesis in vitro. Similar conserved sequences have been reported in a number of plasmids also. However, the relationship between these sites and actual termination is not very clear.

The termination of replication is mediated by a protein, which is coded by the tus gene. This protein recognizes the ter sites and binds there. These, then, interact with DNA polymerase and cause the termination of the replication fork

What will happen if a repressor of gene expression is attached to DNA which is being replicated. It has been found that the polymerase displaces the repressor and continues the replication. Another possible situation can arise if the DNA polymerase encounters a RNA polymerase travelling in the same direction (in E.coli, the movement of DNA polymerase is 10 times faster than the RNA polymerase). Does it displace the RNA polymerase or waits for the RNA polymerase to reach to its terminator. Still more drammatic situation can arise when DNA polymerase collides 'head on' with a RNA polymerase travelling in the opposite dirction. The mechanisms to resolve these situations are not very clear. However, in E.coli most of the transcription units, except for a few very small ones, are oriented in such a way that the chances of head on collisions between the DNA polymerase and the RNA polymerase are minimised.

Replication of small circular DNA molecules

Plasmids, phages and a number of viruses often have circular DNA. Further, the sizes of these circular genomes is much smaller than the bacterial and other DNAs. The fundamental mechanism of the replication of these small circular genome is similar, however, there are certain differences in the mode of their fork movement which are achieved by certain modification of the normal procedure. Some of these alternate modes have been described below.

Theta mode of replication

Majority of the plasmids are relatively small molecules and have only one origin of replication. Same is true for many bacteria such as E. coli. For their replication, the replication bubble is formed at the origin of replication and the DNA synthesis starts at both direction from this point. Thus the shape of DNA looks similar to the Latin letter theta (θ) at the begining of the replication. This region of replication continues to grow until entire DNA is duplicated (Fig. 3.10). This mode of replication of circular DNA is known as Theta mode of replication.

Rolling circle model of DNA replication

In certain phages such as the M13 and φX174, the phage has very specific life cycle. It replicates as a double stranded DNA inside the host cell but is secreted out of the cell as a single stranded DNA molecule.

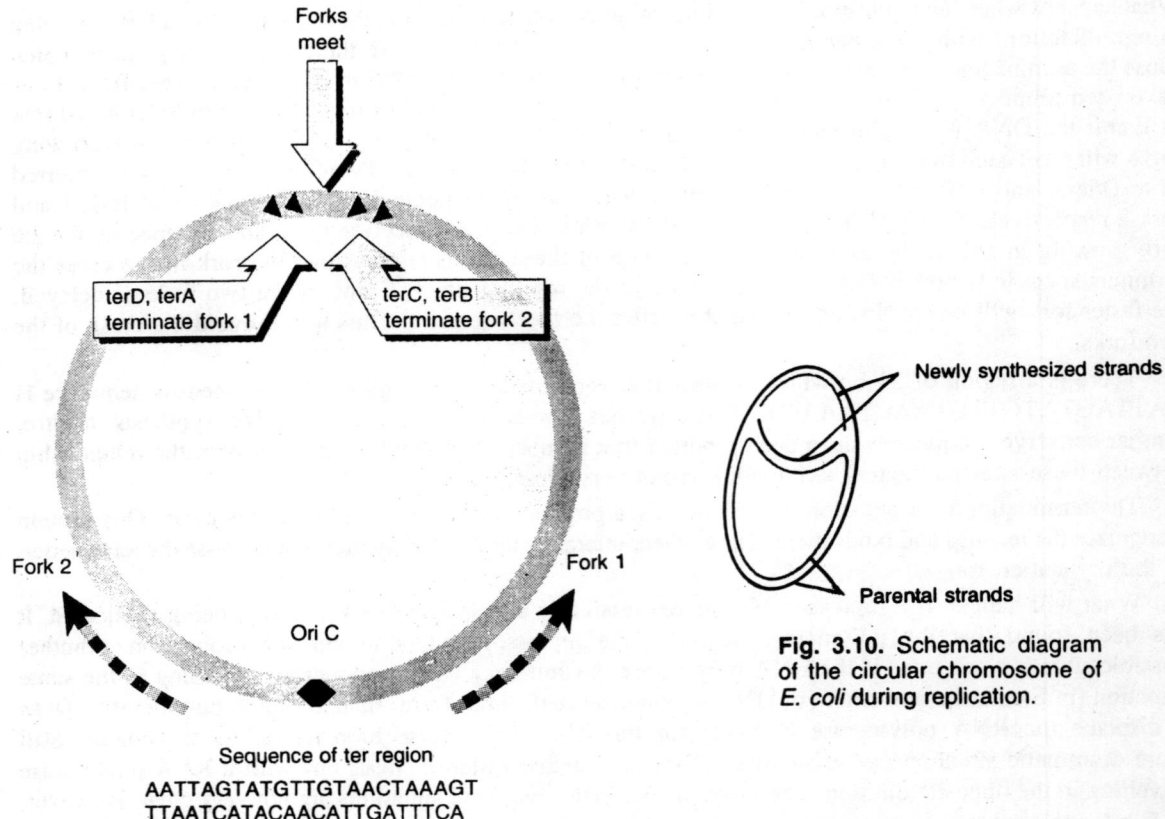

Forks meet

terD, terA terminate fork 1

terC, terB terminate fork 2

Fork 2

Fork 1

Ori C

Sequence of ter region
AATTAGTATGTTGTAACTAAAGT
TTAATCATACAACATTGATTTCA

Fig. 3.9. Termination of replication in E. coli.

Newly synthesized strands

Parental strands

Fig. 3.10. Schematic diagram of the circular chromosome of E. coli during replication.

In such case, all the single stranded phage particles have the copies of only one of the strands and not the copies of the two strands in equal ratio as would be normally expected if these were produced by the melting of the double stranded molecules. The DNA replication takes place in a very special manner in these molecules. First a nick is created in one of the two strands and DNA polymerase starts the DNA synthesis from this nick, using the other strand as template and the nicked DNA as the primer. While the new nucleotides are being added to the 3'-end of this strand, in a simultaneous action the pre-existing nucleotides at the 5'-end of the strand keep on melting from the template strand. Thus the 'old' DNA of the strand is present in single stranded form while the template strand is continuously being copied. The SS DNA binding proteins stabilize the single stranded form. Multiple copies of the template are thus formed in a continuous manner. It gives an impression as if the template strand is rolling along the newly synthesized DNA and new DNA is being produced continuously. This is known as the rolling circle mode of DNA replication. Specific nucleases are present in the host cell which can cleave the DNA at precise position to make DNA segments, each of which represents a single copy of the complete genome. These linear fragments can later become circular. The mechanism of this mode of replication is shown in Fig. 3.11.

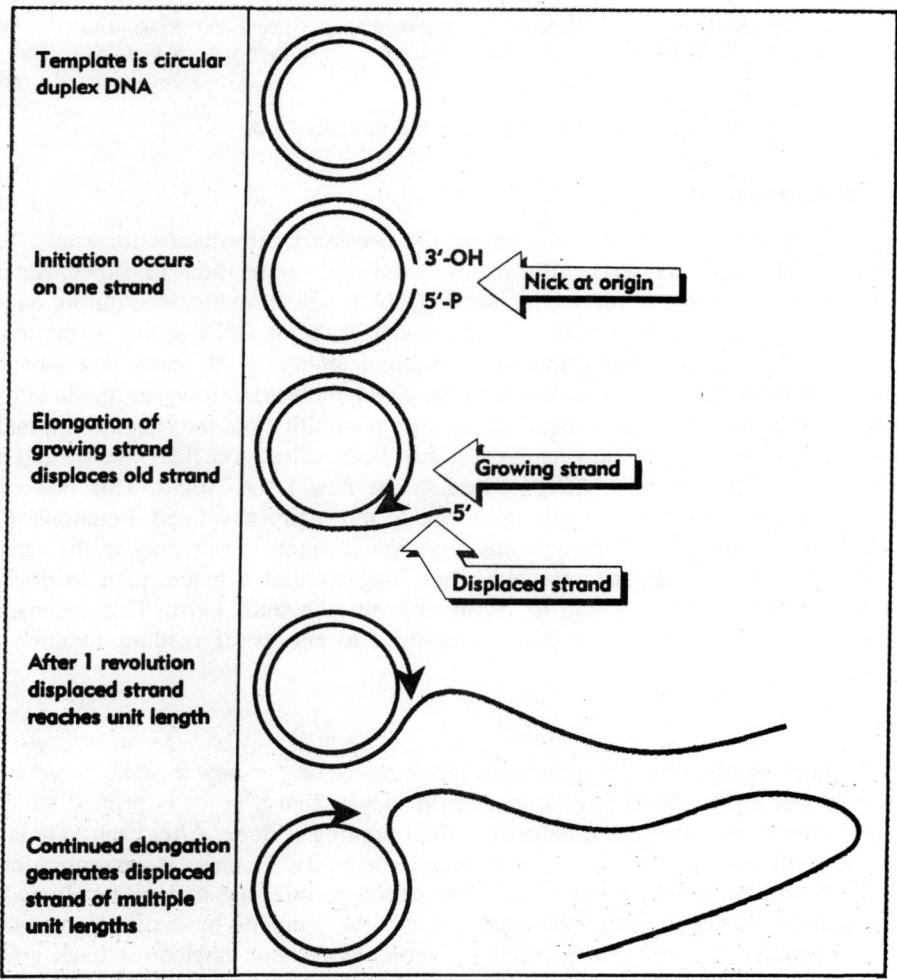

Fig. 3.11. Rolling circle mode of DNA replication.

Based on the life cycle of the organism, the single stranded DNA formed by rolling circle mode may have one of the several fates. The SS DNA, while being formed, may also serve as the lagging strand template and may be copied in a discontinuous manner. This will result in the formation of double stranded DNA molecule. Specific nucleases will cut the ds DNA at right position, so that the size of the genome is maintained. The DNA circularizes and the ends are sealed by the DNA ligase. Thus ds, circular DNA molecules will be formed. Alternatively, the SS DNA may also get circularised and may remain as ss circular DNA. Yet another possibility is that it is first cenverted into ss, circular form and then copied to form ds, circular DNA. Alternatively either the ss or the ds form may remain linear. It is also possible that more than one type of molecules may be formed. The pathway depends on the life cycle of the organism. All these different possibilities have been shown in Fig. 3.12.

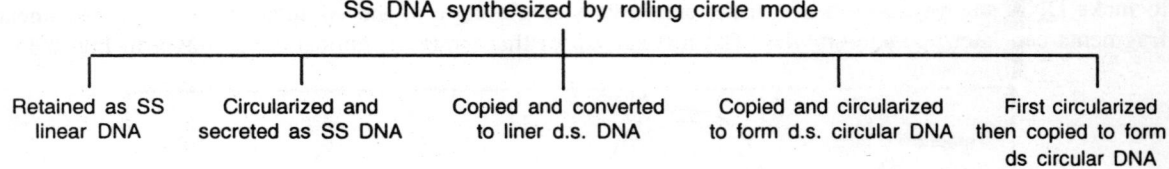

Fig. 3.12. Possible fates of SS DNA.

Fidelity of DNA replication

DNA is the genetic material which not only passes the necessary information for proper functioning of cellular machinery but also transfers information from one generation to other generation. It is, therefore, very important that the primary structure of DNA is strictly maintained during its replication. In the semiconservative mode of DNA replication one strand of the ds DNA serves as the template for the *de novo* synthesis of the other strand and due to complementarity of bases, the newly synthesized DNA copies and maintains the primary sequence of the parent molecule. However, the in vitro experiments and theoratical calculations have shown that there exists a possibility that the enzyme can make ocassional mistakes, resulting in formation of mismatches. It has been calculated that one wrong base may get incorporated for every 10^4–10^5 bases polymerised in the new DNA strand. This rate of error is too high to be acceptable by the cell, as it may give rise to too many unwanted mutations. Further, it has been seen that the observed rate of spontaneous mutation is much lower; only in the range of about 1 change for each 10^{10}–10^{11} bases incorporated. This suggests that a mechanism to double check the added nucleotide for its correctness and to repair any mistake must exist. This mechanism resulting in the increased fidelity of DNA replication is referred as the proof reading function of the DNA polymerase.

Proof reading

The process of checking the newly synthesized DNA molecule for any mistake is very simlar to the procedure adopted during the printing of a manuscript where first a proof is printed which is carefully checked and any mistakes are corrected before the final printing is done. After each base is incorporated, the DNA polymerase checks it for the correct complementarity. If there is incorporation of a wrong base, the mismatch will result in the lack of the base pairing at this base and the newly added nucleotide would remain as single stranded. This mismatch will then be removed by the 3'-5' exonuclease activity of the DNA polymerase. The enzyme in such situation, moves one nucleotide back and incorporates the correct nucleotide (Fig. 3.13). This rechecking for the correctness of the bases by the DNA

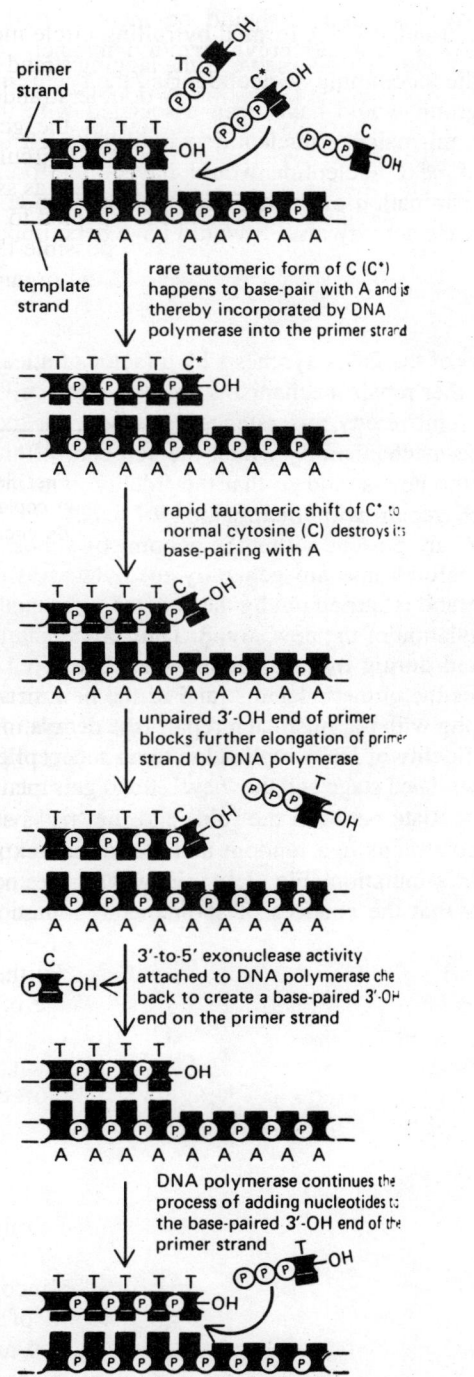

Fig. 3.13. Repair of a mismatch by proofreading function of DNA polymerase.

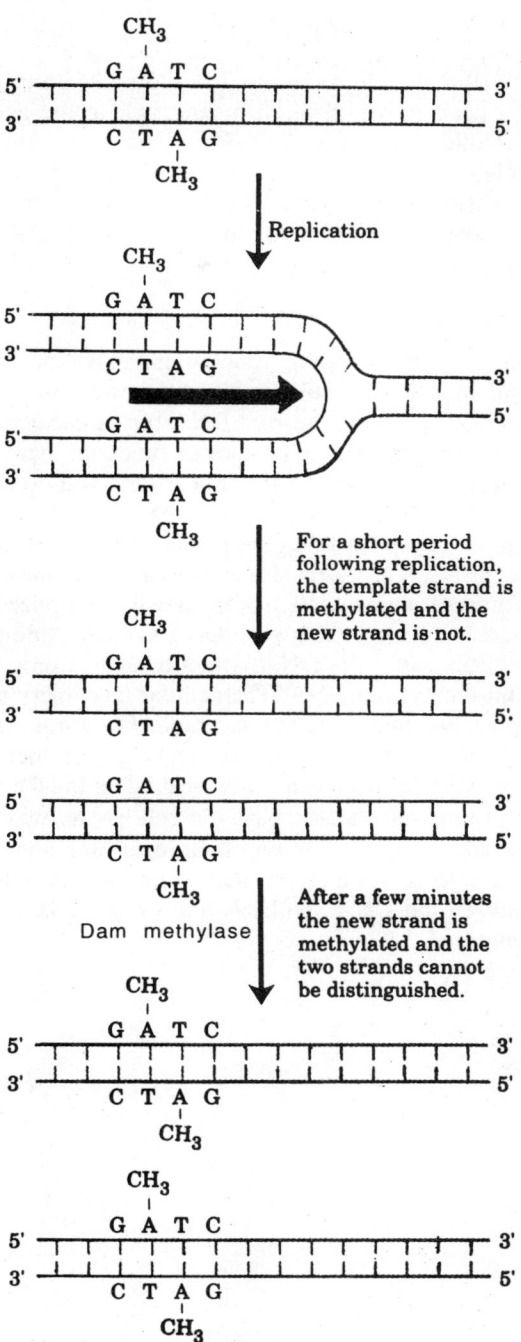

Fig. 3.14. Methylation of DNA strands can serve to distinguish the template strand from newly synthesized strand in *E. coli* DNA, a function which is critical to mismatch repair. The methylation occurs at N^6 of adenines in pallindromic (5') GATC.

polymerase is known as the proof reading function. At this point it should be mentioned that the incorporation of nucleotides in DNA (and also in RNA) is in a tail polymerization manner and the activation of reactive group (the phosphate group) lies in the incomming nucleotide. Had the synthesis been in a head polymerization manner where the activated group would have been associated with the last nucleotide present in the existing chain, the removal of a mismatched nucleotide would have left the last nucleotide without an activated group. The addition of next nucleotide would have, therefore, been impossible. This would have resulted in the premature termination of the growing polynucleotide chain. Similarly, if the DNA polymerase have had 3'–5' polymerase activity also, it would have been impossible to carry out the proof reading function.

Other mechanisms

While the proof reading function increases the correctness of the DNA synthesis by a factor of atleast 10^3, some mistakes are still remained uncorrected. There are other repair mechanisms present in the cell which scan the newly synthesized DNA for its correctness and remove any mismatches. However, for the post-replication repair mechanisms to function, there has to be mechanism by which the cell can differentiate between the 'new' and the 'old' strand and correct only the new strand so that the fidelity is maintained. This is achieved by coupling the process of mismatch repair with methylation of DNA. In fact, a number of repeats of a pallindromic tetranucleotide GATC are present within the genome of almost all the organisms. The A residues in both the strands of this pallindrome are generally methylated at the C6 position. The methylation of the newly synthesized DNA strand is carried out by the enzyme, dam methylase. There is a time gap between DNA synthesis and the methylation of the new strand. Thus immediately after the replication, the DNA is methylated in only one strand during this gap period and is reffered as the hemi-methylated DNA. The cellular machinery recognizes the unmethylated strand as the new strand and repairs any mismatch in this strand. The proof reading along with the mismatch repair (the details of repair mechanism will be discussed later) together, increase the fidelity of DNA replication to an acceptable level. However, if a mismatch is not repaired during the hemi-methylated stage and the 'new' strand gets methylated before the mismatch repair, the cell has no way to differentiate between the 'old' and the 'new' strands. The repair mechanism will then repair any one of the two strands in a random manner to make a perfect base pairing. As a result, half of the repairs will result in a mutation (Fig. 3.14). However, the time gap between the DNA synthesis and its methylation ensures that the chances of spontaneous mutations are minimised.

4

Organization of the Genome

Genome is the term used to define the total genetic material of the cell. The amount of DNA present in any cell is the inherent property of an organism and remains same in all the cells of the an organism as well as in all individuals of a particular species. However, the amount varies from species to species. In general, the eukaryotes have much more DNA than the prokayotes. However, careful analysis of DNA content has revealed that while the number of expressed genes in eukaryotes is about 2-10 times more than that of prokaryotes, the total amount of DNA in an eukaryotic cell is many order of magnitude higher than in a prokaryotic cell. This means, that there is a huge excess of DNA in eukaryotic cells which does not code for any known gene. This DNA is often referred as the junk DNA. Its role, if any, is not fully understood.

The DNA of a cell is present in a highly condensed form. It is packed in long thread like structure, the chromosome. Prokaryotes have their entire genome in a single chromosome. Eukaryotes on the other hand, have many chromosomes. Further, there are generally two copies of each chromosome (diploid, written as 2x) in majority of the organisms. However, occassionally more than two copies may be present (polyploids; 3x, 4x and so on, as the case may be). Polyploidy is more common in the plants than in animals. Similarily, sometimes only one copy may be present when the organism is heploid (1x). The chromosome is thus the ultimate organized form of the genome.

Structure of the chromosome

The total genome of an E.coli cell, in its fully extended form is consist of about 1100 μm long circular DNA. The cell diameter, on the other hand, is only 1–2 μm. This simply means that the DNA is present in a highly coiled and condensed form. It has been found that the bacterial DNA is packed within a dense structure, referred as nucleoid. This is in contrast to the earlier belief that the DNA of bacteria is present as naked DNA and is interspread all over the cell cytoplasm. The earlier pictures which showed DNA as a coiled thread like structure were taken for isolated DNA which was not metabolically active. The later pictures of functional genome have revealed that the bacterial DNA is present as a single chromosome located within the nucleoid of the bacterial cell. The bacterial nucleoid is the folded form of the genome. Its structure can be maintained in the absence of ionic detergents and in presence of high concentration of cations such as polyamines or 1.0 M salt.

Eukaryotic Chromosome

The chromosomes in eukaryotes are compact structure. During interphase, these cannot be seen with light microscope. However, the chemical analysis, electron microscopy and the X–ray defraction studies have revealed their fine structure. The structure of the chromosomes is maintained in a nucleoprotein form where the DNA is present in a complexed form with a number of proteins. The entire structure of chromosome is very compact. Different chromosomes of a cell have different size and shape. For example, there are 46 chromosomes in human, 44 of these are present in 22 homologous pairs while the two chromosomes, the sex chromosomes, are heterologous. The size of these chromosomes varies. The largest of the human chromosomes has about 85 mm of DNA. However, its size is only 0.5 μm × 10 μm. This means that there is about 10^4 fold condensation of DNA. This complex nature of chromosomes presents a number of possibilities.

  (i) The entire DNA present in a chromosome may consist of a number of small DNA molecules. These molecules may be running parallel to each other thus making a compact structure. This type of arrangement will be known as multineme or multistrand (here 'strand' does not mean a single nucleotide chain of a ds DNA, but means a stretch of ds DNA).

 (ii) There is only one large molecule of DNA present which is starting from one end and continues to the other end of the entire genome which is present as a long stretch. This will be the mononeme (or unineme) model of DNA arrangement.

(iii) The DNA may be multineme, however, the multiple DNA molecules present in the chromosome may be joined either from end to end or may be present in any other molecular arrangement.

 (iv) There is a mononeme DNA which is present in a highly coiled form.

   In fact, the total DNA of a chromosome is present in form of a single giant molecule of DNA that extends from one end of the chromosome, through the centromere, all the way to other end of the chromosome. It is present in a highly coiled configuration. Thus the possibility number (iv) in above list is the actual scenario within a cell.

Lamp brush chromosomes

A special chromosome structure is present during prophase I of oogenesis in amphibians and many other eukaryotic species. The chromosome is about 800 μm long. It represents two chromotids formed by the duplication of each of the chromosomes, present in paired form. These have a central axis region of highly condensed chromatid with many lateral loops of DNA arranged in a paired manner. The loops represent the DNA which is transcriptionally active (Fig. 4.1). The integrity of central axis and the loop is DNA dependent and DNase treatment fragments it. RNase and proteases on the other hand, remove the sorrounding matrix but donot distroy the continuity of the structure. The loops have a filament of 20Å diameter which is same as the diameter of ds DNA. It, therefore, reveals that the loops are unineme.

The chromatin structure

The coiling of DNA in the chromosome is in form of a precise and highly organised structure. This is referred as the chromatin. The chromatin is made of a complex of DNA with a number of chromosomal proteins and other chromosomal constituents isolated from nuclei. These may contain a small amount of RNA also.

The proteins of chromatin

Based on their nature, the protein part of the chromatin can be classified into two broad groups.

  (a) The basic proteins: These proteins have a net positive charge at neutral pH. Present in all animal and plant cells, these basic proteins are referred as the histones. Histones are present in almost

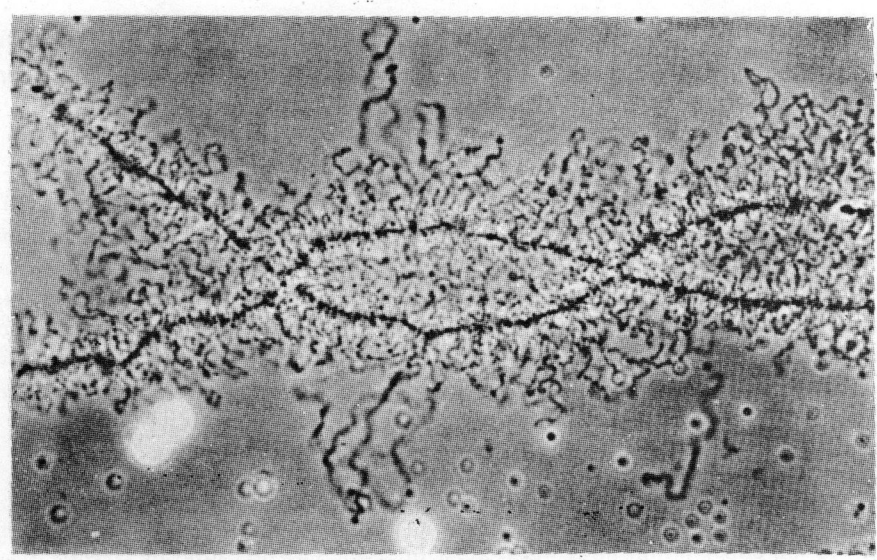

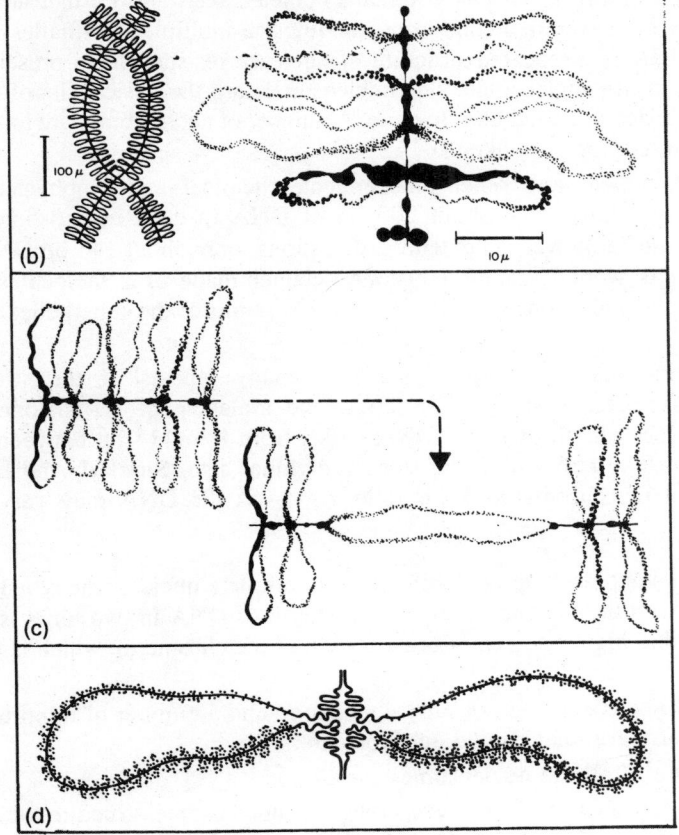

Fig. 4.1. Structure of a lamp brush chromosome.

all the eukaryotic cells and only a few eukaryotic cells which include the sperms of certain species, are the known exceptions where histones are not present. The histones have upto 20-30% Arg and Lys and are highly basic in nature. The analysis has revealed that these are present in almost equal ratio with the DNA (w/w).

The qualitative analysis of histones on acrylamide gels have revealed five different classes of proteins in this fraction. These are referred as H1, H2a, H2b, H3 and H4 histones. The quantitative analysis revealed that these are present in a molar ratio of 1:2:2:2:2 (i.e. for one molecule of H1, there are two molecules each of H2a, H2b, H3 and H4). The histones play an important role in maintaining the structure of chromatin. The structure of chromatin has remained highly conserved during evolution. The histone molecules get complexed with DNA and help it in getting packaged into chromatin.

(b) The acidic proteins: The acidic proteins are heterogeneous in nature, varying in composition and structure from cell to cell and are commonly known as the non-histone proteins.

The organization of chromatin

The electron microscopic studies of chromatin has revealed that it is made up of ellipsoidal beads of 110 × 60Å which are joined by a thin thread at regular interval. The digestion of chromatin with DNase has revealed that a region of 146 bp of DNA remains nuclease resistant. Further analysis revealed that upon partial digestion under sub–optimal conditions, the integral multiples of smallest fragment were obtained. This suggsted that there is a repeated structure of nuclease resistant form present in the chromatin. This structure is referred as the nucleosome. The nucleosomes are the basic units of chromatin structure. The nucleosomes are organized in a bead like structure. A number of nucleosomes are joined together by a nuclease sensitive interbead thread or the linker DNA.

The nuclease treatment and other biochemical, chemical and biophysical studies including the X–ray defraction have shown that about 200 bp of DNA in each nucleosome is protected by partial digestion with nuclease. However, on extended digestions, only about 146 bp DNA fragment is protected. This DNA fragment is wound around a histone octamer made of 2 molecules each of H2a, H2b, H3 and H4. The DNA is wound as one and three fourth ($1^3/_4$) turns of the superhelical DNA around the histone core.

The complete chromatin subunit is made of many repeats of the structure consisted of the nucleosome core associated with a linker DNA, one molecule of H1 histone and some non–histone proteins. (Fig. 4.2). The length of linker DNA varies from 8 to 114 bp between different organisms. Its length varies from cell to cell within the same individual also. Similarly the H1 molecule may not be evenly distributed in the chromatin. Their ratio vis–a–vis the DNA may vary at different loci of the chromatin.

It seems that H1 histones help in stabilizing the complete nucleosome which has two complete turns of superhelical DNA on the histone octamer. The length of DNA in two turns is 166 bp. The H1 histone may also be involved in higher degree of organization of the chromatin, which is the 300Å chromatin fibre (see later).

The structure of nucleosome is not fully understood and a number of important questions still remain unanswered. Some of these unanswered questions are:

(a) Is the structure of all the nucleosomes same?

(b) How does the replication fork move along the nucleosome structure which is highly compact?

(c) Does chromatin structure have any role in the regulation of gene expression, if yes, what is it?

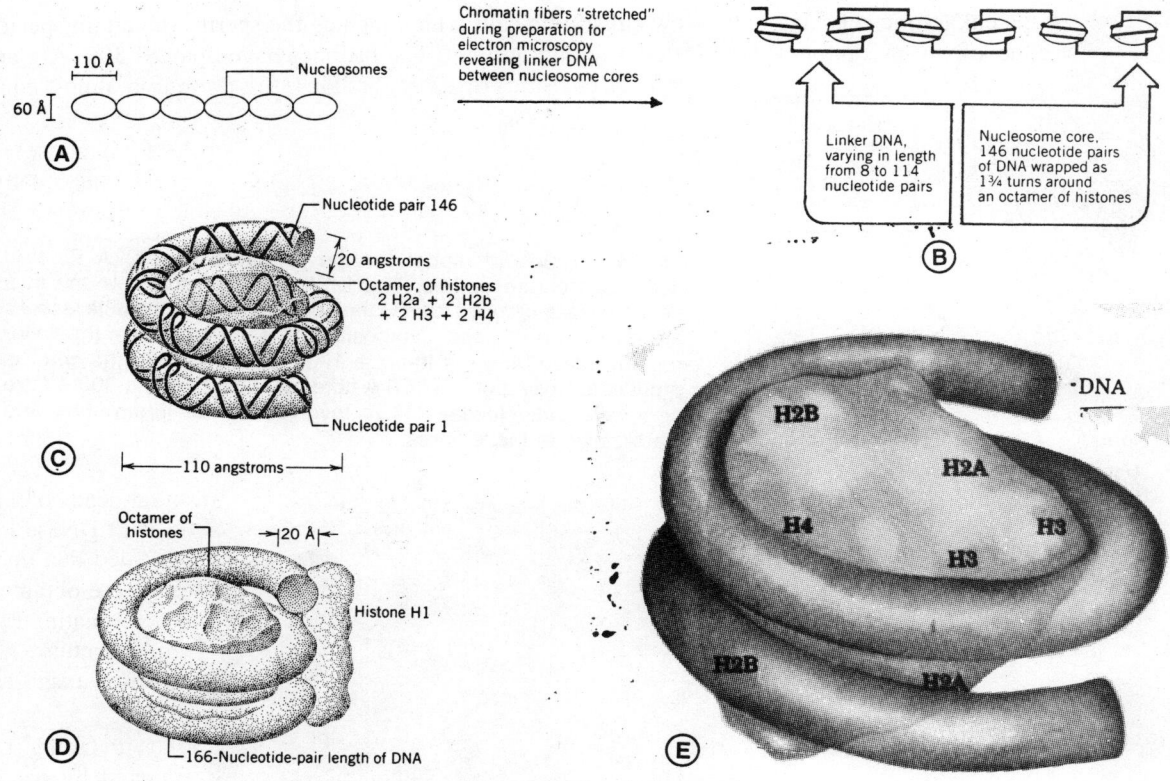

Fig. 4.2. Structure of nucleosomes.

The second degree of organization of chromatin: The 300Å fibres

The electron microscopic studies of isolated metaphase chromosomes revealed that the nucleosomes are futher organized in a highly coiled, lumpy fibres. These fibres have an average diameter of about 300Å. In fact the comparision of E.M. structure with the light microscopic pictures have revealed that what one sees under light microscope during the early stages of meiosis is only the 300Å fibres. Individual nucleosomes are not visible under these conditions. The nucleosomes (~100Å in diameter) are probably in direct contact with each other without detectable large linker regions. These are then wound in a higher order of super coiling or a solenoid structure of 300Å. This structure is shown in Fig. 4.3. However, fine details of the structure of 300Å fibres are not very clear.

Third degree of chromatin organzation

The maximum degree of condensation of chromatin is observed during metaphase. The function of these structures is probably to package the giant DNA molecules in a form which can be segregated into daughter nuclei. It is essential that the DNA molecules donot get entangled with each other during the segregation, so that there is no shearing of the genetic material. This condensation of DNA takes place with the help of non–histone proteins. The histones do not participate in its formation. This condensation results in the formation of scaffold structure (Fig. 4.4). This has a central core sorrounded by huge pool of DNA. No apparent ends of DNA molecule are visible, which supports the theory that the entire chromosome is made up of a single large DNA molecule.

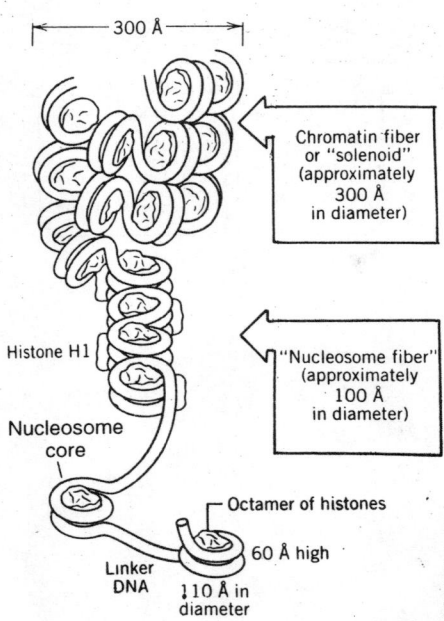

Fig. 4.3. Solenoid model for the structure of 300 Å fibre of eukaryotic chromosomes. The DNA double helix is wound in a negatively supercoiled form in the nucleosome. If the nucleosomes are positioned in close juxtaposition to each other with the linker regions coiled between them, a 100-110 Å "nucleosome fibre" is produced. Coiling of this 100 Å fibre can give rise to a 300 Å fibre or a solenoid. Histone H1 is involved in the information and stabilization of these fibres.

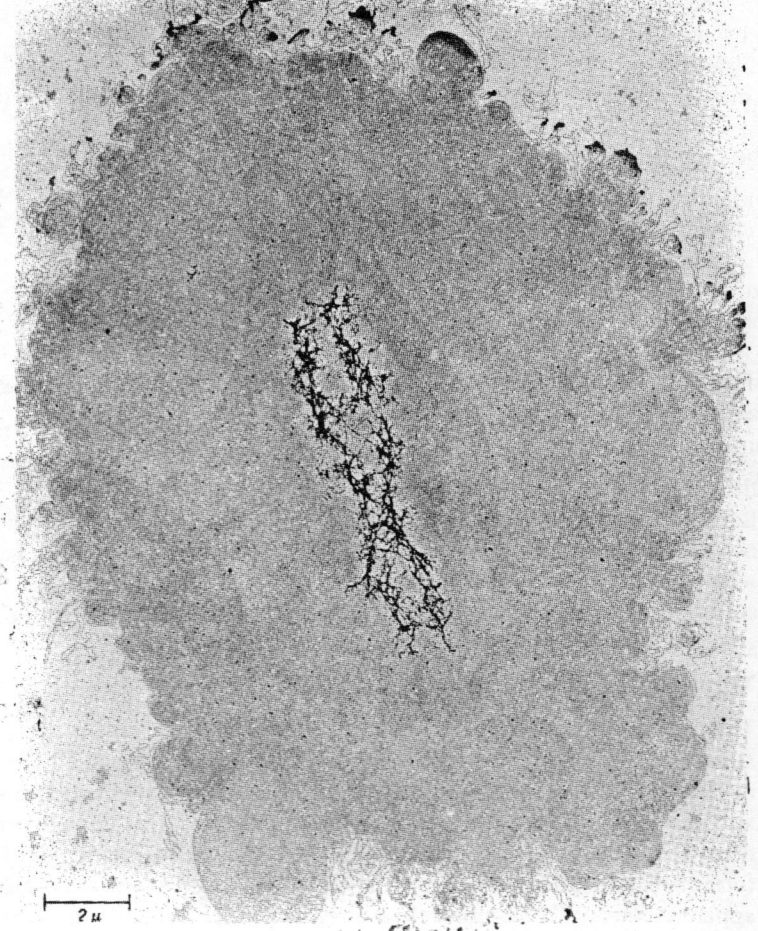

Fig. 4.4. Electron micrograph of a human metaphase chromosome after the histones have been removed. The entire histone-depleted chromosome has been spread on a monolayer of cyto-chrome C, which is floating on an aqueous surface; the chromosome is then picked up on a grid for electron microscopy. The chromosome consists of a central, dense "scaffold" or core surrounded by a huge halo of DNA. Because of the relatively low magnification, individual DNA molecules can be seen only near the periphery. Note the absence of rarity of ends of DNA molecules in the chromosomes.

Thus the chromatin structure has a three tier organization. In first step, the DNA and histone octamers form nucleosomes. The nucleosomes with the help of H1 histone, condenses to form 300Å chromatin fibre and finally these fibres form a scaffold structure with the help of non–histone proteins. After these levels of organization, there is a 10^4 fold condensation of DNA which is arranged to form the chromosomes.

Euchromatin and Heterochromatin

During the cytological studies of chromosomes some characteristic observations were obtained. It was found that when the chromosomes were stained using Fuelgen reaction, two different types of chromatin structures can be seen. A dense structure which receives very intense staining was made of very tightly packed 300Å fibres. Another region which receives relatively weak staining is made up of less tightly packed DNA.

The deeply stained region is referred as the heterochromatin. It has been found that this region is genetically inactive and remains highly condensed throughout the entire life of the cell. Its structure does not vary during different stages of the cell cycle. This region is not transcribed (or poorly transcribed) and is greatly enriched in highly repeatitive tandemely arranged DNA sequences.

The lightly stained region is refered as the euchromatin. This is not visible during the interphase under light microscope. Majority of the known genes are present within this region and the region is actively transcribed. The two types of organizations of chromatin play an important role in regulation of gene expression. The role of the chromatin structure in gene regulation has been discussed elsewhere.

The Satellite DNA

The prokaryotic DNA is relatively simple. It is well established that if a solution of bio–macromolecules is centrifuged through a CsCl gradient, each molecule forms a band in the region where the density of CsCl is same as the density of the molecule. Thus a single band is usually obtained for any one type of molecules. However, when the total cellular DNA is banded though the CsCl gradient, some unexpected results are obtained. It has been found that the prokaryotic DNA generally gives only a single band on CsCl, which is well within the expected lines. As the sequence of a DNA is random, it is expected to have a uniform density and a single band should be obtained. However, when eukaryotic DNA is banded, multiple bands are seen (Fig. 4.5). The predominent band represents the majority of the DNA. Besides, one to several small bands are also obtained. These bands which represent distinct but minor species of DNA are referred as the satellite DNA.

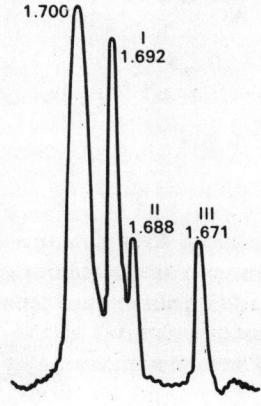

Fig. 4.5. The sedimentation profile of *Drosophila virilis* DNA in CsCl gradient. The satellite DNA shows three prominent bands at ρ = 1.692, 1.688 and 1.671.

It was found that these satellite DNAs represent the species of DNA which is basically composed of the repeats of short sequence of small length. In higher eukaryotes, the repeatitive DNA may constitute a substantial portion of the genome, upto 20–50% of total DNA. Some of the small sequences may be repeated upto 10^6 times. For example in Drosophila virilis, 3 bands of satellite DNA are present. These bands represent the multiple repeats of following three sequences.

1. A |C| A A A |C| T
2. A |T| A A A |C| T
3. A |C| A A A |T| T

As can be seen, these three repeats differ from each other at only two positions which have been boxed. Similar repeats have been found in a related crab species which have 97% A:T rich region. In higher eukaryotes, the length of repeats may be much larger.

These satellite DNAs are present within the heterochromatin region. These are not transcribed and do not have any known function. All efforts to assign any role to these DNAs for the survival of the cell or its replication have met with negative observations. These DNAs are, therefore, quite often referred as the 'selfish' DNA sequences which ensure their own retention during replication but do not contribute anything for the benefit of the cell.

Even though first repeats were discovered by virtue of their unusual sequences, which is very different than the average DNA (for example, highly enriched in A:T) and banded as distinct DNA species, many repeats have now been found which have relatively similar sequence as the average DNA and do not band as separate species.

The satallite DNA have changed in a unusually rapid manner during the course of evolution. It has been found that if one campares two homologous human chromosomes of a pair, some of these repeat sequences are characteristically different. It is in contrast to the general property of DNA that it is highly conserved. Marked differences can be found between setallite DNAs of two closely related species.

Many of these repeated sequences may have been generated by their property to act as transposable element which can get integratead at various regions of the genome. The DNA of the Alu family and the L1 element family of primates represent such repeat sequences, which have multiplied only recently. The Alu family of DNA is the repeat of a sequence of about 300 bp. It may be present in very high copy number, upto 500,000–1,000,000 copies, in human genome and represents upto 5% of the total DNA. It is quite possible that these sequences which are scattered throughout the genome, may have a role in regulation of expression of many genes.

5

The Structure of Gene

A gene is the basic unit of heredity. The entire genome of an organism is made up of a number of genes and a gene usually codes for a single character. The gene has been traditionally defined as a piece of DNA which has necessary information for the synthesis of a protein. However, we now know that there are a number of genes which donot code for a protein but code for an RNA such as the rRNA and the tRNA. In light of these facts, the definition of gene has now been revised. The gene is now defined as a sequence of DNA which codes for a molecule which is transported to another part, other than the site of its synthesis, for its biological action.

The gene has a complex structure having a number of different segments often referred as elements. The composite structure of a typical gene is shown in Fig. 5.1. The prokaryotic and eukaryotic genes differ in their structure, former being simpler than the later. However, there are a number of common features between the two. The eukaryotic genes are monocistronic i.e. they code for a single protein while the prokaryotes have polycistronic genes which code for more than one proteins. Different proteins coded by a polycistronic gene are often functionally related. A typical gene is made of two regions, the regulatory region and the transcriptional unit. The regulatory region contains the sequences essential for the transcription of the gene but are not transcribed themselves while the 'transcription unit' is transcribed to form a RNA molecule. The transcriptional unit starts from a transcription start site. This is the position where RNA polymerase initiates the RNA synthesis during transcription and this nucleotide is traditionally designated as the 1st nucleotide. The nucleotides in the regulatory region which are upstream of the transcription start site are given negative numbers. For example, -10 means a nucleotide 10 bases upstream of the transcription start site while 10 (or, $+10$) means 10th nucleotide from the transcription start site.

The regulatory region

Amongst a number of different elements present in this region, the promoter is the most important regulatory element. It facilitates the binding of RNA polymerase to the gene and directs it to initiate transcription. It is defined as a sequence of DNA having the signal which directs the proper binding of RNA polymerase to DNA and activates it to a form which is capable of initiating the transcription. The promoters are asymmetrical and are orientation and position specific. The structure of eukaryotic and prokaryotic promoters differs from each other considerably. However, there are certain common features of all promoters. Majority of the promoters exhibit a bipartite organization and have two regions of highly conserved sequences. First region which is far from the transcriptional unit, is the recognition site. It is recognized by the RNA

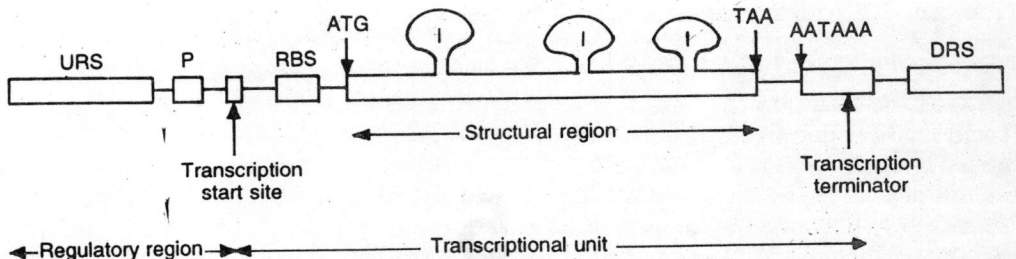

Fig. 5.1. General structure of a gene. URS - Upstream regulator sequences such as activator, silencer, enhancers etc., present only in eukaryotes. P - Promoter. RBS - Ribosome binding site or Shine-Dalgarno sequences, present only in prokaryotes. ATG - Initiation coden. I - Introns present only in eukaryotes. TAA - Stop codon (may be TAG or TGA also). AATAAA - Polyadenylation site, present only in eukaryotes. DRS - Down stream regulatory sequences such as enhancer, present only in eukaryotes.

polymerase and facilitates its binding to the template. The second region, the RNA polymerase binding site, is nearer to transcription initiation site and helps in the initiation of RNA synthesis by opening of the double stranded DNA.

Prokaryotic promoter

In prokaryotes, the first region of promoter is consisted of a hexanucleotide which is highly conserved in most of the promoters. The region has a consensus sequence TTGACA. It is normally present between 30–40 nucleotides upstream of the transcription initiation site and is known as the '−35 region'. The first three nucleotides of the hexamer are highly conserved and are present in more than 80% of the promoters so for studied. The last three nucleotides are relatively less conserved and exhibit certain deviations. The second region is also a conserved hexanucleotide with a consensus sequence TATAAT. It is known as '−10 region' or the 'Prebnow box'. The first two bases and the last base are present in 90% of the promoters. The position of this sequence in relation to transcription initiation site is from −5 to −14, occassionally it may be from −9 to −18. In about 40% of the promoters this hexanucleotide is preceded by another relatively less conserved sequence, ATTTGN. The −10 region (including the preceding sequence, when present) is, thus, highly A:T rich. As the melting of G:C (having three hydrogen bonds) requires more energy than the melting of A:T (having only two hydrogen bonds), this region is easiest to open thermodynamically and is involved in the formation of 'open promoter complex' during the initiation of transcription (see later). The distance between the −10 and the −35 regions varies from promoter to promoter. In 90% of the promoters it is 16 to 19 nucleotides, the optimal being 17 bp. Some of the strong promoters have another A:T rich region at −43. However, this region is not present in all the promoters (Fig. 5.2).

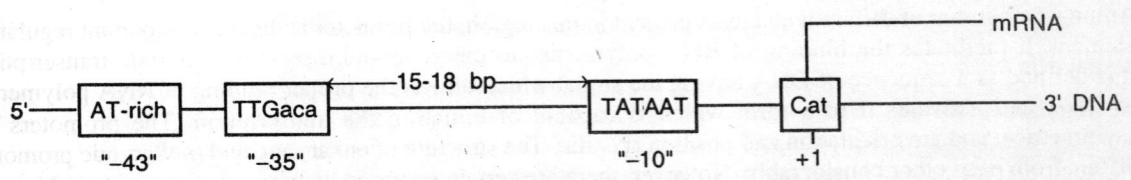

Fig. 5.2A. Structure of a prokaryotic promoter.

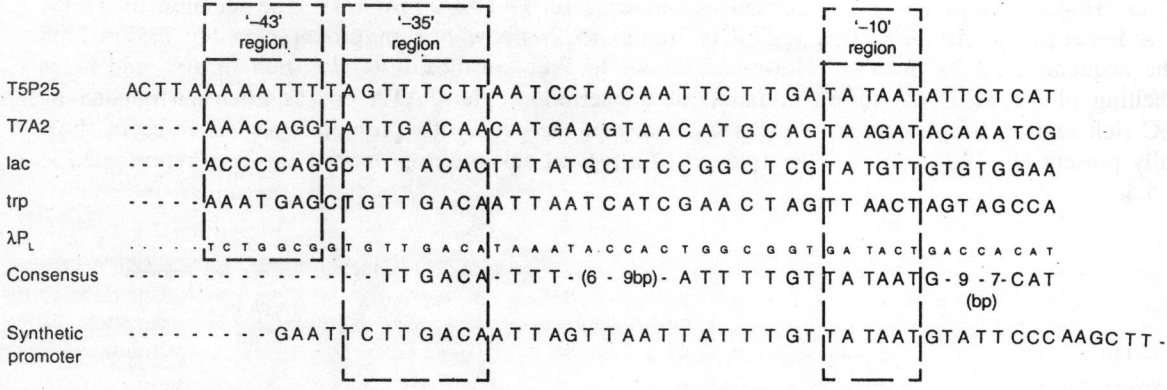

Fig. 5.2B. DNA sequences of promoter regions.

While majority of the promoters have both −10 and the −35 regions, a few promoters may lack either −10 or −35 sequences. The individual promoters have certain degree of variation from the consensus sequence. The promoter of most of the efficiently expressed genes do not deviate much from the consensus sequence. The promoters for the trp (coding for enzymes involved in tryptophan synthesis) and lac (genes coding for β−galactosidase and other enzymes involved in lactose metabolism) genes are some of the strong bacterial promoters. The relative strength of a particular promoter depends on the deviation of the two regions from the concensus and also on the distance between the two regions. A synthetic promoter has been constructed which has −10 region of trp promoter and the −35 region of the lac promoter with a spacer region of 17 bases between the two regions. Known as 'tac' promoter, it is the most potent bacterial promoter. The sequence of −10 region and −35 region and the relative strength of some of the E. coli promoters is given in Table 5.1.

Table 5.1. Relative activity of various promoters

S.No.	Promoter	-10 region	-35 region	Relative Strength
1.	tet	TTTAAT	TTTGAC	100
2.	lac	TATATT	TTTACA	125
3.	trp	TTAACT	TTGACA	360
4.	tac	TATAAT or TTTAAT	TTGACA	440
	Consensus	TATAAT	TTGACA	

Eukaryotic promoter

The regulatory region of an eukaryotic gene is relatively more complex. Two basic regions of the promoter are similar to prokaryotic promoter in structure but differ in their relative positions. The first region (recognition region, similar to the −35 region of bacteria) is known as the 'CAAT box'. Its consensus sequence is GG(C/T)CAATCT and it is present between the positions of −70 to −80. The second region (similar to -10 region of prokaryotes), is a septanucleotide. It is called the 'TATA box' or 'Hogness box' and has a consensus sequence of TATA(A/T)A(A/T). The location of TATA box is between −19 to −27. This region is similar to Prebnow box of prokaryotes but differs both in the sequence and its position. However, similar to Prebnow box it is also rich in A:T and helps in melting of the ds DNA during initiation of transcription. The TATA box is often surrounded by a G:C rich region. Besides these two regions, many of the eukaryotic promoters also have a G:C box, usually present at −120 position. The structure of a typical eukaryotic promoter has been represented in Fig. 5.3.

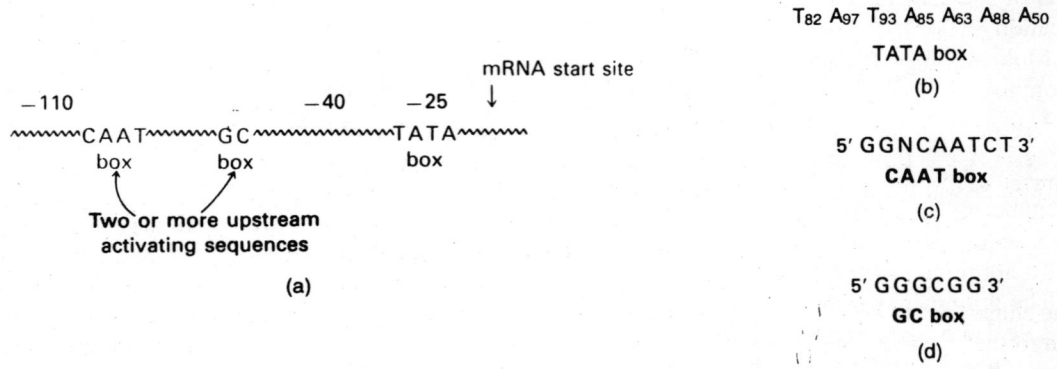

Fig. 5.3. Structure of eukaryotic promoter.

Down stream promoters

As discussed, the position of both the prokaryotic and eukaryotic promoters is relatively conserved and is at a location upstream of the transcription unit. However, in a few genes the promoter may be present downstream of the transcription start site, and is within the transcription unit itself. The promoter of X. laevis 5S RNA gene is a good example of a down stream promoter. It is located between +55 and +80 regions. The promoter itself is transcribed and is represented within the RNA. Other downstream promoters are present in VA gene of adenovirus (+9 to +72) and tRNA met gene (+1 to +72). The presence of such promoters pose a paradox regarding the mechanism of their action. Normally, the RNA polymerase binds to promoter covering about 60 nucleotides (within the −50 to +30 region) and initiates the RNA synthesis at catalytic site (see later). How the downstream promoter will allow this to happen? It is possible that the RNA polymerase binds to promoter, then moves back to transcription start site and starts the RNA synthesis. Alternatively, the DNA folds back in such a manner that it can start the transcription while bound at the promoter region. The precise mechanism is, however, not clear.

Other regulatory elements

Besides the promoter, the eukaryotic genes also contain certain other regulatory elements such as the activators, silencers and enhancers. All these elements are 'cis' acting elements i.e. present on the gene itself and manifest their effect without being expressed in form of either RNA or protein. The function of these elements is to regulate the level of gene expression either all by themselves or with the help of certain other `trans' acting elements. The regulatory mechanisms for their action will be discussed elsewhere. However, it will be appropriate to describe the enhancers in some detail.

The enhancers are present in the genes which are expressed at relatively high level. These elements are position and orientation independent. These sequences can enhance the level of expression many fold. Quite often, these may be present at a distance of thousands of nucleotides from the site of their action. The enhancer of a particular gene, if cloned alongwith another gene, may stimulate the expression of the receiving gene. However, no highly conserved sequences for the enhancers have been found. The precise mode of their action is not very well understood. For example, in SV40 a 72 bp region has been recognized which is repeated twice within the genome. The first stretch is between 109–180 and second at 181–252. It stimulates the transcription of one of the early genes, the 'T' antigen gene, by several fold. The gene starts at position 0/5243 and proceeds in left ward direction. Expression of this gene influences the replication of viral genome. Similar 72 bp repeats have also been found on Polyoma virus, BK virus and Moloney sarcoma virus. It is possible to replace the enhancer of these viruses with SV40 enhancer without compromising on the expression levels. The sequence of SV40 T–antigen enhancer has been shown in Fig. 5.4.

```
CCAGCTGTGGAATGTGTGTCAGTT AGGGTGTGGAAAGTCCCCAG GCTCCCCAGCAGGCAG AAGTATGCAAAGCATGCAT CTCAATTAGTCAGCAAC
GGTCGACACCTTACACACAGTCAA TCCCA CACCTTTCAGGGGGTC CGAGGGGTCGTCCGTC TTCATACGTTTCGTACGTA GAGTTAATCAGTCGTTG
```

Fig. 5.4. Structure of an enhancer element.

As the enhancer elements are position and orientation independent, the relative position of these elements in relation to the the transcription unit of the gene does not make much difference in their activity. If their position is changed by relocting these elements experimentally or by making insertions or deletions in the non–coding region of the gene, these still maintain their activity. Similarly if the enhancer of a gene is cloned near another gene by genetic engineering, the transcription of the recipient gene is enhanced. These elements have proved to be very beneficial in achieving high level expression of foreign genes in heterologous systems using the rDNA technology.

Transcriptional unit

The transcriptional unit of a gene is the portion of gene which starts from the transcription initiation site and ends at the transcriptional terminator. The entire transcription unit is copied to form a RNA as a single entity. The first element in this region is the transcription initiation site which does not have any long conserved region. In majority of the cases (90% or more) it is a purine (A or G), more often a G than an A. In prokaryotes, it is about 6-9 nucleotides downstream of the Prebnow box. Following the transcription start site, there is a spacer region of varying length. There is no rule related to length of this region. In prokaryotes, it is followed by a region which has complimentarity with the 3'-end of the 16S rRNA. This region base pairs with 16S rRNA and thus facilitates the binding of small subunit of the ribosome to the mRNA during the initiation of translation. This region is known as ribosome binding site (RBS) or Shine-Dalgarno (SD) sequences. The SD sequences are normally 4-9 bases long and are present at about 5-11 bases upstream of the initiation codon. These sequences help in positioning the 30S ribosomal subunit to the mRNA. The sequence of RBS of a number of genes has been shown in Fig. 5.5. Any change in RBS site can result in very poor or no translation (Fig. 5.6). Thus two simutaneous but distinct RNA:RNA interactions take place at the time of the initiation of translation, one between mRNA and 16S RNA and the other between mRNA and tRNA (Fig. 5.7). Eukaryotic genes donot have any such region. The mechanism of ribosomal subunit binding is different in eukaryotes and will be discussed later. The genes which are expressed at a very high level usually have a purine rich region with the sequence PuPuPuTTTPuPu which is recognized by one of the ribosomal proteins and thus results in more efficient translation initiation. After about 7-13 base spacer region, the initiation codon ATG is present. The distance between SD sequence and ATG plays an important role in the rate of translation.

Initiation codon

protein	CUG	AGU	AUA	AGA	GGA	CAU	AUG	CCU	AAA	UUA
Phage Q/3 coat	CUU	UCG	GUC	AAU	UUG	AUC	AUG	GCA	AAA	UUA
Phage Q/3 replicase	UUA	CUA	AGG	AUG	AAA	UGC	AUG	UCU	AAG	ACA
Phage γ Cro	AUG	UAC	UAA	GGA	GGU	UGU	AUG	GAA	CAA	CGC
Phage fl coat	UUU	AAU	GGA	AAC	UUC	CUC	AUG	AAA	AAG	UCU
Phage φ X 174 A	AAU	CUU	GGA	GCC	UCC	UUU	AUG	GUU	CGU	UCU
Phage φ X 174 A*	UUG	CUG	GAG	GCC	UCC	ACU	AUG	AAA	UCG	CGU
Phage φ X 174 B	AGG	UCU	AGG	AGC	UAA	AGA	AUG	GAA	CAA	CUC
Phage φ X 174 E	GCG	UUG	AGC	CUU	GCG	UUU	AUG	GUA	CGC	UGG
Lip protein	AUC	UAG	AGG	GUA	UUA	AUA	AUG	AAA	GCU	ACU
RecA	GGC	AUG	ACC	GGA	GUA	AAA	AUG	GCU	AUC	G
GolE	AGC	CUA	AUG	GAG	CGA	AUU	AUG	AGA	GUU	CUG
GalT	CCC	GAU	UAA	GGA	ACG	ACC	AUG	ACG	CAA	UUU
LacI	CAA	UUC	AGG	GUG	GUG	AAU	GUG	AAA	CCA	GUA
LacZ	UUC	ACA	CAG	GAA	ACA	GCU	AUG	ACC	AUG	AUU
Ribosomal L	CAU	CAA	GGA	GCA	AAG	CUA	AUG	GCU	UUA	AAU
Ribosomal L7/L12	UAU	UCA	GGA	ACA	AUU	UAA	AUG	UCU	AUC	ACU
RNA polymerase β subunit	AGC	GAG	CUG	AGG	AAC	CCU	AUG	GUU	UAC	UCC

Fig. 5.5. SD sequences of a number of mRNA. The number of concerned basis and their relative position to initiation codon varies.

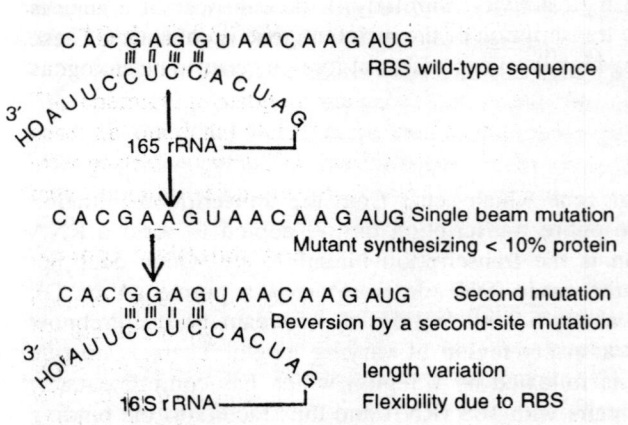

Fig. 5.6. Role of SD sequences in translation.

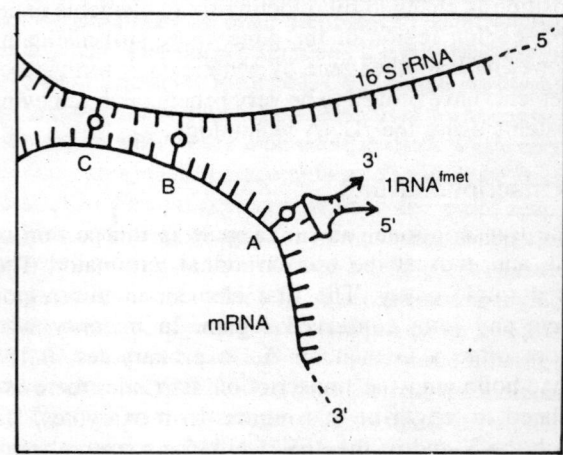

Fig. 5.7. Simultaneous interaction of mRNA with rRNA and tRNA.

The initiation codon is followed by the coding region of the gene. The coding region is a continuous structure in prokaryotes and a single open reading frame is present which ends in a translational stop codon. However, majority of the eukaryotic genes have a number of interveneing sequences interspersed in between the coding region (Fig. 5.8). These sequences donot code for any polypeptide. Known as introns, these sequences are initially copied into RNA (primary transcript) but are later removed from the mature mRNA by a complex post–transcriptional process known as splicing (see later). The coding region ends in one of the three stop codons. This is followed by a region which is not translated but is present in the mature mRNA (the 3'–non coding region).

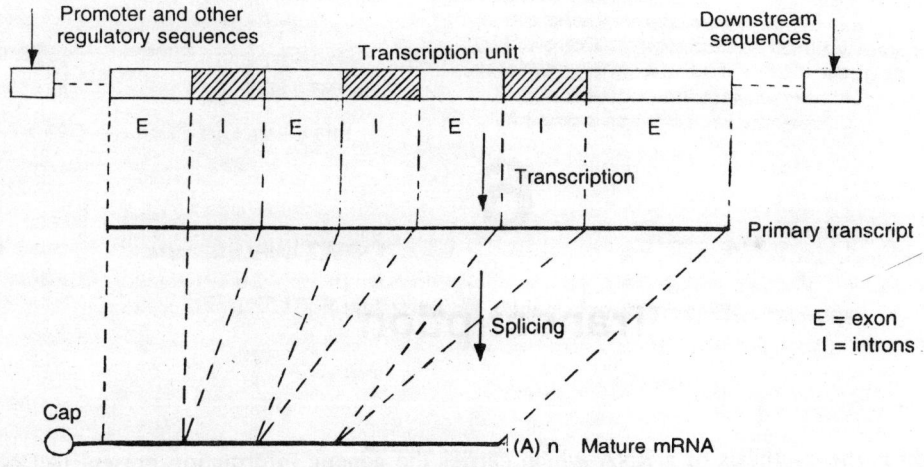

Fig. 5.8. Eukaryotic genes have introns.

The transcriptional unit ends in a transcriptional stop signal. There is no consensus sequences for this element. The mechanism of transcription termination will be discussed later. In eukaryotes, there is a downstream regulatory sequence present 10–20 nucleotide upstream of the transcription terminator. This sequence has a consensus AAATAA and is called as the polyadenylation site. It directs the poly(A) polymerase to add a stretch of A residues (100–200 nucleotides) at the 3'–end of the mRNA. This site also provides a signal for the termination of transcription (see later).

6

Transcription

Transcription is the synthesis of a RNA which carries the genetic information present in DNA. The DNA is double stranded and can theoratically code for two separate RNA molecules. However, it has been found that only one of the two strands of the gene is transcribed. Only in a few exceptional cases both strands are transcribed. This is possible because the promoter is asymmetrical and unidirectional. The DNA strand which have a sequence homology with the RNA is known as the coding strand. The second strand which is complementary to RNA and serves as the template for RNA synthesis is known as the non–coding strand. It is, therefore, a misnomen-clature, as it is the non–coding strand which is in fact transcribed to form the primary transcript.

Enzymes involved in transcription

The principal enzyme involved in transcription is the DNA dependent RNA polymerase (commonly called as RNA pol). The RNA pol is similar to DNA polymerase in most of its requirements, such as the template, Mg^{++} and four ribonucleoside triphosphates (rNTPs). It should be re–imphasised that the sugar in ribonucleotides is ribose rather than the deoxyribose which is present in deoxy-nucleotides which are required for the synthesis of DNA. Three of the four NTPs have same bases (A, G and C) as in dNTPs and the 4th base in RNA is U in place of T of DNA. Similar to DNA polymerase, the RNA polymerase also can not use NDP or NMP as substrate. However, it differs from DNA polymerase in the fact that it does not require a primer and is capable of initiating the RNA synthesis. Another difference between DNA polymerase and the RNA polymerase is that RNA polymerase does not have exonuclease activity. It, therefore, cannot carry out the proof reading function. As a result, the fidelity of RNA polymerase is less (lower by a factor of atleast 10^{-3}) than the DNA polymerase.

To undersatand the transcription, it is necessary to learn a little more about the RNA polymerase. The bacterial RNA polymerase is a multimeric enzyme having 5 different types of subunits, α, β, β', ω and σ. The complete enzyme (holoenzyme) has two α subunits and one each of other four subunits ($\alpha_2\beta\beta'\omega\sigma$). The MW of the complete enzyme is about 450KD. If round in shape, a molecule of this size will have a diameter of about 100Å. This should be able to cover only about 30bp of DNA at the gene (each base in DNA is 3.4Å away from the next base). However, the protection experiments have revealed that during transcription initiation, about 60 bases of the template DNA are covered by the enzyme. It is possible only if the enzyme is elongated in its shape. The size of E. coli RNA polymerase is $95 \times 95 \times 160$Å while in yeast it is about $110 \times 136 \times 140$Å.

The σ factor of the RNA polymerase serves as an ancillary factor and is not needed for the polymerization of nucleotides. However, it is essential for the initiation of transcription. Enzyme without the σ factor is known as core enzyme. The complete enzyme (the core enzyme + the σ factor), on the other hand, is called as the holoenzyme. The core enzyme can bind to DNA in a non–specific manner (see later) which will lead to abortive initiation. For specific binding of the polymerase at the promoter site, the holoenzyme is needed. The number of sigma factors in a cell is about 1/3 of the core enzyme. That means that only about one third of all the enzyme molecules are present as holoenzyme at any given time. Almost all of the holoenzyme molecules are actively engaged in transcription and very little, if any, holoenzyme is present in free form. Similarly, about 50% of total core enzyme molecules are engaged in RNA synthesis. It may be pertinent to state that sigma factor may bear certain degree of promoter specificity also. The importance of this specificity plays a role in the regulation of expression of certain genes and will be discussed later. The properties and the functions of different subunits are described in Table 6.1A.

Table 6.1A. Structure of E. coli RNA polymerase

Subunit	Coding gene	Protein size	Activity
α	rpo A	36.5 KD	Enzyme assembly
β	rpo B	151 KD	Nucleotide binding
β1	rpo C	155 KD	Template binding
α	rpo D	70 KD	Promoter recognition and initiation of transcription
ω		11 KD	Unknown

Table 6.1B. α-aminitin sensitivity of various eukaryotic RNA polymerases.

Enzyme	Localization	Sensitivity to α-aminitin	Function
Pol I	Nucleolus	Insensitive	Ribosomal RNA synthesis
Pol II	Nucleoplasm	Highly sensitive	mRNA synthesis
Pol III	Nucleoplasm	Moderately sensitive	tRNA synthesis, 5S & other small RNA synthesis

The enkaryotes have more than one type of RNA polymerases. Based on the sensitivity to α-aminitin, an antibiotic which inhibits mRNA seynthesis, three classes of RNA polymerases have been identified which are involved in the transcription of different class of eukaryotic genes. Their properties have been summarised in Table 6.1B and described below.

(a) Pol I: Not sensitive to α-aminitin; it is present in nucleolus of the cell and synthesizes the rRNA, about 50-70% of total RNA polymerase of a typical cell belong to this class.

(b) Pol II: Highly sensitive to α-aminitin, it is present in nucleoplasm of the cell and synthesizes the mRNA. This class of RNA polymerase comprises between 20-40% of total cellular enzyme.

(c) Pol III: Partially sensitive to α-aminitin, it carries certain degree of of species specificity also. For example, animal Pol III is sensitive to high doses of α-aminitin while the yeast enzyme is insensitive to the antibiotic. Pol III is also present in nucleolus and synthesizes the tRNA. It accounts for about 10% of total enzyme.

In general, eukaryotic RNA polymerases are large molecules of >500KD in size. It has two large subunits of ~200KD and ~140KD, respectively. The 200 KD subunit is similar to β' subunit of E. coli RNA polymerase and have similar function (the template binding). Besides these two proteins, it also has upto 10 different small subunits. A subunit of Pol II, which has simlarity with one of the subunits present in Pol I and also in Pol III, is similar to the α–subunit of E. coli enzyme and helps in the enzyme assembly. A sigma or sigma like factor is also present in eukaryotic RNA polymerases. However, the efforts to reconstitute the enzyme from individual subunits in an in vitro system have not been successful and it is not very clear if all these proteins are the intrinsic part of the enzyme or not.

The tertiary structure of RNA polymerase of both prokaryotes and enkaryotes is such that it forms a groove and about 20–25 nucleotides of the DNA fit within this groove making a tight fit (Fig. 6.1). Besides the RNA polymerase, a number of other transcription factors are also needed for the transcription. These factors are protein in nature and their role will be discussed along with the details of the transcription process.

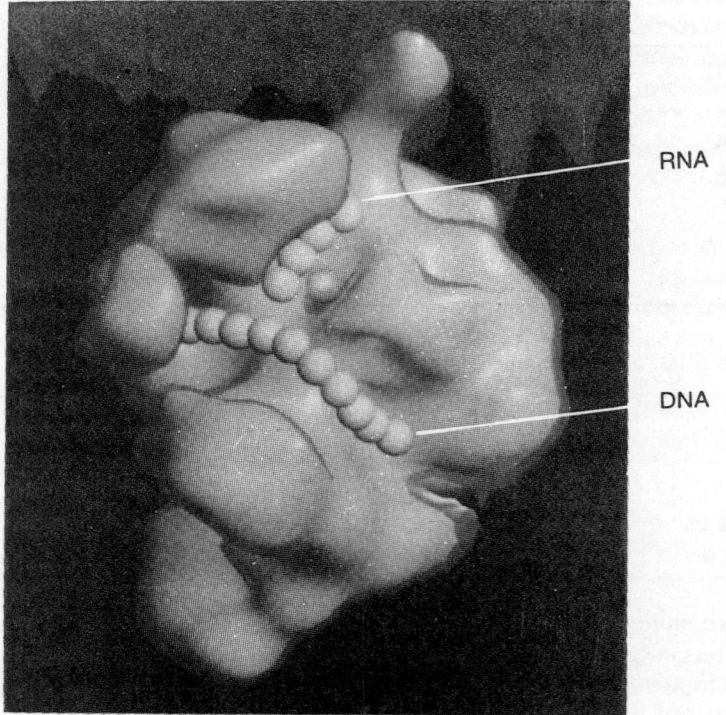

RNA

DNA

Fig. 6.1. Space-filling structure of RNA polymerase : The RNA polymerase has grooves that could be binding sites for nucleic acids. The possible path for DNA is 25 Å wide and 5-10 Å deep. A narrower channel, 12-15 Å wide and 20 Å deep, could hold RNA.

Events in transcription

The entire process of transcription can be divided into following steps.

    (a) Template recognition,

    (b) Initiation,

    (c) Elongation and

    (d) Termination.

The template recognition

The promoter directs the RNA polymerase to recognize the correct region of the gene and to bind at this site. The −35 region serves this function and is recognized by the enzyme. The size of RNA polymerase is such that about 60 nucleotides in the gene are involved in binding of the enzyme to the template. Sigma factor plays an important role in specific binding of the enzyme with the template. The core enzyme without the sigma factor can bind to DNA but the binding is not promoter specific. The binding of holoenzyme to DNA is however, very specific. The sigma factor is, thus, necessary for the formation of promoter–enzyme complex. The binding of RNA polymerase to a site other than the promoter is generally referred as loose binding. In presence of sigma factor, the affinity for loose binding is reduced while the affinity for specific binding is increased. Thus the chances of only the specific binding taking place are enhanced many fold in presence of sigma factor.

The initiation

Once RNA polymerase has bound to the promoter region, the first transcription complex is formed. Having two components (the DNA and the enzyme), it is a binary complex. At this stage the gene (promoter) is still ds and the complex is known as the closed promoter complex. If the binding is specific, it triggers the melting of the −10 region resulting in the opening of a small region of DNA and formation of single stranded DNA. This melting of DNA at the closed–promoter complex changes its configuration and the complex is converted into an open–promoter complex (Fig. 6.2). The melting also results in tight binding of the enzyme. If the sigma factor is not present or if the holoenzyme binds at a site other than the promoter, the melting does not take place and transcription doesnot proceed. Once the tight binary complex is formed and the melting of promoter has taken place, the enzyme proceeds with RNA synthesis. It should be re–emphasized that the RNA polymerase does not require a primer. It initiates the *de novo* synthesis of a new RNA chain. To start with, first two nucleotides are incorporated and the first phosphodiester bond is formed. This complex thus becomes a ternary complex. The first nucleotides to be added are complementary to transcription initiation site of the gene. For proper initiation it is essential that RNA polymerase is covering both the −10 region and the initiation site, the distance between two is thus very important. Any change in the length of the spacer region will adversely affect the rate of transcription. More nucleotides keep on getting incorporated and upto nine nucleotides are added to the growing RNA chain before there is any movement of RNA polymerase along with the DNA template. At this stage, the system scans the complex for a perfect initiation.

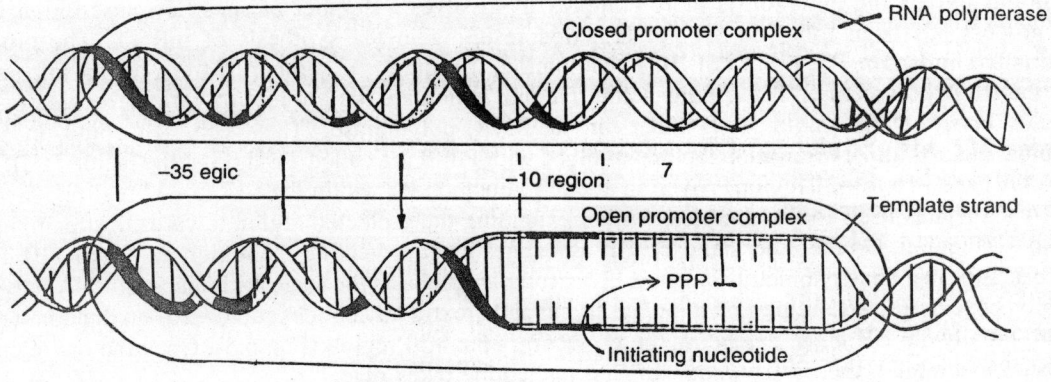

Fig. 6.2. Binding of RNA polymerase to promoter region and formation of open promoter polymerase complex

There is the possibility of premature termination of RNA chain if the conditions are not optimal, Such termination of transcription is referred as abortive intiation. If abortive initiation has taken place, the entire process is repeated. The process has been represented in Fig. 6.3. If the conditions are normal and the initiation is successful, the elongation follows. The exact mechanisms which determine whether the initiation should be abortive or successful, are not well understood. Initiation plays the key role in determining the efficiency of transcription. Once successful initiation has taken place, the sigma factor is released. The sigma factor is thus required only for the initiation and has no role in rest of the processes. It is recirculated by binding to other core enzyme molecule (Fig. 6.4). As discussed earlier, at any time about 1/3 of the total enzymes remain associated with sigma factor. Release of sigma factor changes the enzyme configuration. During the early phase of initiation, upto 75–80 bp of DNA are protected by the enzyme; while only about 60 bp are covered at the begining of the elongation. The process is simpler in bacteria and has been very well understood.

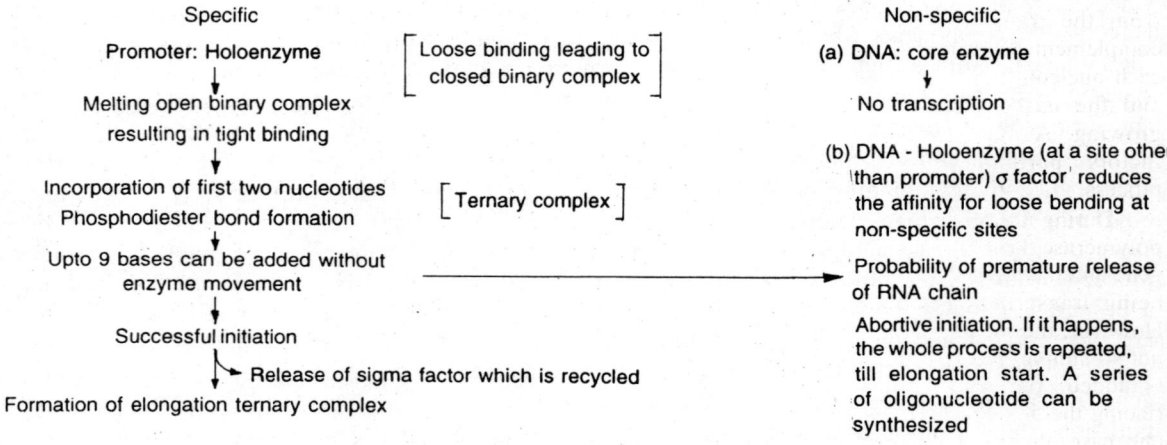

Fig. 6.3. Binding of RNA polymerase to DNA and initiation of transcription.

In eukaryotes the initiation is more complex. It involves a number of specific transcription factors. The process has been followed for pol II action resulting in the synthesis of mRNA. The process is essentially similar for Pol I and Pol III. For initiation, it requires, a number of trans acting factors along with the RNA polymerase. These trans acting factors, which are the product of various regulatory genes, bind to either DNA or to each other or to RNA polymerase. They can also bind in various combinations. All the transcription factors involved with Pol II are called TF II. First the factor TF IID binds to TATA box (−15 to −21 region) covering about 25 nucleotides within the −17 to −42 region. Now factor TF IIA associates itself to the complex, further extending the protected region towards upstream, upto the −55 to −80 region. On the other hand TF IIB associates itself protecting the region at −10 to +10. It binds to two strands in a non−symmetrical manner. This complex prepares the stage for binding of RNA polymerase II which covers upto +15 region on template strand and 5 extra nucleotides (upto +20) on the non−template strand. Finally TF IIE joins, extending the protection upto +30 region (Fig. 6.5). Once the entire complex has been assembled, the incorporation of first nucleotide takes place.

In this chapter we will, discuss the details of bacterial tanscription first and will supplement it with the specific features of eukaryotic system along with it.

Elongation

The elongation is relatively simple process. The RNA polymerase moves along the template DNA. The melting of DNA takes place ahead of the enzyme and simultaneous renaturation of the DNA occurs in the region left by the enzyme. At any given time about 17 bp of DNA remain open. During movement of the enzyme, 30 nucleotides of DNA are covered by it. About 50 nucleotides of growing RNA are in contact with either the DNA or the enzyme. Entire length of RNA except these 50 nucleotides remain hanging from the transcription complex. A complementary nucleotide is added for each nucleotide of the template DNA and the nascent RNA chain keeps growing. A number of trans acting factors participate in elongation process.

During the elongation, the RNA polymerase keeps moving along the gene and the area of the gene which is being transcribed is covered by it. However, the movement of enzyme is not so simple. Every time a new base is added, the back of the enzyme (facing the 5′ side of the gene) moves one base along the DNA. The front, however, remains stationary. Thus there is a change in the configuration of the enzyme. This continues to happen until the addition of 9 nucleotides has taken place. By this time the enzyme has been compressed to its limit and the front portion of the enzyme moves several bases ahead. In other words, it hops in a discontinuous manner. This has been diagrammatically illustrated in Fig. 6,6. The rate of chain elongation is approximately 40 nucleotides/second. This is about 20-fold lower than the rate of DNA replication which is about 800 bases/ second (or ~50,000 bases/min).

Fig. 6.4. Sigma factor and core enzyme recycle at different points in transcription.

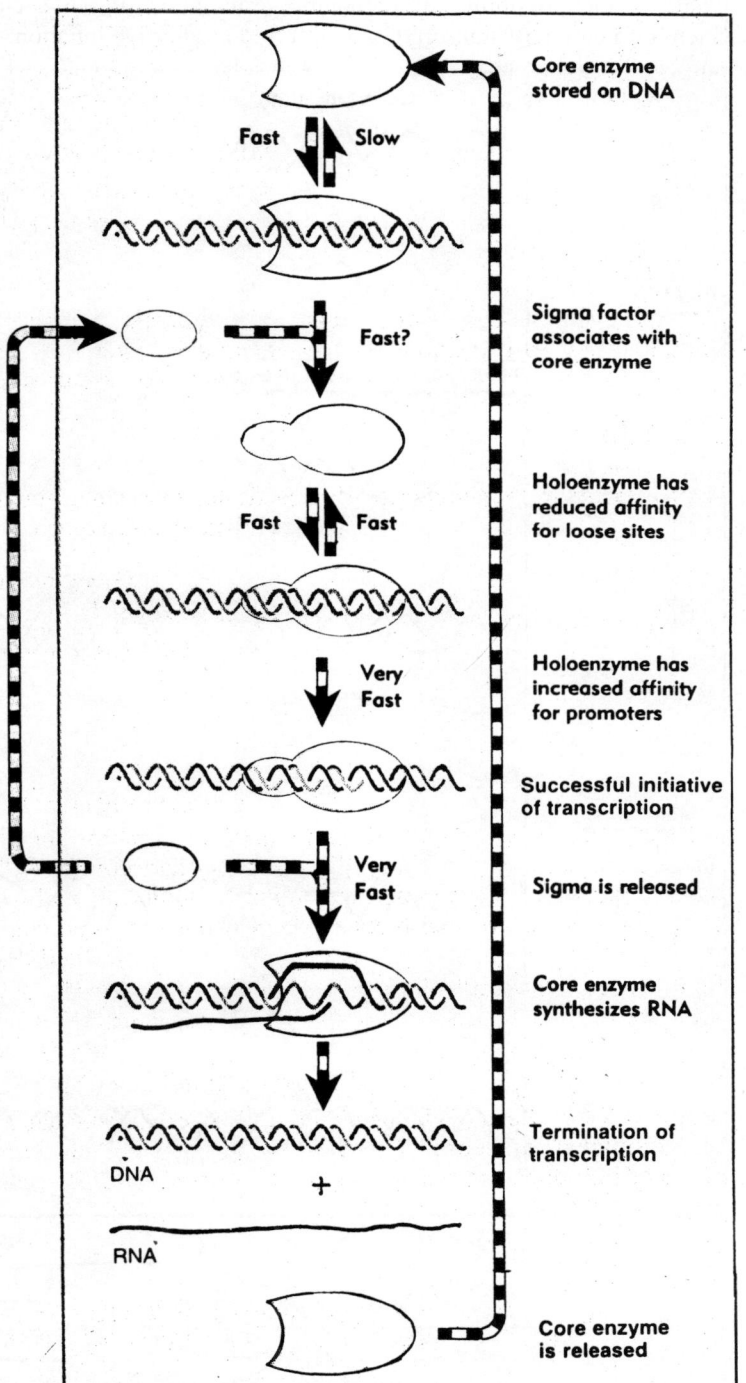

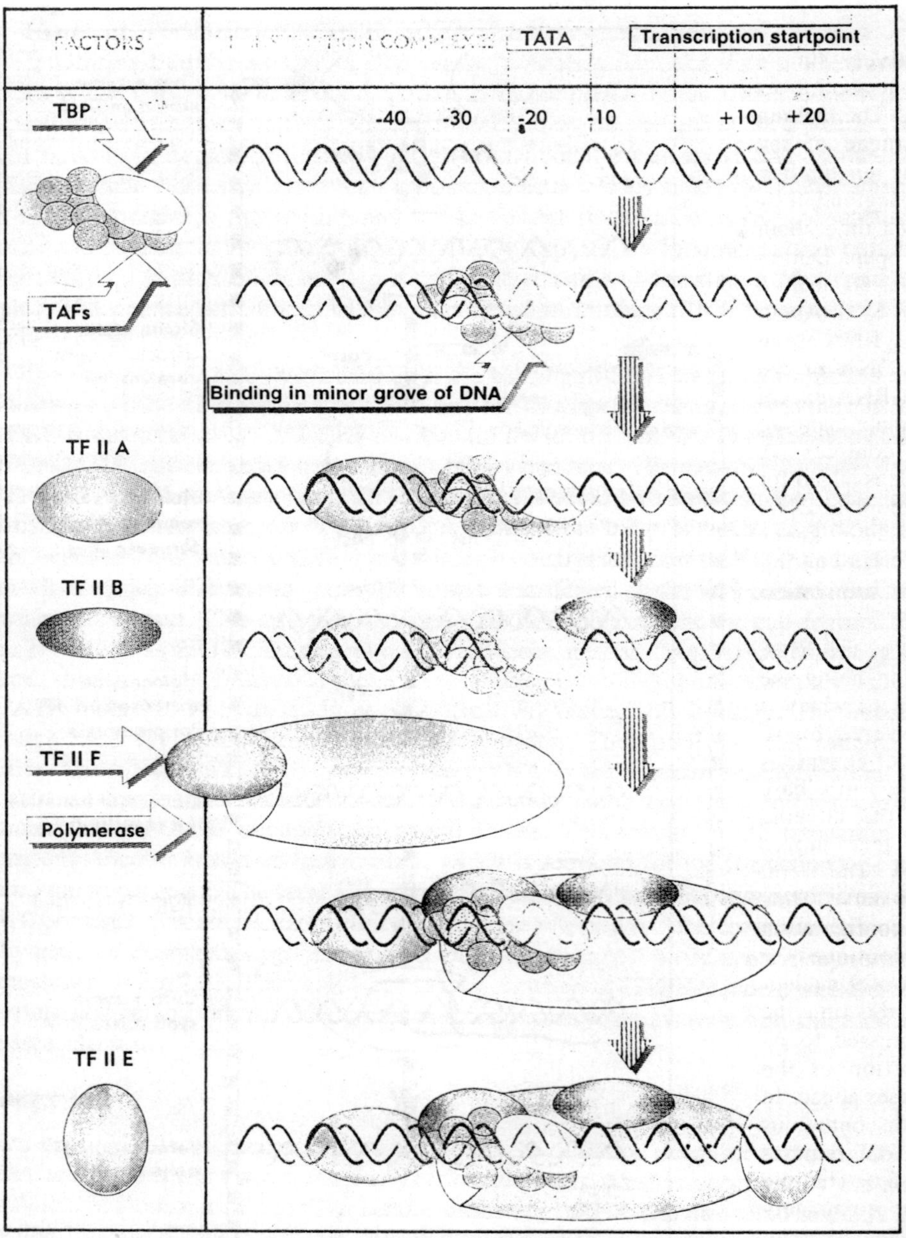

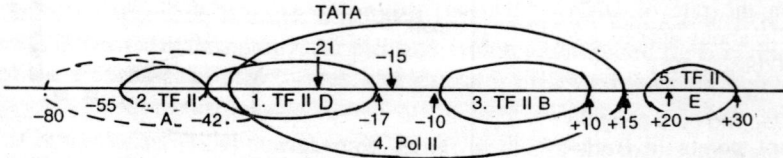

Fig. 6.5A. The initiation complex assembles at promoter in an ordered manner.

Fig. 6.5B. Simplified diagram showing the transcriptor factors during initiation of eukaryotic transcription.

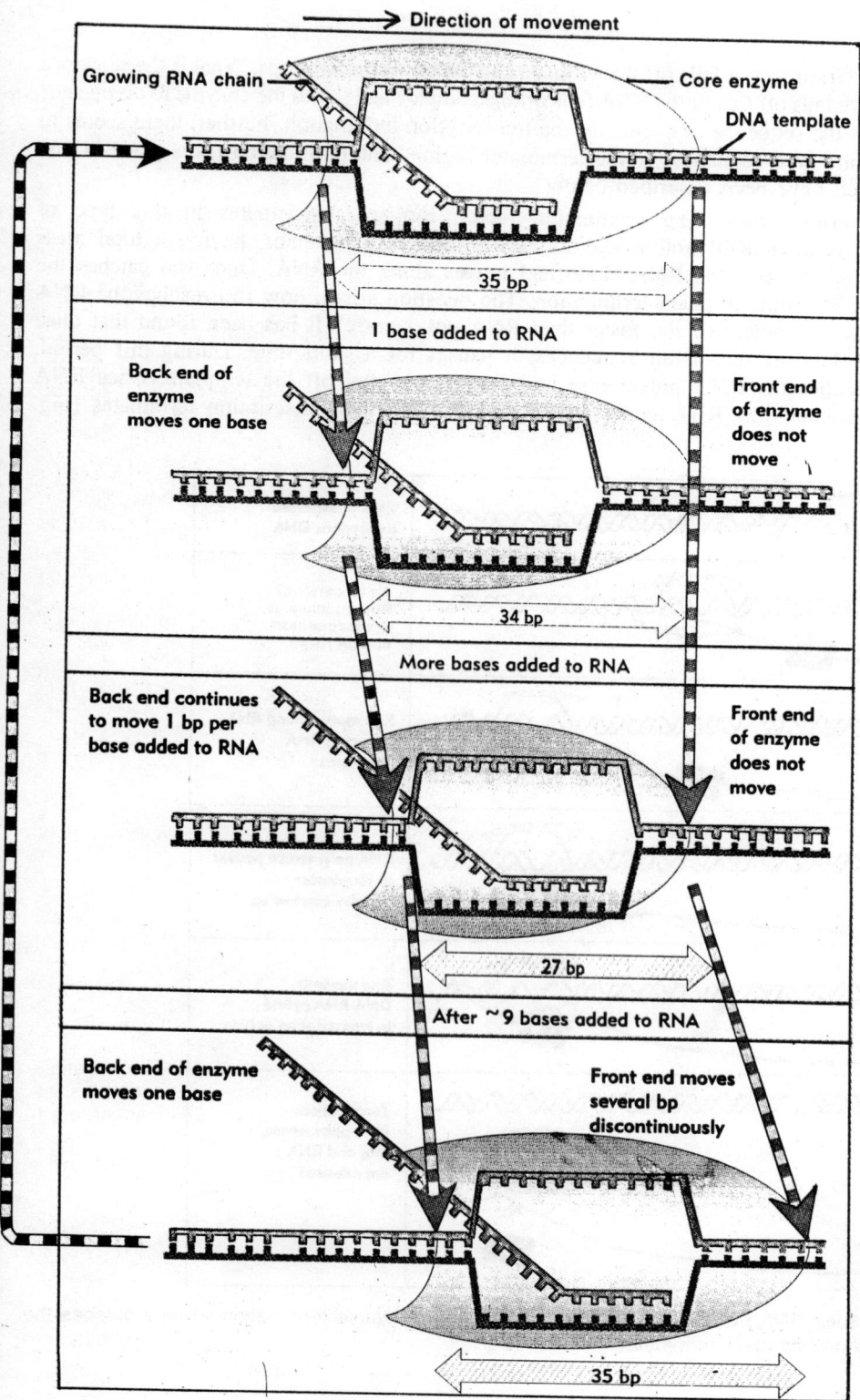

Direction of movement

Growing RNA chain

Core enzyme

DNA template

35 bp

1 base added to RNA

Back end of
enzyme
moves one base

Front end
of enzyme
does not
move

34 bp

More bases added to RNA

Back end continues
to move 1 bp per
base added to RNA

Front end
of enzyme
does not
move

27 bp

After ~9 bases added to RNA

Back end of enzyme
moves one base

Front end moves
several bp
discontinuously

35 bp

Fig. 6.6. Movement of RNA polymerase during elongation. It is compressed from the back end and released from the front end.

Termination

Once the enzyme hits the terminator, it falls off the template and the transcription stops. What is the sequence of events? Whether enzyme falls off first or the RNA falls off the complex and forces the enzyme to disengage? There is no consensus on the sequence of events for the transcription termination. Further, there seems to be no regions of long conserved sequences in the terminator region. The termination takes place in one of the two manners which have been described below.

(a) Rho dependant termination : The termination factor, rho (ρ), participates in this type of termination. Rho is a 46 KD protein and its active form is a hexamer, having a total mass of 275 KD. It binds to growing RNA chain and moves along the RNA. Once rho catches the RNA polymerase, it results in chain termination. The question arises, how rho reaches the RNA polymerase. Is the movement of rho faster than RNA polymerase? It has been found that once RNA polymerase hits the terminator sequences, it pauses for a short time. During this period, the rho factor reaches the RNA polymerase and causes it to fall off the template. Once RNA polymerase is detached, the RNA chain also comes off and the transcription terminates (Fig. 6.7).

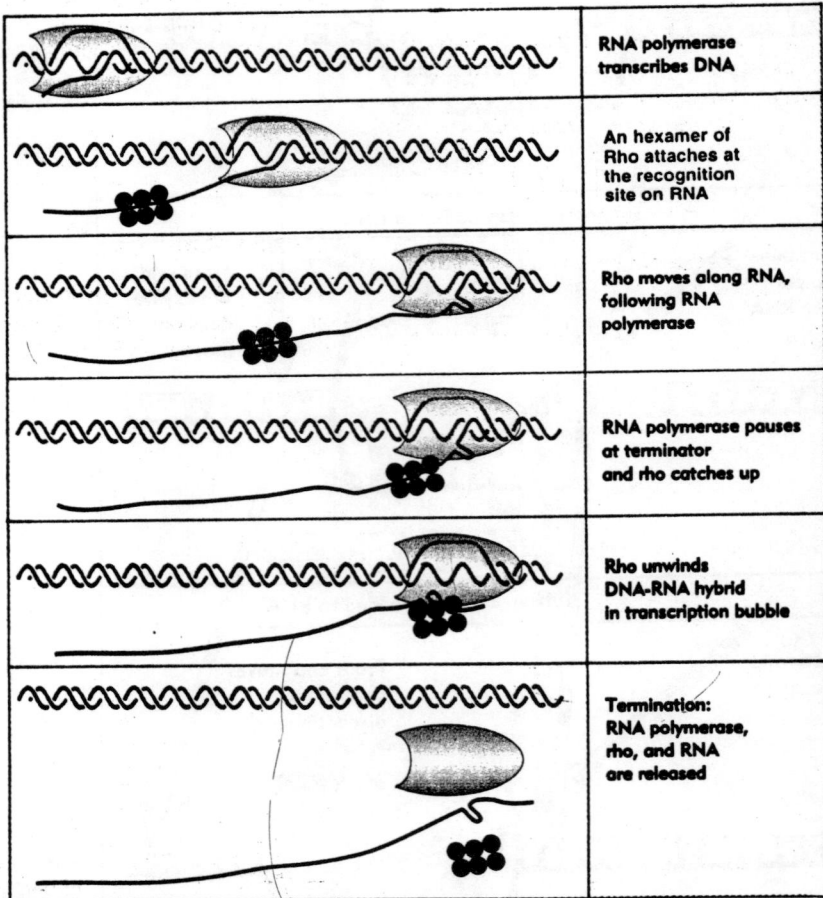

	RNA polymerase transcribes DNA
	An hexamer of Rho attaches at the recognition site on RNA
	Rho moves along RNA, following RNA polymerase
	RNA polymerase pauses at terminator and rho catches up
	Rho unwinds DNA-RNA hybrid in transcription bubble
	Termination: RNA polymerase, rho, and RNA are released

Fig. 6.7. Rho factor pursues RNA polymerase along the RNA and can cause termination when it catches the enzyme pausing at a rho-dependent terminator.

As discussed, there are no conserved sequences at the terminator site. In absence of long conserved sequences, how RNA polymerase gets the signal to pause? It has been found that there is a region with a stretch of C rich and G poor sequence preceding the actual site of termination. This unusual region, known as the terminator, may be responsible for timing the relative movements of RNA polymerase and the rho factor (Fig. 6.8). Next question is what is the recognition site for rho, is it DNA, or RNA or the RNA polymerase. It has been found that rho has an ATPase activity and hydrolysis of ATP is needed for its action. Further, it requires a polyribonucleotide of at least 50 bases for the ATPase activity. It can bind with 5'–PO$_4$ group of polynucleotide. Furthermore, it can dissociate a DNA:RNA hybrid even in the absence of RNA polymerase. This suggests that rho probably acts at the DNA:RNA junction and not at the polymerase. Once the RNA falls off the template, the enzyme also disengages and the termination takes place.

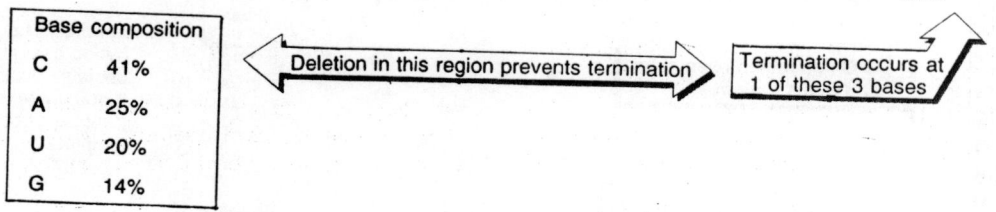

Fig. 6.8. The sequence of rho dependent terminator.

(b) Rho independent termination: In some genes, there is a definite region of intrinsic sequences which causes the termination of RNA chain. This includes two G:C rich stretches at the end of RNA transcript which are complementary to each other. These form a 7-20 bp long intra-molecular hairpin structure. Further, this region is followed by a small stretch of U residues which form relatively weak interaction with dA residues of the gene (Fig. 6.9). Such a structure is highly unstable thermodynamically and causes the displacement of newly synthesized RNA from the DNA template. Once the RNA is detached, the RNA polymerase falls off and the termination of transcription occurs. This type of termination provides an interesting example where the structure of RNA itself can cause its own termination from the DNA chain. As will be seen later, the formation of this structure or prevention of its formation can play an important role in regulation of gene expression.

Thus the sequence of events are different in two types of termination. In rho–dependent termination, a trans acting factor is required. Rho factor causes the RNA to come off the template while in rho–independent termination, the RNA chain detaches itself when a specific three dimentional structure is formed. The enzyme falls off with the detachment of RNA.

The transcription and translation are coupled in bacteria

In prokaryote, the transcription and the translation of newly synthesized mRNA are coupled. The translation of mRNA starts even before the entire RNA chain has been synthesized. Thus a structure similar

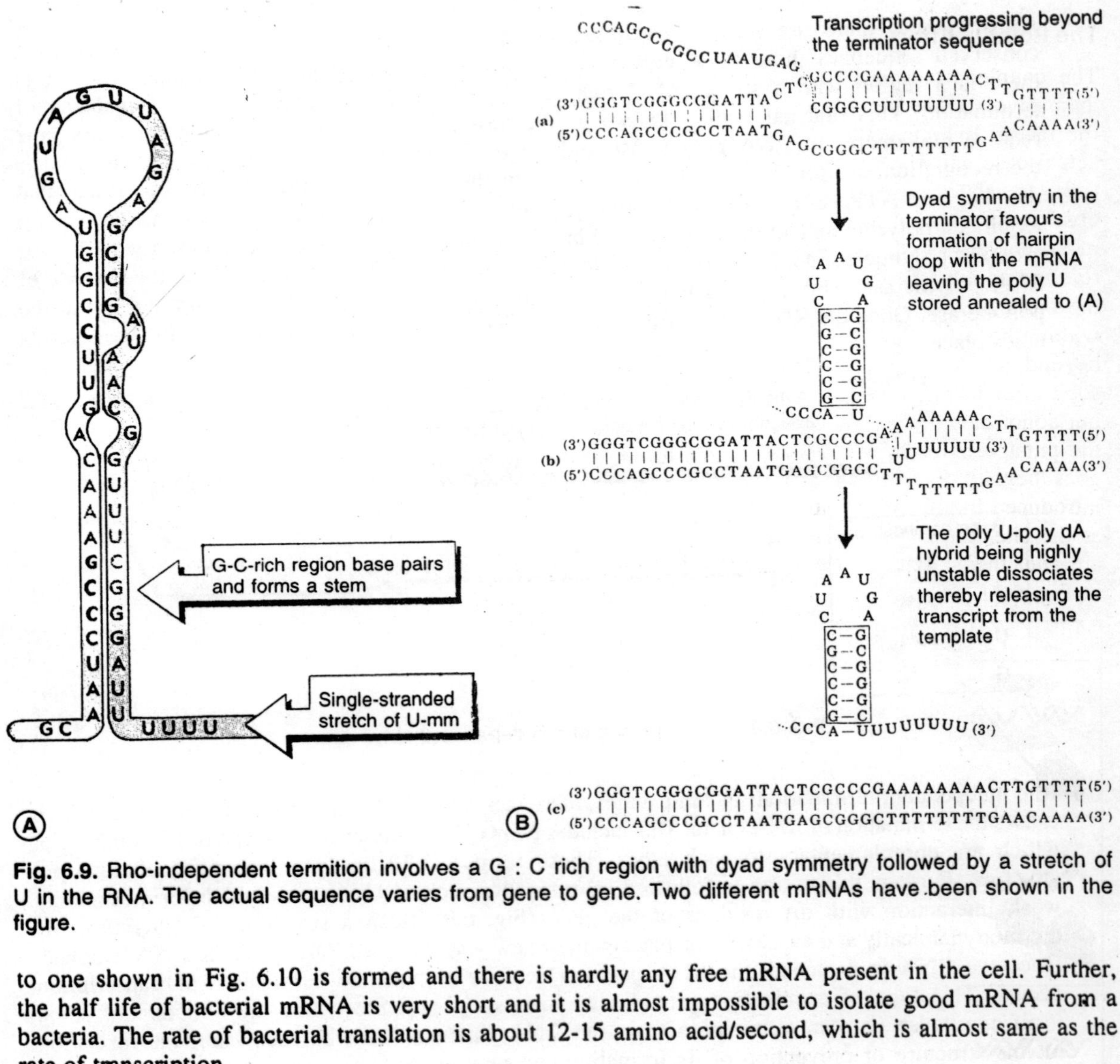

CCCAGCCCGCCUAAUGAG

Transcription progressing beyond the terminator sequence

```
                           GCCCGAAAAAAAAAC
                          TC|||||||||||||||  T
(a)  (3')GGGTCGGGCGGATTA C  CGGGCUUUUUUUU (3')  T GTTTT(5')
      |||||||||||||||||                        |||||
     (5')CCCAGCCCGCCTAATG AG CGGGCTTTTTTTTT G AA CAAAA(3')
```

Dyad symmetry in the terminator favours formation of hairpin loop with the mRNA leaving the poly U stored annealed to (A)

```
           A A U
          U     G
          C     A
          C — G
          G — C
          C — G
          C — G
          C — G
          G — C
     ·· CCCA — U            A A AAAAA C
                          A  |||||| T TGTTTT(5')
(b)  (3')GGGTCGGGCGGATTACTCGCCCGA  UUUUUU (3')  |||||
      |||||||||||||||||||||||||||  U
     (5')CCCAGCCCGCCTAATGAGCGGGC T T TTTTTT G AA CAAAA(3')
```

The poly U-poly dA hybrid being highly unstable dissociates thereby releasing the transcript from the template

```
           A A U
          U     G
          C     A
          C — G
          G — C
          C — G
          C — G
          C — G
          G — C
     ·· CCCA — UUUUUUUUU (3')
```

```
(c)  (3')GGGTCGGGCGGATTACTCGCCCGAAAAAAAAACTTGTTTT(5')
      ||||||||||||||||||||||||||||||||||||||||
     (5')CCCAGCCCGCCTAATGAGCGGGCTTTTTTTTTGAACAAAA(3')
```

G-C-rich region base pairs and forms a stem

Single-stranded stretch of U-mm

Ⓐ   **Ⓑ**

Fig. 6.9. Rho-independent termition involves a G : C rich region with dyad symmetry followed by a stretch of U in the RNA. The actual sequence varies from gene to gene. Two different mRNAs have been shown in the figure.

to one shown in Fig. 6.10 is formed and there is hardly any free mRNA present in the cell. Further, the half life of bacterial mRNA is very short and it is almost impossible to isolate good mRNA from a bacteria. The rate of bacterial translation is about 12-15 amino acid/second, which is almost same as the rate of transcription.

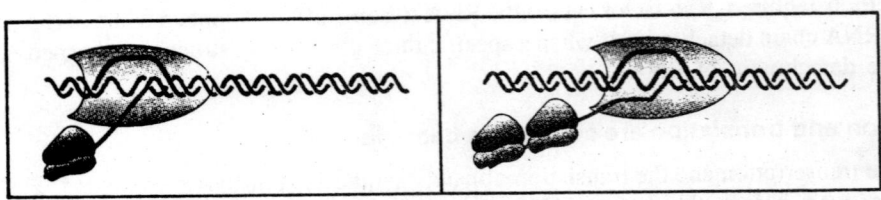

Fig. 6.10. The link between transcription and translation.

The Polarity Effect

The coupled transcription and translation create an interesting situation. The ribosomes must attach themselves while the RNA is being synthesized. Do the ribosomes interfere with the movement of rho factor. Rather, if the movement of rho factor is regulated by the ribosomes. It seems that this is the actual case and rho doesnot get the access to the RNA polymerase site unless the transcript has been fully translated and ribosomes have fallen off. This can explain a very interesting phenomenon observed in certain bacteria. It was found that if a nonsense mutation is introduced in one of the genes of a polycistronic operon, sometimes the transcription of later genes is blocked. This effect is referred as the polarity effect and was very puzzeling for a long time. However, it can be explained on the basis of rho dependent termination. Such an effect can be seen if a putative terminator is present within the coding region of the gene, which is not normally used and the transcription proceeds beyond it. In the wild type bacteria, the ribosomes attach themselves to the nascent RNA chain, soon after it has emerged out of the RNA polymerase. Later, the rho factors also attach to this RNA but donot have the access to RNA polymerase even though RNA polymerase may pause momentarily at the putative terminator, as their movement is impeded by the ribosomes. As a result, the transcription goes beyond this region and the entire operon is transcribed. However, if a nonsense mutation is introduced before the putative terminator site, the ribosome fall apart and when the polymerase pauses at the site, the rho catches with the polymerase and the transcription is terminated. The genes which are after this site are thus not transcribed and become silent. The entire phenomenon has been explained in Fig. 6.11.

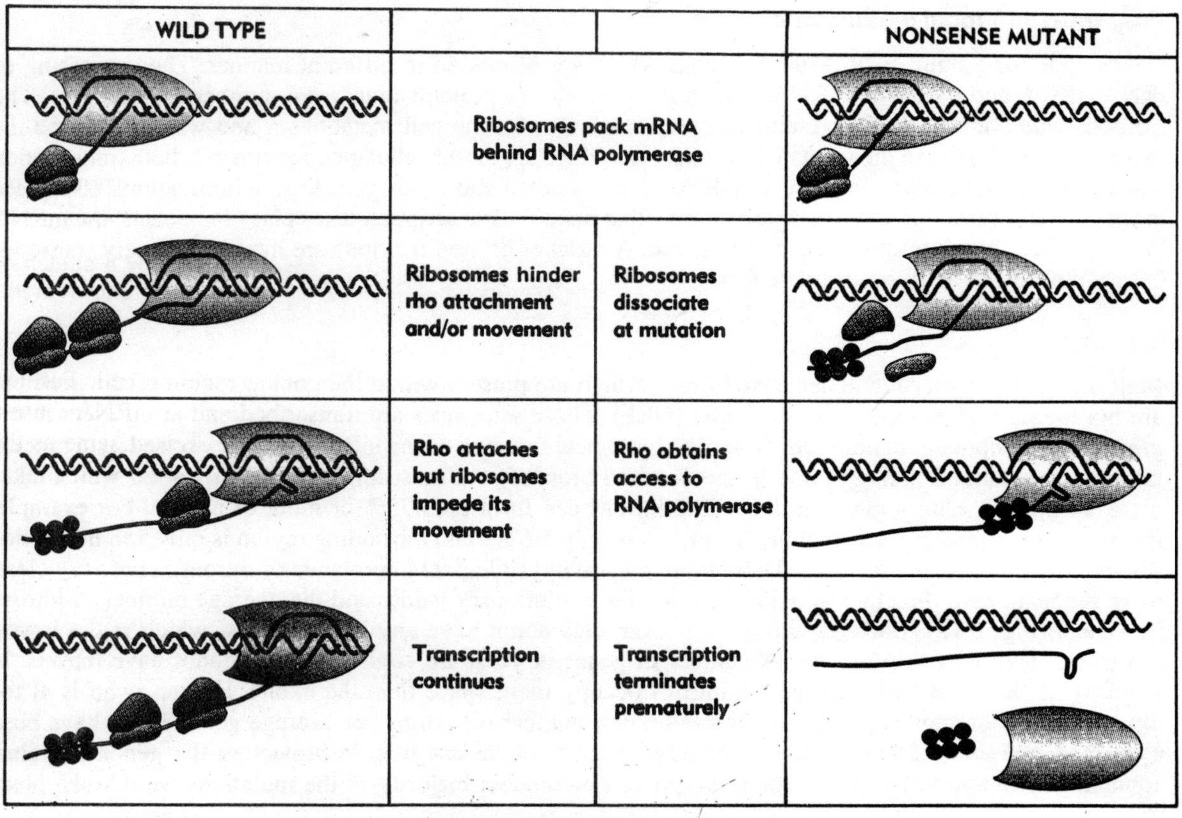

WILD TYPE			NONSENSE MUTANT
	Ribosomes pack mRNA behind RNA polymerase		
	Ribosomes hinder rho attachment and/or movement	Ribosomes dissociate at mutation	
	Rho attaches but ribosomes impede its movement	Rho obtains access to RNA polymerase	
	Transcription continues	Transcription terminates prematurely	

Fig. 6.11. The polarity effect.

Transcription and translation are not coupled in eukaryotes

In eukaryotes the two processes are independent to each other. The transcription takes place in nucleus while the translation occurs in cytoplasm. The RNA has to be transported from nucleus to cytoplasm for its translation. The primary transcript is unstable in its original form and undergoes a number of post–transcriptional modifications before the mRNA attains the mature form and is translated.

Transcripts for rRNA and tRNAs

In prokaryotes, following coupled transcription–translation, the mRNA is degraded. The rRNA and tRNA on the other hand, are synthesized in their precursor forms which are much larger in size. These are processed by a number of specific nucleases. These enzymes, which are endonuclease in nature, produce the mature rRNAs and tRNAs.

In enkaryotes, on the other hand, the precursor form of mRNAs referred as heterogeneous nuclear RNA (hnRNA) is much larger than the mRNA. It is cleaved and is extensively processed before it is transported to cytoplasm. The post–transcriptional modifications of pre–mRNA include splicing, capping, polyadenylation and modification of certain bases. Majority of these modifications take place in nucleus. The mature mRNA is finally translated. The half life of eukaryotic mRNA is relatively long and good quality, biologically active mRNA can easily be isolated. Other RNAs (rRNAs and tRNAs) are also synthesized in precursor form and are cleaved at specific places to give mature RNA molecules.

Post-transcriptional modifications

Genes code for a number of different RNAs which are processed in different manner. The processing of tRNA, rRNA and other small RNAs which do not code for proteins involves a number of nucleases. The mRNAs which code for the proteins are very important for the cell metabolism and we will discuss the processing of mRNAs in great detail. In prokaryotes, there are no subcellular compartments, both transcription and translation take place in close vicinity and are coupled and no or very little modifications take place in the primary transcript. In eukaryotes, on the other hand the transcription takes place in nucleus, the mRNA is transported to cytoplasm and then translated. A number of modifications are made in primary transcript before the mRNA is in translatable form.

Splicing

Majority of the eukaryotic genes have introns which are present within the coding region of the gene but are not the part of the open reading frame (ORF). These sequences are transcribed and are present in the primary transcript but are not required for the biological function of the mRNA and are excised by a process known as splicing. Splicing is one of the first and probably the most important modification which takes place during the maturation of mRNA. The introns can form upto 75% or more of a gene. For example, the mouse dhfr gene is 8.1 Kb while the mRNA is only 1.6 Kb and the coding region is only 558 nucleotide (the protein has 186 aminoacids). Though the precise physiological importance of introns is not very clear, there seems to be a direct co–relation between the evolutionary ladder and the average number of introns in a gene (Fig. 6.12). Bacteria and other prokaryotes donot have any introns, yeast which is the lowest eukaryote have very few introns. A number of genes in yeast are continuous and donot have introns. In majority of the mammalian genes the introns occupy more space than the exons. Human, who is at the top of the evolutionay ladder, probably has highest number of introns per average gene. These have been explained in Table 6.2. The presence of large number of introns help in protecting the genome against spontaneous mutations, since by the principle of randomness majority of the mutations would take place within the introns and should not have any bearing on the coding region of the genome. Usually the introns devide a gene in many functional domains. Often each exon represents a biological or an immunological domain of the protein. In the genes for related proteins from different species, the exons are usually conserved. The sequence of introns, on the other hand, often varies. Not only the sequence, but the size can vary too and often this variation can be very substantial. However, the relative positions of the introns often remain constant. Besides, it is possible that new proteins can be created by alternate splicing of the introns (see later).

Table 6.2. Average size of genes and number of introns in various species.

S.No.	Species	Genome size bp	Size of average gene Kbp	Size of average mRNA Kb	Average No. of introns/gene
1.	Bacteria	1.4×10^6	Polycistronic	-	No introns
2.	Yeast	1.1×10^7	1.6	1.6	-
3.	Fungi	1.3×10^7	1.5	1.4	2
4.	C. elegans	1×10^9	4.0	3.0	3
5.	D. melanogaster	1.1×10^8	11.3	2.7	3
6.	Chicken	1×10^9	13.9	2.4	8
7.	Mammals	1.2×10^9	16.6	2.2	6

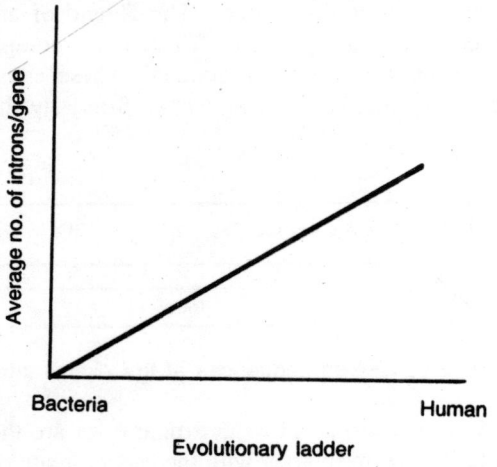

Fig. 6.12. Average number of introns in a gene are related to the position of an organism in the evolutionary ladder.

Considerable debate has taken place regarding the origin of introns. If the introns were present in primordial gene or these have evolved during evolution. The analysis of introns/exons of a number of genes have revealed that many related genes share some of the exons. A particular exon in its totality may be present in more than one gene. Similarly, certain cases have been found where two or more exons of one gene have joined together to form a single exon of another gene. In this case, the intron(s) between these exons has been lost. It seems that the primordial genes contained introns. The presence of multiple exons served an important function where a number of genes could be evolved by joining these exons in various combination. Such recombination of small coding units can explain the assembly of a wide variety of complex genes by relatively few and simple coding sequences which may have been present in the primordial organisms. It is possible that a number of introns were lost from the primordial genes during the course of evolution. Different introns may have been lost during the formation of different lines of descent.

The precursor form of mRNA (hnRNA) is many times bigger than the mature mRNA. An average human hnRNA is 15–25 Kb with 6–8 introns. It is trimmed and the introns are removed by splicing which takes place in nucleus. In order to facilitate the cell machinery to recognize the precise place for the cutting and joining of exons, it was thought that some signals should be present. However, the analysis of a number of hnRNAs has revealed that there are no long conserved sequences in the introns. Also there are no regions of homology or complementarity within or between the two ends of an intron. This rules out the possibility of any type of extensive specific secondary structure in the introns which could be recognized by splicing machinery. The only conserved sequence is at the intron–exon junction and it has been found that all introns start with GT at their 5'–end and finish with AG at the 3'–end. Often it is referred as the GT–AG rule of intron structure. However, in many genes these conserved sequences are further extended by a few more nucleotides which are also conserved but with much less occurance. For example, in many genes upto 9 bases at the 5'–end and 10–15 bases at 3'–end of introns may have some degree of conservation. In about 60% of the known genes an exon ends with trinucleotide C/AAG, followed by intron beginning with GT which is further extended to A/GAGT. Similarily the AG at the end of intron may be preceded by a sequence consist of upto 11 T/C,N (any of the four nucleotides) followed by C/T. The 5'–end of the exon may often begin with G. These sequences have been shown in Fig 6.13. The numbers in subscript refer to percentage of occurance of these nucleotides. The 5'–end of an intron is known as the donor site while the 3'–end is referred as the acceptor site. There is no complementarity between the 3'–site and the 5'–site and the splice sites are thus unidirectional. These sites are generic in nature and do not bear any specificity for any particular mRNA molecule. Similarly there is no tissue specifity in the splicing sites.

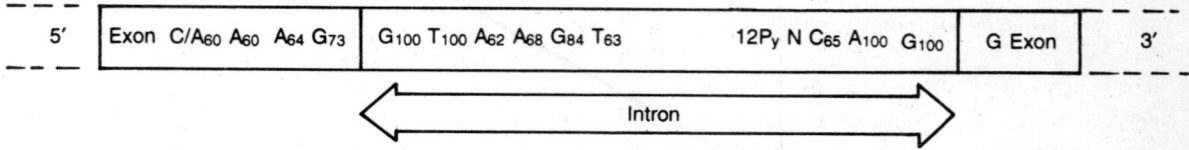

Fig. 6.13. The conserved sequences at the exan : intron boundary.

All the left splicing junctions are similar in their structure, so are the right junctions. It is therefore, probale that a donor site should be able to interact with the acceptor site of either the same or of any other intron of the same gene. However, that is not what actually happens as this will create a confusing situation. If two introns are removed together as a single unit, the exon lying in between these introns will also be removed along with the introns. This will result in loss of the coding region and the cell cannot permit such a situation to arise. A 3'–junction of one intron always interacts with the 5'–junction of the same intron. Thus an intron is always removed as a singe entity and the exons are protected. Further, there are many introns in a typical mammalian gene. This may result in many possibilities for their removal. Are all introns removed simultaneously? If yes, this will result in many exons available for the ligation which will increase the chances of mistake in ligation. It has been found that the introns are removed one at a time and the removal of one intron is always coupled with the ligation of two exons which are freed by its removal.

Is there a definite sequence in which the introns are removed from a gene or it is entirely a random process? If the process was random, the number of splicing intermediates will increase tremendously. The study of many genes have shown that only few of the possible intermediates can be detected. It has been found that the removal of introns follows what is referred as a 'preferred pathway'. In this case, while there is not a very strict order for the removal of multiple introns within a gene, the process is not totally random. It is a definite pathway with built in flexibility. For example, the ovomucoid hnRNA has 7 introns (and 8 exons). It was found that either intron V or VI is removed as the first reaction, its removal is followed by the other introns. Intron III is never lost in the first three steps. The sequence of removal of introns seems to follow the following order, V/VI, VII/IV, II and finally III/I. The splicing is primarily intramolecular, however, the possibility of intermolecular splicing exists. Though it is more an exception than the rule.

Nuclear splicing is a complex and multistep process. First there is a cut made at the 5' splicing junction and the exon at the 5'–end of an intron is separated. The 5'–end of the intron then recognizes a site at about 18–40 nucleotides upstream of the 3'–splice junction. This site, referred as the branch site, has a small highly conserved recognition sequence. The sequence at the branch site in yeast is TACTAAC. in higher eukaryotes the specificity is relatively less and the sequence is PyNPyPyPuAPy. The intron structure can thus be extended to accomodate this site. It has been shown in Fig. 6.14. It has been found that any mutation in branch site results in the loss of splicing activity. The freed 5'–PO$_4$ group of the intron reacts with the 'A' residue at the branch site and forms a unusual 2'–5' phosphodiester bond. As there is no free –OH group at the 2' position in DNA, such bond formation can not take place in DNA and no splicing of a DNA molecule can take place. This bond formation results in the formation of a specific loop like structure of the intron part of the RNA, which is referred as the 'lariat'. Once the lariat has been formed, the exon located at the 3'–end of the intron is excised off. The 3'–end of first exon and the 5'–end of second exon are then joined by the RNA ligase and the lariated intron is spliced out. This is followed by the debranching of the lariat shaped intron and the production of a linear RNA molecule which is degraded by the cell. This has been shown in Fig. 6.15.

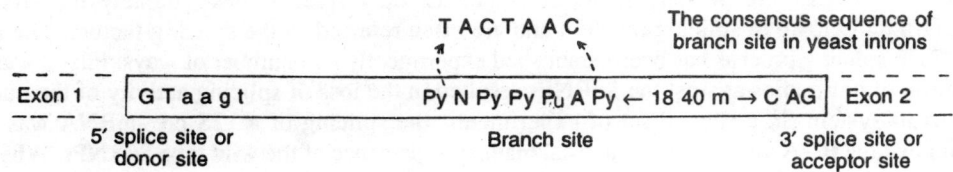

Fig. 6.14. The Structure of intron.

The nuclear splicing takes place in a self contained manner, mediated by the RNA itself and without the involvement of any enzyme or other proteins. This is a case which shows that the RNA can act as the catalyst and the concept that all enzymes are proteins is no longer true. These RNAs with catalytic activity are known as the ribozymes. The nuclear splicing requires the bringing of donor site to the branch site and to the 3'–end of the first exon to 5' end of the second exon for their interactions. Many introns are too large to permit such possibilities without the aid of some factors. It has been found that under in vivo conditions, this is facilitated by the participation of a number of small RNA molecules present in nucleus. These RNAs, referred as the small nuclear RNA (SnRNA), are of about 100–300 bases long, though some of these may be upto 1000 bases in length. Some of these may contain a cap like structure at the 5'–end which is similar to cap structure of mRNA (see later). Usually these are not present as free RNA but are present in a protein associated form and are known as small nuclear ribonucleoprotein particles (snRNPs, pronounced as snurps). Some

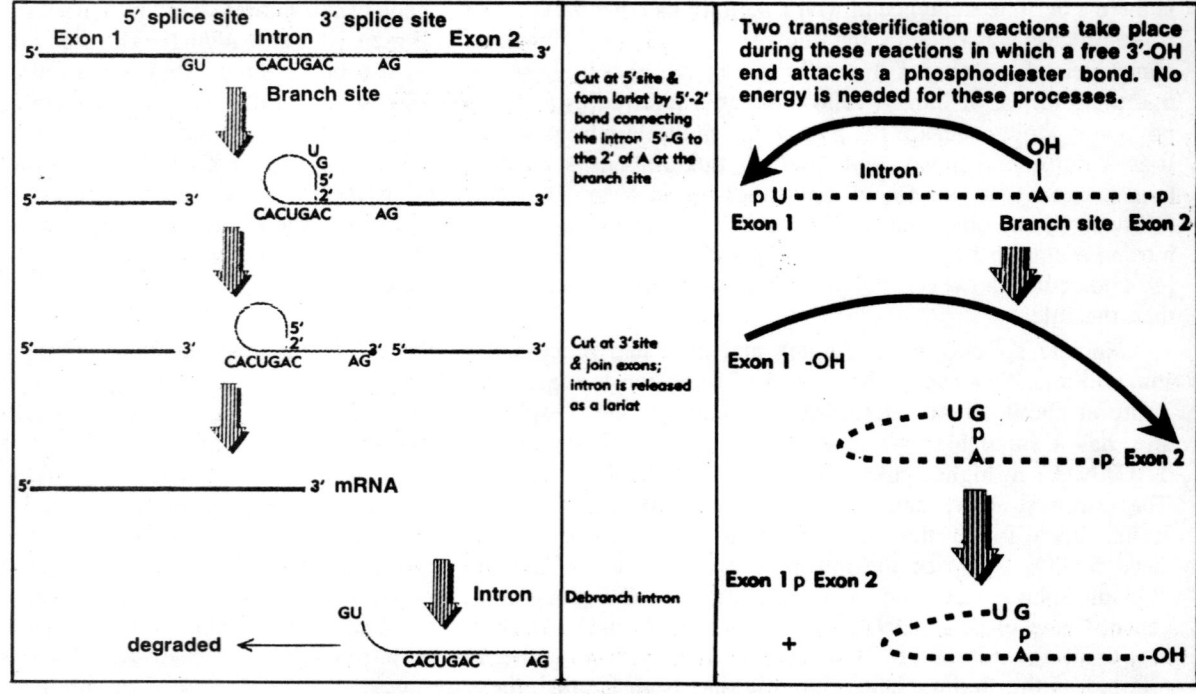

Fig. 6.15. The nuclear splicing.

of the SnRNP like molecules are also present in the cytoplasmic compartment of eukaryotic cells. These are then called small cytoplasmic ribonucleoprotein particle or ScRNP (pronounced as scurps). While a number of SnRNPs are present in the cell nucleus, only five of these, namely the U-1, U-2, U-4/ U-6 and U-5 participate in splicing reaction and are often referred as the splicing·factors. The involvement of SnRNPs in splicing process has been established experimentally in a number of ways. First it was established that addition of antibodies against the SnRNPs resulted in the loss of splicing activity of the nuclear extract in an in vitro system. In a second set of experiments, the splicing of a 12S pre–mRNA was followed. It was found that the RNA was spliced in normal manner in presence of the wild type SnRNPs. When a mutation was introduced in the RNA which abolished the splicing donor site, its splicing was impaired. However, introduction of a complementary mutation at the 5'–end of the U–1 SnRNP, which resulted in a complementarity with mutated donor site of 12S RNA, was able to restore the splicing of the substrate RNA. This established the role of U–1 SnRNP in recognizing the.donor site of the pre–mRNA. The detailed characteristics of the splicing factors are given below. The role of various SnRNPs has been established by various immunological and protection and RNA mapping experiments.

U-1 SnRNP

The U-1 SnRNPs have a number of regions of internal homology and form a secondary structure with a number of double stranded stems. The structure of U-1 SnRNP is shown in Fig. 6.16. Their presence has been demonstrated in animals, birds and insects. At least 11 nucleotides at the 5'-end of the.RNA donot have any intermolecular comlimentarity and are present in single stranded form. However, this region has a complementarity with the splicing donor site of the intron. The length of complementarity between U-1 SnRNP and the donor site is 4-6 nucleotides. However, the actual number of bases present in this complementarity is not very important.

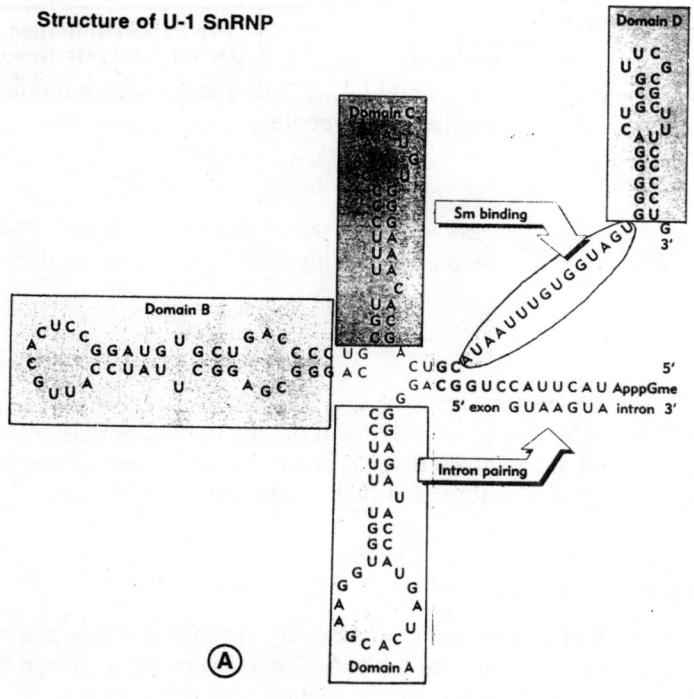

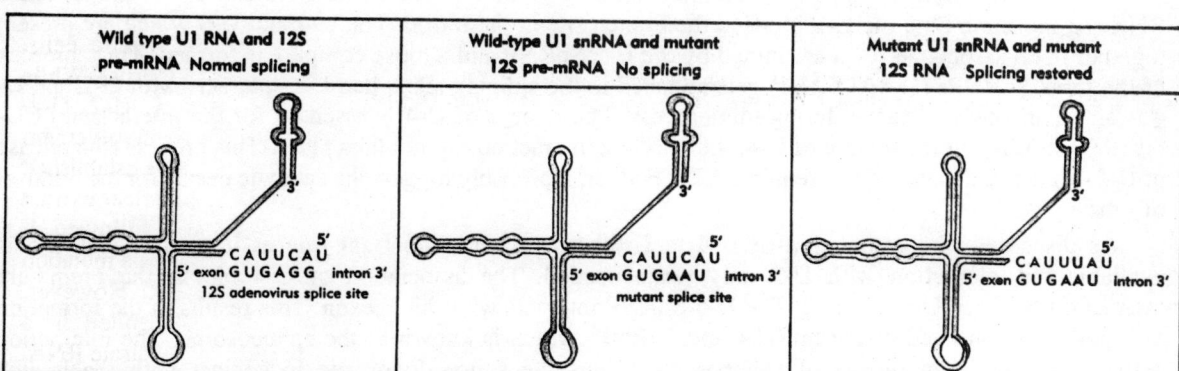

Fig. 6.16. U-1 snRNA has a base paired structure that creates several domains. The 5' end which has complementarily with 5' splice site remains single stranded and can base pair with the 5' splicing site. A. Structure of U-1 snRNA. B. Mutations that abolish function of the 5' splicing site can be suppressed by compensating mutations in U1 snRNA that restore base pairing.

U-2 SnRNP

The U-2 SnRNPs have two regions of complementarity which are important for splicing reaction. The first region is complementary to the branch site of the intron and the second region has the complementarity with a region in the U-6 SnRNP (see later).

U-4 SnRNP

These SnRNPs have a region of complementarity with U-6 SnRNP. It plays an important role in ensuring that the U-6 SnRNP is free and available to pair with U-2 SnRNP only when required (see later). Normally the U-4 and U-6 SnRNPs are present togather as a complex.

U-5 SnRNP

It binds to 3' region of the exon and later shifts to the 5'-end of the intron. There are no regions of complementarity in the RNA part and the binding of this SnRNP may involve the proteins present in the SnRNP.

U-6 SnRNP

It also has two regions of complementarity, one with U-2 SnRNP and the other with U-4 SnRNP. The binding of U-4 SnRNP with the U-6 SnRNP results in masking of the site for U-2 SnRNP binding. Thus U-6 SnRNP can bind either to U-2 or to U-4 at any given time. This ensures the correct timing for complex formation (see later). The binding sites of U-6 SnRNP and their interaction with U-2 and U-4 SnRNPs have been shown in Fig. 6.17.

The Mechanism of Lariat Formation

The SnRNPs play an important role in the entire process. By virtue of the base pairings, the SnRNPs react among themselves and also with the substrate hnRNA. These interactions change the structure of RNAs in such a manner that the reacting groups come in contact with each other.

The first step in the splicing reaction is the binding of the U-1 SnRNP to the donor site of the substrate RNA. At the same time the U-2 binds at the branch site in the intron. The U-4 and U-6 which are present together in an associated form are joined by the U-5 SnRNP and a loose complex is formed. This complex of the three SnRNPs (U-4/U-6.U-5) gets attached to the splicing site when U-6 interacts with U-2 and U-4 is simultaneously released during this process. The release of U-4 is essential for the interaction of U-6 with U-2. Without the release of U-4, the U-6/U-2 interaction can not take place. This process (the release of U-4) is energy dependent and requires ATP. Further, it probably triggers the catalytic events for the removal of intron.

As discussed, the association of U-4 to U-6 plays a very important role as it ensures that U-6 is available for interaction with U-2 only when needed. The association of U-4 blocks the premature interaction between U-6 and U-2. The U-5 SnRNP interacts with the 5' exon. This results in the formation of a complex consisted of the hnRNA and SnRNPs which is known as the spliceosome. The interaction between various components of spliceosome brings the splice donor site in contact with the branch site. Now the 5' exon is excised and the 2'-5' phosphodiester bond between the 5'-end of intron and 2'-OH of the 'A' residue at the branch site is formed resulting in the lariat formation. This phosphodiester bond formation does not require any energy as it is not a new bond but is the shifting of the bond from one position to another position, involving the melting of the phosphodiester bond between the exon-intron junction and simultaneous formation of bond at the branch site. This process is known as trans-esterification which is probably catalysed by the RNA structure achieved by the interaction of U-2 SnRNP with the U-6. The binding of U-1 and U-2 SnRNPs to the hnRNA is essential for the cleavage but does not control the actual cleavage of the bond. Now the 3'-end of intron is excised off. The binding of U-5 probably triggers the cleavage of the 3' exon. However, precise mechanism of this cleavage is not very clear. The intron alongwith the SnRNPs is released. The two exons are ligated and are now

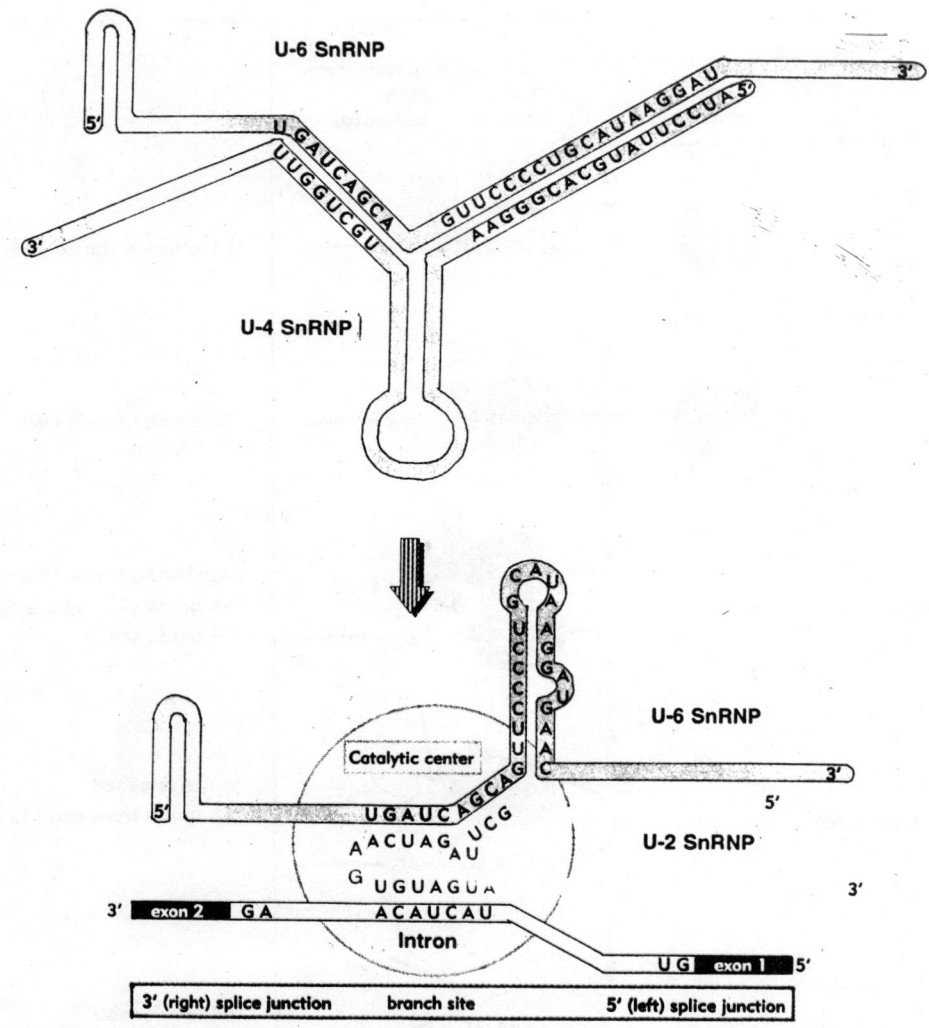

Fig. 6.17. U6-U4 pairing is incompatible with U6-U2 pairing. When U6 joins the spliceosome it is paired with U4. Release of U4 allows a conformational change in U6; one part of the released sequence forms a hairpin (dark grey) and the other part (black) pairs with U2. Because an adjacent region of U2 is already paired with the branch site, this brings U6 into juxtaposition with the branch. Note that the substrate RNA is reversed from the usual orientation and is shown 3'-5'.

joined together. Again this is a tran-esterification reaction. Finally, the intron is degraded. The events in splicing are shown in Fig. 6.18. The entire splicing process is thus self contained and does not require any energy.

It has been demonstrated that the nuclear extract can carryout the splicing of a preformed pre-mRNA. Thus the transcription and the splicing are two independent processes which are not coupled to each other. The simultaneous transcription is not necessary for splicing.

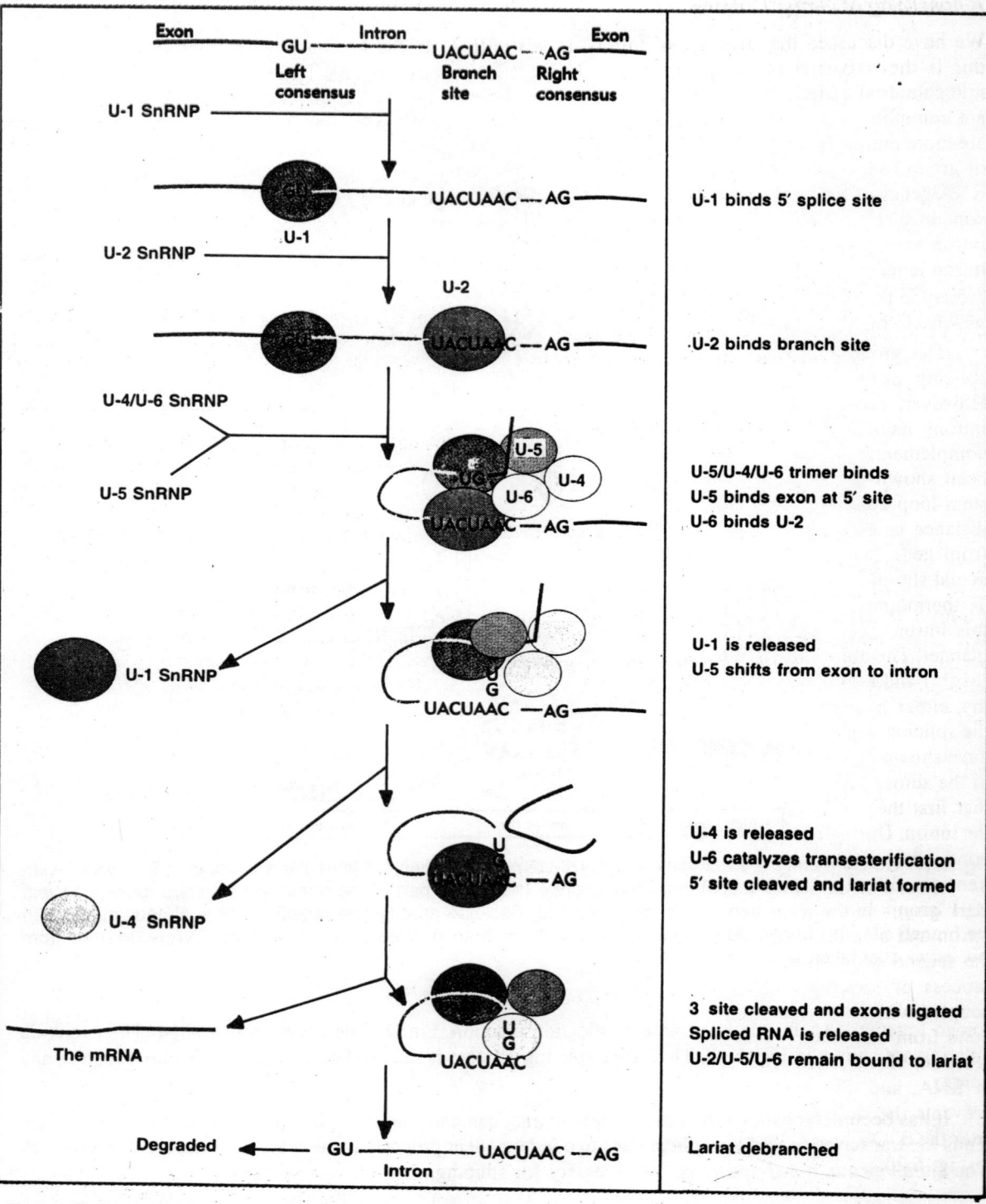

Fig. 6.18. The splicing reaction proceeds through discrete stages in which spliceosome formation involves the interaction of components that recognize the consensus sequences.

Autosplicing of Group I introns

We have discussed the structure of introns in pre-mRNA. In the begining it was thought that probably this is the universal structure of introns. However, two other types of introns were identified in the mitochondrial genes of certain fungi which have a different and very specific internal organization. These are commonly referred as the group I and group II introns. Out of these two classes, the group I introns are more predominant than the group II introns. Though originally recognized in mitochondria, the presence of group I introns has also been shown in a number of other genes of very diverse origin. The ribosomal RNA genes of Tetrahymena thermophila, Physarum polycephalum and certain other lower eukaryotes also contain such introns. Group I introns differ from pre-mRNA in not having the conserved sequences at the intron-exon junction. As a result, the group I and group II introns do not follow the GT-AG rule of exon-intron junction which is present in the pre-mRNA. Similarly, the sequences at the branch site are also not present in these introns. These introns, however, carry certain elements of small sequences within the introns which are highly conserved.

The group I introns are characterized by the capability of the RNA to splice all by itself (self splicing or autosplicing) without the requirement of any other factor(s), in the in vitro reactions. However, certain trans acting protein factors may assist the splicing under in vivo conditions. These introns have a characteristic secondary structure which is achieved by virtue of a number of short complementary sequences within the intron. The structure of a group I intron of Tetrahymena has been shown in Fig. 6.19. It has 9 short regions of intramolecular complementarity forming a complex stem-loop structure. This structure allows the positioning of the two ends of the intron within striking distance to each other. However, the location and length of the regions of complementarity may vary from gene to gene and sometime such sequences may be present at a considerable distance from the actual site of splicing. For example, the precursor (primary transcript) for 26S RNA and a small rRNA of T. thermophila is 35S in size. The 26S RNA is interrupted by a single intron. It has been found that this intron can be spliced off as a single circular RNA (approx 400 bases) in vitro in an autonomous manner. The only requirement seems to be the presence of monovalent cations such as Na^+, a divalent cation (Mg^{++}) and a guanine residue. The guanine residue serves as the cofactor. The experiments have shown that either free guanosine or any of its nucleotides, i.e. GMP, GDP or GTP can serve as the co-factor for the splicing. However, no other nucleotide (or nucleoside) can replace guanine for splicing. Further studies have shown that this seems to be the general mechanism for the splicing of group I introns. The mechanism of the autosplicing using a G residue was later established by radiolabelling experiments. It has been found that first the 3'-OH of this guanosine (or its nucleotide) attacks the exon-intron junction at the 5'-end of the intron. During this process, the exon is excised and the 'G' residue (the cofactor) forms a phosphodiester bond with the terminal phosphate group of the intron. This phosphodiester bond is formed by the trans-esterification reaction. The excised exon, on the other hand, has a free 3'-OH group. This free -OH group is highly reactive and attacks the phosphodiester bond at the junction of 3'-end of the intron and 5'–end of the second exon. This results in the formation of a bond between the first exon and the second exon. This bond formation also takes place by a trans-esterification reaction. Thus the entire process of splicing is energy independent and the breakage of bond at the intron-exon junction is coupled with the formation of bond at the exon-exon joint. Thus, this is the shifting of the phosphodiester bond from one place to another place. The thermodyanamics tells that the reaction should be a reversible reaction. However, the concentration of G nucleotide in the cell is much higher than the concentration of RNA, and it drives the reaction in forward direction. Further, the secondary structure of RNA also prevents the reverse reaction. During splicing the intron is excised off as a linear molecule. However, later the 3'-OH at the intron attacks the 5'-PO_4 group and forms a circular molecule. This has been shown in Fig. 6.20.

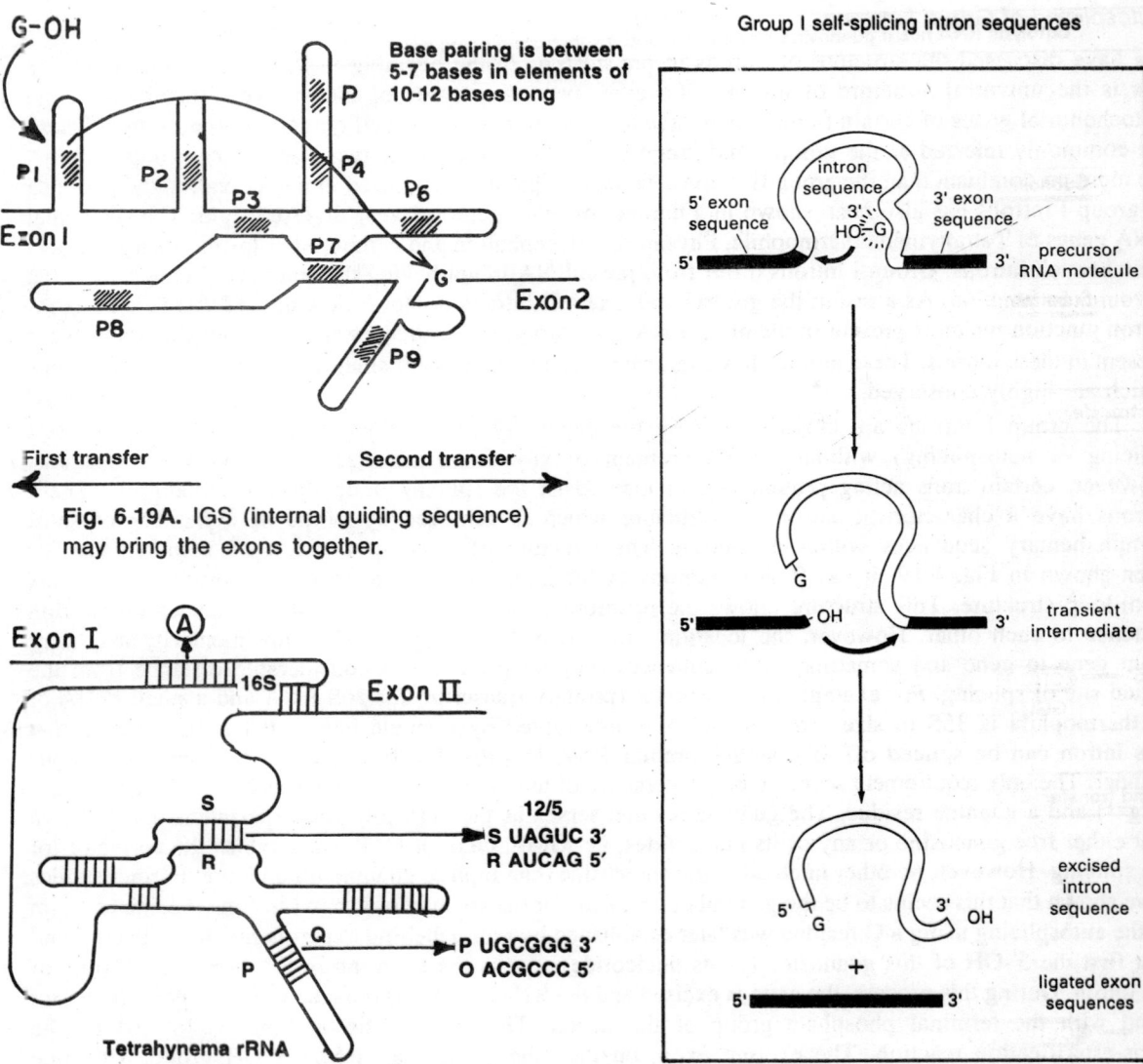

Fig. 6.19A. IGS (internal guiding sequence) may bring the exons together.

Fig. 6.19B. Structure of Tetrahynema rRNA introns.

Fig. 6.20. Splicing of group I introns.

The general process of the splicing of group I introns is not as simple as described above. Within the introns, there are certain specific regions which serve as binding site for the G residue. Fig. 6.21 shows the intron of Tetrahymena rRNA gene. There is a site near the 3'-end of intron, referred as the guanosine binding site, where the G residue gets attached in a non-covalent manner and later attacks the splicing site at the exon-intron junction. Similarly, it has a site known as the substrate binding site. This region has certain degree of complementarity with the 3'-end of exon 1. As a result, a secondary structure is formed which facilitates the interaction between the 'G' cofactor and exon-intron junction. Such sequences within the intron which can pair with exon are also referred as the internal guiding sequences

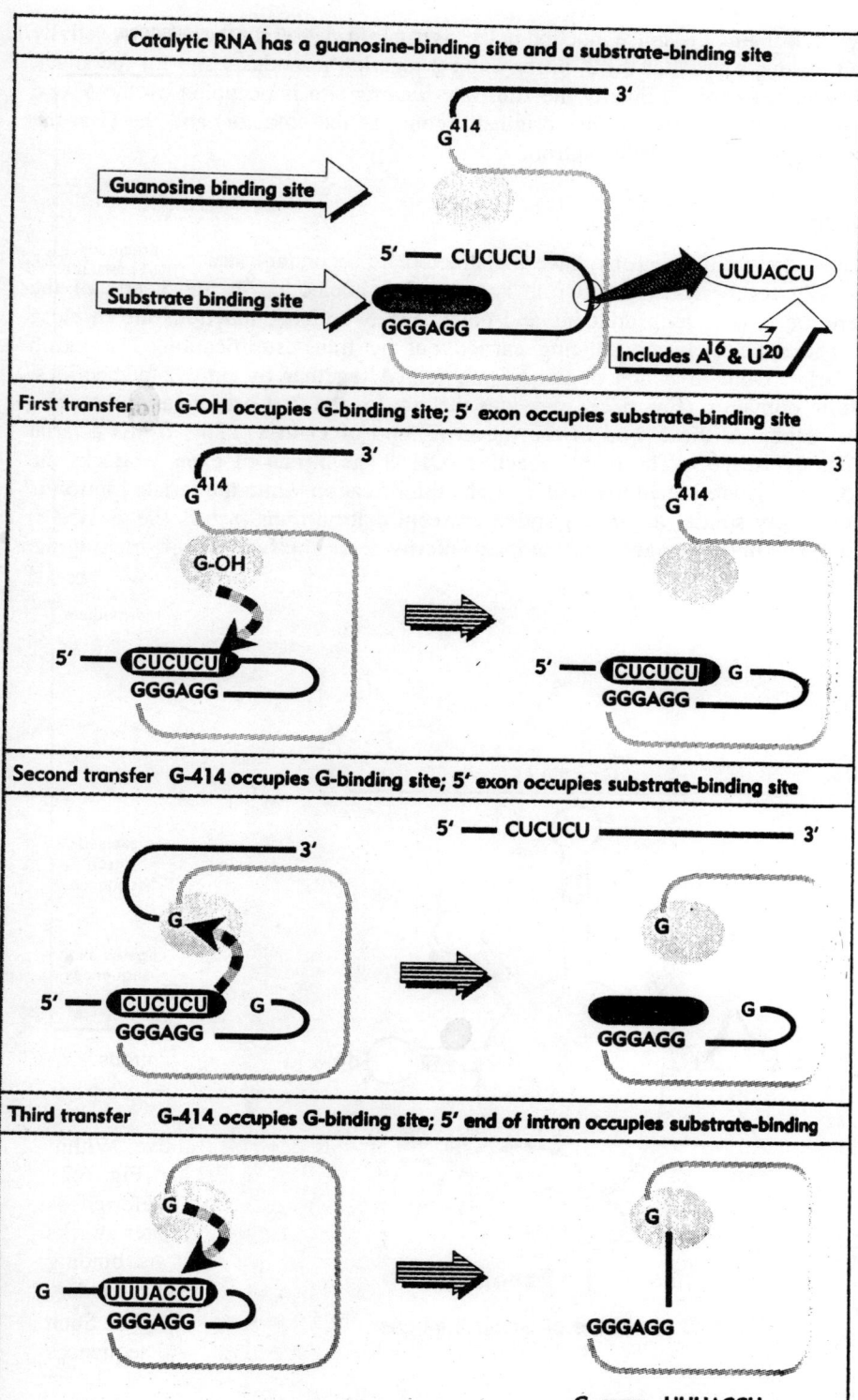

Fig. 6.21. Excision of the group I intron in Tetrahynema rRNA occurs by successive reactions between the occupants of the guanosine-binding site and substrate-binding site.

or IGS. The IGS are involved in bringing the splice junction in the right confirmation for the catalytic activity of the ribozyme. Another G residue present at the 3'-intron-exon 2 junction provides a site for the attack by free 3'-OH group of the cleaved exon 1. Finally the substrate binding site is occupied by the 5' end of the intron (which now has the G residue, that has originally come as the cofactor) and the G at the 3'-end of intron reacts with it to form the circular intron.

Splicing of Group II introns

The group II introns also, like the group I introns, have a characteristic secondary structure (Fig. 6.22). However, these introns usually follow the GT-AG rule and the first nucleotide at the 5' end of the intron is a G residue. There are 6 stem loop domains and the 5' and 3' splicing junctions are in close vicinity with each other. The splicing is autosplicing carried out by trans-esterification. The intron is removed in form of a lariat. Domain 5 and domain 6 are joined together by only 2 nucleotides. An 'A' residue present within domain 6 (Fig. 6.23), provides the site for the first esterification between its 2'-OH group and the G residue at the 5' end of the intron (3' end of exon 1). This forms a lariat structure when the exon 1 is excised off. The highly reactive -OH at the 3' end of exon 1 attacks the 3'-splice junction and the two exons are joined together by trans-esterification while the lariated intron is given out. The process is thus very similar to nuclear splicing except that no trans factors (i.e. SnRNPs) are required for this splicing. The internal regions of complementarity serve the function of bringing the reactive sites near to each other.

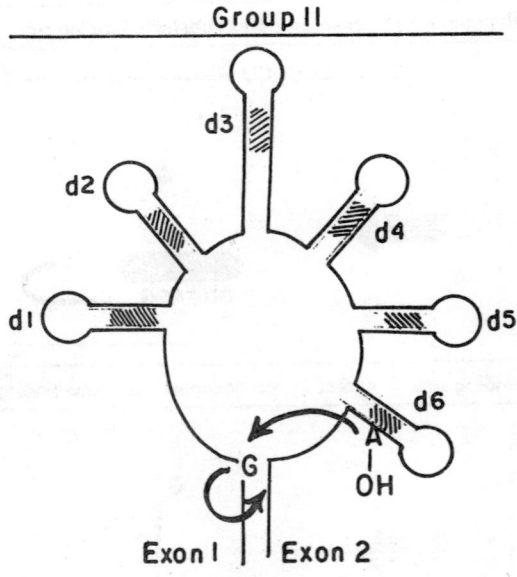

Fig. 6.22. Structure of Group II introns.

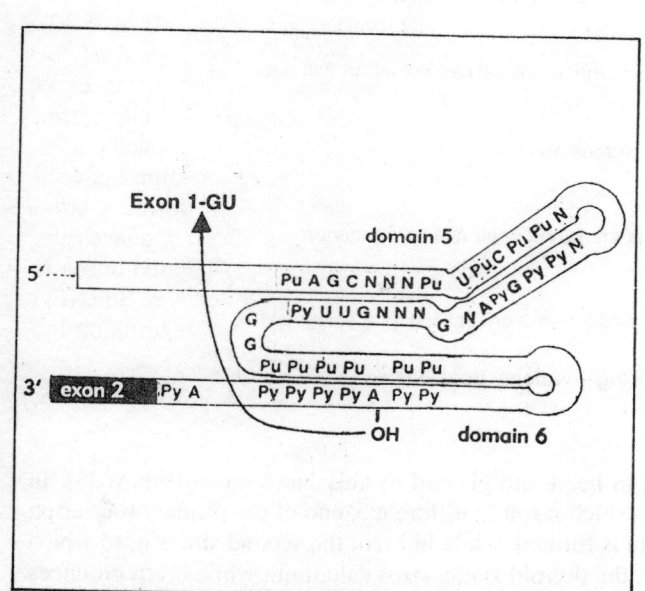

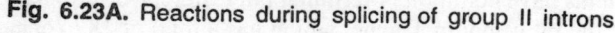

Fig. 6.23A. Reactions during splicing of group II introns.

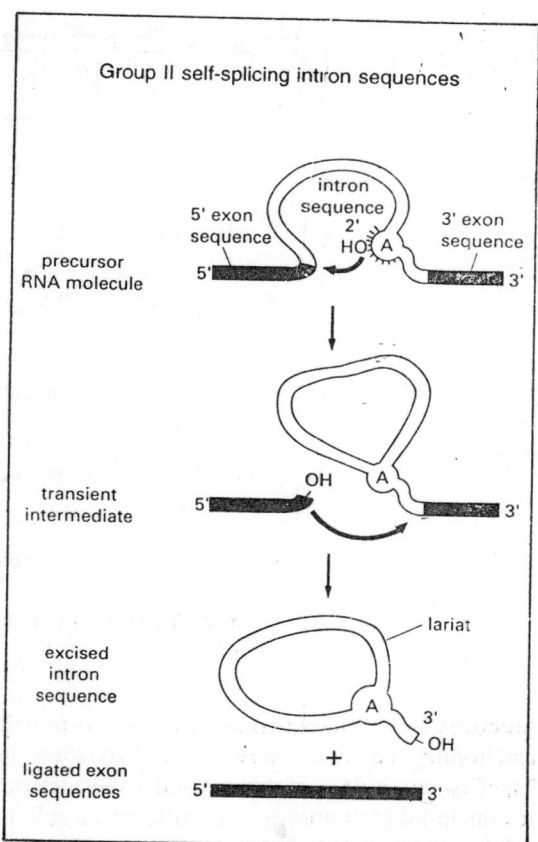

Fig. 6.23B. Self splicing of group II introns.

Alternate Splicing

A gene usually codes for only one mRNA in eukaryotes. However, sometimes a primary transcript may produce more than one mRNA by alternate splicing. This takes place either by the removal of only a few and not all of the introns or by the alternate ligation of the exons (Fig. 6.24). In the first case, the removal of various cambination of introns will produce a number of different mRNAs. Thus different mRNAs may have different size due to the presence of different introns in some of these. It should be noted that not only the size of some of the mRNAs may be increased due to the presence of an (or more) intron in the mature mRNA, the meaning of all the exons which are present after the intron will also change if the intron changes the reading frame. In the second case where all the introns are removed but the sequence of exons is changed (i.e. the exon 3 may come before exon 2, for example), then the sequence of mRNA will change, though its size will remain same. However, the change in reading frame may take place.

Occcasionally there are multiple promoters in a gene, each of which transcribes different region of the gene and produce multiple species of mRNAs. In such an event, the mRNAs will be related to each other and will have stretches of common sequences. For example, the myosin alkali light chain gene of chicken

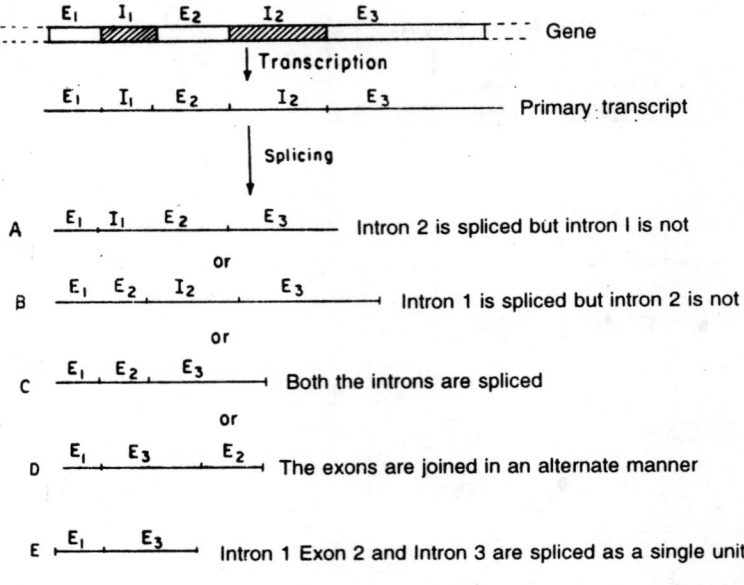

Fig. 6.24. Alternate splicing—various possibilities.

produces two different tissue-specific iso-proteins in heart and gizzard by this mechanism (Fig. 6.25). In calcitonin gene, there are two polyadenylation sites which result in different 3' end of the primary transcript. The first site is used in thyroid and a short transcript is formed, while in brain the second site is used which results in longer transcript. By differential splicing, the thyroid synthesizes calcitonin while brain produces calcitonin gene related peptide (CGRP). The two proteins have common N-terminal but different C-terminal (Fig. 6.26). Other examples for alternate splicing are the rat troponin T gene, which has a total of 18 exons separated by 17 introns. By differential splicing, 32 different species of mRNAs are produced. All these mRNAs code for various isoforms of troponin T. It was found that exons 1, 2, 3, 9, 10, 11, 12, 13, 14,

Two promoters and different splicing patterns : the chicken myosin alkali light-chain gene

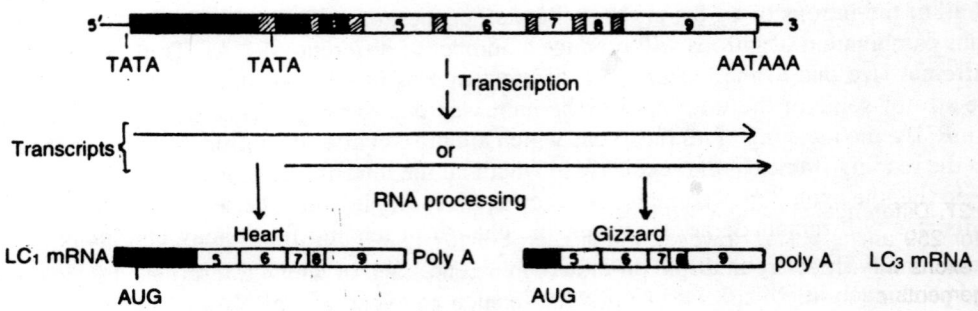

Fig. 6.25. Different mRNAs are produced from the same gene in different tissues.

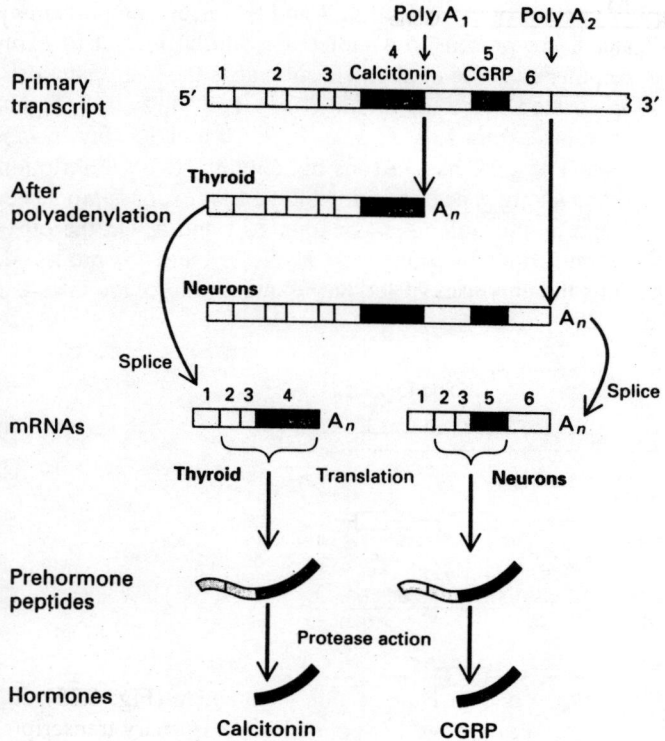

Fig. 6.26. Differential processing of primary transcript from calcitonin gene results in two products, calcitonin in the thyroid gland, and calcitonin gene-related product (CGRP) in certain neurons. Choice of the poly A site and the subsequent splicing choices are co-ordinated.

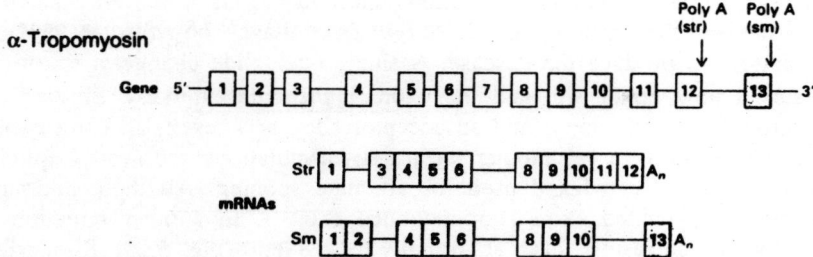

Fig. 6.27. Differential splicing in synthesis of muscle functions (a) The rat troponin T gene has 18 exons which code for 259 amino acids. However, the length of this protein varies in different muscles of the body. Eleven of the exons will appear in all the mRNAs; exons 4-8 appear in various combinations giving rise to 32 possible arrangements such as 4, 7, 8; 7, 8 etc.); exon 16 or 17, but not both, is in one mRNA. Thus, there is a total of 64 possible mRNAs. (b) The α-tropomyosin gene has 13 exons that are variably spliced in different muscle tissues; shown are the predominant splices found in striated (str), or skeletal, muscle and smooth (sm) muscle, which is found, for example, in arterial walls.

15, and 18 are always present in all these mRNAs but out of exon 4, 5, 6, 7 and 8, various combinations such as 4, 6, 8 or 4, 5, 7 or 4, 7, 8 or only 7 and 8 are present in a molecule. Similarily, out of exon 16 and 17 only one exon is present in a molecule. Another example of alternate splicing is the α–tropomyosin gene. It has 13 exons out of which the mRNA in striated muscles contain exons 1, 3, 4, 5, 6, 8, 9, 10, 11 and 12 while the mRNA in smooth muscle contains exons 1, 2, 4, 5, 6, 8, 9, 10 and 13 (Fig. 6.27). A different scenerio is presented by α–amylase gene. The gene has 4 exons but contains two transcription start sites. In salivary gland the first start site is used and a long gene containing all the four exons is produced. However, during splicing the exon 2 is removed and mature mRNA has exons 1, 3 and 4. On the other hand, in liver the second start site is used and short transcript containing only exons 2, 3 and 4 is produced. All the three exons are retained during splicing. Thus the amylases of salivary gland and liver are different enzymes though product of the same gene (Fig. 6.28).

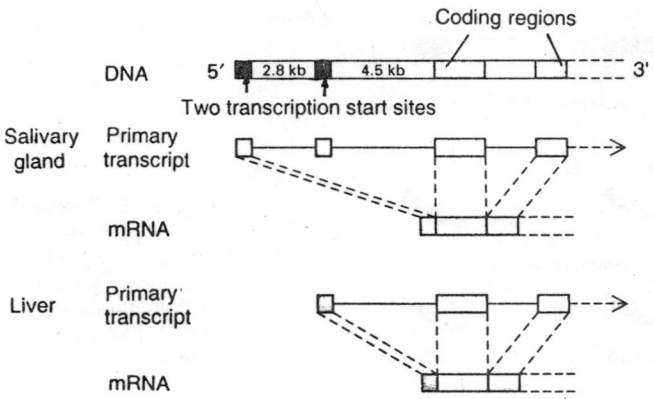

Fig. 6.28. Overlapping transcription units for α-amylase and the primary transcripts produced preferentially in salivary gland and liver. Transcription starting from the salivary gland start site in more frequent than that from liver start site. The coding regions in the α-amylase mRNA in both tissues are the same.

The molecular basis of β-thalassemia presents another example where alternate splicing plays an important role in the formation of a number of different mRNAs, all coding for different forms of β-globin. The normal β-globin gene contains three exons and two introns which are spliced to produce the normal mRNA. However, the mapping of defective genes have shown some mutations which can alter the splicing pattern to produce the desease. A single nucleotide change at intron 1, upstream of its donor site creates a new donor site and the exon 2 becomes extended. Similarily two other known mutations in intron 2 create a donor and an acceptor sites as a result, an extra exon is formed between the exon 2 and the exon 3. In yet another set of known mutations, the normal splicing sites are altered while cryptic sites are activated and used for alternate splicing. All these alternate splicings result either in shortened or extended exon 1 or extended exon 3. In another mutation the normal polyadenylation site is lost which results in an abnormally long 3'-end (Fig. 6.29). Similarily a number of splicing related changes are found in human hemophilia factor VIII gene which result in hemophilia (Fig. 6.30).

Some viruses have a different scenario. The primary transcript codes for multiple mRNAs, however, only one has the cap. By differential splicing the position of cap structure changes which results in translation of different peptides (Fig. 6.31).

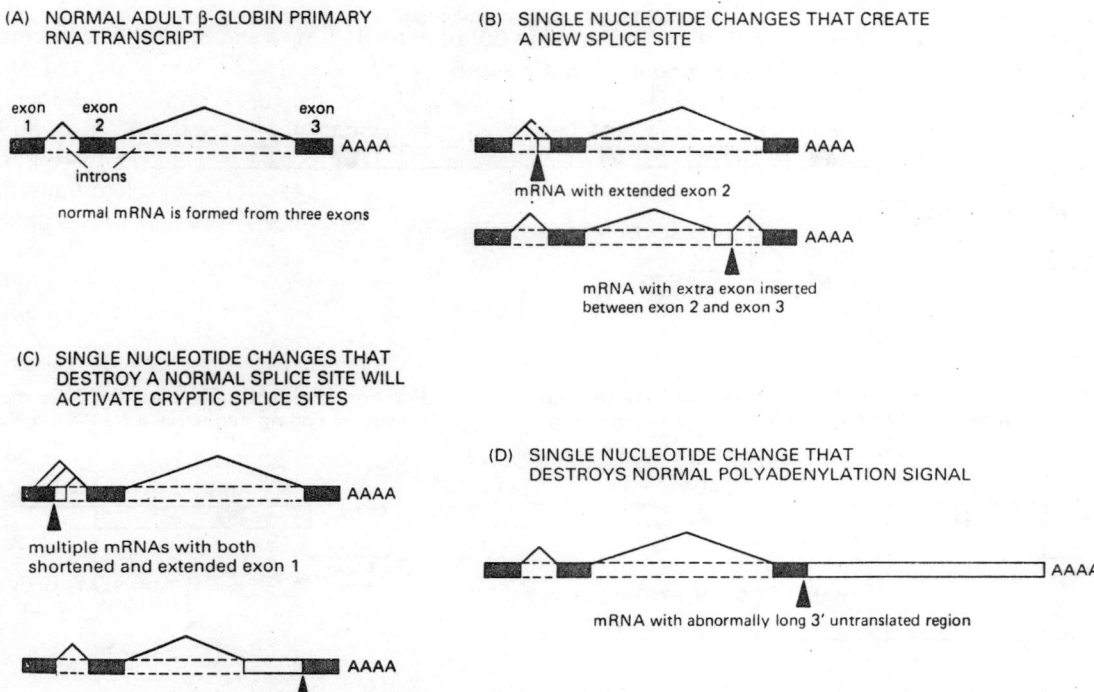

(A) NORMAL ADULT β-GLOBIN PRIMARY RNA TRANSCRIPT

exon 1 exon 2 exon 3

introns

normal mRNA is formed from three exons

(B) SINGLE NUCLEOTIDE CHANGES THAT CREATE A NEW SPLICE SITE

mRNA with extended exon 2

mRNA with extra exon inserted between exon 2 and exon 3

(C) SINGLE NUCLEOTIDE CHANGES THAT DESTROY A NORMAL SPLICE SITE WILL ACTIVATE CRYPTIC SPLICE SITES

multiple mRNAs with both shortened and extended exon 1

mRNA with extended exon 3

(D) SINGLE NUCLEOTIDE CHANGE THAT DESTROYS NORMAL POLYADENYLATION SIGNAL

mRNA with abnormally long 3′ untranslated region

Fig. 6.29. β Thalassemia is produced by a number of splicing related changes in the gene.

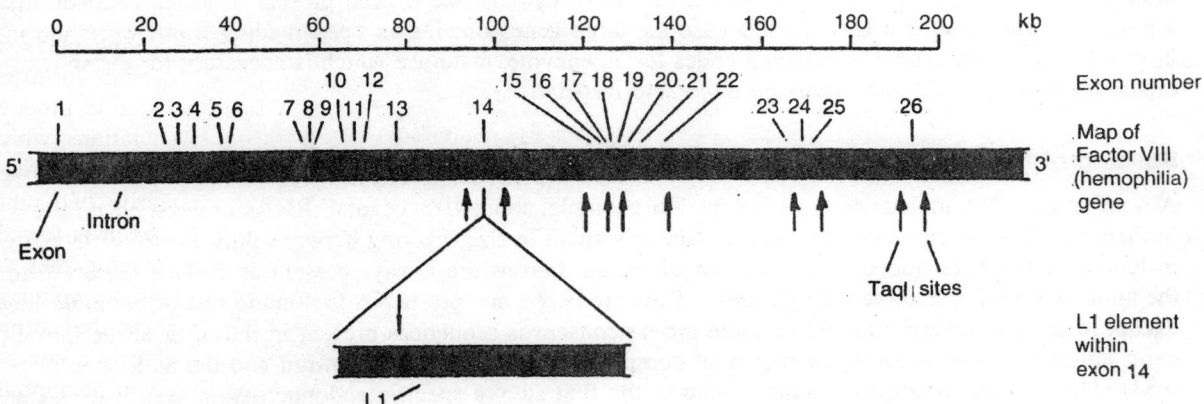

Fig. 6.30. The mutation in the hemophilia (Factor VIII) gene caused by the insertion of an L1 element.   A map of the hemophilia gene, showing the location of its exons (numbered 1-26) and TaqI sites (arrows). The L1 element lies within exon 14 and contains one TaqI site (arrow).

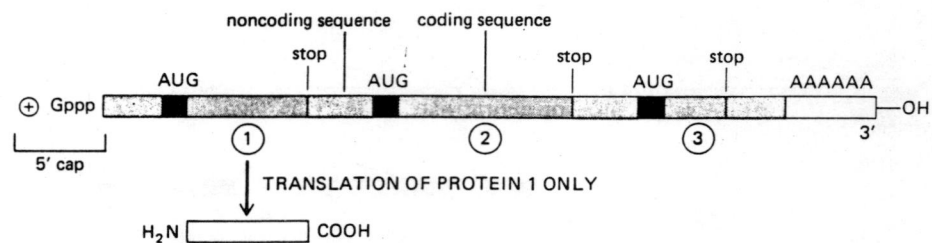

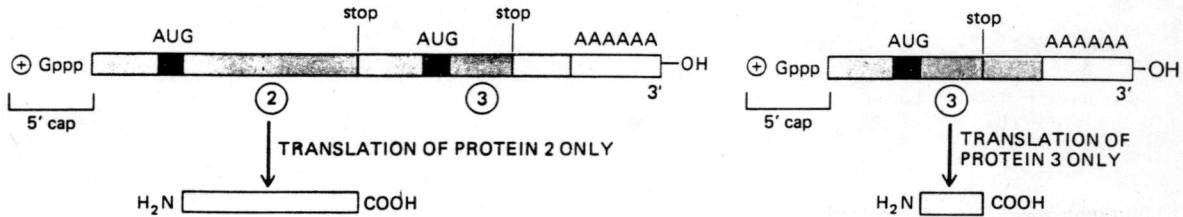

Fig. 6.31. For some viruses the same primary RNA transcript is spliced in several ways to produce three (or more) different mRNA molecules, each coding for a different protein. In each case, only the coding sequence closest to the 5' cap is translated from the mRNA molecule.

Ocassionally the introns may code for biologically active proteins

While introns by definition donot code for a protein, there are certain cases where a biologically active molecule is coded by the part of an intron. The yeast cytochrome b gene present in its mitochondria is a good example of such a case. In this case the large gene contains an open reading frame in its intron 2, which along with exon 2 and exon 3 codes for an enzyme, maturase which is necessary for the splicing of the intron (Fig. 6.32 and discussed elsewhere in detail).

Splicing of tRNA molecules

A number of tRNA molecules have introns. for example, about 10% ot total tRNAs in yeast have introns in them. In all these cases the introns are relatively small in size, varying between only 14-46 nucleotides in length. It has been found that in all the cases, the introns are always present at a place adjacent to the anticodon region and the configuration of mature tRNA and pre-tRNA is same in rest of the molecule except in the anti-codon arm. While there are no consensus sequences present in intron or at the intron-exon junctions, there is always a region of complementarity between the intron and the anticodon (Fig. 6.33). The splicing is enzyme mediated and in the first step, a specific endonuclease makes two cuts at both ends of the intron. Thus the intron is removed in a single step. This excision results in the formation of two half tRNA molecules along with the excised intron, present in form of a linear molecule. The entire molecule of tRNA except the anticodon arm is in correct configuration. The two half molecules are held together by the intra-molecular hydrogen bonds in the acceptor, the Ψ and the D arms. At this stage the

(a)

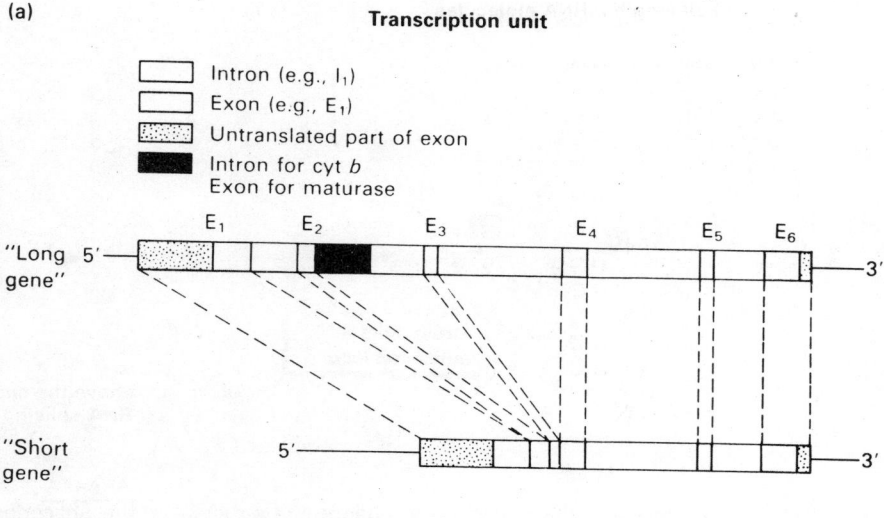

Transcription unit

Intron (e.g., I₁)
Exon (e.g., E₁)
Untranslated part of exon
Intron for cyt *b*
Exon for maturase

(b)

Synthesis of cytochrome *b* mRNA

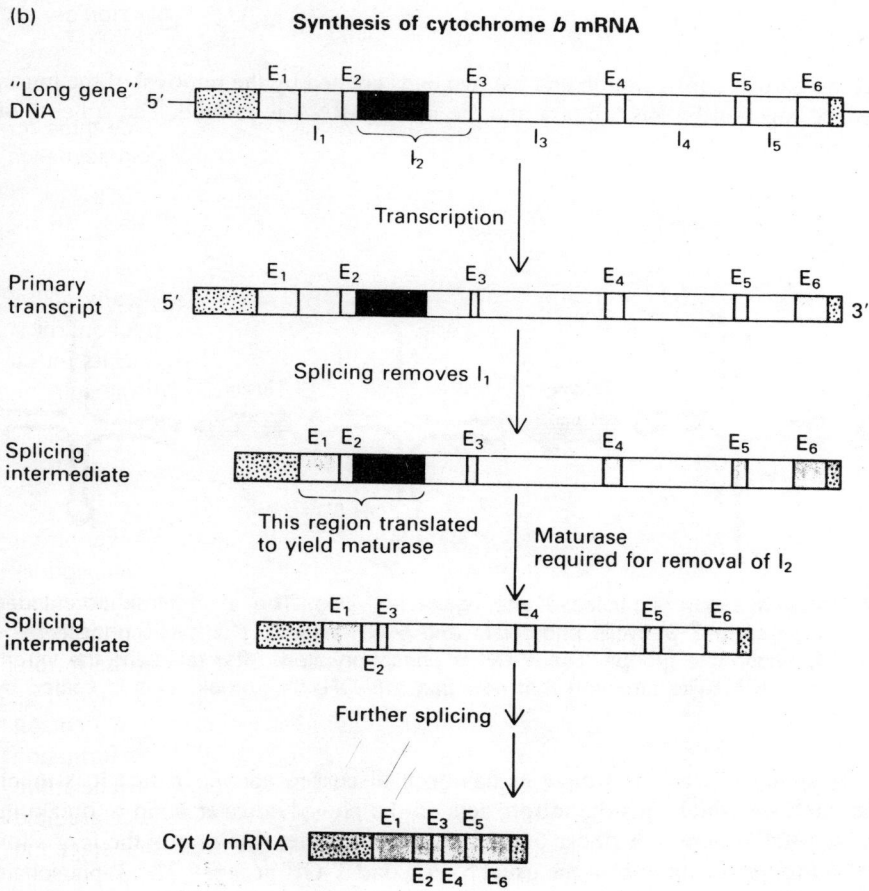

Fig. 6.32. The cytochrome of gene of yeast. (a) The mtDNA of "long-gene" yeast strains contain 6 exons for cytochrome b. The DNA the closely related "short-gene" yeast strains contain only three exons. Two of these correspond to exons E_5 and E_6 of the long gene strain; the other sends a fusion of exons E_1, E_2, E_3 and E_4 with the precise deletion of the introns present in the long gene strain. (b) Production of cytochrome in the "long-gene" strain involves several novel splicing stages. Intron 1 is removed from the primary RNA transcript by splicing; a protein catalysing this reaction is encoded by nuclear DNA. The resulting RNA (the splicing intermediate) is translated into a protein with sequence at its N-terminus that are encoded by exons E_1 and E_2 of cytochrome b and a sequence at its C-terminus that is encoded in intron I_2 of cytochrome b. Only the splicing activity of this chimeric protein (maturase) can remove intron I_2. Other splicing reaction generate mature cytochrome b mRNA I_2 is a type II intron; in cell-free reactions. RNA which contain such an intron undergo self catalyzed splicing similar to that as in its *Tetrahymena* rRNA.

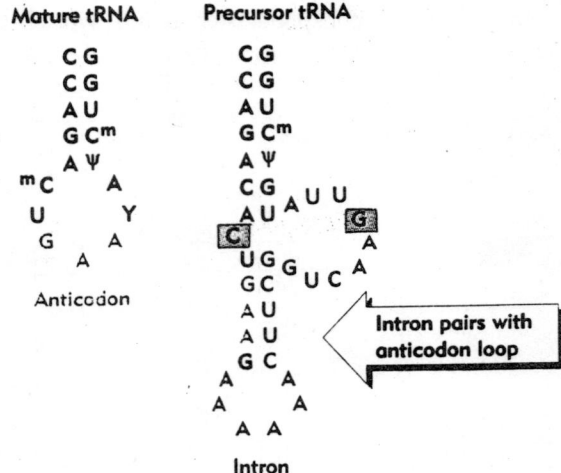

Fig. 6.33. The intron in yeast tRNA^{Phe} base bairs with the anticodon to change the structure of the anticodon arm. Pairing between an excluded base in the stem and the intron loop in the precursor may be required for splicing.

anticodon region also attains the correct configuration and the two ends created by the removal of the intron come together. These are joined together by RNA ligase and the mature tRNA is formed. The splicing of yeast tRNA$_{Phe}$ is shown in Fig 6.34.

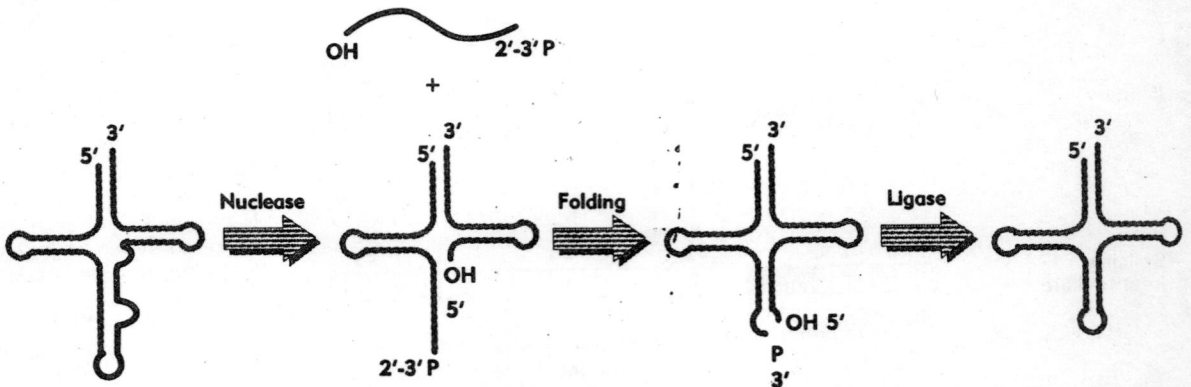

Fig. 6.34. Splicing of tRNA requires separate nuclease and ligase activities. The exon-intron boundaries are cleaved by the nuclease to generate 2'-3' cyclic phosphate and 5'-OH termini. The cyclic phosphate is opened to generate 3'-OH and 2' phosphate groups. The 5'-OH is phosphorylated. After releasing the intron, the tRNA half molecules fold into a tRNA-like structure that now has a 3'-OH, 5'-P break. This is sealed by a ligase.

The mechanism of tRNA splicing is not as simple as has been discussed above. In fact it is much more complex. In yeast, the nuclease which cuts the intron, acts on the phosphodiester bond to break the linkage of phosphate group with the 5' carbon of ribose of the tailing nucleotide, resulting in the formation of free 3'-phosphate and 5'-OH groups (in contrast to the usual 5'-PO$_4$ and 3'-OH groups). The 3'-phosphate group simultaneously forms a cyclic phosphodiester bond with 2'-OH of the same nucleotide. This 2',3'-cyclic phosphodiester bond is then digested by a specific phosphodiesterase which forms 2'-phosphate and 3'-OH groups. The 5'-OH group of the exon 2 is phosphorylated by a kinase in an ATP dependent manner. The ATP molecule serves as phosphate group donor. The resultant 5'-phosphate then gets ligated to the 3'-OH of exon 1 by a ligase and the RNA is sealed. However, the original 5'-end of the now sealed exon 1 still has the extra PO_4 group at the 2'-position. A specific phosphatase removes the 2'-phosphate group and the mature tRNA is synthesized. The phosphate group for the formation of phosphodiester bond is thus provided by exogeneous ATP molecule and is not of tRNA origin. The entire process is shown in Fig. 6.35.

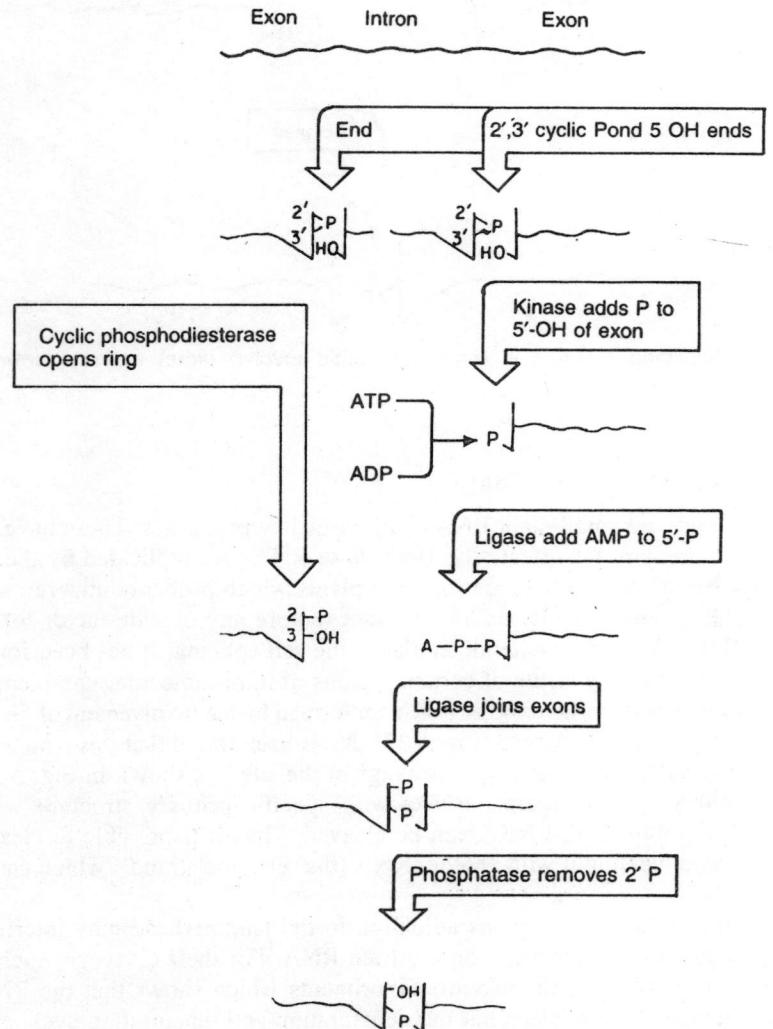

Fig. 6.35. Splicing of yeast and plant tRNAs involves a series of reactions that rely on unusual 5' and 3' termini in the RNA.

It has been found that in plants, the tRNA splicing takes place in a similar manner. However, the mammalian tRNA splicing follows a different pathway. The early steps and the cleavage of the intron are similar to the splicing of yeast tRNA and the exon 1 with a 2',3'-cyclic phosphate group and the exon 2 with a 5'-OH group are obtained. However, in the next step a specific ligase joins the two groups without the need of decyclisation or phosphorylation. As a result, the mature tRNA molecule is formed. The phosphate group which is used for phosphodiester bond formation comes from the tRNA itself and not from the ATP as is the case with in yeast (Fig. 6.36).

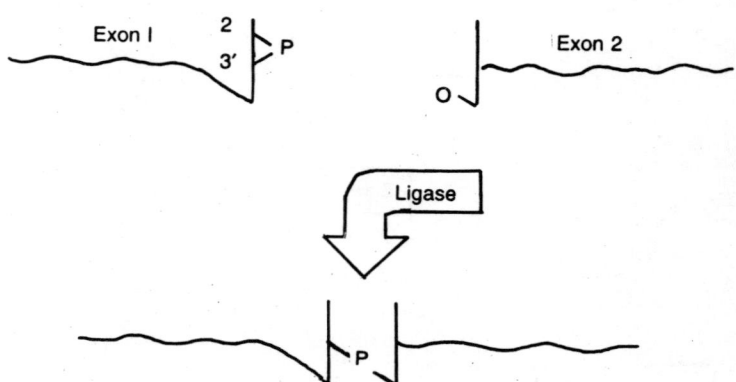

Fig. 6.36. The tRNA-splicing reaction in mammals could involve direct reaction between the 2', 3'-cyclic phosphate and a 5'-OH group.

Self cleavage of viroids and virusoids

The viroids and virusoids are small plant RNAs with virus like properties. These have similar organization but differ in their requirement for infectivity. Both these RNAs are replicated by the rolling circle mode. A number of multimers of these RNAs are found in plants which probably undergo self cleavage to form the monomers. Under in vitro conditions, these donot require any outside factor for their cleavage. The cleavage of these RNAs is, to some extend, similar to the self splicing. It has been found that these RNAs form a very specific structure by virtue of certain regions of intra-molecular complementarity within their sequences. The structure has three stem-loops which are formed by the involvement of 58 nucleotides. Thirteen of these nucleotides are highly conserved (Fig. 6.37). It has been found that this structure, which is referred as the hammerhead, is sufficient to undergo cleavage at the site. As shown in Fig. 6.38, if a hybrid RNA is created by annealing of two separate RNAs with specific primary structure which can produce a hammerhead like configuration, this RNA can be cleaved. Thus it is possible to cleave a substrate RNA with a cleavage site by annealing it with another RNA (the 'enzyme strand') which can provide the correct confirmation.

Addition of extra bases in the regions adjoining to the hammerhead may interfere with the specific configuration and also with the cleavage of substrate RNA. For their cleavage, such RNAs may require a cycle of heating and cooling in the in vitro experiments which shows that the RNA probably did not have correct configuration in first place but the denaturation and renaturation cycle can bring it to proper confirmation.

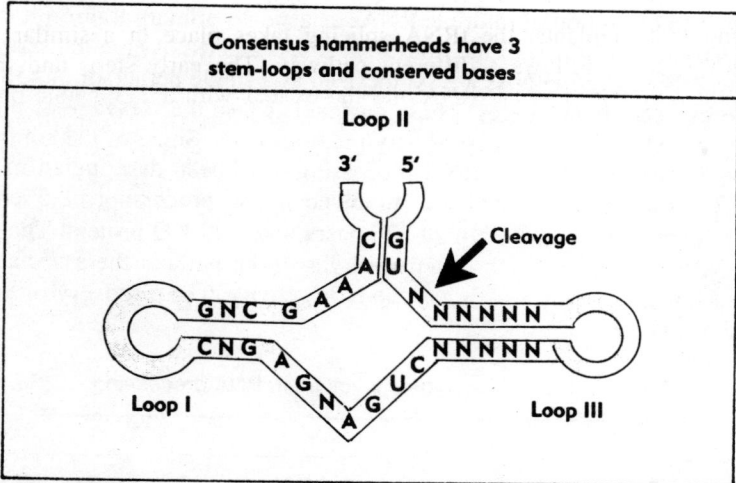

Fig. 6.37. Self cleavage sites of viroids and virusoids have a consensus sequence and form a hammerhead secondary structure by intramolecular pairing.

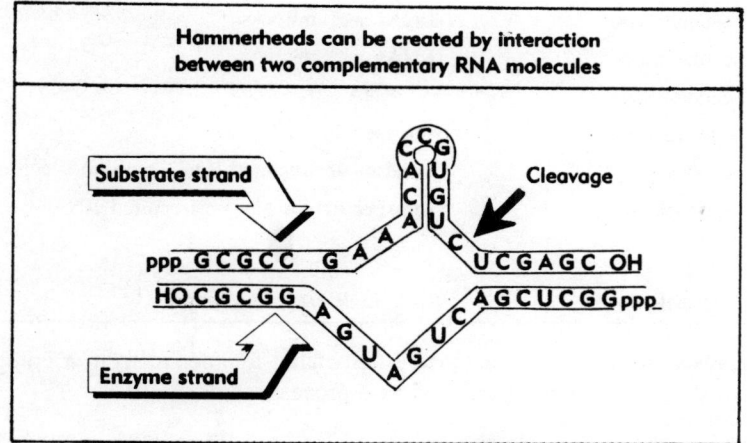

Fig. 6.38. Hammerheads can also be generated by pairing between a "substrate" strand and an "enzyme" strand.

RNA processing

Many primary transcripts represent more than one RNA molecules which are often separated from each other by a stretch of polynucleotides. This region is referred as the spacer region. This spacer very clearly differs from the introns of the eukaryotic genes. The intron is present in between the sequences of a single RNA molecule and its removal is necessary for obtaining the mature RNA. The removal of intron is always associated with the joining of two pieces of RNA (the exons). The spacer on the other hand, is the region between two separate RNAs with independent and complete structure and functions which are, however, transcribed together as a single primary transcript. The removal of a spacer results in the formation of two mature RNAs. There is no simultaneous ligation of the two RNA fragments. The removal of spacer is referred as RNA processing.

This phenomenon of transcription of multiple RNAs as a single primary transcript is more common in prokaryotes than in eukaryotes. Majority of the ribosomal RNAs and tRNAs are transcribed in this manner. Even in eukaryotes, the 28S and 18S rRNAs are synthesized as a single percursor of 45S in size. The RNA processing takes place by specific nucleases. These nucleases cause the cleavage of the transcript. Some of these nucleases are very specific and digest at very precise points. Some of the common nucleases and their site of action involved in prokaryotic RNA processing have been descibed in Table 6.3. It may be pertinent to point out that RNase P which is involved in the processing of 5'-end of tRNAs, is a nucleoprotein in nature containing a 10S RNA of 375 bases and a 20 KD protein. The enzymatic activity of RNase P lies in the RNA moiety, which is active in vitro even without the association of the protein. It was the first isolated RNA molecule which has catalytic activity. The discovery of this RNA has given rise to the concept of ribozymes.

Table 6.3. E. coli enzymes involved in RNA processing

Enzyme	Nature	Site of action
RNase P	Endonuclease	5'-end of tRNA
RNase BN	Exonuclease	3'-end of tRNA
RNase D	exonuclease	3'-end of tRNA
RNase T	exonuclease	CCA at the 3'-end of tRNA
RNase III	endonuclease	rRNAs and mRNAs
Rnase R	exonuclease	rRNAs and mRNAs
RNase E	endonuclease	5S rRNA
RNase I	endonuclease	Non-specific
RNase II	exonuclease	3'-end of unstructured RNAs with no specificity for type of RNA
Polynucleotide phosphorylase (PNPase)	exonuclease	Non-specific for any unstructured RNA
RNase H	exonuclease	RNA in RNA:DNA hybrid

Many of these RNases are present in a loosely associated manner to form a complex of large size. Sometimes this type of complex has been referred as a processosome.

Cap formation and polyadenylation

The cap formation at the 5'-end and the additon of a 100-200 bases long poly (A) tail at the 3'-end of the mRNA are other post-transcriptional events in eukaryotes. The addition of cap takes place in the nucleus. The cap is a very specific structure which have some unusual features. The most striking feature is the addition of a 7-methyl guanosine residue at the 5'-end of the hnRNA. This addition of methylated G doesnot take place by the usual 3'-5'-phosphodiester bond rather the ^{7m}G is attached to the terminal nucleotide of the primary transcript by a 5'-5' condensation of phosphates present at the 5'-end of the hnRNA and the 5'end of ^{7m}G. In this condensation not only the α-PO_4 but all the three phosphates are preserved, and these participate in this bonding. Thus the bond is 5'-$^{7m}G_{ppp}N$ (Fig. 6.39). Another striking feature of the cap is that either one or two terminal nucleotides of the transcript (which now become the 2nd and the 3rd nucleotide after the addition of the ^{7m}G residue) are also methylated. However, the methylation is not in the base (which is the normal site of methylation in nucleic acids), but is at the 2'-OH of the sugar. The

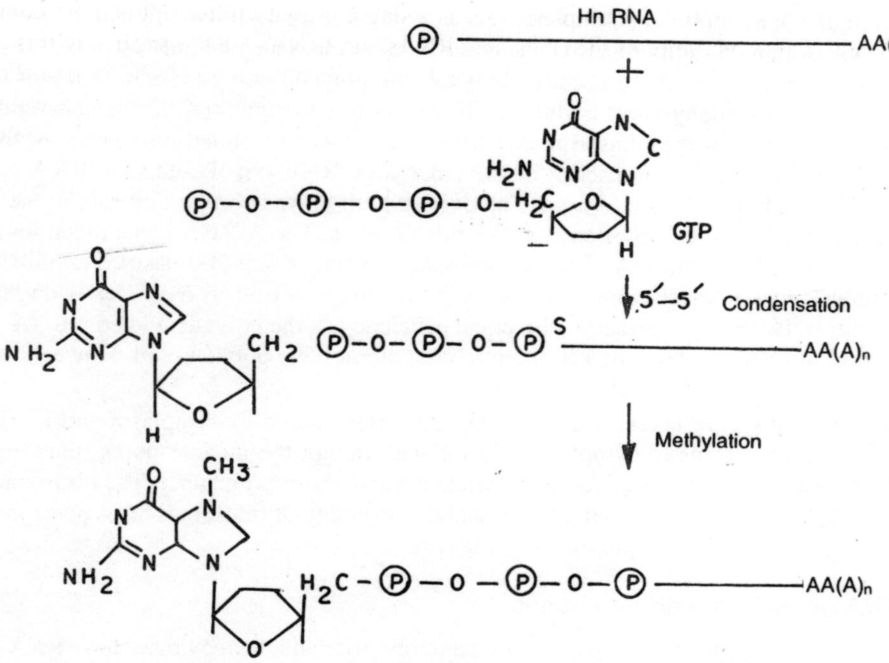

Fig. 6.39. Cap formation.

cap structure is thus $^{7m}G_{ppp}NmN(m)N$ which has been shown in Fig. 6.40. It plays an important role in the recognition of initiation codon by the eukaryotic ribosomes (see later) and is essential for the translation. Besides it may also play some role in the stability of the mRNA.

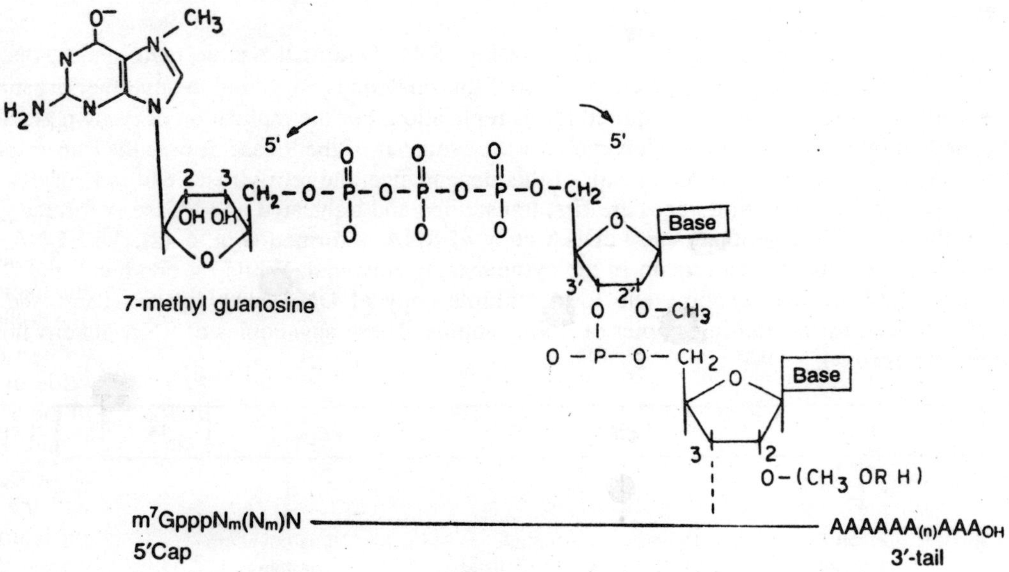

7-methyl guanosine

$m^7GpppN_m(N_m)N$ ——————————————————— $AAAAAA_{(n)}AAA_{OH}$
5'Cap   3'-tail

Fig. 6.40. Structure of the 5'-cap of mRNA.

In the same manner a long stretch of A residues (commonly known as poly(A) tail), is also added at the 3'-end of the mRNA. Again this addition also takes place in the nucleus and the hnRNA is polyadenylated. The poly (A) addition is carried out by a specific enzyme, the poly(A) polymerase which is a template independent enzyme. The polyadenylation is directed by the poly (A) signal (AAATAA) present 10-20 nucleotide upstream of the end of the transcript. As discussed earlier this signal also plays an important role in defining the 3'-end of primary transcript of the eukaryotic RNA pol II catalysed RNA synthesis. This signal codes for the addition of poly (A) tail. The poly (A) tail plays an important role in the stability of the mRNA. The length of poly A is shortened as the mRNA ages. The hnRNA has a much longer poly (A) tail than the tail present in the mRNA. The average length is about 100-200 bases. Previously it was thought that it also plays a role in translatability of mRNA but in vitro experiments have clearly demonstrated that the deadenylated mRNA can be translated with equal efficiency as the polyadenylated mRNA. Besides some of the eukaryotic mRNAs such as the histone mRNAs, donot have poly (A) tail. However, the poly (A) tail has an important role in the stability of mRNA.

Once these modifications have taken place, the mRNA is transported to cytoplasm and is translated. The transport of RNA from nucleus to cytoplasm takes place through the nuclear pores (the structure of nuclear pores has been discussed later) in an energy dependent active transport manner. The ribosomal RNAs, on the other hand, combine with the ribosomal proteins and the assembly of ribosomes takes place in nucleus. The assembled ribosomes are then transported to cytoplasm. .

Replication of RNA genome of certain viruses

It has already been discussed that certain viruses such as the retroviruses and the reoviruses have RNA genome. How the RNA synthesis in these viruses takes place. The two types of viruses follow separate route. In retroviruses, first the RNA is copied to DNA by a virus coded enzyme, the reverse transcriptase. This DNA is then replicated and transcribed to produce multiple copies of the RNA genome. The reoviruses on the other hand multiply without the synthesis of DNA by a RNA dependent RNA polymerase (RNA replicase) and form new progeny.

RNA synthesis in retroviruses

The structure of a typical retrovirus has been shown in Fig. 6.41. One of the three main genes, the pol gene codes for the reverse transcriptase. The counterpart of this enzyme is not found in any other organism. Thus the virus itself codes for the enzyme required for its replication. For the replication of its own genome, the virus is dependent on its own genome. However, for the synthesis of the RTase, it uses the transcription and translation machinery of the host. As a result of this dependance, the retroviruses can not survive out side the host. After infection, the viral genes are first transcribed and translated and RTase is formed. The enzyme acts on the viral RNA genome and a cDNA copy of RNA is formed (Fig. 6.42). This DNA can get integrated to host genome or can remain in the cytoplasm as episomal. While on one hand, the DNA will replicate alongwith the host genome and form multiple copy of DNA, on the other hand, the the transcription of the DNA forms multiple copies of RNA genome. These new copies of RNA get envaloped and new virions are formed.

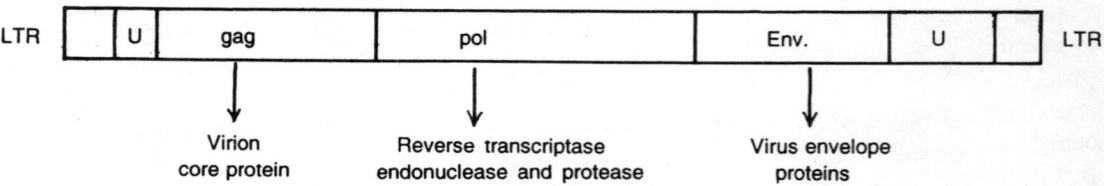

Fig. 6.41. General structure of a retrovirus.

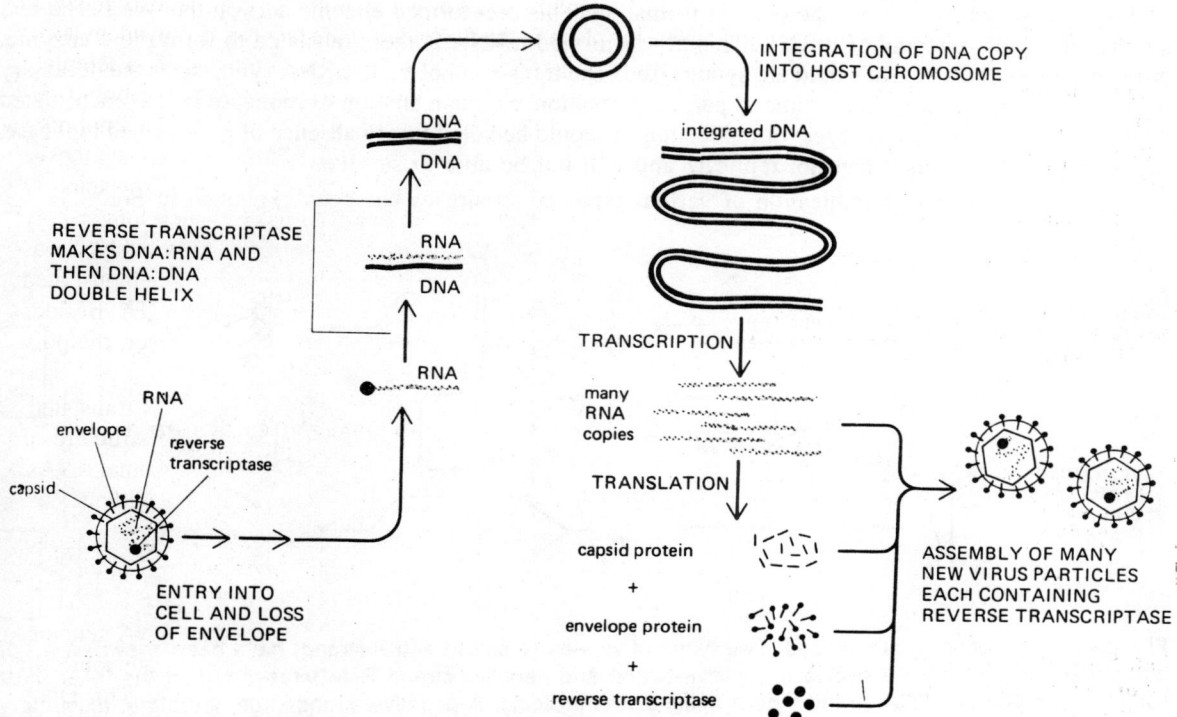

INTEGRATION OF DNA COPY
INTO HOST CHROMOSOME

integrated DNA

DNA
DNA

REVERSE TRANSCRIPTASE
MAKES DNA:RNA AND
THEN DNA:DNA
DOUBLE HELIX

RNA
DNA

RNA

TRANSCRIPTION

RNA

many
RNA
copies

envelope

reverse
transcriptase

capsid

TRANSLATION

capsid protein
+
envelope protein
+
reverse transcriptase

ENTRY INTO
CELL AND LOSS
OF ENVELOPE

ASSEMBLY OF MANY
NEW VIRUS PARTICLES
EACH CONTAINING
REVERSE TRANSCRIPTASE

Fig. 6.42. The life cycle of a retrovirus. The retrovirus genome consists of an RNA molecule of about 8500 nucleotides : two such molecules are packaged into each viral particle. The enzyme reverse transcriptase is a DNA polymerase that first makes a DNA copy of the viral RNA molecule and then a second DNA strand, generating a double-stranded DNA copy of the RNA genome. The integration of this DNA double helix into the host chromosome, catalyzed by a viral protein, is required for the synthesis of new viral RNA molecules by the host cell RNA polymerase.

RNA synthesis in reoviruses

The reoviruses multiply without synthesizing the DNA intermediate. Here again, the enzyme RNA replicase is coded by the viral genome. For the synthesis of replicase the host machinery is used by the virus. Once the enzyme has been synthesized it copies the RNA genome and multiple copies are formed which are envaloped and released.

Based on the nature of the virus, it may be either a double stranded RNA genome or a single stranded genome. The synthesis of replicase from the double stranded genome and the replication of RNA is straight forward. The single stranded genome is of two kind. It is either a positive strand (i.e. the genome is made of the coding strand) or a negative strand (i.e. the genome is consisted of the non-coding strand). The synthesis of replicase from +ve strand RNA is straight forward. The enzyme then copies the genome and –ve strand is formed. Multiple copies of this negative strand are formed by replicase which are then envaloped.

The replication of –ve strand virus, on the other hand, poses a very tricky situation. The genome being non–coding strand, cannot be translated to form the enzyme. What is the source of enzyme. It has been found that for its replication, the virus should have some pre–formed enzyme which is encapsulated along with the RNA genome during the particle formation. This pre–formed enzyme acts on the –ve strand and synthesizes the +ve strand of mRNA. This newly formed mRNA is then translated to form more enzyme. Now multiple copies of –ve strand are synthesized. The translation of viral mRNA synthesizes the necessary proteins for encpsulation. At the time of particle formation, a certain amount of replicase is also encpsulated which will carry out the next cycle of replication. It should be noted that in absence of pre–formed replicase, the –ve strand reoviruses can not replicate and will not be able to survive.

The entire process of replication of various types of reoviruses has been explained in Fig. 6.41.

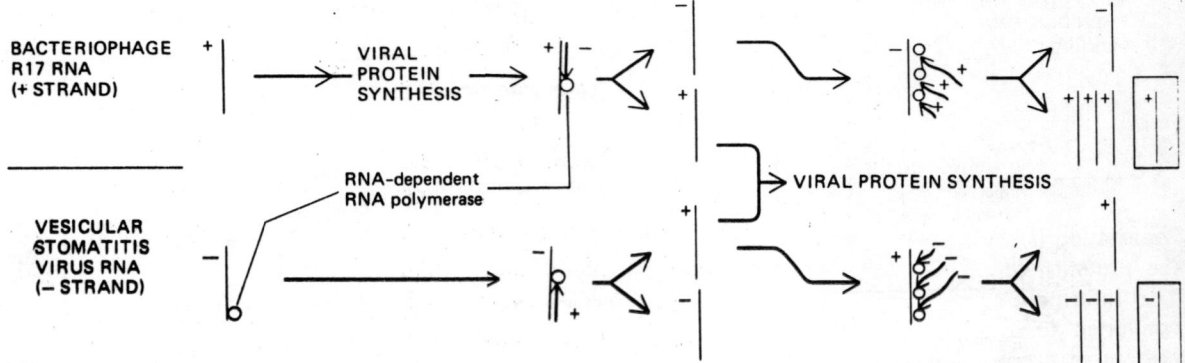

Fig. 6.43. Replication of reo viruses. Two types of viruses (+ strand and – strand) have been shown. A major difference between the life cycles of positive-strand and negative-strand RNA viruses is that the latter must synthesize a positive RNA strand before making viral proteins. A negative-strand virus, therefore, must carry within its capsid one or more molecules of the viral RNA-dependent RNA polymerase (replicase).

7

Translation

Translation is the final step in the transfer of genetic information from the DNA to its ultimate product, the proteins which are the functional molecules for majority of the metabolic processes in the cell. The information present in the genes in form of the sequence of four deoxynucleotides is finally converted to a sequence of entirely unrelated compound, the amino acids (aa). This information, present in a coded language in the DNA, is recognized and decoded by the cellular machinery. This coded language is known as the 'genetic code'. The aa contains two active groups, a −COOH group and a −NH₂ group. Condensation of two aa takes place by interaction of these groups and a bond between the carboxyl group of the first aa and the amino group of the next aa is formed. This bond (−CONH bond) is known as the peptide bond. A water molecule is given out during this condensation. This process is repeated a number of times and a protein or a polypeptide chain is synthesized. Thus the first aa of a protein contains a free amino group (the N-terminal end) while the last aa contains the free carboxyl group (the C-terminal end). The protein synthesis takes place from the N-terminal to the C-terminal. The formation of the peptide bond has been shown in Fig. 7.1. The protein synthesis or the translation, as the process is known, is a complex multistep multi-enzyme process. A cellular mechanism is required for reading the genetic code and bringing the appropriate aa to the site of protein synthesis. Both these roles are played primarily by the tRNA, a small (4S) RNA molecule which serves as the adopter molecule. The synthesis of proteins take place at the ribosomes, which are the largest cytoplasmic particles in a cell. Ribosomes are nucleoprotein in nature and have a complex molecular structure. Besides these two main particles, a number of different factors are also essential for these reactions which facilitate the protein synthesis. These factors are classified as the translation factors.

In order to understand the process of translation, it is essential that the structure and the functions of all these molecules are fully understood. We will, therefore, first discuss all these molecules in detail.

The mRNA

The mRNA is the template for protein synthesis. It transfers the genetic information which was originally stored in DNA to its final recipient, the proteins. The mRNA, in terms of its actual quantity, is relatively minor class of cellular RNA and represents only about 2% of the total cellular RNA. It is also the least stable amongst all the RNAs. The prokaryotic mRNAs have a half life of only few miniutes while the average eukaryotic mRNA has a half life of about 20 h. It is, therefore, very difficult to isolate good quality mRNA from prokaryotic cells. The purification of unbroken, biologically active bacterial mRNA

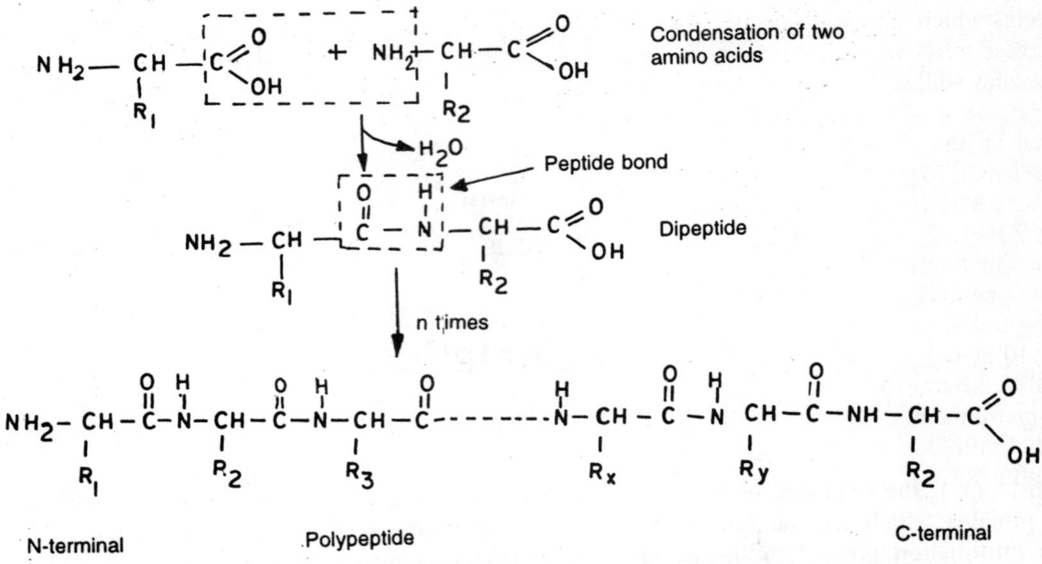

Fig. 7.1. Condensation of amino acids and formation of a peptide bond.

for molecular biology studies is almost impossible. One has to take extreme precautions in isolating the mRNA from eukaryotic cells also. The eukaryotic mRNAs are very heterogeneous in size (varying from less than 4S to more than 30S), however, 7-15S is the predominant size class. These have certain specific characters such as the presence of a methylated cap at the 5'-end and a stretch of A residues (poly A tail) at the 3'-end. These characteristic features have already been discussed. The coding region of mRNA which has the necessary information for the primary structure of proteins start from the initiaton codon AUG and ends in one of the three stop codons (UAA, UAG, UGA). Besides the coding region, there are some sequences upstream of AUG as well as downstream of the stop codon. These regions, referred as 5' and 3' noncoding regions or untranslated regions (5'-UT and 3'-UT), vary considerably in length and may have regulatory function. The role of SD sequences present in 5'-UT region of prokaryotic mRNAs have already been discussed. There are a number of secondary structures present in mRNAs specially at the 5' noncoding region. These have certain specific functions including in the translatibility of mRNAs. The structure of a typical mRNA has been shown in Fig. 7.2.

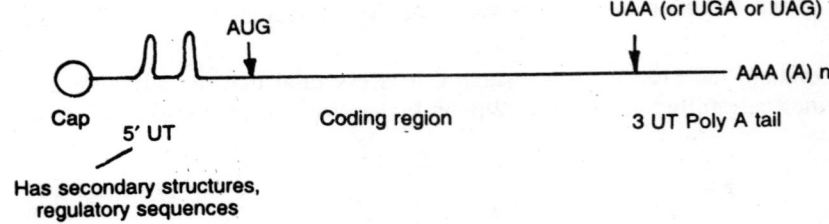

Fig. 7.2. Structure of eukaryotic mRNA.

Abundance of mRNAs

There are thousands of different mRNAs present in a cell. Some of these mRNAs code for the proteins which are present in all the cells, primarily the structural proteins. Some other mRNAs code for the proteins which are tissue specific. The transcription of certain other mRNAs is developmentally regulated. All these mRNAs are not present in equal copy number. Some of the mRNAs have very large number of molecules while others have relatively low copy number and some have only single or a very few molecules. It may be a good idea to discuss the relative abundance and distribution of mRNAs at this stage. Based on the copy number, the cellular mRNAs may be divided into three classes. (a) High abundant class which includes the mRNAs which are present in very high copy number (upto 12,000 copies/cell). These are very few (less than 10) in actual number and thus constituite only the minor species (less than 0.1%). However, in terms of the total mass, these represent upto 15% of the mRNAs. (b) Intermediate class which comprising about 5% of mRNA species (about 500-1000 mRNAs) and are present at about 300 copies/cell. Thus these represent about 40% of total cellular mRNA mass. (c) Rare class represents most of the mRNAs (about 10,000 or more or about 95% of total cellular mRNA species) and are present in only 10-20 copies/cell. Some of these mRNAs have only a single copy/cell. These thus represent only about 45% of the total mass of mRNAs in the cell. It may be pointed out that in most of the cases, the copy number of the mRNA of a specific species is directly proportional to the copy number of the proteins coded by that mRNA species. The typical distribution of various mRNAs in a mammalian cell has been shown in Table 7.1.

Table 7.1. Distribution of various classes of mRNAs in mammalian cells

S.No.	Class of mRNA	Copies/cell	mRNA species in the class		Total no. of mRNA molecules	% of total
			Absolute number	%		
1.	High abundant	upto 12,000	~4	~0.05%	48,000	~15%
2.	Intermediate	Average of 300	~500	~4.5%	15,000	~42%
3.	Rare	15 or less	~11,000	~95.5%	165,000	~43%

The Genetic Code

The analyses of a large number of proteins from various organisms have shown that there are 20 primary aminoacids which constitute most of the proteins. As there are 4 bases present in the mRNA, if each base had coded for one aa then it could code for only 4 aa; if two bases were to code for an aa then $4 \times 4 = 16$ aminoacids can be represented. A basic code of 3 nucleotides for each aa will result in $4 \times 4 \times 4 = 64$ codons. Thus a minimum of three nucleotides are required for forming a single codon. The experiments aimed at decifering the code using synthetic polyribonucleotides as mRNA have confirmed that an aa is represented by a set of three nucleotides (triplet), which is recognized by a specific tRNA. Each triplet is known as a codon and the entire arrangement is called as the genetic code. The genetic code has certain salient features. The first property of genetic code is that it is universal in nature i.e. a particular triplet always represents the same aa in all known organisms, from bacteria to primates. The only known exceptions are in mitochondrial and chloroplast genome and in some ciliates. However, there are no deviations in nuclear genome in other organisms. Thus it is possible to translate the mRNA from one organism by the cellular machinery of another organism. If genetic code was not universal, it would have been impossible to express a foreign gene in heterologous system which is presently being done routinely by genetic engineering route. As discussed earlier, the possible number of codons is 64. However, there are only twenty aa which constitute all the known proteins. It is therefore, possible that some of the aa will have more than one codon. In fact, this is the actual scenerio. In other words, the genetic code is degenerated. The entire genetic code has been decoded by M. Nirenberg who have shown that out of the 64 codons, 61 code for 20 aa while the three codons, UAA,

UAG and UGA, code for the termination of translation (terminator codon or the stop codon also referred as nonsense codons). AUG which codes for Met also serves as the initiation codon. Only in rare cases, alternate codons, GUG and UUG, can code for the initiation of translation. The universal genetic code has been shown in Table 7.2. The analysis reveals that two aminoacids (Met and Trp) have only one codon each, nine aminoacids (Phe, Tyr, Asp, Asn, Glu, Gln, His, Lys and Cys) have two codons each, Ile has three codon, five aminoacids (Val, Gly, Pro, Thr and Ala) have four codons each, while three aminoacids (Ser, Arg and Leu) have six codons each. The analysis of the aa composition of a number of proteins have revealed an interesting relationship between the number of codons for an aminoacid and the frequency of its occurance in the proteins. As shown in Fig 7.3, the aminoacids which have maximum number of codons are present more often than the aminoacids which have only one or two codons. Further, it has also been found that all the codons for a particular aminoacid are not used with equal efficiency. Different organisms seem to have preference for a particular codon. This phenomenon is known as the 'codon bias'. The codon bias is directly reflected in the presence of tRNAs containing the anticodon for the codon in that organism (see later).

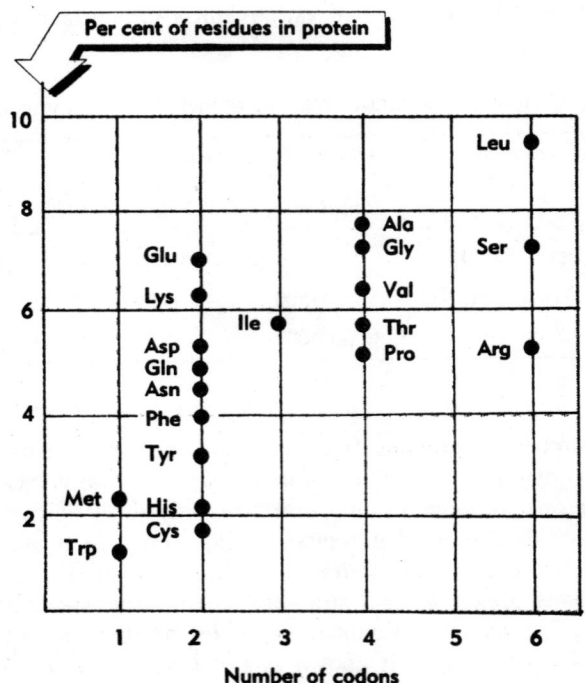

Fig. 7.3. The number of codons for an amino acid and its frequency of use in proteins show certain degree of correlation.

As discussed, the initiator codon, ATG, codes for Met also. In other words, the first aa to be incorporated in any protein is always a methionine. It is known that many of the proteins donot have Met as the N–terminal aa. How can this be explained? It has been found that the cleavage of the N–terminal methionine takes place in these proteins as one of the post–translational events. However, all proteins have methionine as their first aminioacid at the time of their synthesis. Occassionally GUG and UUG can serve as the initiation codon. Even when GUG or UUG is used as the initiator codon, the N–terminal

Table 7.2. Genetic code for chromosomal genome

First position (5'-end)	Second position			Third position	
	T	*C*	*A*	*G*	*(3'-end)*
T	Phe	Ser	Tyr	Cys	T
	Phe	Ser	Tyr	Cys	C
	Leu	Ser	Stop	Stop*	A
	Leu	Ser	Stop	Trp	G
C	Leu	Pro	His	Arg	T
	Leu	Pro	His	Arg	C
	Leu	Pro	Gln	Arg	A
	Leu	Pro	Gln	Arg	G
A	Ile	Thr	Asn	Ser	T
	Ile	Thr	Asn	Ser	C
	Ile*	Thr	Lys	Arg*	A
	Met (Initiator)	Thr	Lys	Arg*	G
G	Val	Ala	Asp	Gly	T
	Val	Ala	Asp	Gly	C
	Val	Ala	Glu	Gly	A
	Val	Ala	Glu	Gly	G

* These codons differ in mitochondria and chloroplast genome, TGA codes for Trp, ATA codes for Met, AGA and AGG code for Stop codon

Aminoacid	Number of codons	Aminoacid	Number of codons
Met (M)	1 (ATG)#	Val (V)	4 (GTT, GTC, GTA, GTG)
Trp (W)	1 (TGG)	Gly (G)	4 (GGT, GGC, GGA, GGG)
Phe (F)	2 (TTT, TTC)	Pro (P)	4 (CCT, CCC, CCA, CCG)
Tyr (Y)	2 (TAT, TAC)	Thr (T)	4 (ACT, ACC, ACA, ACG)
Asp (D)	2 (GAT, GAC)	Ala (A)	4 (GCT, GCC, GCA. GCG)
Asn (N)	2 (AAT, AAC)	Arg (R)	6 (CGT, CGC, CGA, CGG, AGA, AGG)
Glu (E)	2 (GAA, GAG)		
Gln (Q)	2 (CAA, CAG)	Ser (S)	6 (TCT, TCC, TCA, TCG, AGT, AGC)
His (H)	2 (CAT, CAC)		
Lys (K)	2 (AAA, AAG)	Leu (L)	6 (TTA, TTG, CTT, CTC, CTA, CTG)
Cys (C)	2 (TGT, TGC)		
Ile (I)	3 (ATT, ATC, ATA)	Stop	3 (TAA-Ochre, TAG-Amber, TGA-Opal)

Also serves as initiator codon.

aa of the nascent protein is always a methionine. The GUG and UUG which normally code for Val and Leu, respectively in the middle of the chain, will code for Met when used as the initiator coden. Further, the use of these codons as initiator codon is only an exception and is also very rare. Eukaryotes donot use UUG as initiation codon and in prokaryotes its use is extremely rare, many times less than GUG.

Machinery for protein synthesis

In order to understand translation, it is essential that we discuss the cellular machinery involved in protein synthesis. The protein synthesis takes place in cytoplasmic compartment of the cell, the genetic information is carried from nucleus to cytoplasm by the mRNA; the site of translation is the ribosome which is a complex ribonucleoprotein molecule and serves as a protein synthesizing factory; the aa are brought to the site of synthesis by the tRNA (4S in size) molecule, which also contains a mechanism to read the codons present in mRNAs. The attachment of the amino acid to the tRNA molecule is mediated by an enzyme, the aminoacyl tRNA synthetase.

Ribosomes

Ribosomes are one of the largest cellular entities. However, these are not a single molecule but are made by the non-covalent, but very specific, association of a number of macromolecules to form a complex structure. Their size is 70S (molecular weight 2.52×10^6D) in prokaryote and 80S (4.22×10^6D) in eukaryotes. These have complex nucleoprotein structure and are made of two subunits, the small subunit and the large subunit. In prokaryotes, the small subunit (30S, 930KD) has one RNA (the 16S RNA, 1541 bases) and 21 proteins (S-1 to S-21), while the large subunit (50S, 1590KD) has two RNAs (the 23S RNA, 2904 bases and the 5S RNA, 120 bases) and 31 proteins (L-1 to L-31). In eukaryotes, the subunits are bigger than the prokaryotic ribosomal subunits. The small subunit (40S, 1400KD) has one RNA (the 18S RNA, 1874 bases) and 33 polypeptides (S-1 to S-33) while the large subunit (60S, 2820KD) has three RNAs (the 28S RNA, 4718 bases; the 5.8S RNA, 160 bases and the 5S RNA, 120 bases) and 49 proteins (L-1 to L-49). The detailed composition of ribosomes is given in Table 7.3. The three dimensional structure of prokaryotic small subunit is elongated and asymetrical having a plateform like structure on one side and a head and a base on other side. There is a depressed cleft between the head and the plateform. The large subunit is more compact having a base, a stalk and a protuberance. During the assembly of ribosomes, the plateform region of the small subunit sits on the base of the large subunit and the mRNA fits in between the two subunits. During translation, the ribosomes move along the mRNA. The size of the ribosome is big enough to bind with two tRNA molecules and about 40 bases of mRNA at the same time. The complete ribosome has three distinct functional sites; the acceptor site (A site, also called as the aminoacyl tRNA site or the entry site), the donor site (P site, also called the polypeptidyl tRNA site) and the exit site (E site or the deaminoacylated tRNA site). The diagramatic representation of ribosomal subunit structure and the size of ribosome in relation to other components of protein synthesizing machinery is shown in Fig. 7.4.

The assembly of ribosomal subunits takes place in a well defined and sequential manner. Both the RNA-protein and protein- protein interactions participate in ribosome formation. The rRNAs have a number of regions of intramolecular complementarity which form double stranded regions. These ds stems provide a complex secondary structure to rRNAs with a number of functional domains. However, due to many regions of complementarity a number of possible structures for all these RNAs are possible. A number of chemical and enzymatic reactions such as the reaction with ketoxal which specifically binds with free G residue and with psoralin which cross-links the double stranded regions, have helped in determining the secondary

Table 7.3. The structure of ribosomes

S.No.	Property	Ribosome	Small Subunit	Large subunit
A. PROKARYOTIC RIBOSOMES				
a. Physical characteristics:				
1.	Size	70S	30S	50S
2.	Mass	2,520 KD	930 KD	1,590 KD
b. RNA moiety:				
3.	Major RNA		16S	23S
			1541 bases	2904 bases
4.	Minor RNA			5S
				120 bases
5.	RNA maas	1,664 KD	560 KD	1,104 KD
6.	RNA proportion	66%	60%	70%
c. Protein moiety:				
7.	Proteins molecule		21 polypeptides	31 polypeptides
8.	Protein mass	857 KD	370 KD	487 KD
9.	Protein proportion	34%	40%	30%
B. EUKARYPTIC RIBOSOMES				
a. Physical characteristics				
10.	Size	80S	40S	60S
11.	Mass	4,220 KD	1,400 KD	2,820 KD
b. RNA moiety:				
12.	Major RNA		18S	28S
			1874 bases	4718 bases
13.	Minor RNA			5.8S, 160 bases
				5S, 120 bases
				respectively
14.	RNA maas	2,520 KD	700 KD	1,820 KD
15.	RNA proportion	60%	50%	65%
c. Protein moiety:				
16.	Proteins molecule		33 polypeptides	49 polypeptides
17.	Protein mass	1,700 KD	700 KD	1,000 KD
18.	Protein proportion	40%	50%	35%

structure of rRNAs. The nuclease protection studies and the protein binding experiments have further added to our knowledge about these structures. It has been found that even a small molecule like the 5S RNA can have a number of possible secondary structures. In the large subunit of eukaryotic ribosomes, an extra RNA (5.8S) is present which does not have a counterpart in prokaryotes. Its primary structure has revealed that it has extended homology with the 5'-end of prokaryotic 23S RNA. It is justified to conclude that 23S RNA of prokaryotes serves the function of both the 28S and 5.8S RNA of eukaryotes. The comparision of RNA structure in subunits and in complete ribosomes and also in free as well as in mRNA-bound ribosomes

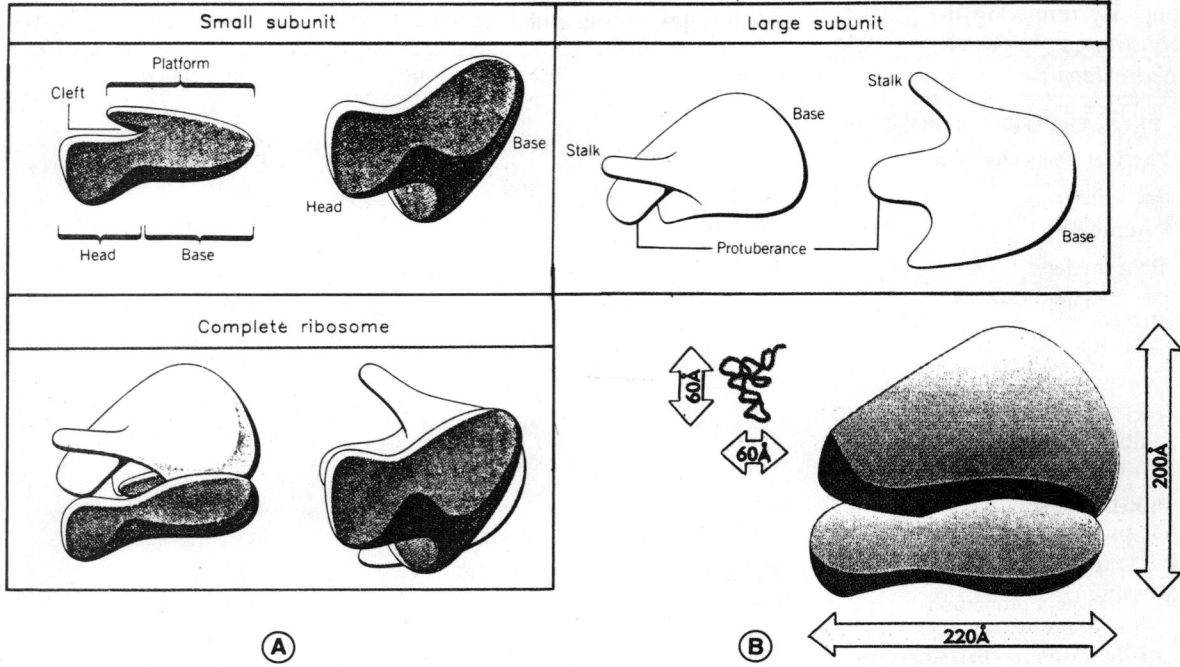

Fig. 7.4. The 30S subunit is elongated and asymmetrical in shape, the 50S subunit is fairly compact from which a "central protuberance" and a "stalk" stick out, and the 70S ribosome may be held together by associations between discrete areas of the two subunits. A. Structure of ribosome. B. Sizes of ribosome shows that it is large enough to bind two tRNAs (as well as 40 bases of mRNA).

has revealed that the secondary structure of RNA is variable. Various associations result in some changes in the secondary structure. The structures of these rRNAs are shown in Fig. 7.5.

There are a number of methylated bases present in the rRNAs. In an average, the 16S RNA has 10 methylated bases and 23S RNA has 20 methylated bases. Eukaryotic rRNAs have much higher number of methylated bases, about 2% of total bases are methylated, almost three times more than in prokaryotes. For example, there are 43 methylated bases in 18S and 74 in 28S RNA. The precise role of methylation is not very clear. However, majority of the methylated bases are present in the regions which are well conserved. The primary structure has also revealed that large portions of bases in rRNAs have remained well conserved during evolution.

Addition of proteins to RNA results in ribosome formation. Some of the proteins bind directly to RNAs at specific binding sites. This results in folding of the structure and exposure of other binding sites where other proteins can associate to these proteins. Different proteins have different affinity of binding and dissociate under different stringent conditions. The dissociation and reconstitution studies have shown that centrifugation of ribosomes in presence of CsCl results in separation of a group of proteins. These proteins, known as the split proteins, are most loosely associated. The dissociation of these proteins results in a core structure which is 23S and 42S respectively for the 30S and the 50S ribosomal subunits. Increasing the concentration of CsCl or LiCl results in the loss of certain other proteins. However, the loss of proteins is in groups and not one at a time. This suggests that there is co–operativity between different groups of proteins and removal of one protein of a particular group results in the removal of all the proteins of that group. By removing the CsCl (by dialysis) and adding MgCl$_2$, it is possible that the ribosomes can be reconstituted. In fact Mg^{++} is necessary for maintaining the structure of ribosomes. The reconstitution experiments have suggested that the formation of 30S subunit takes place in phases. In the first phase which takes place at 4°C, about 15 proteins approach and bind to the 16S RNA and form a nucleoprotein structure referred as the RI particles. In the in vitro experiments, the RI particles have to be warmed before other proteins can bind to it. The warming probably results in the change in configuration of RI particles to form the RI* particles. Rest of the 6 other proteins can now get associated to the RI* particle and the complete 30S subunit is reconstituted. Some temperature sensitive mutant bacteria have been isolated which can not assemble the subunits. Known as sad$^-$ (for subunit assembly defficient) mutants, these have helped in understanding the sequence of subunit assembly. The process for the assembly of ribosomes has been illustrated in Fig. 7.6. The process can be reversed by the treatment with EDTA. It has been found that some of the proteins associate with rRNAs soon after their transcription, even before the RNA molecules are processed. For example, the studies aimed at understanding the formation of 30S subunit have revealed that a precursor form of 16S RNA (p^{16} RNA) gets associated with about 50% of the proteins to form a 21S molecule which results in change of its confirmation. Some of the methyl groups are then added and 10–20% more proteins get associated. This is followed by the processing of the precursor RNA to form mature 16S RNA and the addition of rest of the methyl groups to form a structure similar to the RI particles. Other proteins are later associated to the RI particle and finally the complete 30S subunit is assembled. These experiments suggest that the addition of certain ribosomal proteins may also play a role in the processing of rRNA.

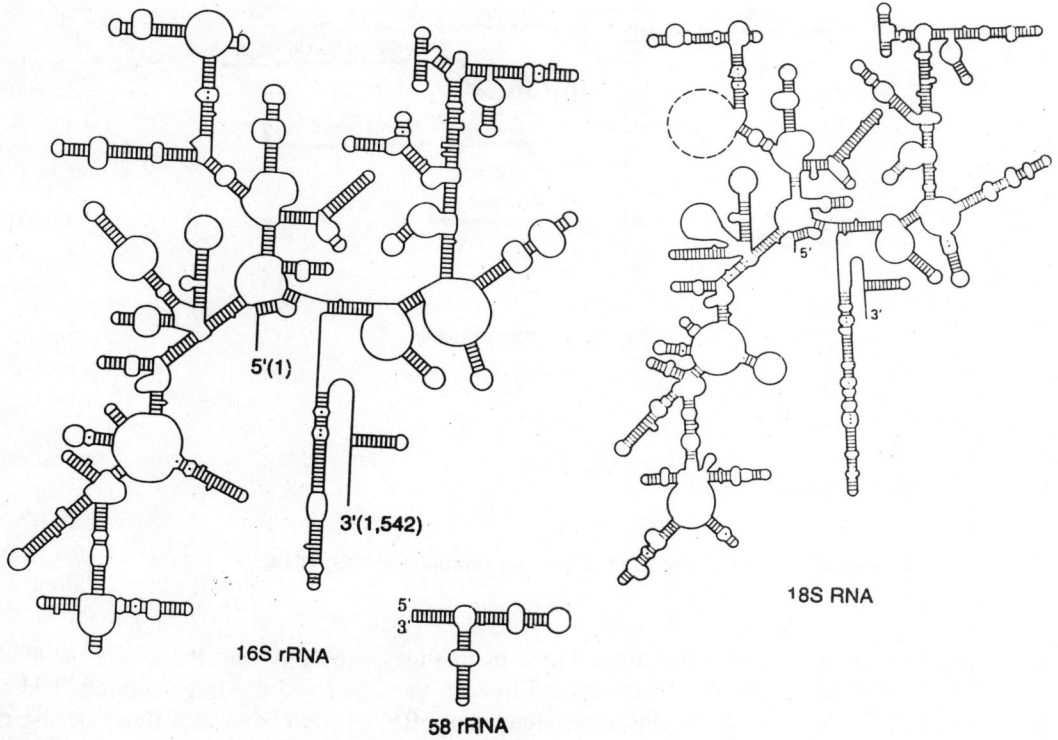

Fig. 7.5. A. Structure of ribosomal RNAs.

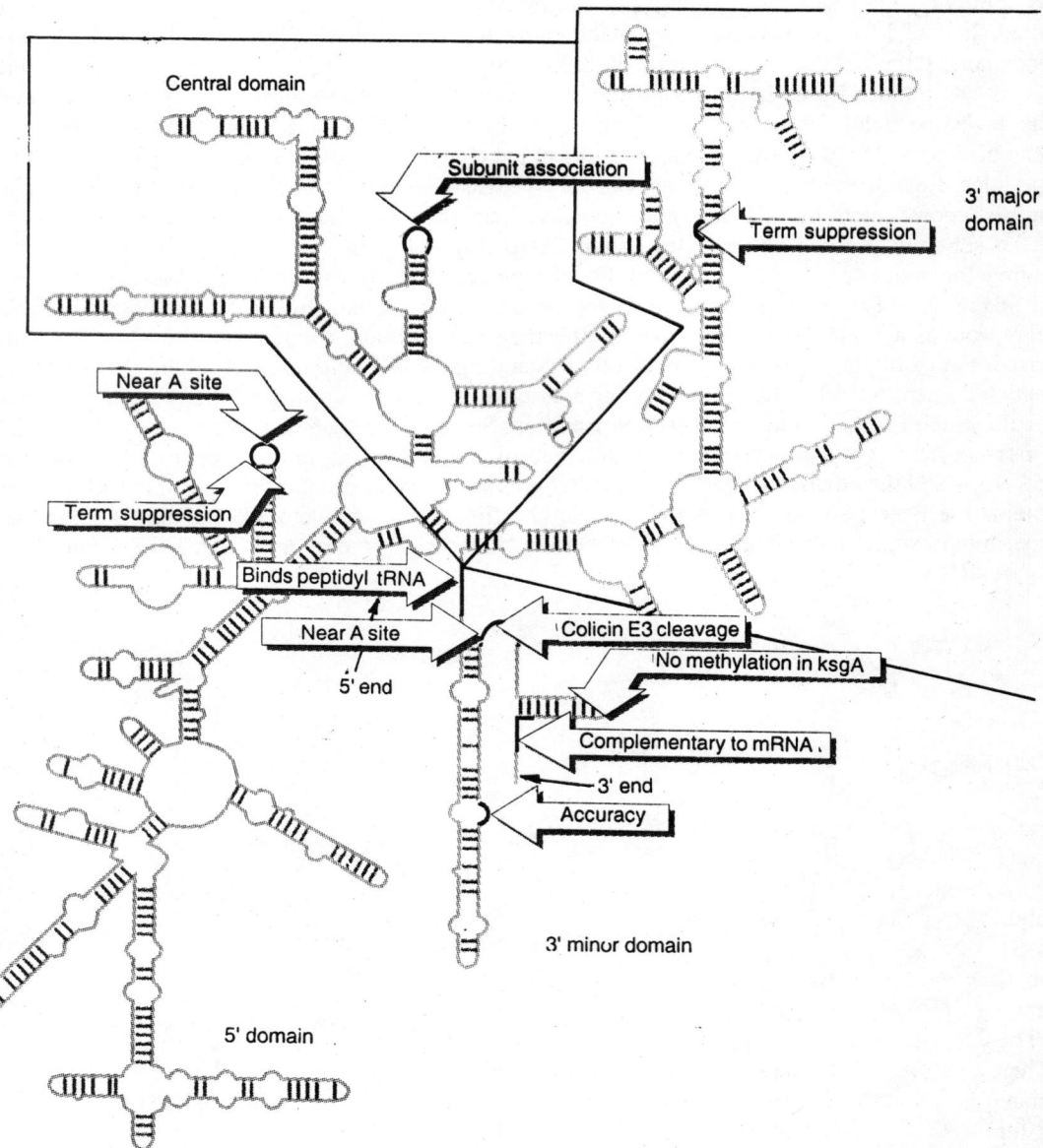

Fig. 7.5. B. The functions of various domains of 16S RNA.

The ribosomes have a number of active sites. Three main sites, namely A site, P site and the E site have already been discussed. The A and P sites extend to both the small and the large subunits and are adjacent to each other. The movement of ribosome along the mRNA (one codon at a time) during the translation (elongation of polypeptide chain) shifts the tRNA occupying the A site to P site and a new tRNA comes to join the A site. However, this shifting of tRNA from one site to another site poses some

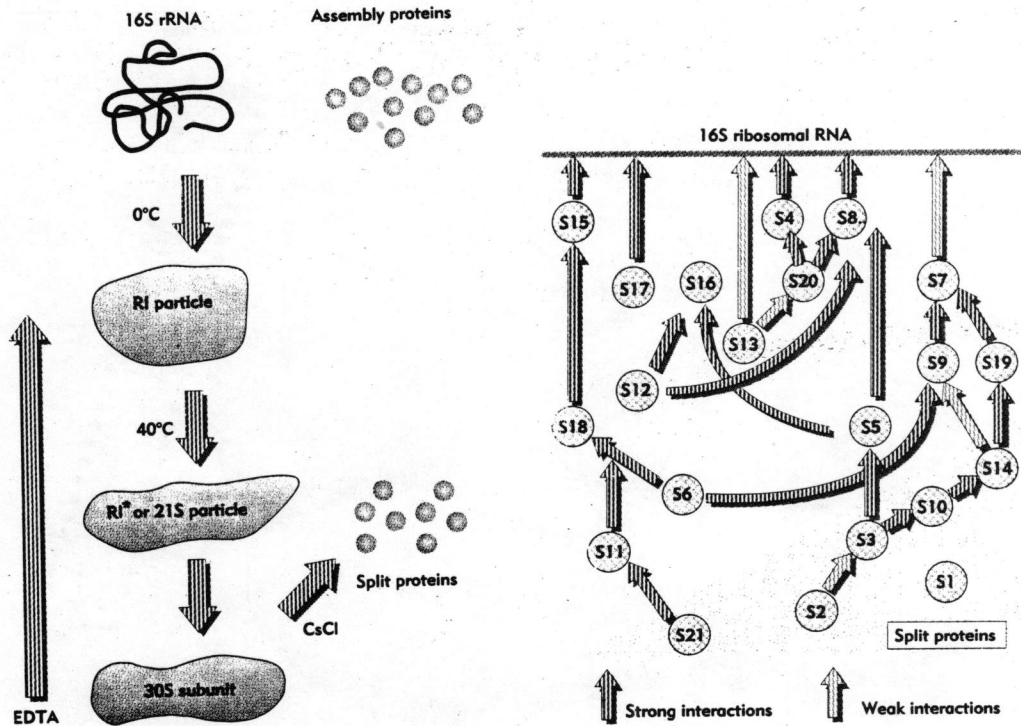

Fig. 7.6. Assembly of ribosomal 30S subunit.

configurational problems. The distance between two codons is not more than 10Å (3 bases, 3.4A each) while the diameter of tRNA is about 20Å. How two tRNAs attach to mRNA at adjacent codons? One of the possible mechnisms may be that they are angled in such a manner that both are easily accomodated. The small subunit has the site for binding of mRNA which lies near the cleft of the small subunit. Ribosomal proteins S1, S18 and S21 participate in the binding of mRNA to small subunit. The site for binding of initiation factors lies in its vicinity. In prokaryotic ribosomes, the 3' end of 16S rRNA which has the complementarity with the SD sequences in mRNA base and pairs with these sequences is located in this region. The ribosomes also have the site for the binding of the elongation factors, EF–G and EF–Tu. (see later). There is also a site for the enzyme peptidyl transferase which transfers the growing peptide which is associated with the peptidyl tRNA at P site to the aminoacid bound to aminoacyl tRNA that is present at the A site, and forms a new peptide bond during the polypeptide elongation. These binding sites together constitute about 2/3rd of the total area of the ribosome and are jointly known as translational domain. The other 1/3rd part of ribosome, which contains the E site is referred as exit domain. The structure of these sites is given in Fig. 7.7. The attachment of membrane bound ribosomes (see later) with the membrane is through the exit domain. The 5S RNA is attached to the large subunit in association with the proteins L5, L8 and L25. In fact these proteins form a complex with the 5S RNA which associates with 23S RNA for the assembly of 50S subunit in prokaryotes. The precise mechanism of the binding of small subunit with the large subunit is not very clear. However, in prokaryotes, a mutation in one of the loops of 16S RNA at position 791 affects the subunit association. Also, there is a region of complementarity between a region in 23S RNA and 3'–end of the 16S RNA.

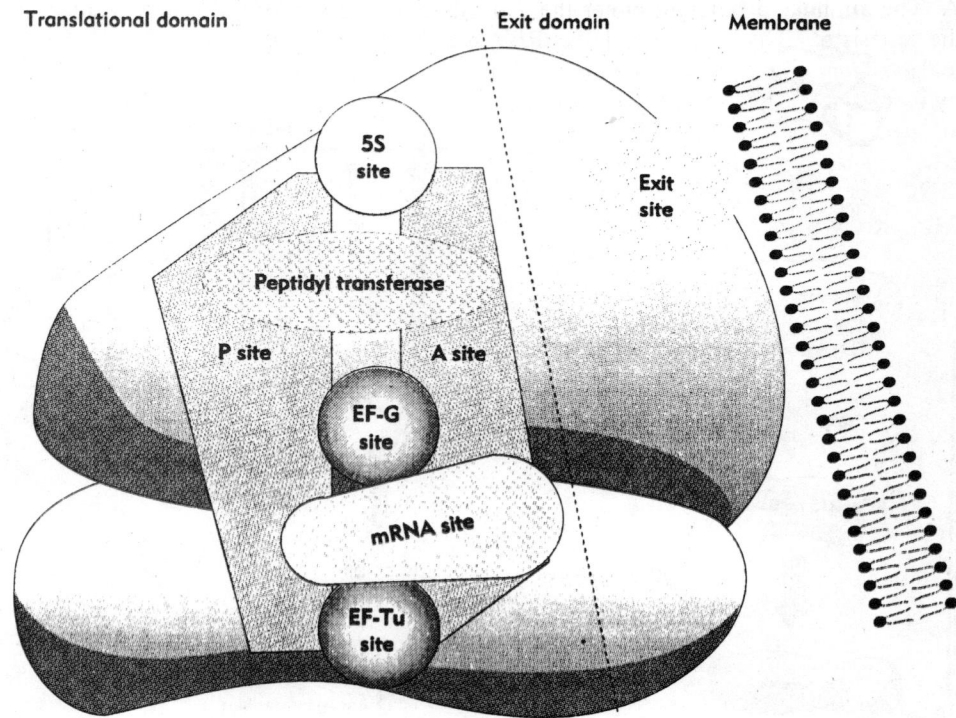

Fig. 7.7. The functional sites of ribosomes.

Besides providing the backbone for ribosomal assembly and various catalytic sites, the ribosomal RNAs play important and active role in protein synthesis. These have several specific interaction with mRNA and tRNAs. In prokaryotes, the 16S RNA binds with mRNA to start the formation of the initiation complex. The 16S RNA also interacts with the anticodon arm of tRNA in both A and P sites and facilitates the codon–anticodon interaction as well as translocation of tRNA from A site to P site. The 23S RNA interacts with the trinucleotide CCA present at the 3' terminus of peptidyl tRNA at the P site. These functions have been assigned to various regions of RNA with the help of different mutants which are defective at a particular step. No direct catalytic or enzymatic function has been assigned to rRNAs. However, it has been found that any change in the configuration of rRNAs affects the function of ribosomes. It is believed that the scenerio is similar in eukaryotes also and the rRNAs play direct role in protein synthesis though only little information about these is available.

Transfer RNA

The tRNA is the acceptor molecule which selects the correct aa from the cytoplasmic pool and brings it to the ribosomes for incorporation into the growing polypeptide chain. It is relatively small in size (4S) with only 74-95 bases. There are a number of regions of intramolecular sequence complementarity which are base paired to form at least four separate double stranded portions and provide a specific three dimensional structure to it. It has a clover leaf like structure with 4 arms (Fig. 7.8). The 5' and 3' ends form a ds region, known as the acceptor arm. The aa attaches here and is transported to the ribosome. The acceptor arm has a ds stem of seven base pairs and 3-4 protuding bases at the 3'-end. The last three bases are always 3' OH-

ACC-tRNA. The aminoacid binds to either the 2'or the 3'-OH group of the last A residue at its 3'-end. Based on the genesis of CCA at the 3'-end, the tRNA are referred as type I and type 2. As discussed earlier many of the tRNA genes are clustered and the primary transcripts have the sequences for a number of tRNAs separated by the spacer regions. These spacers are removed during processing to provide individual tRNAs. The CCA of type I tRNA is coded by gene itself and is present in the primary transcript (or the precursor form of the tRNA) and after processing the mature tRNA contains these three bases at its 3'-end. However, in type II tRNAs the genes donot code for the CCA and the primary transcript does not contain these bases. As a result the tRNA formed by processing reaction is without these three bases. These bases (CCA) are later added to the 3'-end of these tRNAs as a post-transcriptional modification by a template independant enzyme, the tRNA nucleotidyl transferase (Fig. 7.9). However, all the mature tRNAs have CCA at the 3'-end. E. coli tRNAs are of both type I and type II while majority of the eukaryotic tRNAs are of type II. Some phages code for type II tRNAs. When the ss region of the acceptor arm is 4 bases long, CCA is usually preceded by a purine; more often by an A than by a G.

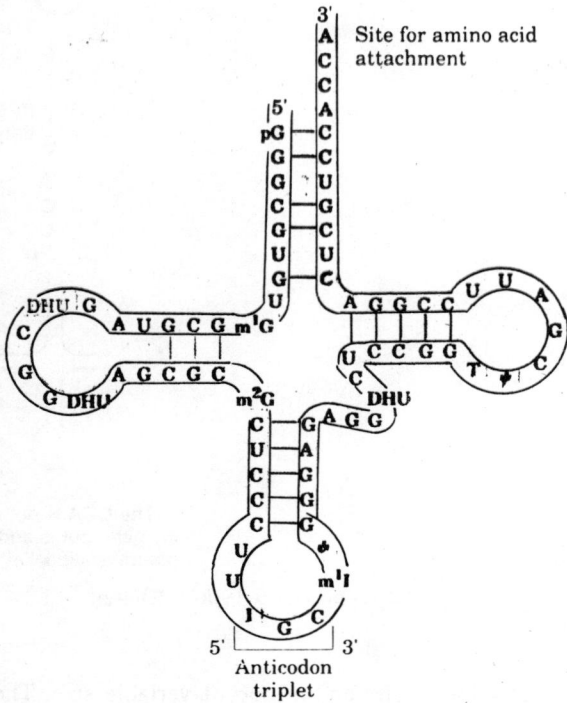

Fig. 7.8. Clover leaf structure of tRNA.

All the other arms of the tRNA are made of a paired stem and the unpaired loop. The arm opposite to aa stem is the anticodon arm. The stem usually has 5 base pairs and the loop is usually 7 bases long. The three bases at the centre of the loop have complementarity to one of the codons present in mRNA. These bases are known as the anticodon. The anticodon region base pairs with the codon and transfers the right aminoacid for polymerization. A tRNA is thus specific for a particular codon. The arms towards the 5' of anticodon arm is D arm (so called because of the presence of a modified base the dihydrouridine or

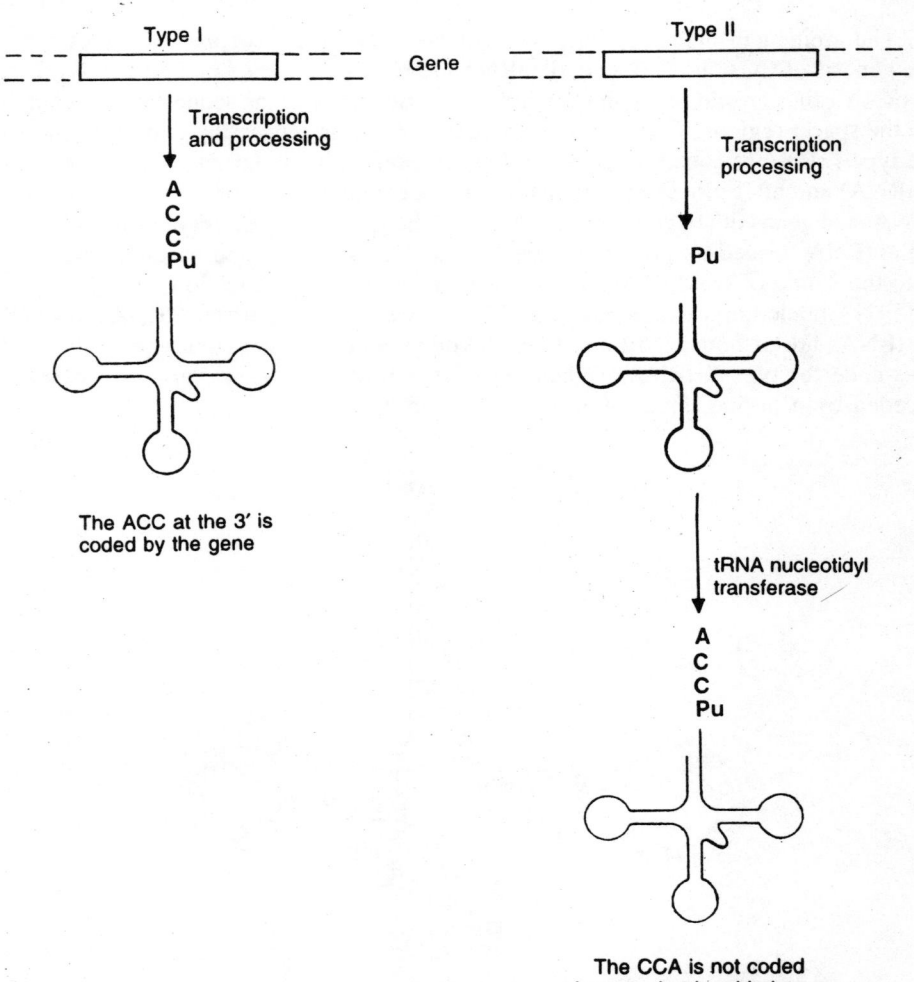

Fig. 7.9. Type I and Type-II tRNAs.

D) which usually has a stem of 4 base pairs and a loop of variable size. The arm opposite to D arm is TΨC arm or Ψ arm (Ψ is pseudo uridine). Besides these four primary arms, an extra arm may also be present in some tRNAs. The extra arm is between the anticodon arm and the TΨC arm (see the Fig. 7.10). The length of the extra arm varies in different tRNAs. The size variability of different tRNAs is primarily due to variation in the length of extra arm. Based on the length of extra arm the tRNAs are classified as class 1 and class 2 tRNAs. Relatively smaller tRNAs containing only 3–5 bases in extra arms are known as class 1 tRNAs. About 75% of all the tRNAs fall in this category. The tRNAs which have an extra arm of larger size, usually 13–21 bases, are referred as the class 2 tRNAs. The functional importance of extra arm is not known. However, the tertiary structure of tRNAs is very important and the length of extra arm plays very important role in maintaining the correct three dimensional structure (see later).

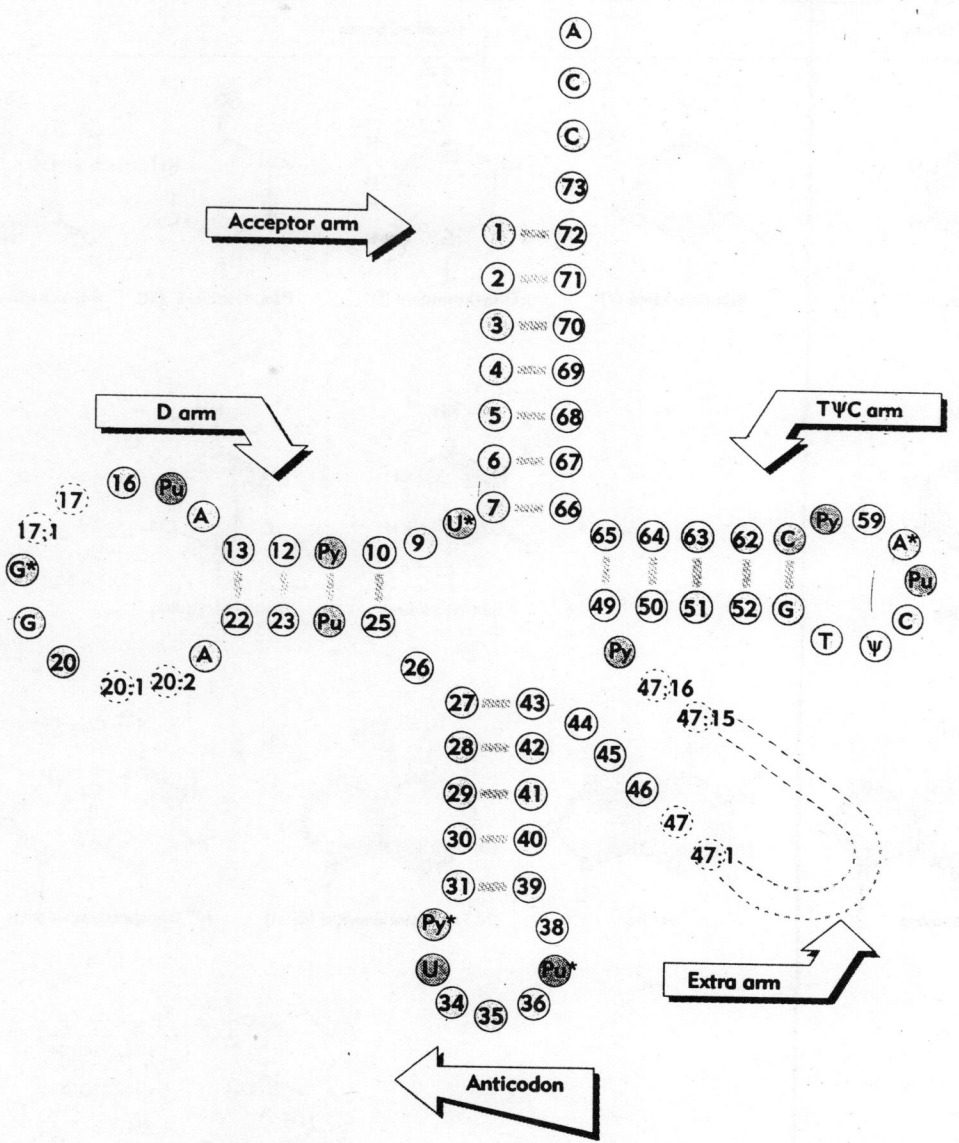

Fig. 7.10. tRNA has a variable extra arm.

The tRNAs are unique RNA molecules in the fact that these contain a number of modified and unusual bases. Some of the modified bases normally present in tRNAs are shown in Fig. 7.11. The tRNAs also have some unconventional base pairing like G:U and A:G. The modifications in the bases help in formation of unusual hydrogen bonds. Even three base bonds are also present in tRNA which provide the specific tertiary structure. Some of the unconventional bonds are shown in Fig. 7.12.

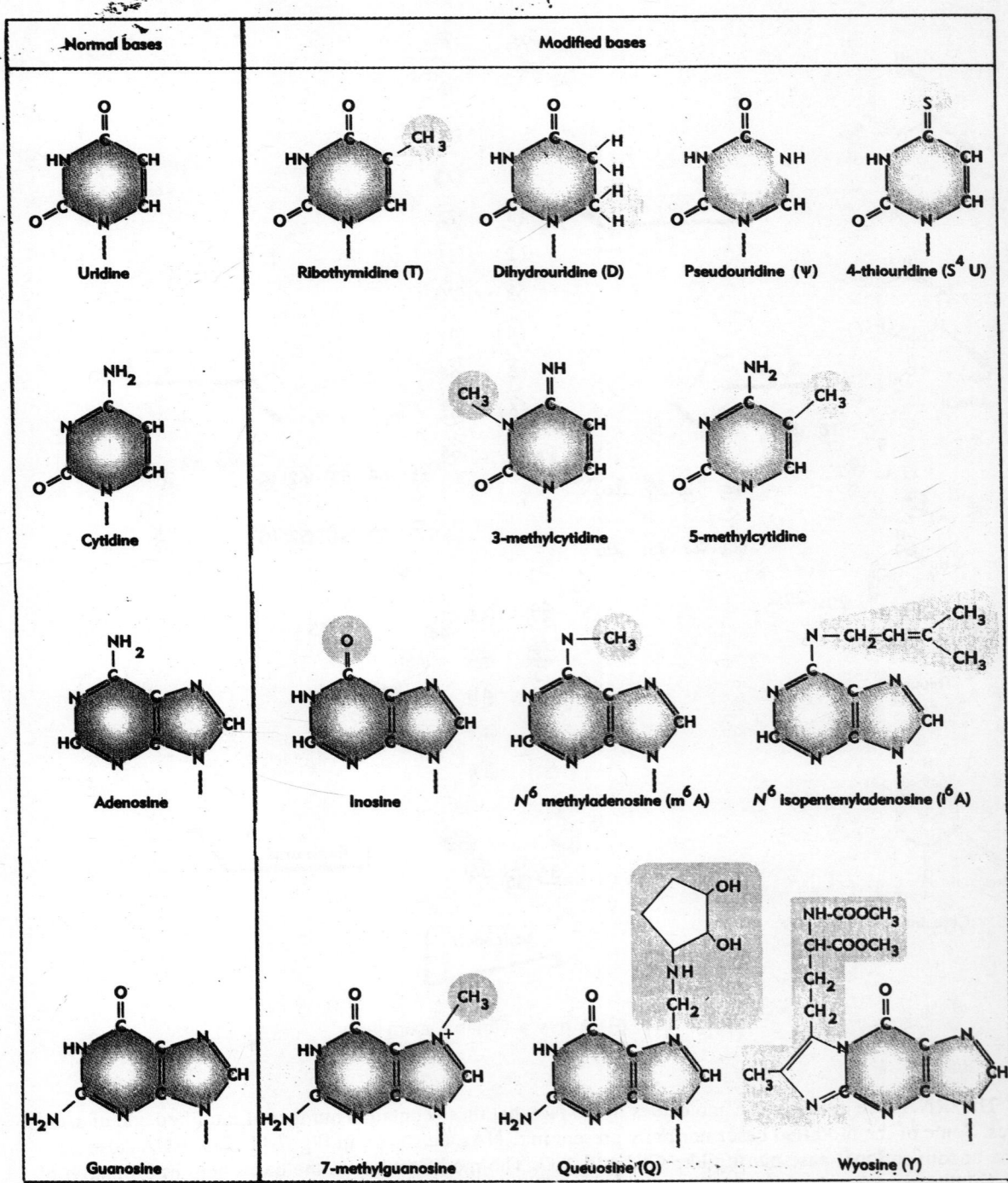

Fig. 7.11. Some of the modified bases found in tRNA.

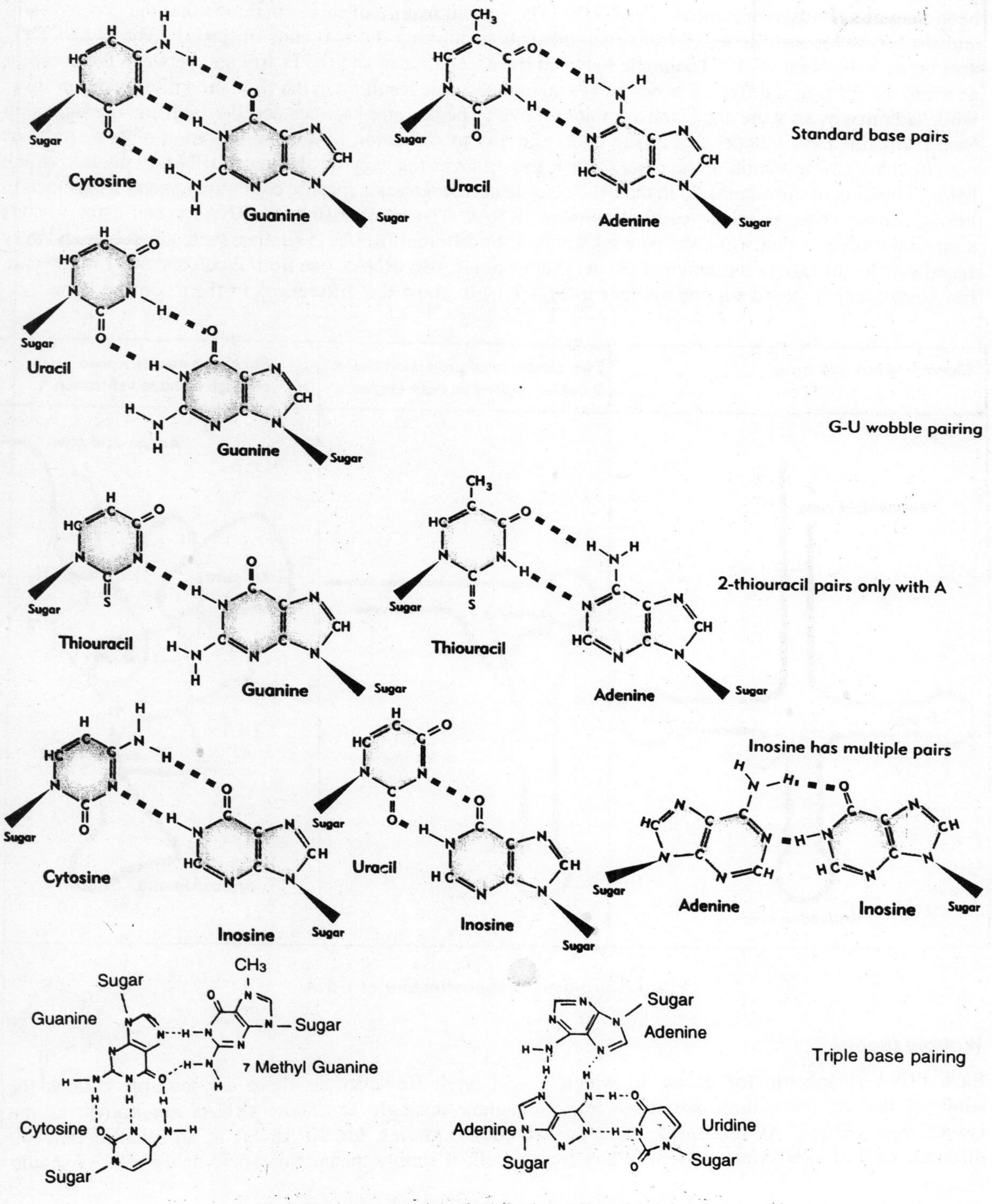

Fig. 7.12. Unusual base pairing in tRNA.

While the secondary structure of tRNA is clover leaf like, the tertiary structure is 'L'–shaped. This has been diagramatically represented in Fig. 7.13. The special feature of this structure is that the acceptor arm and the anticodon arm lie away from each other, both forming the two ends of the 'L'. The D and TΨC arm lie near the bend of 'L'. The angle between the acceptor arm and the D arm and between the acceptor arm and the TΨC arm differs. Former makes an obtuce angle resulting in the formation of a 'major groove' while later makes an acute angle and a 'minor groove'. The distance between acceptor arm and the anticodon loop maintains their independence (see later) and any modification in the configuration of one arm does not affect the configuration of the other. This is important as the enzyme aminoacyl tRNA synthetase which helps in binding of the aminoacid to the tRNA (see later) recognises a specific configuration and its interaction brings certain changes in the configuration of tRNAs. The comparision of tRNAs specific for various aminoacids reveals that while the general structure of different tRNAs is similar, there are subtle and very specific differences between different tRNAs. For example, two tRNAs, one from E.coli and other from yeast, has been super-imposed on one another in Fig. 7.14 to show the differences in their configuration.

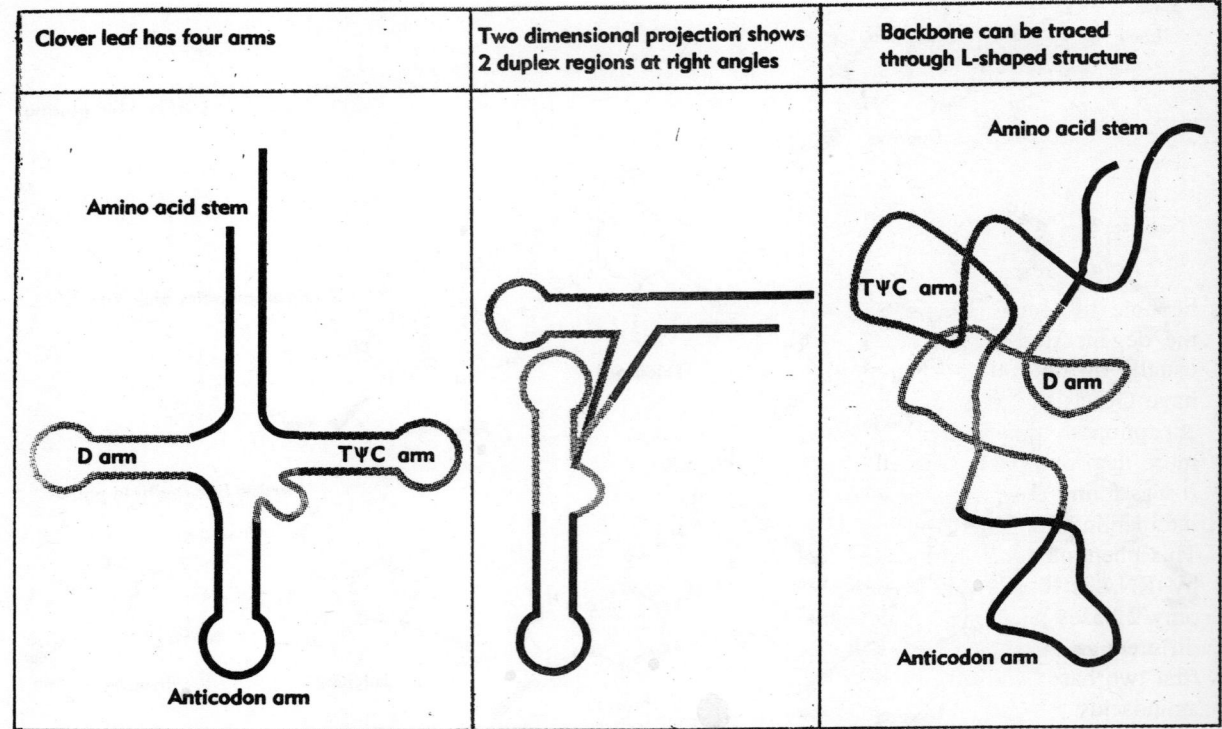

Clover leaf has four arms	Two dimensional projection shows 2 duplex regions at right angles	Backbone can be traced through L-shaped structure

Fig. 7.13. 3-dimensional structure of tRNA.

Wobble theory

Each tRNA is specific for an aa, to which it will bind. However, as there are multiple codons for some of the aa, more than one tRNA may recognize a single aa. These tRNAs are known as the iso-acceptor tRNAs. As discussed, there are 61 codons coding for 20 aa but at an average only 40 different kind of tRNAs are present in any typical cell. It simply means that some of the tRNAs should

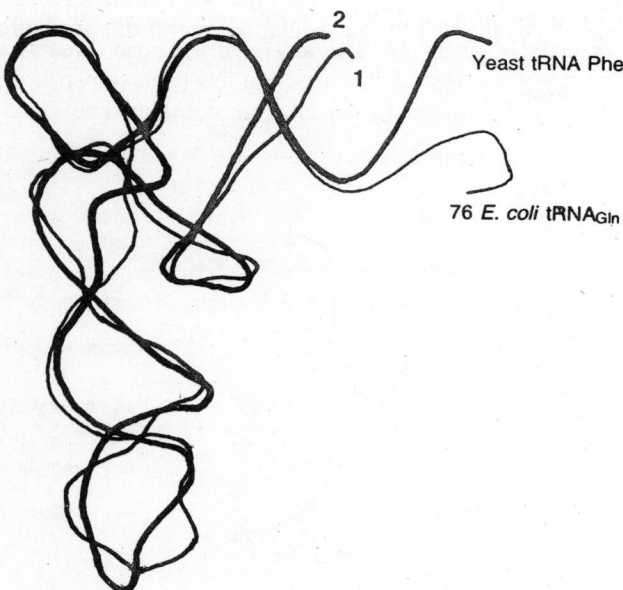

Fig. 7.14. Different tRNAs differ in their 3-D structure.

be able to recognize more than one codons. A careful glance at the genetic code will reveal that the degeneration of genetic code, in majority of the cases, is at the third base. The first two bases usually do not vary in the multiple codons of an aminoacid. For example all the four codons for Val have GU as the first two bases while third base may be any one of the four bases. However, there are exception to this general rule, for example Leu and Arg, both have 6 codons each which differ in more than one bases. Also the same bases in first two position donot always represent same aminoacid. It was found that in many cases, only first two bases of the codon participate in strong codon-anticodon interaction. The interaction with third base can be loose or even unconventional like the G:U pairing. This phenomenon is known as 'wobble effect'. The efficiency of recognizing only 2 bases of the codon by tRNA is 10-100 fold less than the recgnition of all the three bases. Further, this process of recognizing only 2 bases takes place only between multiple codons for the same aa and not between the codons for different aa. A single tRNA will never recognize the codon for two different aa even if they have the same first two bases and differ only in the third base. The wobbling is, thus, between the codons of the same aminoacids.

Charging of tRNA molecule

The binding of aa to tRNA is called 'charging' and a charged tRNA is known as the aminoacyl tRNA. To differentiate between different tRNAs, the name of the specific aa is written as a subscript at the right hand side which specifies that the tRNA is specific for that particular aminoacid. After tRNA is charged with the aa, the name of the aa is written before tRNA in superscript. For example 'tRNA$_{Met}$' is the tRNA specific for methionine and ^{Met}tRNA$_{Met}$ or simply ^{Met}tRNA (sometimes also written as Met-tRNA) means that a tRNA which is specific for methionine has a methionine molecule bound to it (also known as methionyl tRNA$_{Met}$). The charging of tRNA is energy dependent and the first step is the activation of aa by interaction with ATP. AMP gets associated with aa to form aminoacyl AMP and inorganic pyrophosphate is given out. The activated aminoacid reacts with its specific tRNA to form aminoacyl tRNA. The AMP is released. The reaction has been shown in Fig. 7.15. This charging of tRNA is an enzymatic reaction facilitated by an enzyme complex known as the aminoacyl tRNA synthetase.

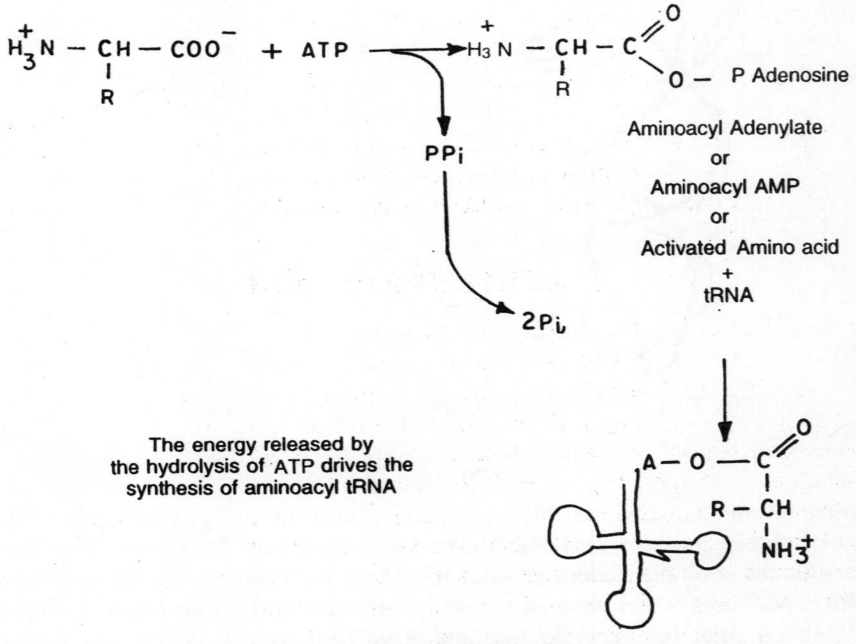

Fig. 7.15. The 'Charging' of an tRNA.

Aminoacyl tRNA synthetase

This is a complex enzyme system which vary in its size. The molecular weight of an aminoacyl tRNA synthetase varies between 40KD and 100KD. However, all the molecules have the common function, namely the charging of tRNA with the specific aa. There are 20 different aminoacyl tRNA synthetases in the cell. Each enzyme is specific for an aa and a single enzyme recognizes all the iso-acceptor tRNAs for this particular aa. However, an enzyme does not recognize the tRNAs for different aminoacids. All the tRNAs which are recognized by an aminoacyl tRNA synthetase are known as 'cognate tRNAs' for that enzyme.

Based on the size and structure of various aminoacyl tRNA synthetases, these have been classified in two groups, the class 1 and class 2 aminoacyl tRNA synthetases. Each group contains 10 enzymes. The class 1 aminoacyl tRNA synthetase contains a large catalytic domain, which includes the sites for binding of aminoacid and the ATP. This constitutes the N–terminal end of the enzyme and contains two short stretches of aminoacids which are highly conserved. These sequences are known as the 'signature sequences'. This region forms the part of ATP binding site. The domain is interrupted by a region which has the domain for the recognition and binding of the acceptor arm of tRNA molecule. The entire region (the catalytic domain along with the recognition site for acceptor arm of the tRNA) is folded in a common structure present in all the enzymes of this class and is referred as the 'nucleotide–binding fold'. This consists of alternating β–strands and the α–helices present in a parallel fashion. This is followed by a domain for the association of anticodon region of the tRNA. The C–terminal end of class 1 aminoacyl tRNA synthetase is consist of a domain which facilitates the oligomer formation. The class 1 aminoacyl tRNA synthetase are generally oligomer of this basic structure.

The class 2 aminoacyl tRNA synthetases have similar domains and show a number of similarities with the class 1 enzyme in their basic stucture. However, they differ in having the tRNA anticodon binding site as their N-terminal domain. The nucleotide fold has antiparallel β-sheet sorrounded by α-helices. The binding domain for acceptor arm of tRNA differs between individual enzymes of this class. The oligomerization domain, if at all present, varies widely between different molecules of class 2 enzymes, both in size and in location. Many enzymes of this class are monomers (Fig. 7.16).

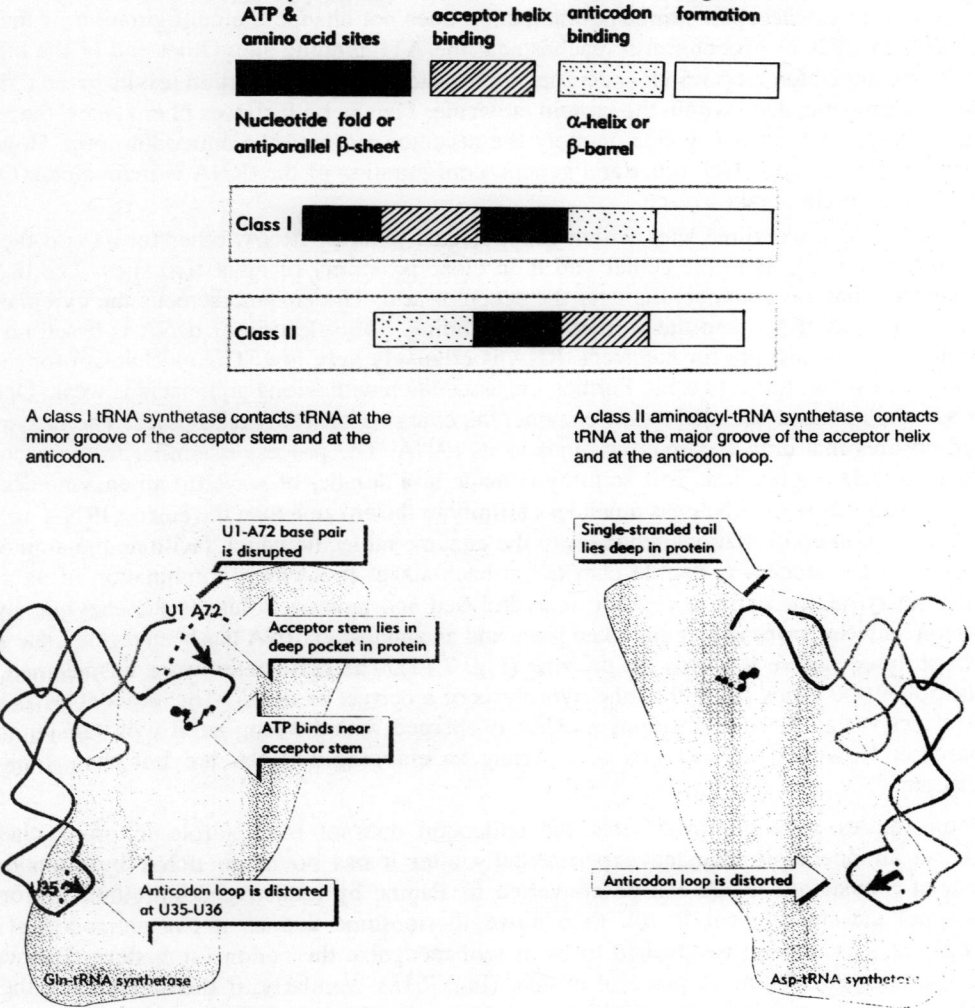

Fig. 7.16. Structure of aminoacyl tRNA synthetase.

Both class of enzymes bind the tRNA along the side of the 'L' shaped structure. Only the acceptor arm, the anticodon arm and the D–loop is in close association with the enzyme. However, the three dimensional structure of the aminoacyl tRNA synthetases of class 1 and class 2 varies considerably. Thus the enzymes of both the classes approach the tRNA in different manner. The class 1 enzymes approach the tRNA from the D–loop side. It associates with the acceptor arm from its minor groove at one end of the binding site while the anticodon arm makes contact with other end of the tRNA binding site. This interaction changes the configuration of tRNA and certain distortion in the structure of anticodon loop takes place. The anticodon is pulled in and gets embeded inside the enzyme. Similarly, considerable distortion of acceptor arm also takes place. The base pairing between the first nucleotide and its complementary nucleotide in the acceptor stem is broken and the single stranded end increases in length. This elongated end is present in the embeded state, deep inside the enzyme and reaches near to the ATP binding site.

The class 2 enzyme on the other hand, contacts the tRNA from the variable loop side. It recognizes the major groove of the acceptor arm. The interaction does not change the configuration of the acceptor arm. The terminal CCA of acceptor arm reaches near the ATP binding site. Other end of the binding site interacts with the anticodon loop which undergoes some distortion. This distortion results in the tight binding of the loop with enzyme, deep within the protein molecule. Thus in both classes of enzymes, the interaction of enzyme with tRNA is at two points, namely the acceptor arm and the anticodon loop. However, the two regions remain far from each other and general configuration of the tRNA is maintained. Only some distortion in these regions takes place.

The enzyme, thus, has three sites within the molecule, one for tRNA, other for aa and the third for ATP. The aa binding site is at the center and is in close proximity of other two sites. The tRNA binds in such a manner that the aminoacid is near the acceptor arm. The enzyme screens the cytoplasmic pool and selects the correct tRNA and the correct aa for binding. The selection of tRNA is based on its shape and configuration. The affinity for incorrect tRNA is relatively very low. The mechanism for recognition of correct aa is, however, not very clear. Further, the association with wrong aminoacid is weak. Once correct pair of tRNA and aa has associated to the enzyme, the charging of tRNA takesplace. The enzyme double checks and ensures that only a correct aa binds to its tRNA. The process is similar to the proof reading function during DNA replication. This scrutiny is made in a number of ways (a) an enzyme accepts only a correct aa, (b) an incorrect tRNA has much less affinity to the enzyme than the correct tRNA, (c) a correct tRNA triggers certain confirmational changes to the enzyme molecule which facilitate the aminoacylation of tRNA and (d) the process is double checked at each stage. If a wrong combination of aa and tRNA has bound to enzyme, the aminoacyl AMP is hydrolysed and aminoacid leaves the enzyme. Even if the eststerification between a wrong pair has taken place and an aminoacyl tRNA has been formed, the aminoacyl tRNA is hydrolysed before it leaves the enzyme (Fig. 7.17). The dissociation of a mismatched aa:tRNA takes place 500–1000 times faster than the hydrolysis of a correct aa:tRNA. The anticodon has no role at this stage. If despite all these precautions a tRNA is charged with a wrong aa, it will transfer this wrong aa to ribosome. However, the chances of a wrong aa charging a tRNA are less than 1 mistake/10^5 aminoacylations.

Mutation studies have confirmed that the anticodon doesnot have a role in proof reading. For example if an aminoacid is changed experimentally after it has bound to tRNA by chemical means (the cystein of a cysteinyl tRNA can be converted to alanine by reductive desulfation), the aminoacyl tRNA does not get hydrolysed. It will then move to ribosome and as it has anticodon for cystein (even though now an alanine is attached to it), it will recognize the codon for cystein. This will result in the incorporation of alanine in place of cystein (Fig. 7.18). Similarly, if the anticodon of a tRNA is changed through mutagenesis it will still bind to the aminoacid it originally represented. As charging of

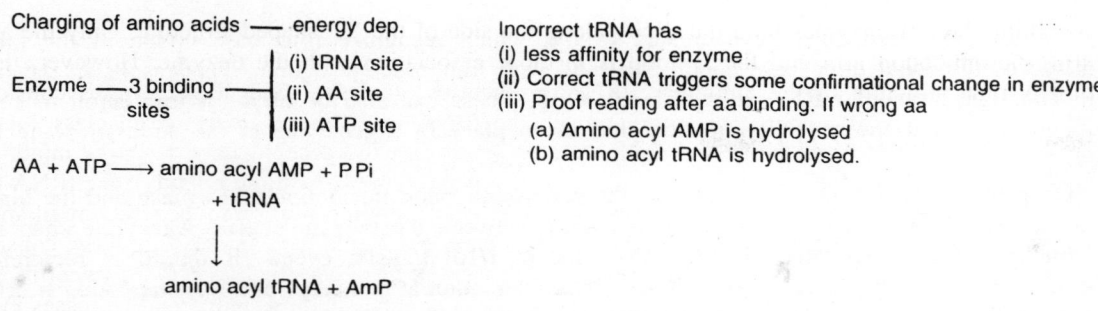

Charging of amino acids —— energy dep.

Enzyme ——3 binding sites
| (i) tRNA site
| (ii) AA site
| (iii) ATP site

Incorrect tRNA has
(i) less affinity for enzyme
(ii) Correct tRNA triggers some confirmational change in enzyme
(iii) Proof reading after aa binding. If wrong aa
    (a) Amino acyl AMP is hydrolysed
    (b) amino acyl tRNA is hydrolysed.

AA + ATP $\longrightarrow$ amino acyl AMP + PPi
+ tRNA

$\downarrow$

amino acyl tRNA + AmP

Fig. 7.17. 'Proof reading' during charging of tRNA molecule.

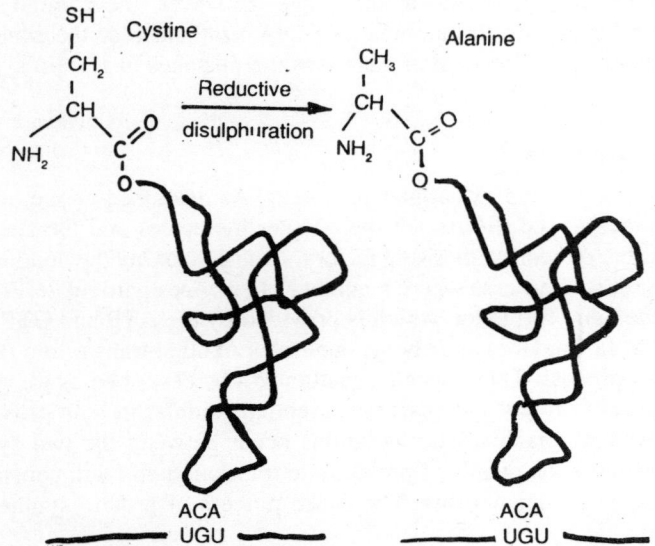

A tRNA with a wrong amino acid will incorporate the wrong amino acid as at ribosomes no scrutiny of amino acid is done.

Fig. 7.18. A tRNA with a wrong aminoacid will result in a mistake during protein synthesis.

tRNA is independent of the anticodon, but is a function of other regions, the mutation in anticodon will not change the specificity of tRNA. This property of tRNA specificity is used for the creation of 'supressor tRNAs', which can overcome the mutation in a gene. If a mis-sense mutation is created in the gene and a complementary mutation is made in the anticodon tRNA region of the specific tRNA for the original aminoacid (the codon for which has been mutated in the gene), the mutated tRNA will still be charged with the correct aminoacid and deliver it to ribozome for incorporation. Such tRNAs are referred as mis-sense supressor tRNAs. However, as the tRNA which has the anticodon complimentary to the mutated codon will also recognize this codon and deliver the 'wrong' aminoacid at this codon. The correction will thus be in only half of the molecules. In a similar manner tRNAs which can recognize a stop codon can be created. These will result in the 'read-through' of a stop codon. This will result in the incorporation of an aa for stop codon and will lead to the synthesis of an unusually long polypeptide. This type of tRNAs are known as non-sense supressor tRNAs. These tRNAs can also be used to overcome a non-sense mutation in the gene.

Certain other mutations have created tRNAs which recognize four base codon in the mRNA in place of the usual three base codon and bind with four bases at a time. This results in the frame shift and translation of mRNA in a different ORF. These can also be used for translation in correct reading· frame if a 'frame shift mutation' has taken place in a gene due to ·the addition of an extra base.

Once the tRNA reaches the ribosome, the codon-anticodon interaction takes place and the binding of a correct tRNA is ensured by the base pairing between the two molecules. Again the chances of the binding of a wrong tRNA are less than one in $1/10^5$ transfer events. It should be remembered that there is no scrutiny of aa at the mRNA:tRNA interaction at this stage but only the codon:anticodon interaction (i.e: recognition of correct tRNA irrespective of which aminoacid it carries) is checked. If at RNA has been charged with an incorrect aa by escaping the scrutiny at the aminoacyl tRNA synthetase level, it can not be hydrolysed at this stage. However, the combination of two checkings, namely, the scrutiny carried out by the aminoacyl tRNA synthetase at the time of charging of tRNA and the fidility of codon:anticodon interaction maintains the mistakes in protein synthesis to an acceptable level.

The events in protein synthesis

Translation is one of the most complex cellular processes. As discussed above, the mRNA serves as the template for protein synthesis. The tRNAs are the adopter molecules and the site of protein synthesis is ribosome which serves as the protein synthesising factory. Amino acids are the building blocks of the proteins. The entire process is a multistep process where a number of enzymes participate. A large amount of energy is required for the peptide bond formation which is provided by the ATP and GTP molecules. Besides the mRNA, ribosomes, tRNA, aa, enzymes and energy, a number of other trans acting factors are also necessary for the completion of this process. These specific factors will be described as we discuss the details of the process. The basic features of protein synthesis are essentially similar in both prokaryotes and eukaryotes. However, certain striking and characteristic variations occur between the two systems. For the sake of simplicity, first we will discuss the details of prokaryotic translation and will consider the specific features of eukaryotic translation to supplement this. The entire process of protein synthesis can be divided into following four basic steps.

(a) Activation of aa and formation of aminoacyl tRNA
(b) Initiation of protein synthesis
(c) Elongation of polypeptide chain and
(d) Termination of translation and release of the nascent polypeptide chain.

Activation of aminoacids and aminoacyl tRNA formation

Some details of this step have already been discussed briefly earlier. This is an enzymatic process catalysed by aminoacyl tRNA synthetase. There are separate enzyme molecules for each of the 20 aminoacids. The aminoacyl tRNA synthetase binds with its cognate tRNA molecule, the right aa and an ATP molecule at different sites. A cognate tRNA has very high affinity for its enzyme, binds very rapidly and dissociates slowly. A non-cognate tRNA on the other hand, binds slowly and dissociates very rapidly. The association of cognate tRNA triggers certain configurational changes in the confirmation of the enzyme which are necessary for the catalytic activity of the enzyme. Without these confirmational changes, the enzyme will either not carry out the assigned task or the rate of aminoacylation will be very slow. It is pertinent to mention that if a wrong tRNA gets associated with the enzyme, either no confirmational change in enzyme will take place or it will not be the correct change. As the first step during the charging of tRNA, the ATP reacts with aa to form aminoacyl

AMP (activated aa) and inorganic pyrophosphate is released. If the aminoacid is not the correct aminoacid, the hydrolysis of aminoacyl AMP takes place and the aa is dissociated. If correct aminoacid has been activated then the next step follows. The activated aminoacid is esterified either at the 2' or at the 3' position of the A residue present at the 3'-end of the tRNA, AMP is released and aminoacyl tRNA is formed. The enzyme once again scrutinizes for the correct pairing. If pairing is wrong and a wrong aa (which some how escaped the earlier scrutiny) is esterified with tRNA, the aminoacyl tRNA dissociates and aminoacid is released. If the combination is correct only then the aminoacyl tRNA leaves the enzyme and is transported to ribosome. In this manner, the fidility is maintained to ensure that only correct aminoacyl tRNA is released from the enzyme complex. Should a wrong pairing between tRNA and aa take place and incorrect aminoacyl tRNA is released from the enzyme, the wrong aminoacid will be incorporated as there will not be any further scrutiny for this step. The energy for charging is provided by the ATP molecule and one ATP is used for the charging of each tRNA. The reaction has been diagramatically represented in Fig. 7.19.

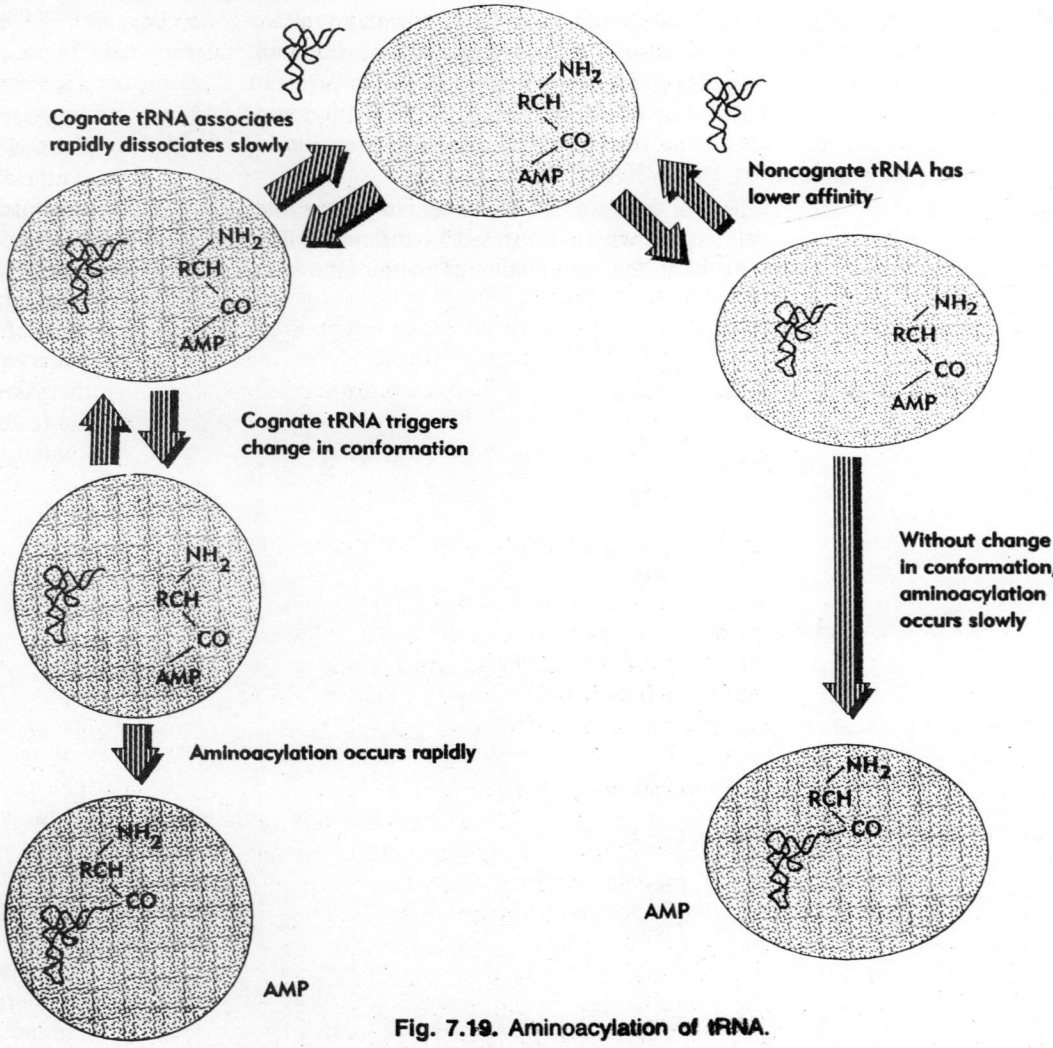

Fig. 7.19. Aminoacylation of tRNA.

Initiation

All the steps and reactions which precede the formation of first peptide bond are referred as the initiation of translation. This is, probably, the most complex process in protein synthesis and requires a number of trans acting protein factors, referred as the initiation factors (IF). Atleast three factors, IF1, IF2 and IF3, participate in initiation of translation in prokaryotes. First of all the 30S subunit of ribosome binds to the mRNA at the RBS sequences by virtue of the complementarity between 16S RNA and SD sequences of the mRNA. In case of some of the mRNAs which are very efficiently expressed, this binding may be further facilitated by the specific interaction of some of the ribosomal proteins with mRNA. This binding positions the small subunit in such a mannner that the initiation codon of mRNA is at the 30S subunit part of the P site. It has already been discussed that the first AUG after the RBS acts as the initiator codon. An initiation factor, called IF3 is essential for this binding. The IF3 plays two distinct roles. First it acts as an anti-association factor and prevents the binding of the free 30S subunit with the free 50S subunit. The 30S subunit without IF3 can bind to 50S subunit to form the 70S ribosome. Thus the 70S ribosome formation can take place either with mRNA (as part of translation process, see later) or without mRNA (free ribosome). However, the free ribosome can not initiate the translation, it will have to dissociate into individual subunits. In presence of IF3, the 30S cannot associate with 50S and thus the individual subunits remain available for translational initiation. Secondly, it facilitates the binding of 30S to mRNA. However, it doesnot play any role in selecting the site of binding of 30S to mRNA. The selection of proper site is exclusively due to complementarity between the SD sequences and the 16S rRNA.

The initiator codon, AUG, codes for methionine. However, in prokaryotes the initiator aa is always formylated (i.e. it is N–formyl methionine) which is formed by the reaction of the methionyl tRNA with 10–formyl tetrahydrofolate. This results in the formylation of methionine at the amino group and release

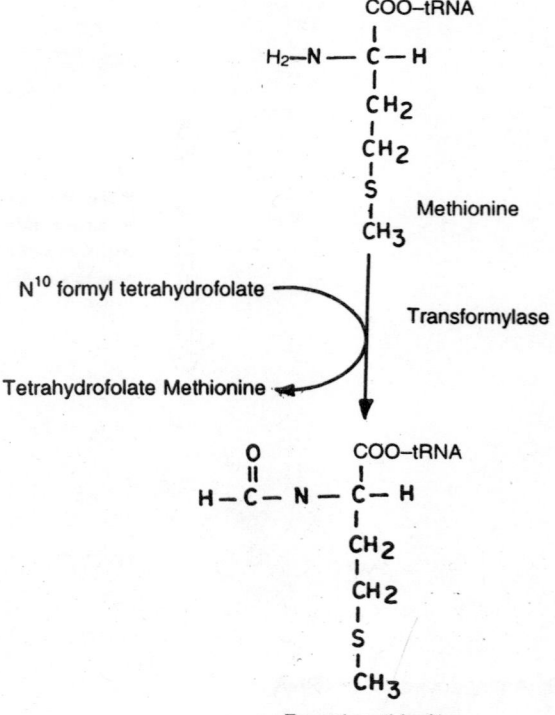

Fig. 7.20. Formation of fMet-tRNA.

of tetrahydrofolate. (Fig. 7.20). A specific initiator tRNA (tRNA$_i$) is required for this purpose. A tRNA which incorporates methionine in the middle of the chain (the methionyl tRNA) cannot serve as initiator tRNA, even though both have the same anticodon. The initiator tRNA is specific for initiation only and can not transfer a methionine residue in the middle of the chain. The tRNA$_i$ has a few characterisitc structural properties which make it unique. Firstly, the first base at its 5'-end is not paired with a base in the 3' region and is not the part of the stem of the acceptor arm. In all the other tRNAs it remained base paired and no single stranded nucleotide is present at the 5'-end of tRNA. A mutation to form the base pair and change the 5'-end in ds, converts the tRNA$_i$ as tRNA$_{met}$ which can transfer a methionine in the middle of the chain. Secondly there are atleat 3 G:C base pairs at the end of the stem in the anticodon arm. A mutation here results in inactivation of tRNA$_i$ which can not occupy a partial P site. Finally it is charged with a N–formyl methionine which lacks a free amino group. However, if an initiator tRNA is charged with normal methionine, it has the capability to initiate the chain. It is therefore, unlikely that formylation of methionine is responsible for the specificity of tRNA$_i$ for initiation codon. Rather, it is reverse and the Met–tRNA$_i$ undergoes formylation. It may be pointed out here that if one of the alternate initiation codons, GUG or UUG (only in extremely rare cases) is used for begining the protein synthesis, it is also recognised by the same initiator tRNA. Even though in the middle of the chain GUG will be recgnized by tRNA val. Thus the initiating aminoacid is always a N–formyl methionine.

The charged initiator tRNA, fMet-RNA$_i$, reacts with another initiation factor, IF2, and forms a binary complex. Initiation factor IF2 is specific for tRNA$_i$ and does not bind to any other tRNA. This specificity, thus plays an important role in ensuring that only the fMet-tRNA$_i$ can initiate the protein synthesis. This factor is also required for the hydrolysis of GTP (see later) as it seems to be responsible for a ribosome-associated GTPase activity. The precise mechanism of GTPase action is not very clear. Though IF2 itself does not seem to possess the GTPase activity, its association with ribosome results in specific confirmational change in the structure of the ribosomal proteins which in turn activates one of the r-protein bearing GTPase activity. The fMet-tRNA$_i$:IF2 binary complex reacts with GTP (which provides energy for initiation) and forms a ternary complex. The process is GTP specific and ATP (or any other NTP) can not subsitute for GTP as the source of energy for initiation. This ternary complex now moves to the mRNA.30S.IF3 complex and occupies the partial P site (both the small and the large ribosomal subunits contribute for the formation of the binding sites in the ribosome and as the large subunit of ribosome is not present at this stage, therefore, the P site is incomplete or partial). The codon-anticodon interaction between the tRNA and the mRNA takes place. It is not very clear whether first the association of GTP to binary complex takes place and the ternary complex binds to mRNA : 30S; IF3 complex or the binary complex and the GTP, both react simultaneously and associate with the mRNA : 30S; IF3 complex. However, in both the cases the initiation complex of mRNA : 30S : IF3 : fMet-tRNA$_i$: IF2 : GTP is formed. It should be re-emphasised that no other aminoacyl tRNA except the initiator tRNA can occupy the partial P site and initiate the protein synthesis.

This complex formation sets the plateform for the association of large subunit. The 50S subunit binds to this complex. GTP is hydrolysed to GDP (and the inorganic phosphate) and provides the energy required for the formation of this complex. The mechanism of GTPase activity have already been discussed. Both the initiation factors, IF2 and IF3, are released and the complete ribosome:mRNA complex consisted of mRNA.70S. fMet-tRNA$_i$ is formed. IF1, another initiation factor, is involved at this stage which gets associated with the 30S subunit of the ribosome. The precise role of IF1 is not very well understood. It probably provides the stability to the initiation complex. After successful initiation, the complex is ready to accept subsequent aa and elongation of the polypeptide chain takes place. The entire process of initiation of prokaryotic protein synthesis has been diagramatically represent in Fig. 7.21.

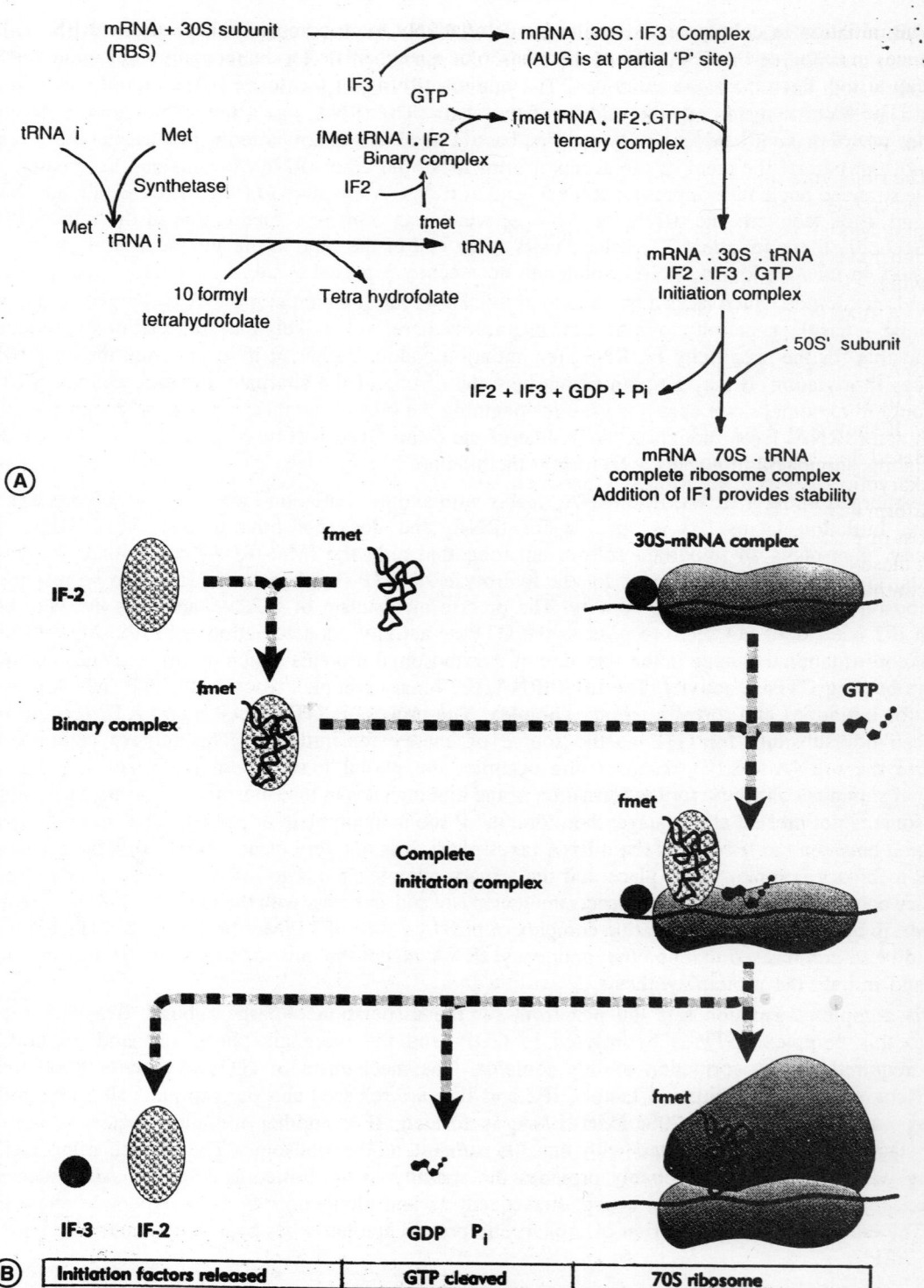

Fig. 7.21. Initiation of prokaryotic translation. A. Flow chart. B. Diagramatic representation.

The initiation in eukaryotes is similar but is relatively more complex. There are no RBS or the SD sequences in eukaryotic mRNAs. Thus, there has to be a mechanism for the recognition of initiation codon. The cap at the 5'–end of eukaryotic mRNA helps in positioning the small (40S) subunit to the initiator codon. The 40S subunit associates with the cap of the mRNA. This assocaition is facilitated by certain cap binding proteins (CBP) which attach to the cap and help the 40S subunit to position itself.

The ribosomal subunit now slides through the mRNA. It scans the mRNA until it finds an AUG codon. This procedure of finding the initiation codon was proposed by M. Kozak and is known as the Kozak's Scanning Model. Usually the first AUG of the mRNA serves as the initiator codon. However, certain other criterion have to be fulfilled before the AUG is accepted as the initiator codon. These criterion are as following:

1. A functional AUG is usually flanked by a purine (more often an A than a G) at the −3 position from the A in AUG.
2. A guanosine residue should be present at the +4 position.
3. In yeast, an U is generally present at +6 position.
4. It should lead to an open reading frame.

Based on above considerations, a consensus sequence which is very often present at the initiation site of eukaryotic mRNAs is CCA/GCCAUGGGU. The close examination of this sequence will reveal that in DNA form this sequence will have a NcoI site (CCATGG) at the initiation codon. Thus the coding sequences of most of eukaryotic genes can be isolated by digestion with NcoI (Fig. 7.22). Should the first AUG not fulfill these criterion, it will be usually ignored by the 40S subunit which will proceed further on the mRNA and continue its search for another AUG codon.

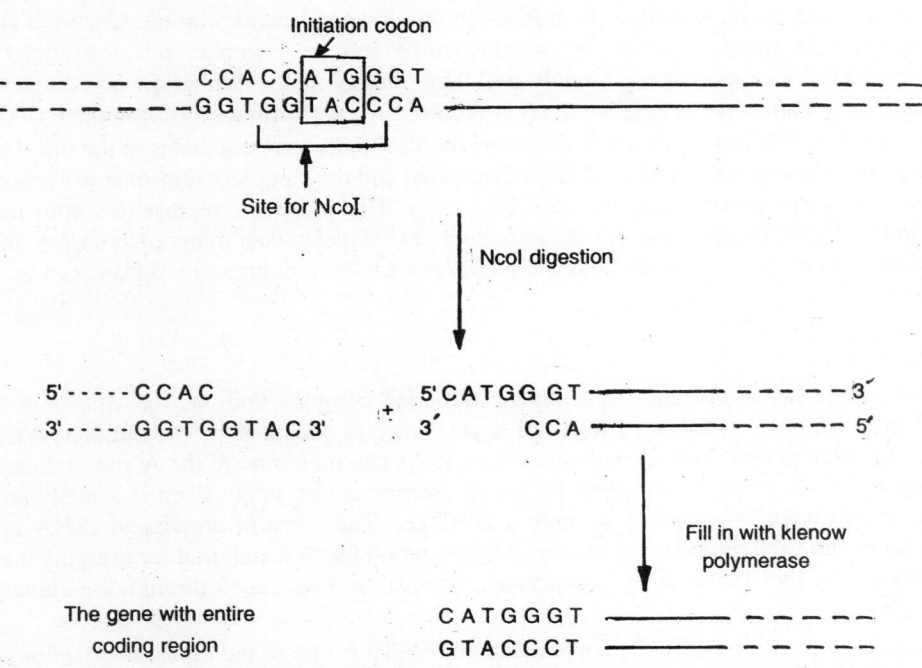

Fig. 7.22. Isolation of coding region of eukaryotic gene by NcoI digestion.

There are 9 different initiation factors in eukaryotes. These are referred as eIFs to differentiate with prokaryotic initiation factors (the prefix 'e' stands for eukaryotic). The function of some of these factors is not very well understood. Initiation factor eIF4A binds with the mRNA at the cap region and helps in unwinding any tertiary structure which may be present at its 5'-end. The eukaryotic mRNAs often have high degree of tertiary structures and for the smooth sailing of the ribosomal subunit, it is obligatory that these structures are unwound. Factor eIF4B helps in further unwinding. In eukaryotes, the first aminoacid is methionine and not N-formyl methionine as in prokaryotes. However, similar to prokaryotes, there is a distinct initiator tRNA capable of binding to the partial P site. This differs from tRNA$_{met}$ (which binds only to a complete A site and transfers a Met residue at the middle of the chain). The precise differences in the structure of an initiator tRNA from the tRNA$_{Met}$ in eukaryotes are not very clear.

The first step in eukaryotic initiation is the binding of CBPs to the cap structure at the 5'-end of mRNA. Following this, the initiation factors eIF4A and eIF4B associate themselves to the cap region. Prior association of CBP is essential for the binding of these eIFs with the mRNA. On the other hand, the initiation factor eIF2 and GTP associate togather to form a binary complex. The met-tRNA$_i$ binds with this binary complex (GTP.eIF2) and the ternary complex is formed. It should be noted that the sequence of events during the formation of ternary complex in eukaryotes differs from the prokarotes. In prokaryates, first the IF2 binds with f-met-tRNA, then the GTP joins while in eukaryotes, first the GTP and eIF2 join together then the Met-tRNA joins. The ternary complex is now transferred to the 40S subunit and a 40S:aminoacyl tRNA complex is formed. This complex moves to mRNA and binds at the cap region. Initiation factor eIF3 is required for this (mRNA:aminoacyl tRNA:40S complex) binding. Association of CBP to the cap helps in proper positioning of the complex. The binding of 40S subunit complex is energy dependent and an ATP molecule is hydrolysed to ADP (and Pi) during this binding. The entire complex then slides through the mRNA and scans for initiation codon. The details of this scaning have been discussed earlier. The eIF4A and eIF4B maintain the mRNA in the unwound configuration. Once the complex has located an appropriate intiator codon, the scaning stops and the complex positions itself in such a manner that the AUG occupies the partial P site. This results in the formation of complete initiation complex. Another initiation factor, eIF5, which is required for the formation of complete ribosome joins the initiation complex. The large subunit of ribosome (60S subunit) now associates to the mRNA:40S: Met-RNA$_i$ complex. Initiation factors eIF2 and eIF3 are released and the complete ribosome is formed. The GTP is hydrolysed during this process and provides the energy. The schematic representation of initiation has been shown in Fig 7.23. The basic steps in the formation of GTP dependent initiation complex and ribosome are thus similar in both the eukaryotes and the prokaryotes even though some differences exist between the two classes.

Elongation

Once the initiation is successful and the complete initiation complex and the 70S ribosome are formed, the A and P sites are now complete. The P site at this stage is occupied by the aminoacyl tRNA$_i$ while the A site of ribosome is free. The second aminoacyl tRNA can now bind to the A site. It should be noted that the initiator tRNA cannot be accepted by the ribosomes at this stage. Even if a methionine is to be incorporated, it will have to approach through a tRNA$_{Met}$. The entry of aminoacyl tRNA is an energy dependent process and GTP provides the energy. An elongation factor is required for bringing the aminoacyl tRNA to the A site of the ribosome. In prokaryotes, elongation is mediated through the elongation factor EF-Tu (see later).

The mechanism of action of EF-Tu is complicated. EF-Tu is one of the most abundant proteins of the cell, comprising at an average, about 5% of the total cellular proteins. An average of about 70,000 molecules

A. Flowchart

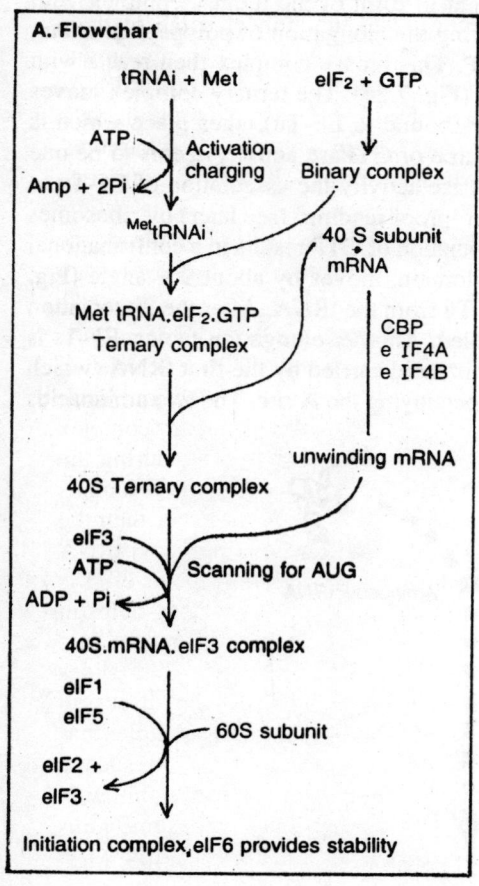

tRNAi + Met   eIF₂ + GTP

ATP → Activation charging   Binary complex

Amp + 2Pi

Met tRNAi

Met tRNA.eIF₂.GTP
Ternary complex

40 S subunit
mRNA

CBP
e IF4A
e IF4B

unwinding mRNA

40S Ternary complex

eIF3
ATP   Scanning for AUG

ADP + Pi

40S.mRNA.eIF3 complex

eIF1
eIF5   60S subunit

eIF2 +
eIF3

Initiation complex, eIF6 provides stability

B. Diagrammatic representation

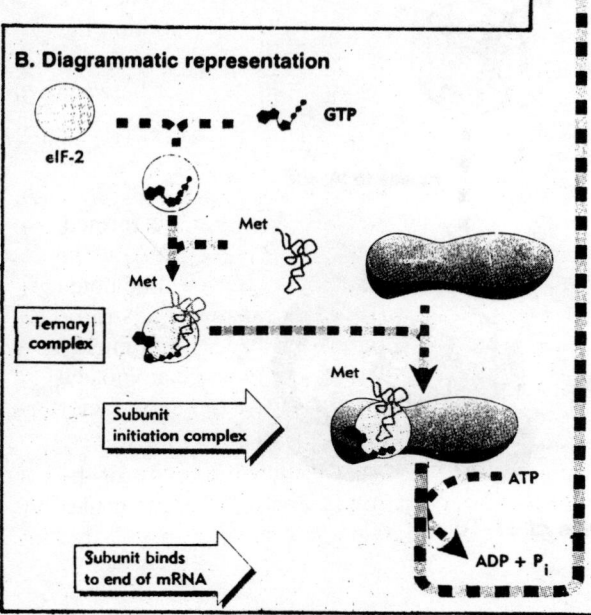

GTP

eIF-2

Met

Ternary complex

Subunit initiation complex

Subunit binds to end of mRNA

ATP

ADP + Pᵢ

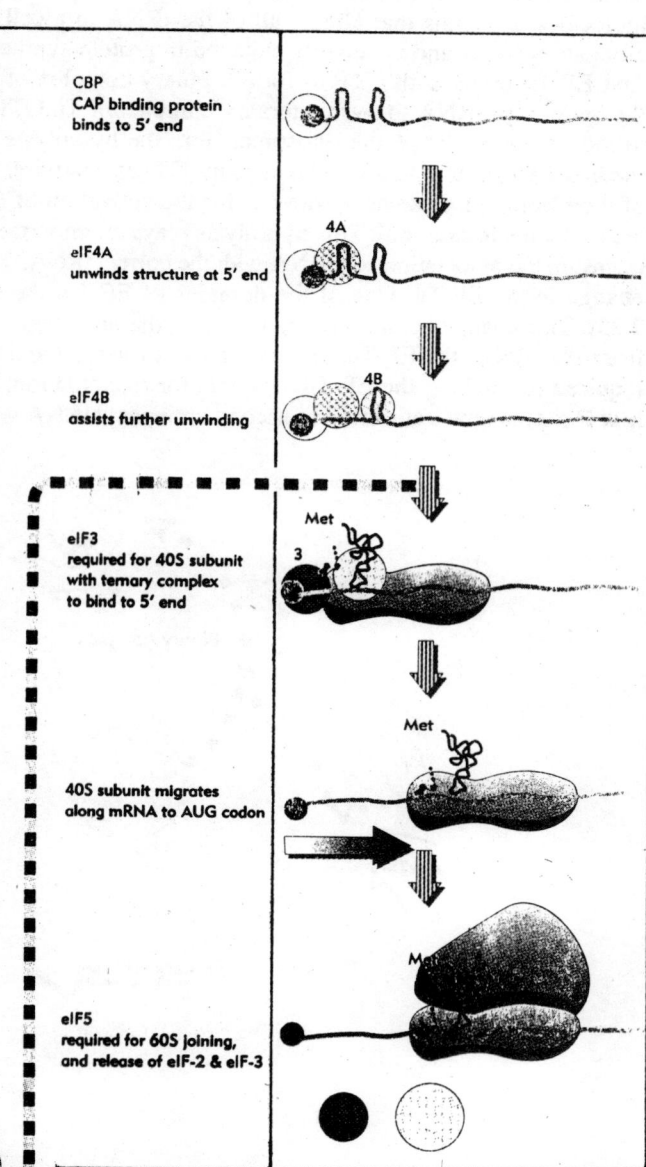

CBP
CAP binding protein binds to 5′ end

eIF4A
unwinds structure at 5′ end

4A

eIF4B
assists further unwinding

4B

eIF3
required for 40S subunit with ternary complex to bind to 5′ end

Met

3

40S subunit migrates along mRNA to AUG codon

Met

eIF5
required for 60S joining, and release of eIF-2 & eIF-3

Fig. 7.23. Initiation of eukaryotic translation. A. Flowchart. B. Diagrammatic representation.

of EF-Tu are present in each cell, which is roughly in equimolar ratio with the abundance of the tRNA molecules. It means that almost all of the tRNA in a cell is present in form of the ternary complex with elongation factor and is actively engaged in protein synthesis. During the elongation of polypeptide chain, first EF-Tu binds with GTP to form a binary complex of Tu.GTP. This binary complex then reacts with the aminoacyl tRNA to form a ternary complex of Tu.GTP.tRNA (Fig. 7.24). The ternary complex moves to the vacant A site of the ribosome. Here the hydrolysis of GTP (bound to EF-Tu) takes place which is mediated through a ribosome dependent GTPase activity. The source of GTPase activity seems to be one of the ribosomal proteins. However, for the activation of this GTPase activity the association of EF-Tu to the ribosome is essential. This hydrolysis plays an important role in 'proof reading' (see later) by ribosomes to ensure the association of mRNA with the correct tRNA. The dissociation of GTP results in a confirmational change in the EF-Tu. One of the domains of EF-Tu, the switch domain, moves by about 90° angle (Fig. 7.25). This changed configuration results in the dissociation of EF-Tu from the tRNA. After the dissociation from the tRNA, the EF-Tu.GDP complex is released and is recycled. Another elongation factor, EF-Ts is required for making the EF-Tu available for recirculation. The aminoacid carried by the first tRNA (which is at P site) is now transferred to second aminoacyl tRNA which is occupying the A site. The two aminoacids

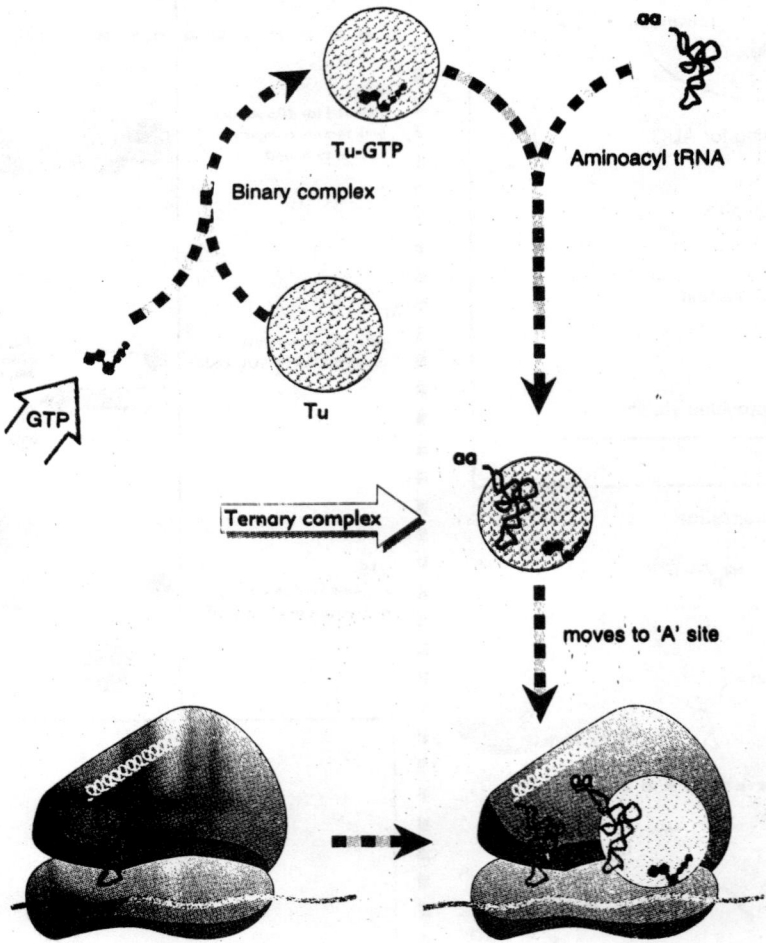

Fig. 7.24. The role of EF-Tu.

join together through the covalent linkage (the peptide bond). The release of EF-Tu:GDP complex is obligatory for the peptide bond formation. The aminoacyl tRNA can not accept the peptide from the peptidyl tRNA as long as the EF-Tu remains associated with it. One of the antibiotics, kirromycin, which is a potent inhibitor of protein synthesis, blocks the release of EF-Tu:GDP complex. The peptide bond is formed between the −COOH group of Ist aa and −NH$_2$ group of 2nd aminoacid (Fig. 7.26). Enzyme petidyl transferase is required for this esterification. The peptidyl transferase activity is a function of the ribosomes. The search for the site of peptidyl transferase activity has revealed that it is located in the 50S subunit (60S in eukaryotes). Further analysis has shown that stripping of 50S with most of the proteins (when less than 5% of total proteins remain) does not result in loss of enzyme activity. It is, therefore, believed that the peptidyl transferase activity is located in the 23S RNA and not in the ribosomal proteins. However, direct evidence for this hypothesis has not been obtained. The formation of peptide bond is energy dependent and the energy is provided by GTP.

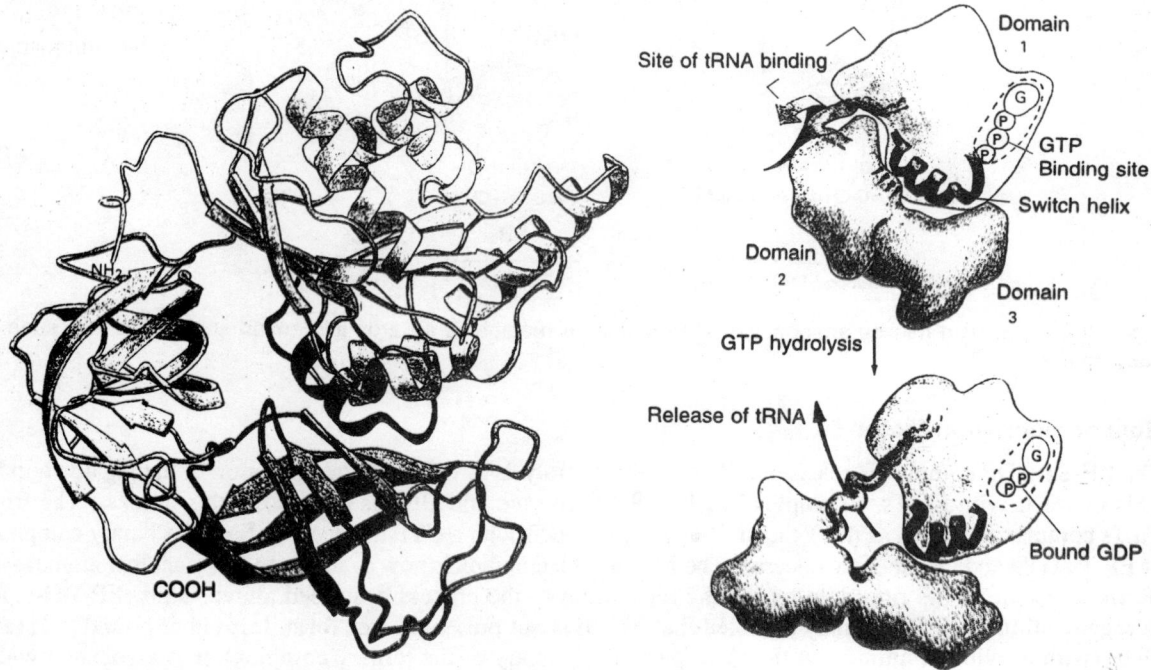

Fig. 7.25. GTP hydrolysis causes confirmational change in EF-Tu molecule.

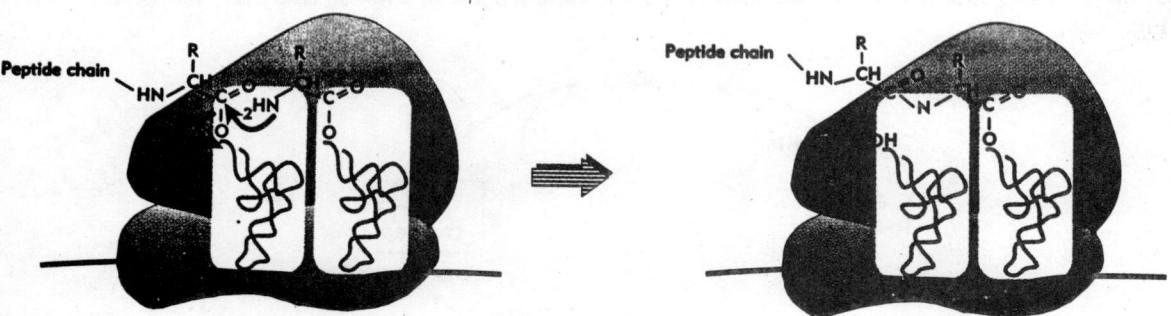

Fig. 7.26. Peptide bond formation takes place by reaction between the polypeptide of peptidyl-tRNA in the P site and the amino acid of aminoacyl-tRNA in the A site.

Puromycin, which is one of the most potent inhibitors of protein synthesis, has a structure which resembles with aminoacyl tRNA and is recognised by EF-Tu as well as by ribosome. It gets incorporated in the growing polypetide chain in place of an aminoacyl tRNA. However, its incorporation blocks further elongation of the chain as the next aminoacid cannot from the peptide bond with puromycin. It results in premature release of the polypeptide chain (Fig. 7.27).

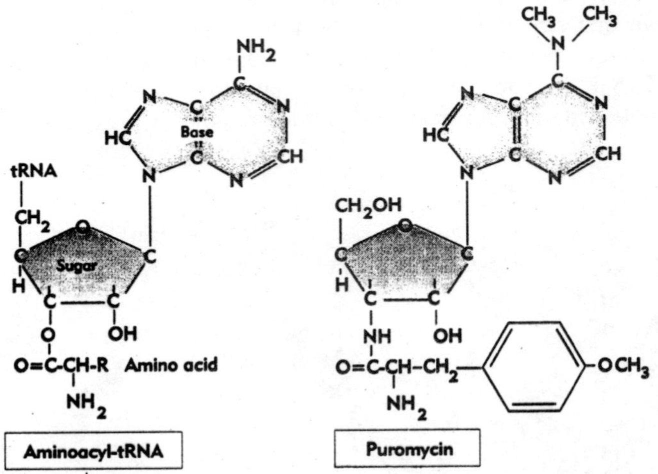

Fig. 7.27. Puromycin mimics aminoacyl-tRNA because it resembles an aromatic amino acid linked to a sugar-base moiety.

Role of elongation factor Ts

The EF-Tu-GDP complex is released following the hydrolysis of GTP and the formation of the peptide bond. This interacts with EF-Ts, a complex of EF-Tu.Ts is formed and GDP is released in this process. The EF-Tu.Ts complex is known as the T factor. The T factor reacts with a GTP molecule to form the binary complex of EF-Tu.GTP and the EF-Ts is released. The EF-Tu.GTP complex is now available to bring another aminoacyl tRNA molecule to the ribosome by the the repeatition of the process described above. Thus, EF-Ts helps in regeneration of EF-Tu. It may be noted that EF-Tu is not present in free form. It is either bound to GTP/GDP (with or without aminoacyl tRNA as part of the binary or the ternary complex) or is associated with EF-Ts as T factor. EF-Ts, on the other hand, is present either as free Ts or as Tu-Ts complex (the T factor). Both these factors shuttle between different forms and form a cycle of events. This cycle has been shown in Fig. 7.28.

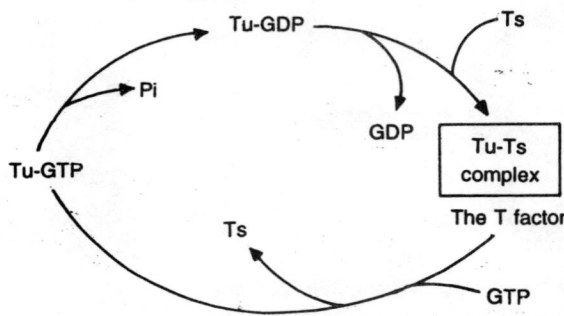

Fig. 7.28. Formation of T factor.

In eukaryotes, the elongation is carried out by the elongation factor eEF1. This works in the same manner as the EF-Tu and is present in high abundance in all the cells. The basic events of elongation are similar between eukaryotes and prokaryotes.

Translocation of the ribosome

Once the aminoacid carried by the tRNA at P site has been transferred to the tRNA at A site and the peptide bond is formed, the deacylated tRNA (presently at the P site) moves out of the ribosome through the E site. The tRNA present at the A site now carries the growing polypeptide chain and becomes the peptidyl tRNA (the tRNA having a growing polypeptide chain). The ribosome moves forward on mRNA by three nucleotides (one codon) at this stage, so that the next codon will now occupy the A site. The location of peptidyl tRNA which was earlier at A site, now shifts to P site. This movement of ribosome (referred as translocation) is an energy dependent process and the energy is provided by GTP. ATP can not substitute the GTP. A number of elongation factors also participate in this process. In prokaryotes, the translocation of ribosome is facilitated by elongation factor EF-G also known as the translocase. EF-G is also a major constituent of the cell. About 20,000 molecules of EF-G are present in each cell, which translates into approximately 1 molecule of EF-G/ribosome. EF-G can bind to ribosome only after the EF-Tu has been released and the peptide bond has been formed. Simultaneously to the binding of EF-G, GTP also binds. The movement of ribosome is coupled with the hydrolysis of GTP. The movement of ribosome is a two step process. In the first step, the peptidyl tRNA which is still at the A site is moved to P site by one of the two manners (Fig. 7.29). In first mode, the tRNA itself moves from A site and reaches to P site, The A site becomes free. The entire ribosome (along with the peptidyl tRNA, now present at the P site) then translocates to the next codon as discribed earlier. The alternate approach is that first the 50S subunit moves forward (tRNA does not relocate) and the peptidyl tRNA automatically occupies the P site of 50S subunit. The 30S subunit now joins the 50S subunit and translocation is complete. In E.coli the movement of 50S subunit precedes the movement of 30S. This suggests that probably second mode operates in E. coli. Once both the subunits of ribosome have moved by one codon, the EF-G is released. Fusidic acid, one of the inhibitors of protein synthesis, blocks the release of EF-G and arrests the ribosome at the post-translocation state (Fig. 7.30).

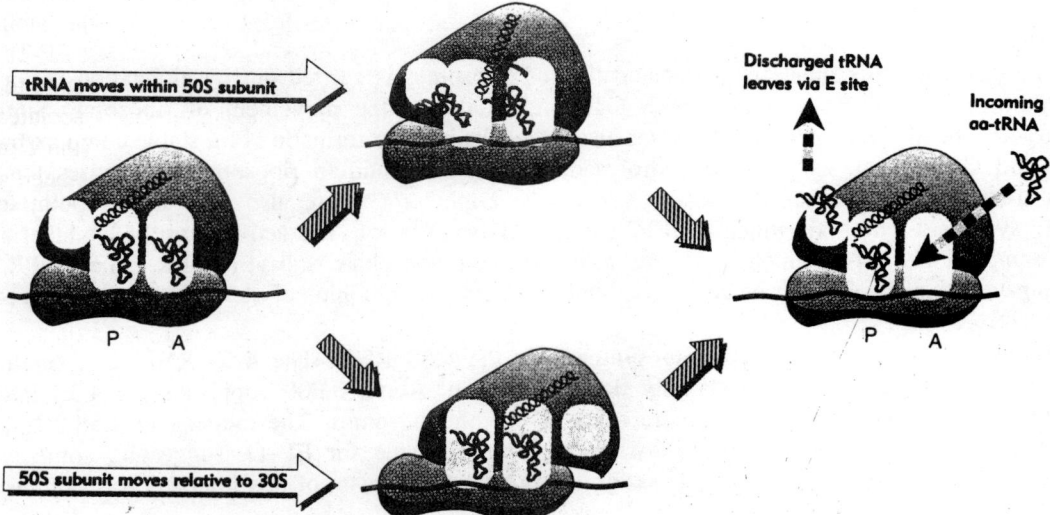

Fig. 7.29. The movement of ribosome can be in two different manner.

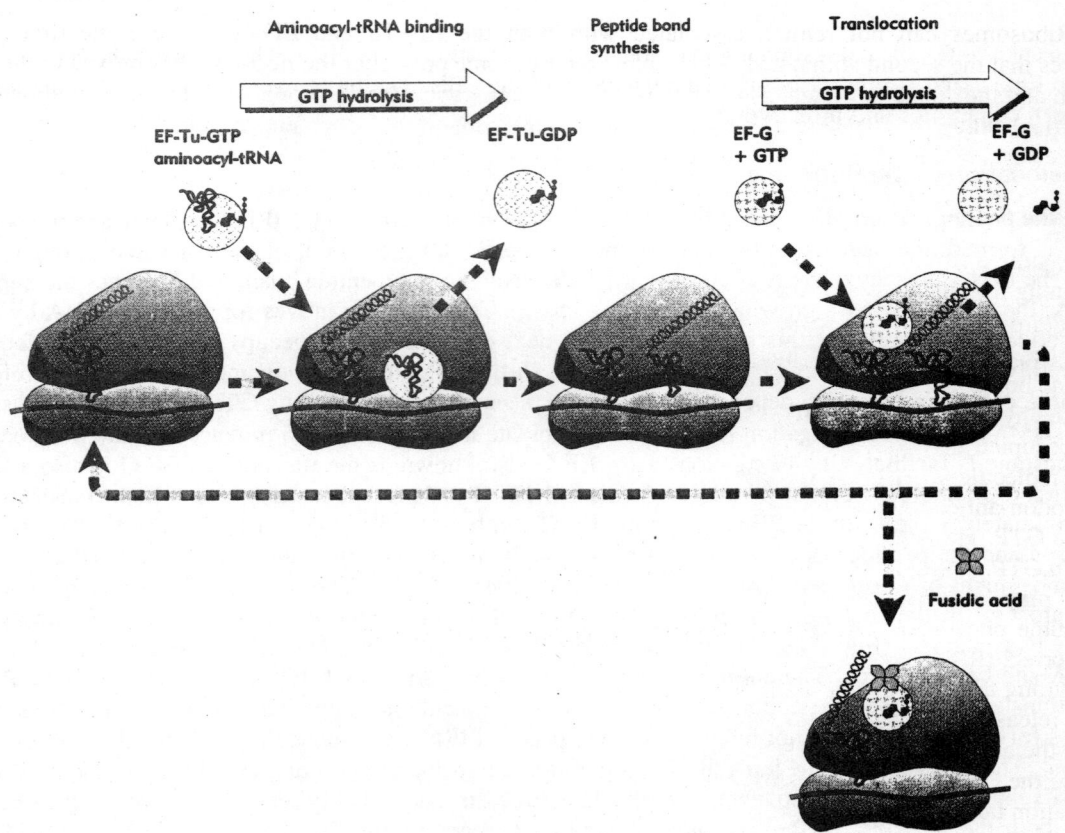

Fig. 7.30. Binding of factors EF-Tu and EF-G alternates as ribosomes accept new aminoacyl-tRNA, form peptide bonds, and translocate. Fusidic acid diverts the ribosome into a post-translocation state that is jammed with EF-G-GDP.

In eukaryotes, this function of translocation of ribosomes is carried out by elongation factor eEF2 which binds to the ribosome alongwith GTP and facilitates the movement of ribosome. Similar to prokaryotes, fusidic acid affects eukaryotes also. It results into the formation of a stable complex between eEF2 and GTP which can not be hydrolysed. It remains bound to ribosome and causes the arrest of its translocation. One of the deadly toxins, the Diphtheria toxin, also acts at this point to stop protein synthesis. The toxin binds to eEF2 using NAD as cofactor. The active form of Diphtheria toxin is its complex with NAD which is referred as adenosine diphosphate ribosyl (ADPR). The ADPR forms a conjugate with eEF2 which is inactive resulting in the complete inhibition of ribosome translocation causing lethal effect.

Another factor required in protein synthesis is the 4.5S RNA. The 4.5S RNA is a small RNA molecule of 114 bases which is largely double stranded. About 3,000 copies of the 4.5S RNA are present in a cell and a few of these are associated with ribosomes. The mutants in 4.5S RNA grow very poorly. This can be suppressed by mutation in the gene for EF–G, suggesting some type of interaction between the two factors. However, the precise mechanism of this interaction is not very well understood.

Ribosomes can not remain associated with both the EF–Tu and EF–G at the same time. This ensures that the second aminoacyl tRNA enters the ribosome only after the ribosome has moved to the next codon and the A site is vacant. The fact that only one elongation factor (along with the attached molecules it carries) binds to ribosome at any given time is the property of ribosome and not that of the factors themselves.

GTPase timer

Every time a tRNA enters the A site of ribosome, it is screened to ensure that it is the correct tRNA. The screening for correct codon-anticodon interaction at this stage is the proof reading function of the ribosome. It requires a few milliseconds. As discussed above, the hydrolysis of GTP present in the ternary complex, EF-Tu.GTP.tRNA and the dissociation of EF-Tu.GDP are obligatory steps for the formation of peptide bond. The hydrolysis of GTP is caused by a ribosome mediated GTPase activity. It has been found that the hydrolysis of GTP does not take place immediately after the complex has moved to ribosome and has occupied the A site. The enzyme seems to pause for a few milliseconds before the hydrolysis of the GTP molecule takes place. This pausing provides the time needed by the ribosomes to check and recheck the codon-anticodon interaction. If the interaction is correct, only then the GTPase carries out hydrolysis of the GTP. However, if the interaction is wrong, the GTP is not hydrolysed and the ternary complex of EF-Tu.GTP.aminoacyl tRNA is aborted. This pausing of enzyme is referred as the 'GTPase timer'. The GTP-timer plays an important role in maintaining the fidility of translation. After the hydrolysis of GTP, the ribosome once again ensures that the interaction of the codon in the mRNA has taken place only with the correct tRNA. If interaction is right, only then elongation factor Tu.GDP is released (and is recycled). If a wrong tRNA is found, The EF-Tu.GDP.tRNA complex is aborted. However, once the EF-Tu.GDP has been released, the aminoacyl tRNA can not be released and the formation of the peptide bond takes place. Thus the authenticity of tRNA bound to A site is double checked. A wrong tRNA leaves the A site either before the GTP hydrolysis or after GTP hydrolysis but before the dissociation of EF-Tu. The peptide bond formation takes place only after the dissociation of EF-Tu. However, if a wrong tRNA has escaped the two step check, it will result in the incorporation of a wrong aminoacid into the protein. These possibilities have been summarised in Fig. 7.31.

As discussed above, the tRNA present at the A site which is containing the growing polypeptide chain moves to P site, ribosome moves one codon forward and another tRNA comes and binds to A site. Again the ribosome cannot bind to the EF–Tu and EF–G at the same time. Release of EF–Tu.GDP is essential for the binding of EF–G. As the release of EF–Tu.GDP is coupled with the peptide bond formation, the premature movement of ribosome is prevented. The ribosomal translocation to next codon takes place only after the formation of the peptide bond. Similarly, the EF–Tu (in the form of ternary complex) can not bind to the ribosome until EF–G has been released, which is coupled with the translocation movement of ribosomes. In this manner the correct timing for the entry of new tRNA is ensured. The process is repeated till entire coding region of mRNA has been translated.

Termination of Translation

Once the ribosome reaches to any of the three termination codons (also called as the non-sense codons, the three stop codons are UAG or the Amber codon, UAA or the Ochre codon and UGA or the Opal codon), the chain termination occurs. No tRNA with anticodons for any of the stop codons is present in the cell. As a result, when the last tRNA with complete polypeptide chain has moved to the P site and the A site is sitting over a stop codon, there is no tRNA which can be accepted by the ribosome. Thus the A site remains unoccupied. A protein factor, referred as the release factor (RF) enters the ribosome in this situation.

It mediates the transfer of polypeptide chain from the peptidyl tRNA but in absence of an aminoacid the incorporation of only a water molecule takes place in place of the aa. This results in the dissociation of the peptide from the peptidyl tRNA molecule and release of the completed polypeptide chain to the cell cytosol (Fig. 7.32). There are two different RFs in prokaryotes. The RF1 recognizes UAA and UAG and causes the termination while RF2 recognizes UGA and UAA. In eukaryotes a single eRF is present which recognizes all the three termination codons. There are about 600 molecules of RF/cell (approx 1 RF/50 ribosomes). Following the hydrolysis of polypeptidyl tRNA and release of the polypeptide chains, the ribosome falls off the mRNA and are dissociated to individual subunits. In eukaryotes, the dissociation of 80S ribosome into individual subunits is mediated by an initiation factor, eIF6. The ribosomal subunits are then recycled.

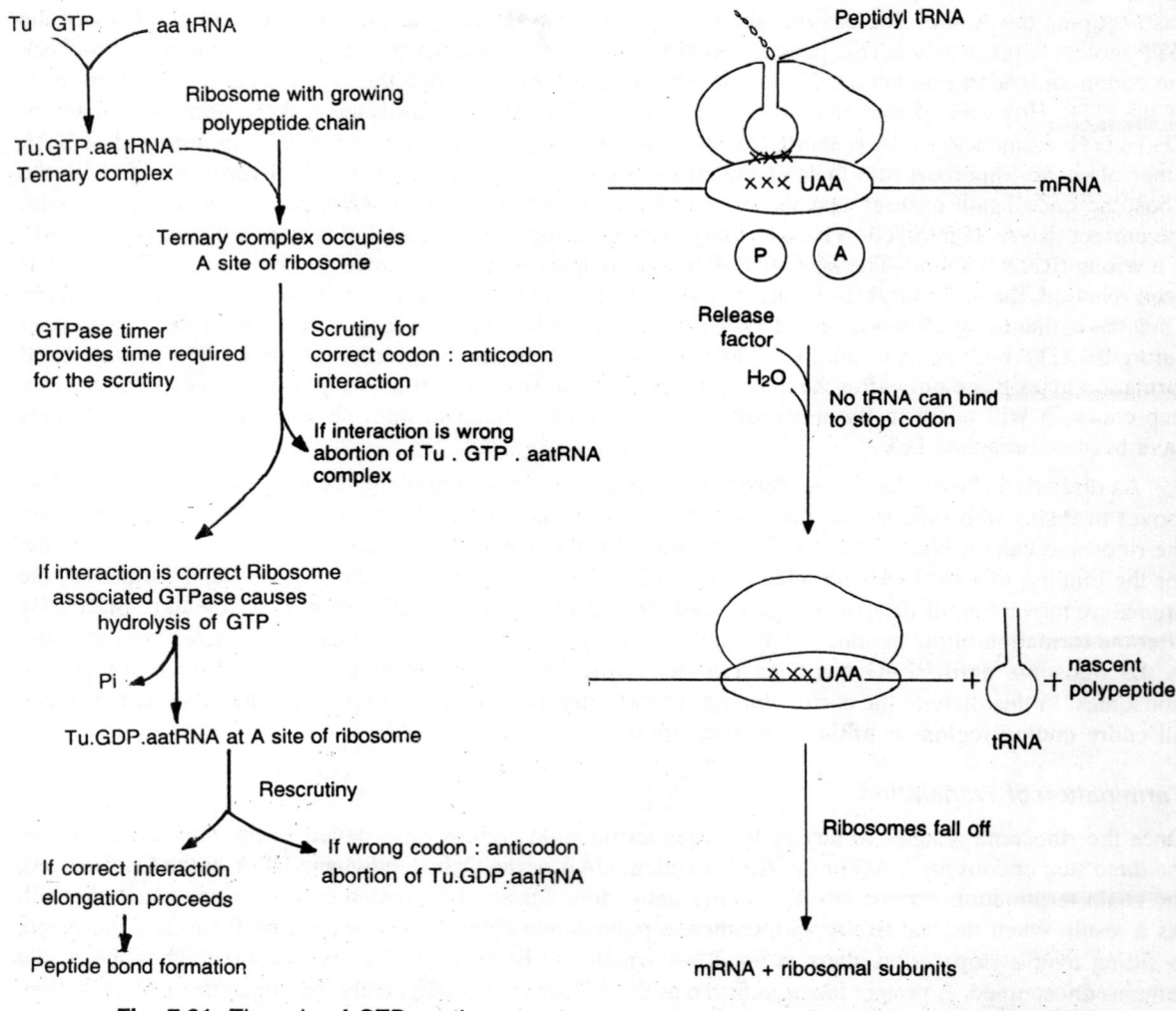

Fig. 7.31. The role of GTPase timer.　　　　**Fig. 7.32.** Release of polypeptide.

The entire process of protein synthesis has been shown in a schematic manner in Fig. 7.33.

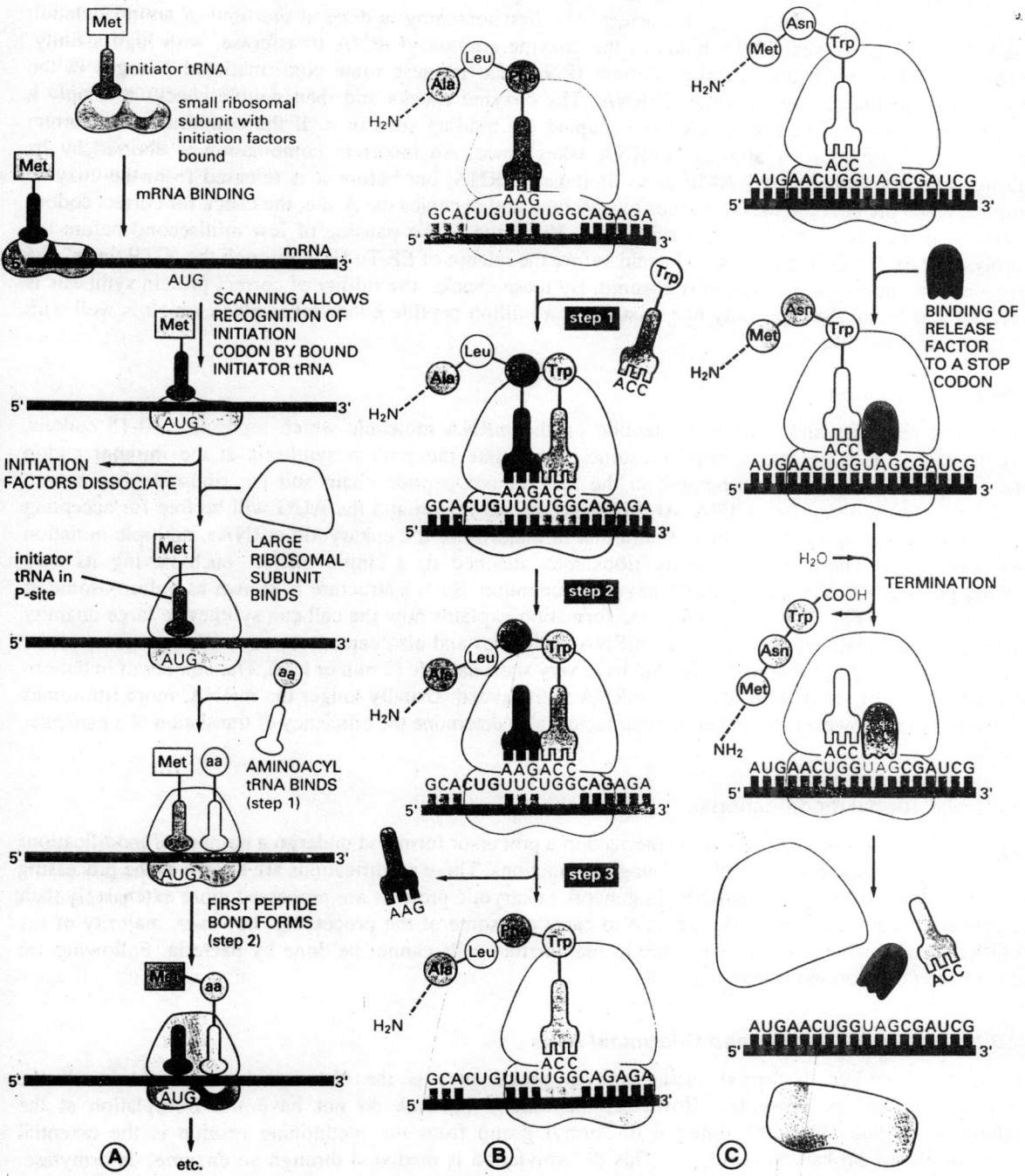

Fig. 7.33. Schematic representation of protein synthesis. A. Initiation. B. Elongation. C. Termination.

Fidility of protein synthesis

As discussed, various checks are made at every stage to ensure that the sequence of aa constituting the primary structure of the protein is correct. The first screening is done at the time of aminoacylation of tRNA. Only the correct tRNA binds to the enzyme aminoacyl tRNA transferase, with high affinity. Wrong tRNA has much less affinity. Correct tRNA also triggers some confirmational changes in the enzyme that facilitates the charging of tRNA. The enzyme checks and then double checks that only a correct combination of aa and tRNA has occupied the binding sites in it. If the combination is correct only then the formation of aminoacyl tRNA takes place. An incorrect combination is aborted by its hydrolysis either as aminoacyl AMP or as aminoacyl tRNA, but before it is released from the enzyme complex. Once the charged tRNA reaches to ribosome and occupies the A site, the check for correct codon-anticodon interaction is made by the ribosomes. By virtue of the pausing of few millisecond before the hydrolysis of EF-Tu.GTP complex and again before the release of EF-Tu.GDP through the 'GTP timer', the correct codon:anticodon interaction is ensured. By these checks, the fidility of correct protein synthesis is increased and on an average, only one mistake in a million peptide bonds takes place which is well with in acceptable limit for the cell.

Polysome formation

A ribosome occupies about 30-40 nucleotide on the mRNA molecule which represents 10-15 codons. It is therefore, possible that a new ribosome can initiate the protein synthesis at the initiator codon once 15-20 aa have been incorporated in the nascent polypeptide chain and the ribosome has moved about 50-60 bases along the mRNA. At this stage the SD region and the AUG will be free for accepting a new initiation complex. It has been found that in majority of the eukaryotic mRNAs, multiple initiation does take place. There may be many ribosomes attached to a single mRNA each having its own growing polypeptide chain at different stage of elongation. Such a structure is known as polyribosome or simply polysome (Fig. 7.34). The polysome formation explains how the cell can synthesize large quantity of proteins with relatively few copies of mRNA molecules and also can survive even though some of the mRNAs (specially the prokaryotic mRNAs) have very short half life (2 min or less). The number of initiations determines the efficiency with which an mRNA is translated. Usually longer the mRNA, more ribosomes are attached to it. However, a number of other factors also determine the efficiency of translation of a particular mRNA.

Post-translational modifications

Majority of the proteins are usually synthesized in a precursor form and undergo a number of modifications before they are ready to perform their biological functions. These modifications are known as the processing and the maturation of the polypeptide. In general, eukaryotic proteins are processed more extensively than the prokaryotic proteins. Bacteria are able to carry out some of the processing, however, majority of the modifications which routinely take place in mammalian cells cannot be done by bacteria. Following are some of the common modifications.

Modification of N-terminal and C-terminal ends

As discussed earlier, N-formyl methionine in prokaryotes is the N-terminal aminoacid in all the newly synthesized polypeptides. However, the mature proteins do not have the formylation at the methionine residue. Thus the removal of formyl group from the methionine residue is the essential feature of all the prokaryotic proteins. This deformylation is mediated through an enzyme, deformylase. Deformylase catalyses the hydrolysis of N-formyl methionine to methionine and acetaldehyde is given out.

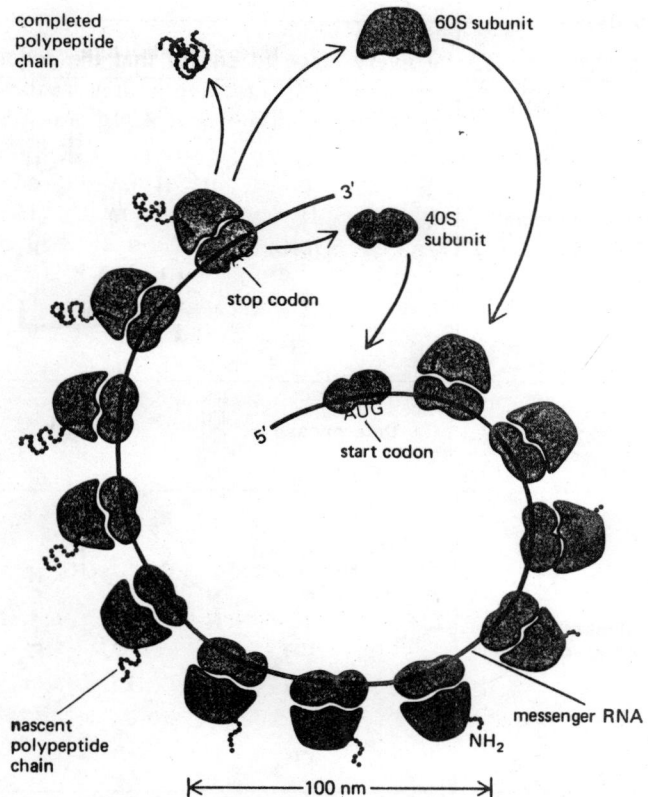

Fig. 7.34. Schematic drawing of a polyribosome showing that a series of ribosomes simultaneously translates the same mRNA molecule. For each polypeptide chain being synthesized from an mRNA molecule in a eucaryotic cell, protein synthesis begins with the binding of a small ribosomal subunit to the single appropriate site on the mRNA molecule and proceeds from the 5' end to the 3' end of the mRNA chain. When a polypeptide chain is completed, the two ribosomal subunits dissociate from the mRNA.

If methionine is the N-terminal aminoacid of the mature protein, this is retained. In such cases, the deformylation alone is sufficient enough to generate mature protein. However, in majority of the mature proteins methionine is not the the N-terminal aminoacid. In such proteins, the methionine has to be cleaved off and another enzyme, aminopeptidase is required to cleave the methionine residue. The second aminoacid then becomes the N-terminal residue. When both steps are required, these take place in a sequential manner, first the N-formyl Met is converted to Met and then the Met is cleaved off. The N-formyl Met cannot be removed in a single step. The reactions are shown in Fig. 7.35. In eukaryotes, N-terminal methionine is not formylated, therefore, there is no need for deformylase activity. Aminopeptidase is the only enzyme needed in eukaryotes.

In many of the proteins certain extra aminoacids, other than the terminal Met, are also removed from the N-terminal end before the protein attains its mature form. Specific peptidases carry out this function. Many times, these proteins may be removed as an oligopeptide in a single step. In almost half of the eukaryotic and in many prokaryotic proteins, the N-terminal aminoacid is acetylated. The acetyl group is attached to

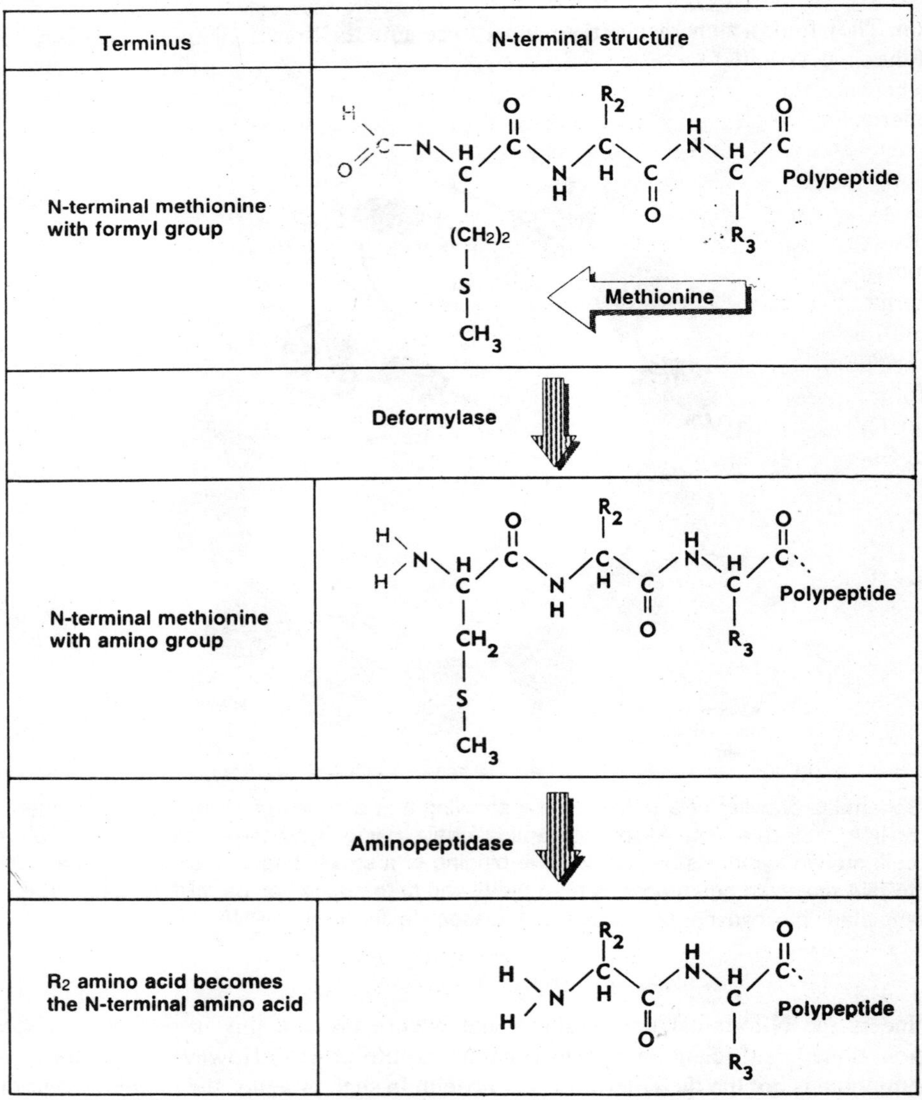

Terminus	N-terminal structure
N-terminal methionine with formyl group	
	Deformylase
N-terminal methionine with amino group	
	Aminopeptidase
R2 amino acid becomes the N-terminal amino acid	

Fig. 7.35. Modification of N terminal of a polypeptide.

the free amino group. Some of the proteins which have glycine as their N-terminal aa, have myristoyl group attched to it via an amide bond (see later).

Similarly the carboxyl group of some of the proteins is modified during processing. This includes the removal of some residues and addition of certain groups to the C-terminal aminoacid.

Formation of disulphide bonds

The ribosomes catalyse the polymerisation of aminoacids in form of a long chain like structure during the protein synthesis. However, most of the proteins are not linear molecules but have a specific three dimensional configuration. They fold in a characteristic manner to acquire this special shape and these specific foldings are, most of the time, essential for its biological activity. These foldings are stabilized primarily by intrachain S-S bridges between the Cys residues. In the proteins which have multiple subunits, the subunits are often joined by interchain S-S bridges. The disulphide bridges are formed in the lumen of the rough ER, either during or after the protein synthesis. A number of proteins contain more than one disulfide bonds. These bonds are both intrachain and interchain (in case of multimeric proteins). In the cases where a number of Cys residues are present, there may be multiple possible positions for the formation of S-S bridges. In the lumen of ER, where the environment is non-reducing and there is a pool of newly synthesized polypeptide chains, the possibility of wrong disulfide bond formation increases. However, only correct disulphide bonds provide a thermodyna-mically stable structure to the protein. The enzyme protein disulfide isomerase (PDI) is responsible for the formation of S-S bridges at correct position. PDI has a free Cys residue in it. If a wrong S-S bridge is formed, the Cys residue of the enzyme reacts with it. PDI gets associated with the protein by forming S-S bridge with one of the two Cys residues involved in the formation of wrong bond and the other Cys becomes free. Now PDI looks for correct Cys to create S-S bond with Cys to which it is attached. Once correct S-S bond has been formed, the enzyme is released (Fig. 7.36). Thus the molecules

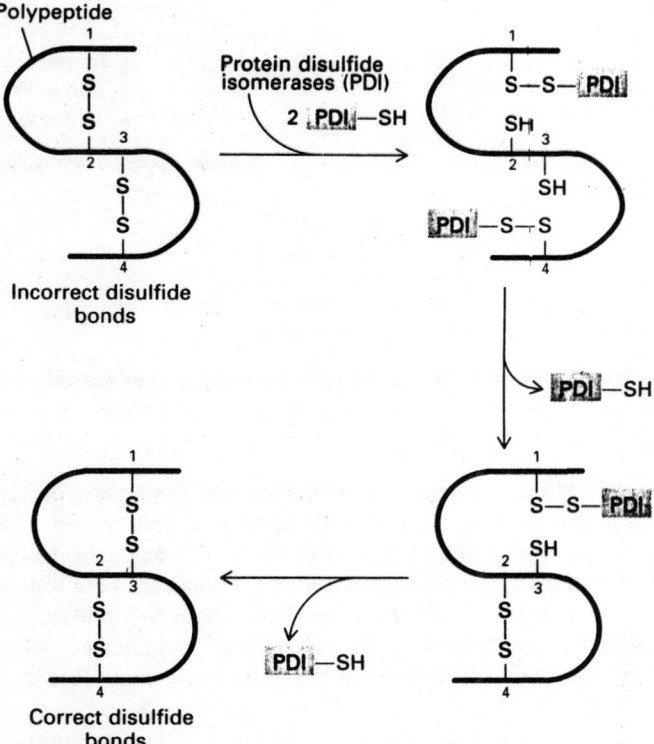

Fig. 7.36. Protein disulfide isomerase (PDI) catalyzes the breakage and reformation of disulfide bonds and, in doing so, accelerates the refolding of proteins containing multiple disulfide bonds. In the oxidizing environment of the ER lumen, disulfide bonds form spontaneously in newly made secretory proteins but are often incorrect. PDI contains an active-site cysteine residue with a free reduced sulfhydryl (S—S) bonds on newly made proteins to form as S—S bond between PDI and the protein. This bond, in turn, can react with a free SH on the protein to form a new S—S bond. In this way, the disulfide bonds on a protein can rearrange themselves until the most stable configuration for the protein is achieved.

with wrong configuration are not formed. Usually a protein leaves the ER only after it has achieved the correct folding. The cytosolic compartment has a number of thiol compounds which provide a reducing environment and formation of any new S-S bridges is not possible here. Should a protein with wrong configuration leave the ER, it can not be repaired.

Oligomerization

A number of proteins are madeup of more than one polypeptide chains, commonly known as the subunits. The protein may either be a homopolymer in which case all of its subunits are same and only the polymerization of more than one molecule of the same polypeptide is needed. Alternatively, the protein may be a heteropolymer and various subunits may be different polypeptides. Immunoglobulins and gonadotropins are good example of heteropolymeric proteins. The individual polypeptides are coded by different genes and are synthesized independently. These are then annealed together as a post-translational event. Different chains are usually held together by inter-chain disulphide bonds (Fig. 7.37).

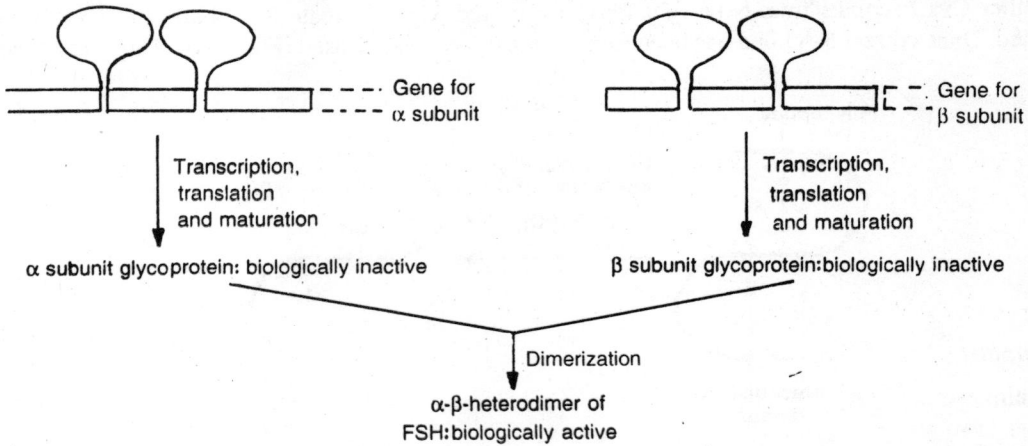

Fig. 7.37. Formation of bioactive FSH by heterodimer formation.

Proteolytic cleavage

Some of the proteins are synthesized as a much larger molecule than the mature protein, the precursor form of the protein is known as the pro-protein. A number of hormones and certain viral proteins as well as some of the enzymes are good examples of this type of proteins. For example, mature insulin is made up of two chains, A and B of 21 and 30 aminoacids, respectively. These are held together by two interchain S-S bonds and the configuration is maintained by a single intra-chain S-S bridge in the chain A. A single gene codes for the precursor form of the insulin which is a much larger molecule, referred as pre-proinsulin. In pre-proinsulin the chain A forms the carboxyl end of the protein and chain B is at the N-terminal region. Two chains are joined together through a third peptide, the chain C. Associated with the amino end of the chain B is the signal peptide (which is necessary for the secretion of the hormone). The newly synthesized protein thus have following structure:

$$NH_2\text{-signal peptide-B chain-C chain-A chain-COOH.}$$

By specific proteolytic cleavage, first the signal peptide is removed (see later) and the proinsulin is formed. This is followed by specific cleavage which removes C chain and also separates the A and B chains.

While C chain is degraded, A and B chains are annealed together by S–S bridges and the mature insulin is obtained. This is represented in Fig. 7.38. Similar precursor forms for glucagon, somatostatin, trypsin and chymotrypsin are also processed by proteolytic digestion to produce bioactive proteins (Fig. 7.39).

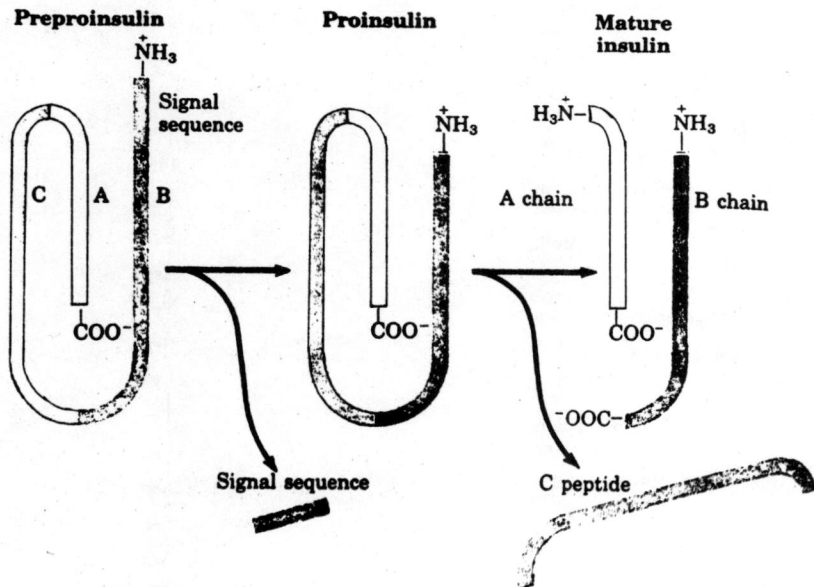

Fig. 7.38. Formation of Insulin by proteolytic cleavage of chains.

Detatchment of signal peptide

The proteins which are secretory in nature and have to cross the membrane to reach their final destination (see later) have a specific tag attached to them which directs the protein to its final destination across the membrane. This tag is in the form of a small peptide of 20-30 aa which is present at their NH_2-end. This region is known as the signal peptide and is responsible for the secretion of the protein. Once the protein has crossed the membrane, the signal peptide has served its purpose and is no longer required. It is, therefore, cleaved from the mature protein. The removal of signal peptide is mediated through specific peptidases, known as 'signal peptidase'. The details of signal peptide will be discussed elsewhere.

Modification of individual aminoacids

A number of proteins have either modified aminoacids or have the aminoacids with different side chains associated with it. The aa like Tyr, Ser and Thr have free –OH group, Asp and Glu have a free –COOH group and lysine has an extra NH_2 group which can react with different radicals and get modified. One of the common modifications is the addition of a (or more) phosphate group. The addition of phosphate group adds a net negative charge to these proteins. The functional importance of the phosphorylation is very wide. For example, casein in milk contains several phosphoserine residues which bind to calcium. Thus milk provides Ca and P along with the proteins to the suckling youngs. The phosphorylation is carried out by a number of different protein kinases and ATP serves as the phosphate group donor. Many of the regulatory proteins are present in both phosphorylated and dephosphorylaed forms and the phosphorylation

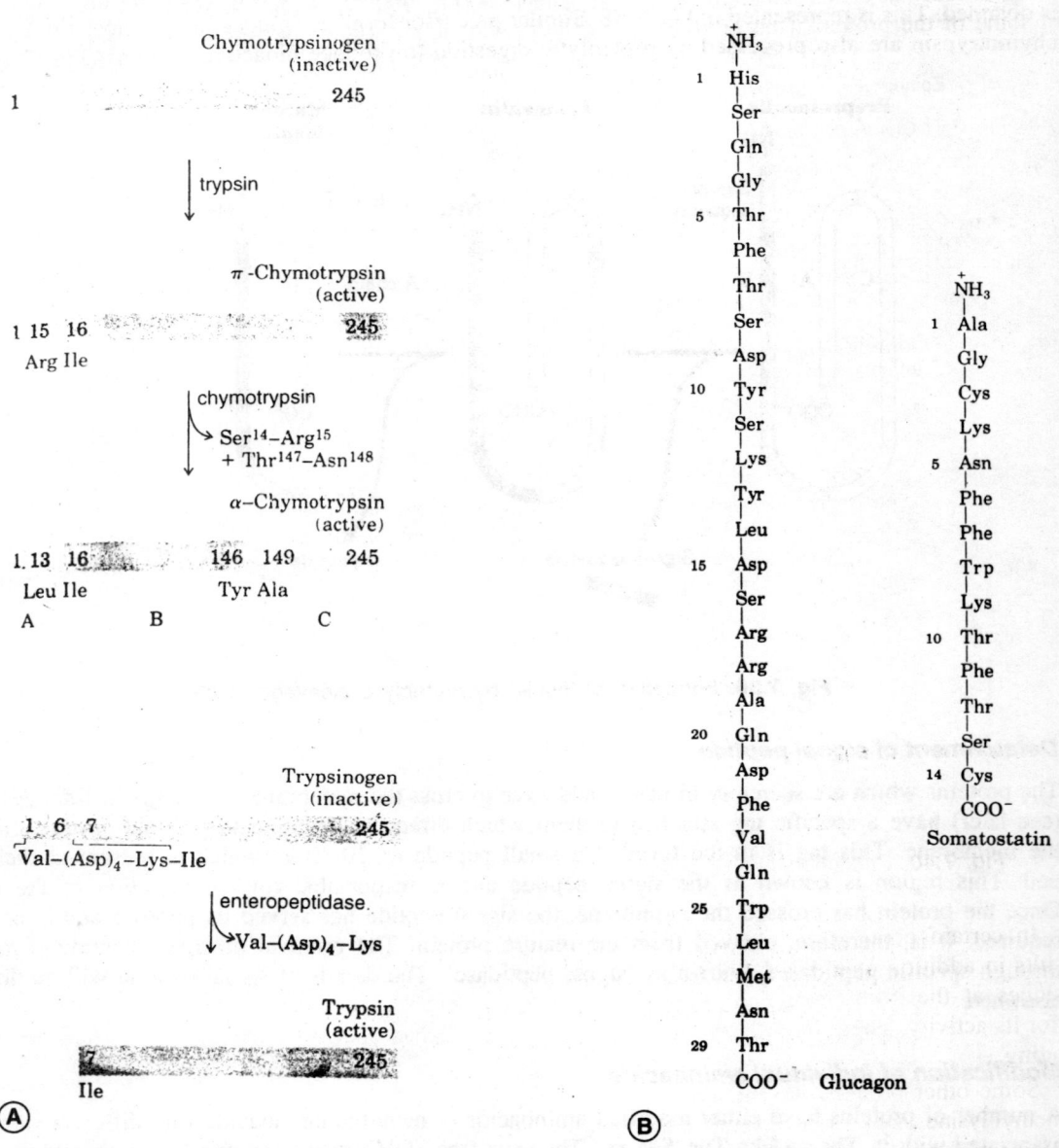

Fig. 7.39. A. Activation of the zymogens of chymotrypsin and trypsin by proteolytic cleavage. The bars represent the primary sequence of the poly-peptide chains. Amino acids at the termini of the polypeptide fragments generated by cleavage are indicated below the bars. The numbers represent the positions of the amino acids in the primary sequence of chymotrypsinogen or trypsinogen. (The amino-terminal amino acid is number 1.), **B.** Structures of glucagon and somatostatin. These are also formed by the proteolytic digestion of their precursors.

by specific protein kinases acts as the modulator of their activity. For example, the concentration of glucose and its conversion to glycogen is maintained by two enzymes, glycogen phosphorylase and glycogen synthetase. The activity of these enzymes is regulated through a cascade of phosphorylation and dephosphorylation reactions. This is mediated through protein kinases which are controlled by a number of factors such as cAMP, calcium, insulin and glucagon (Fig. 7.40). The phosphorylation of tyrosine residues in some of the proteins (the proto-oncoproteins) converts a normal cell into a cancer cell.

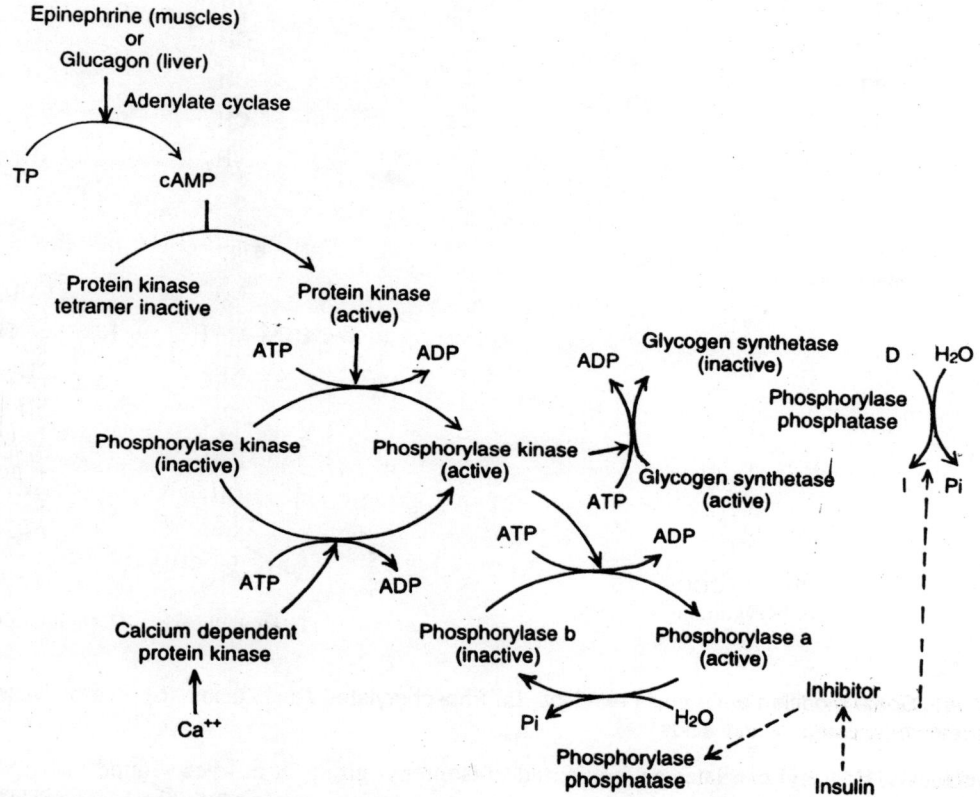

Fig. 7.40. Phosphorylation plays an important role in regulating the activity of many proteins.

In certain other proteins the glutamate has an extra carboxyl group attached at γ-position. This results in addition of a negative charge. For example, prothrombin has a number of γ-carboxyglutamate residues at the N-terminal end. These residues are modified by an enzyme which requires vitamin K for its activity. These modified residues are responsible for the binding of Ca which regulates the blood clotting.

Some other proteins are methylated, for example cyt C has methylated Lys. Both monomethyl and dimethyl lysines are present in some of the muscle proteins. Calmodulin, a protein important in cell signalling, contains trimethyl lysine. The free carboxyl group of glutamic acid can undergo methylation to form methylglutamate which is present in some proteins. This helps in removal of negative charge from the protein. Certain other proteins are acetylated. The structures of some of the modified aminoacids have been shown in Fig. 7.41.

Similarly relatively large side chains like fernasyl group or isoprenyl group are also attached to certain proteins such as proto-oncoproteins, G-proteins and the nuclear matrix protein, lamins. The fernasylation of ras protein takes place by the formation of a thioether bond between Cys residues of the protein and fernasyl pyrophosphate. Fernasyl pyrophosphate is produced during the cholesterol

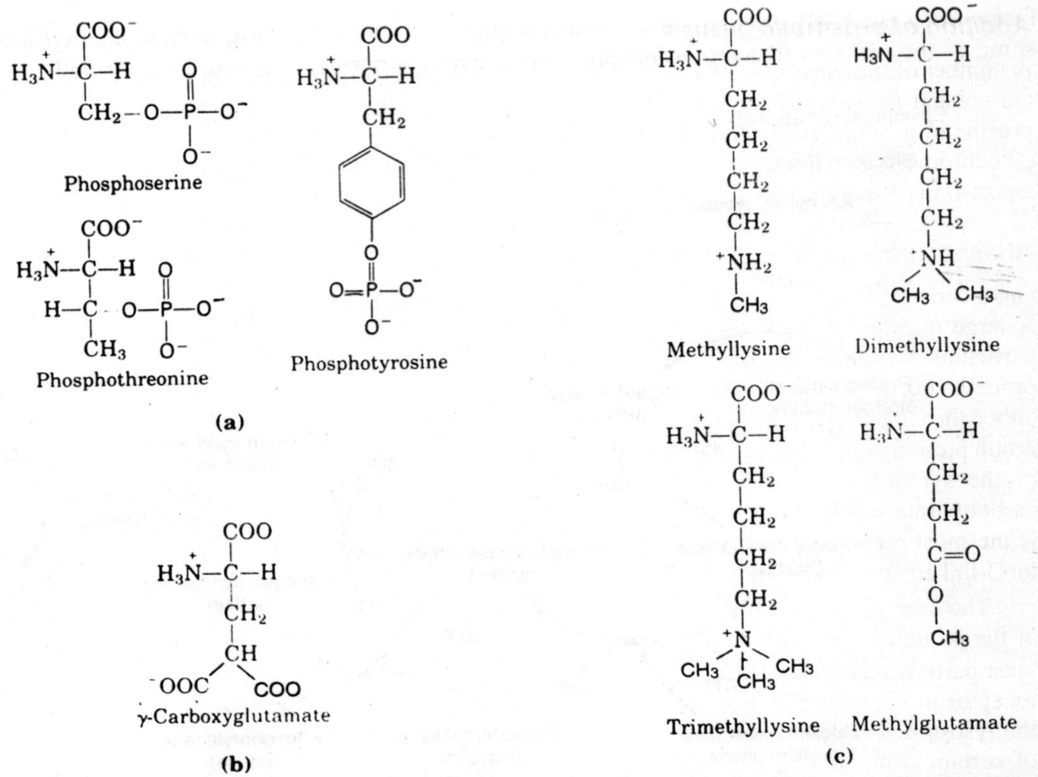

Fig. 7.41. Some modified amino acid residues. (a) Phosphorylated amino acids. (b) A carboxylated amino acid (c) some methylated amino acids.

biosynthesis. Fernasyl can later get converted to isoprenyl group. It has been found that isoprenylation of certain proto-oncoproteins (such as the ras protein) leads to oncogenicity. The blockage of this addition results in inhibition of carcinogenecity of these proteins. The study of this post-translational modification is of great interest.

The fattyacids can also modify some proteins. For example, N-terminal glycine residue of some of the proteins gets myristoylated through an amide bond. This addition is caused by the enzyme N-myristoyl transferase. Similarly palmitate, stearate and oleate can get attached to cystein residue through a thioester bond. Fig. 7.42 shows the attachment of a number of commonly present groups to the amino acids.

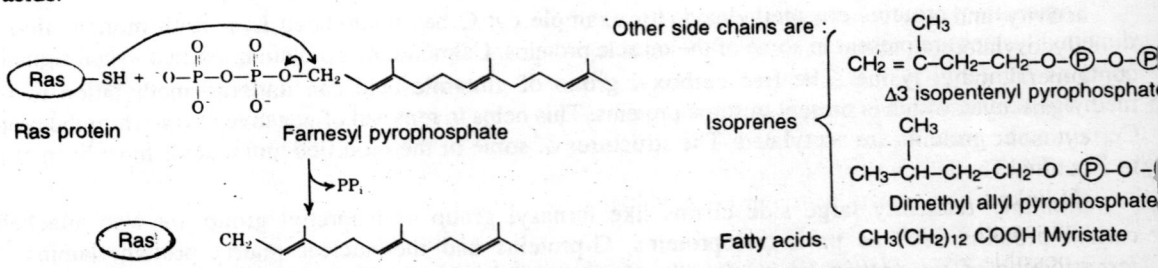

Fig. 7.42. Farnesylation of a Cys residue in a protein. The thioether linkage is shown; ras protein is the product of the ras oncogene.

Addition of prosthetic groups

A number of proteins, specially the enzymes, have prosthetic groups attached to them. These type of proteins are present in both eukaryotes and in prokaryotes. For example acetyl coA carboxylase has biotin as the prosthetic group, hemoglobin has Fe^{+++}, Zn finger motifs of DNA binding proteins have Zn^{++} and the cytochrome C has heme as their prosthetic group. The attachment of the prosthetic group takes place in a post-translational manner.

Attachment of carbohydrate moieties

One of the most important post-translational modifications is the addition of carbohydrates to the proteins. A large number of eukaryotic proteins are glycosylated. The carbohydrate moiety is very specific for a particular protein and is often essential for its biological activity. Glycosylation is a complex, multistep process and will be discussed separately in detail. In short, the oligosaccharides are attached to the proteins either through an $-OH$ group present in the hydroxy aminoacids such as serine and threonine or a $-NH_2$ group present on glutamine and asparagine (O-linked and N-linked carbohydrates, respectively). The initiation of the synthesis of N-linked carbohydrates take place in ER. However, further addition of complex carbohydrate residues and the addition of O-linked carbohydrates take place in the Golgi apparatus. Asn is the most common site for the attachment of a N-linked carbohydrate moiety. While serine is involved in O-linked glycosylation.

The carbohydrates play a number of different important functions. These include the correct folding of the proteins, blockage of sites where other unwanted macromolecules can get associated, protection (at least partial) against protease digestion, thus increasing the stability of the proteins and recognition of the receptor proteins by the ligands. For example, mannose-6-phosphate is recognized by receptor proteins in the lysosomes which shuttle back and forth between specific membranes. These also help in the transport of certain compounds, in cell to cell interaction and in molecular targetting.

Other modifications

A number of other post-translational modifications also take place, these include the addition of lipids to form lipoproteins and proteolipids, binding with nucleic acids to form nucleoproteins etc.

Glycosylation

As discussed, glycosylation is one of the most important post-translational modifications. A large number of eukaryotic proteins are glycosylated. Bacteria donot have the necessary machinery to carry out glycosylation which is an exclussive feature of the eukaryotic proteins. Ocassionally a few bacterial proteins may contain some simple sugar residues attached to them. Many of the hormones and other regulatory proteins are glycoprotein in nature. In these proteins, the carbohydrate moiety is essential for their biological activity and deglycosylation leads to loss of biological activity. Many of the membrane proteins are glycosylated. In these proteins the sugars are localised at the exoplasmic facet of the membranes. In general, majority of the proteins synthesized in endoplasmic reticulum are also glycosylated while very few of the cytosolic proteins have carbohydrate moiety. Further, when glycosylated, the carbohydrates of cytosolic proteins are relatively simple. The ER glycoproteins, on the other hand, are more complex in nature. The attachment of sugar residue is either at the $-OH$ group of serine, threonine and hydroxylysine (O-linked glycosylation) or with the $\gamma-NH_2$ group of asperagine (N-linked glycosylation). In general an aminoacid sequence Asn-X-Ser or Asn-X-Thr (where X represents any aminoacid except proline) represents a possible glycosylation site. However, the presence of this sequence doesnot necessarily means that there has to be the glycosylation.

The O-linked and N-linked sugars differ considerably in their primary structure. Usually the N-linked glycosylation is more complex than the O-linked glycosylation. The O-linked glycosylation is generally carried out in Golgi apparatus while the N-linked glycosylation is initiated in the ER where a part of the chain is synthesized. It is then tranferred to Golgi apparatus where the synthesis of the chain is completed. A number of simple and complex sugars are involved in the synthesis of carbohydrate moieties, these include mannose (man), glucose (glc), fucose (fuc), N-acetyl glucosamine (GlcNAc), N-acetyl galactosamine (GalNAc), and N-acetyl neuraminic acid (NANA or the sialic acid). The structure of these sugars in given in Fig. 7.43.

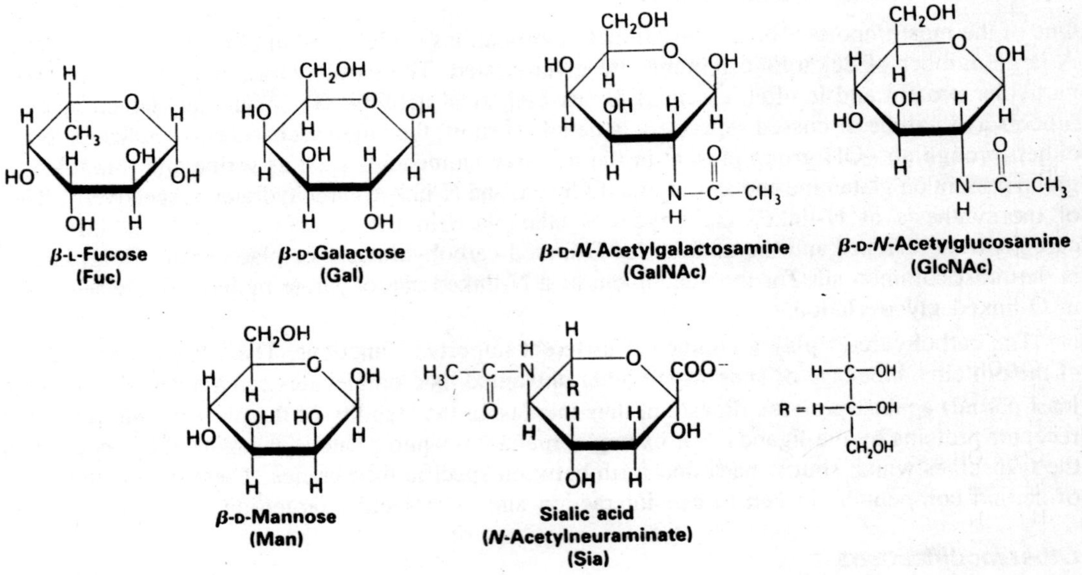

Fig. 7.43. Sugar residues commonly found in glycoproteins.

The sugars are generally not permeable to membranes of Glogi apparatus and can not be taken in as such. These are transported inside the Golgi in the form of sugar nucleotides. For example, mannose is transported as GDP-mannose, NANA is transported as CMP-NANA while glucose, galactose, GlcNAc and GalNAc are transported as their UDP derivatives. The structure and the schemes for the synthesis of common sugar nucleotides are shown in Fig. 7.44.

The entry of sugar nucleotides to Golgi apparatus is through specific antiports. Inside the Golgi, the UDP–sugars are converted to respective sugars and UDP is broken to UMP and Pi by the action of a specific phosphatase. The UMP goes out in exchange for the sugar through the antiport while Pi is transported out by a permease mediate action. The transport process is shown in Fig. 7.45.

O-linked glycosylation

The O-linked sugars are synthesized in ER or Golgi vesicles. The process is energy dependent and the energy is provided by the hydrolysis of the high energy intermediates. The addition of sugars is in a step wise manner and only one sugar residue is added at a time. The addition is catalysed by the enzyme glycosyl transferase. There are specific transferases for different residues. These glycosyl transferases are the integral part of the membranes and their active sites face the lumen of Golgi (or ER). While majority of the sugar

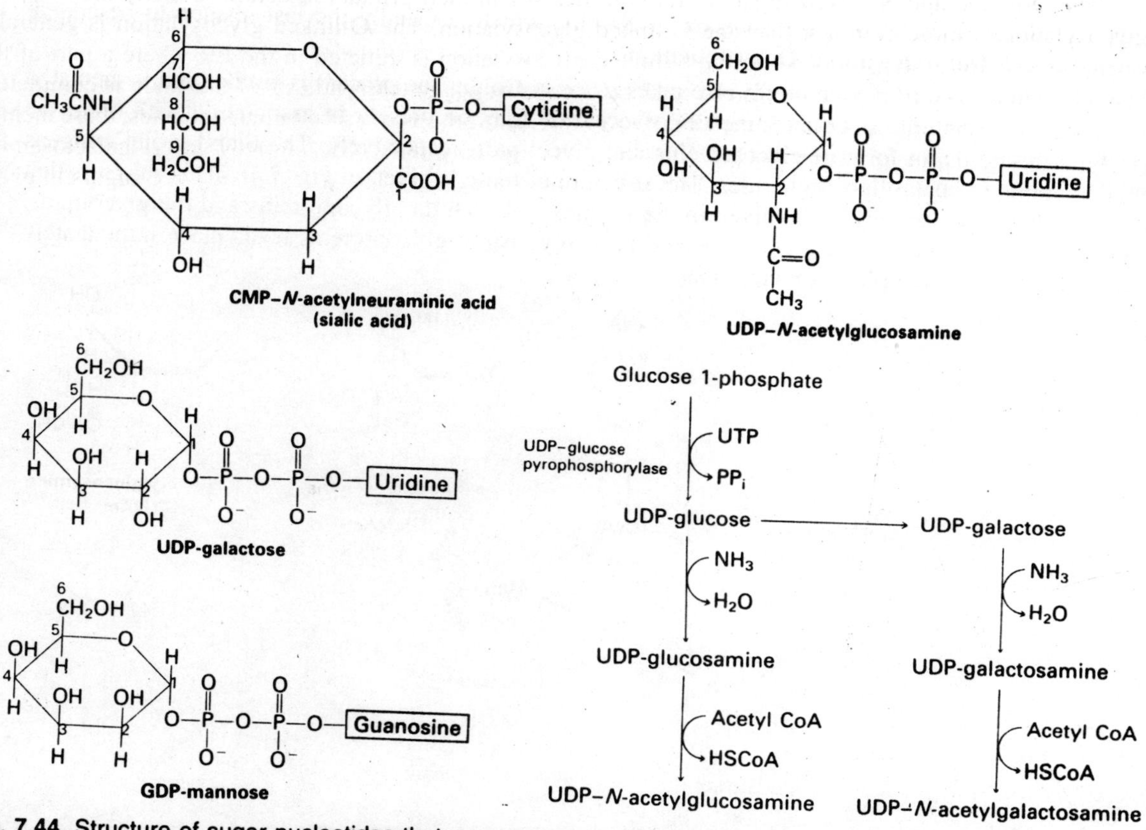

**CMP–N-acetylneuraminic acid
(sialic acid)**

UDP–N-acetylglucosamine

UDP-galactose

GDP-mannose

Glucose 1-phosphate

UDP–glucose
pyrophosphorylase

$\overset{\displaystyle\frown}{}$ UTP

$\searrow$ PP$_i$

UDP-glucose $\longrightarrow$ UDP-galactose

$\overset{\displaystyle\frown}{}$ NH$_3$ $\overset{\displaystyle\frown}{}$ NH$_3$

$\searrow$ H$_2$O $\searrow$ H$_2$O

UDP-glucosamine   UDP-galactosamine

$\overset{\displaystyle\frown}{}$ Acetyl CoA $\overset{\displaystyle\frown}{}$ Acetyl CoA

$\searrow$ HSCoA $\searrow$ HSCoA

UDP–N-acetylglucosamine   UDP–N-acetylgalactosamine

Fig. 7.44. Structure of sugar nucleotides that are precursors of the carbohydrate residues in glycoproteins and schematic outline of the synthesis of some sugar nucleotides.

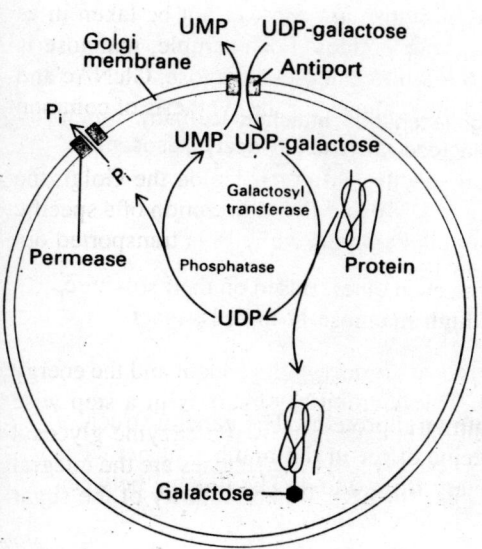

Fig. 7.45. The uptake of nucleoside sugars into Golgi vesicles, UDP-galactose enters from the cytosol in exchange for UMP, using an antiport located in the Golgi membrane. UMP is produced by phosphatase action on UDP, a product of the galactosyl transferase reaction. A permease allows the inorganic phosphate formed from UDP to exit the Golgi vesicle. Other known antiports allow CMP-N-acetylneuraminic acid to enter in exchange for CMP and UDP-N-acetylglucosamine to enter in exchange for UMP.

residues are added in the lumen, the addition of NANA, which is usually the last residue to be added, takes place in the trans Golgi and Golgi reticulum.

The addition of sugars to glycolipids also takes place in Golgi. The process is similar and is mediated through glycosyl transferases. Often same oligosaccharide may be present in association with both, the proteins and the lipids, in form of glycoproteins and glycolipids, respectively. The blood group antigens are good example of such oligosaccharides. The structure of these is given in Fig. 7.46. This suggests that same glycosyl transferase may be involved in the synthesis of both the glycoproteins and the glycolipids. The addition of carbohydrates to glycolipids and probably also to glycoproteins takes place immediately before these appear on the plasma membranes.

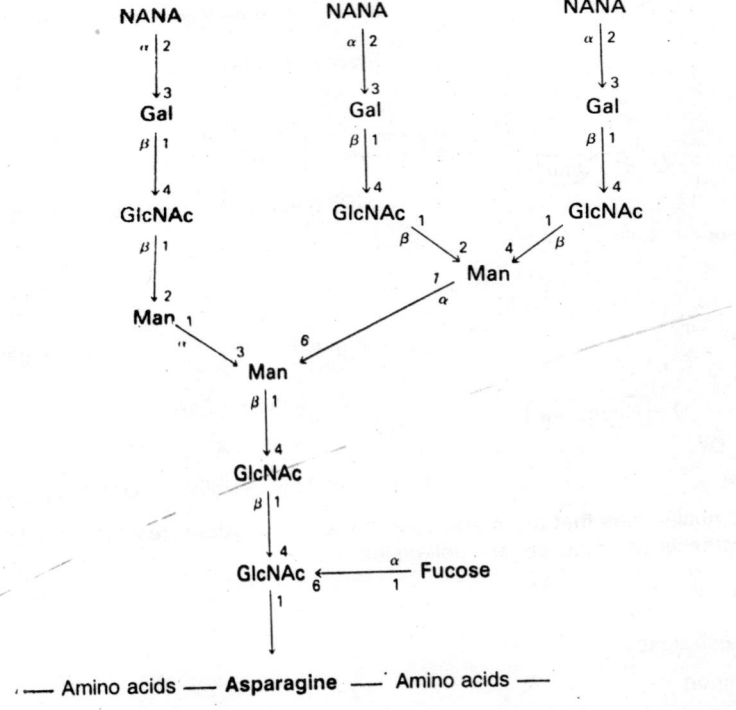

Fig. 7.46. The structure of a typical N-linked (asparagine-linked) oligosaccharide attached to many serum proteins, such as antibodies. (NANA = N-acetylneuraminic acid, Gal = galactose, GlcNAc = N-acetylglucosamine, and Man = mannose).

N-linked Glycosylation

The N-carbohydrate chains of different glycoproteins widely differ from each other. Based on their structure, the carbohydrates are referred as complex N-linked sugars and the high mannose N-linked sugars.

Complex N-linked sugars

These are associated with a number of serum proteins and with certain viral proteins. The general structure of these is given in Fig. 7.47. The sugars attached to different proteins differ in the number of branches associated with the chains. Also the number of sialic acid residues vary from 0 to 4. The linkage between

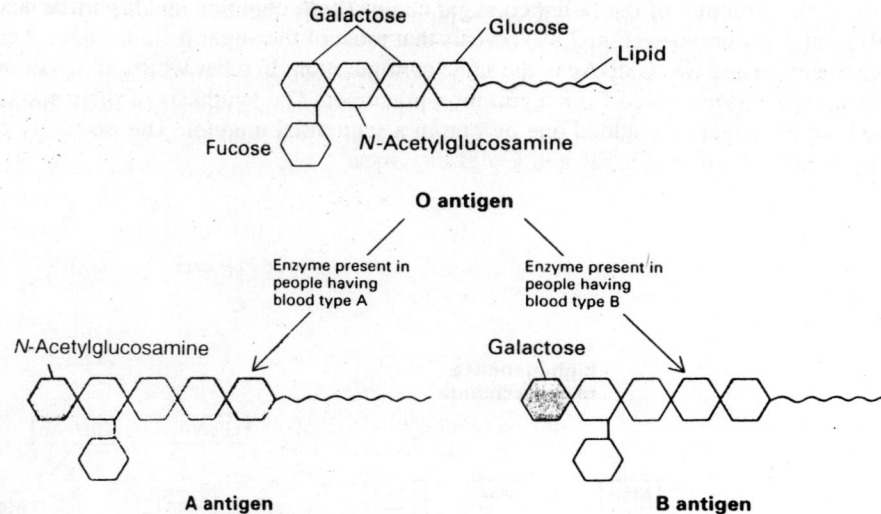

Fig. 7.47. The structures of the human blood-group antigens.

NANA and Gal is either a 2-3 or a 2-6 glycosidic bond. The branches thus formed, some times have a long stretch of NANA residues in place of only one NANA. The linkage between NANA in such cases is α2-8. In certain other cases there are no NANA but a stretch of repeats of a disaccharide, Gal-GlcNAc, joined together by a β1-4 linkage is present. All the sugars present in glycoproteins are neutral in nature except for NANA which is the only sugar moiety with a net charge.

High mannose N-linked oligosaccharides

Only mannose and GlcNAc are present in these sugars. The structure of a typical carbohydrate moiet is given in Fig. 7.48. Different carbohydrates of this class differ in the number of mannose residues present in the chain.

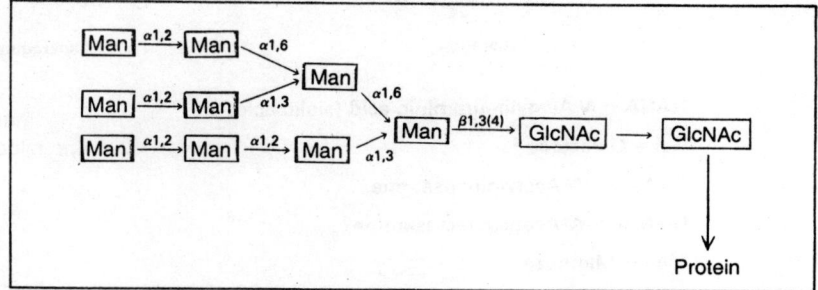

Fig. 7.48. Structure of the oligosaccharide precursor of N-linked oligosaccharides.

Many highly glycosylated proteins have sugar chains attached to more than one aminoacid residues. In such cases, the glycoproteins may have only one type of sugar associated to all the chains. However, some proteins have one type of chain associated with one Asn and another type of chain with different structure attached to a second Asn. Also a protein may have both O-linked as well as N-linked carbohydrates associated with them.

A careful scrutiny of the structure of the N-linked sugar chains (both complex and high mannose type) from a number of different glycoproteins (Fig. 7.49) reveals that most of the sugar residues have a common core consisted of three mannose and two GlcNAc in the same configuration. In other words, it can be assumed that all the N-linked sugars are synthesized from a common precursor. The synthesis of different sugars is a multistep process where the sugars are added one by one in a sequential manner. The assembly of these sugars is catalysed by a number of rough ER and Golgi enzymes.

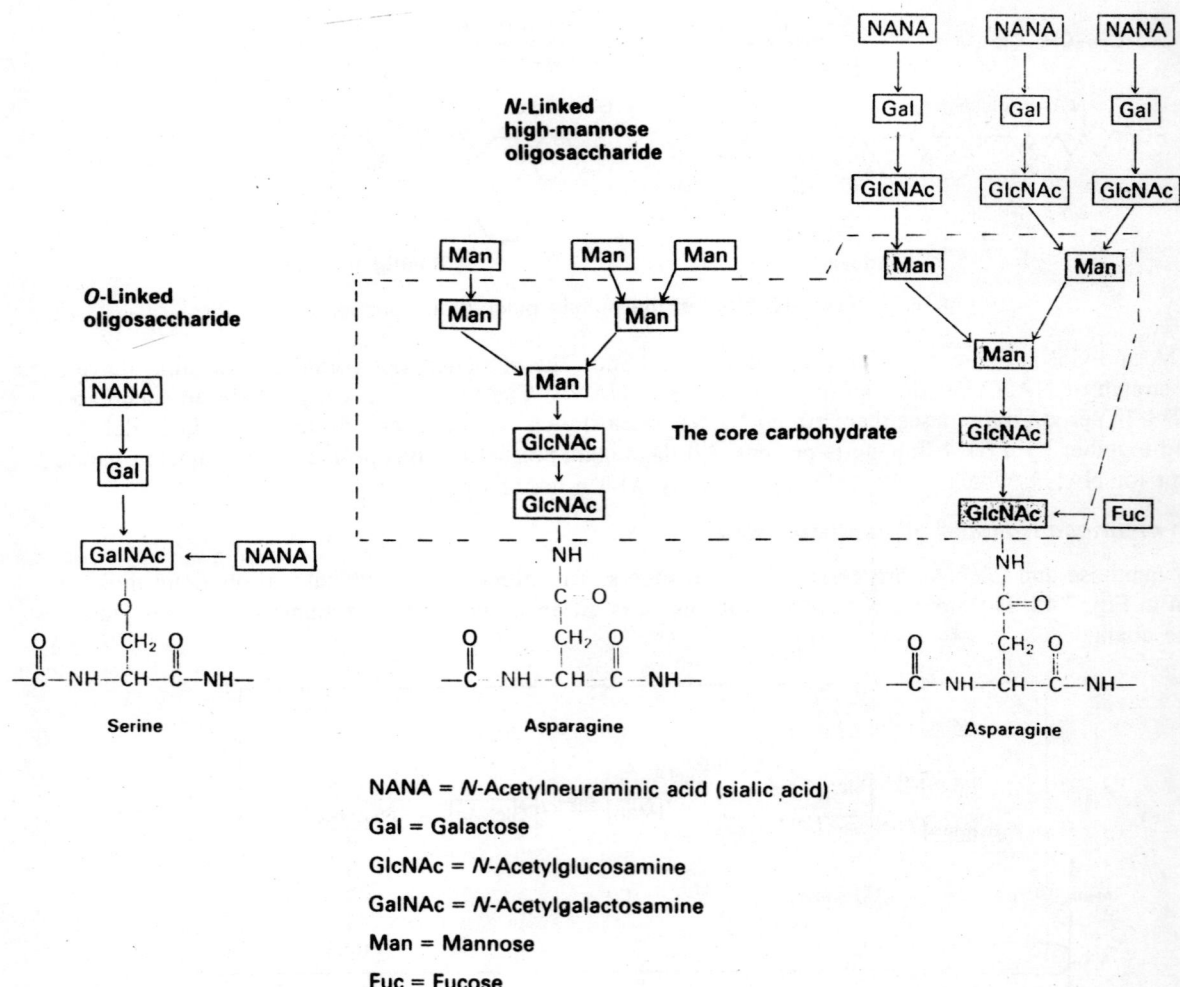

NANA = N-Acetylneuraminic acid (sialic acid)

Gal = Galactose

GlcNAc = N-Acetylglucosamine

GalNAc = N-Acetylgalactosamine

Man = Mannose

Fuc = Fucose

Fig. 7.49. Structure of typical N-linked and O-linked oligosaccharides. (a) Structure of the O-linked oligosaccharide, linked to serine and threonine hydroxyl groups, in proteins such as glycoprotein and the LDL receptor. As shown here, one negatively charged N-acetylneuraminic acid (sialic acid) is attached to the galactose and one is attached to the N-acetylgalactosamine, although only one of these is present in some cases. (b) Structure of typical "high-mannose" and "complex" N-linkied oligosaccharides, linked to residues in a variety of mammalian serum glycoprotein as immunoglobulins. The five residues always found in N-linked oligosaccharides are in green. High-mannose charides can have a few as three mannose oligosa residues are as many as 60 in protozoans and yeast.

A complex lipid which is the constituent of the ER membrane, dolichol, plays an important role in the synthesis of a common precursor of carbohydrate chain which is also referred as the core carbohydrate. Dolichol is a long chain polyunsaturated lipid containing 75-95 carbon atoms. Its structure is given in Fig. 7.50. Dolichol is present in an embeded form in the ER membrane and is large enough so that it criss-

Long chain polymers of isoprene

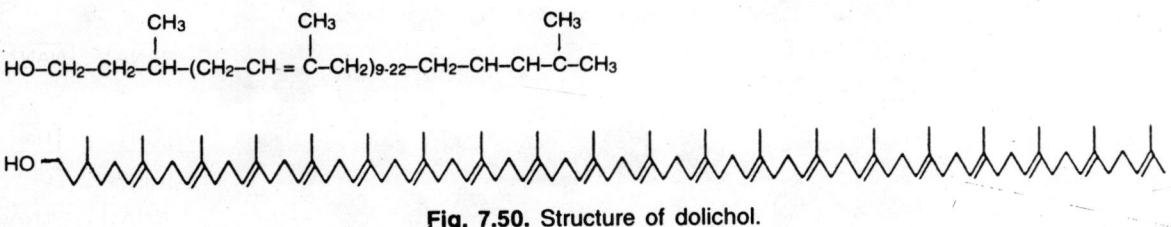

HO–CH2–CH2–CH–(CH2–CH = C–CH2)9-22–CH2–CH–CH–C–CH3

Fig. 7.50. Structure of dolichol.

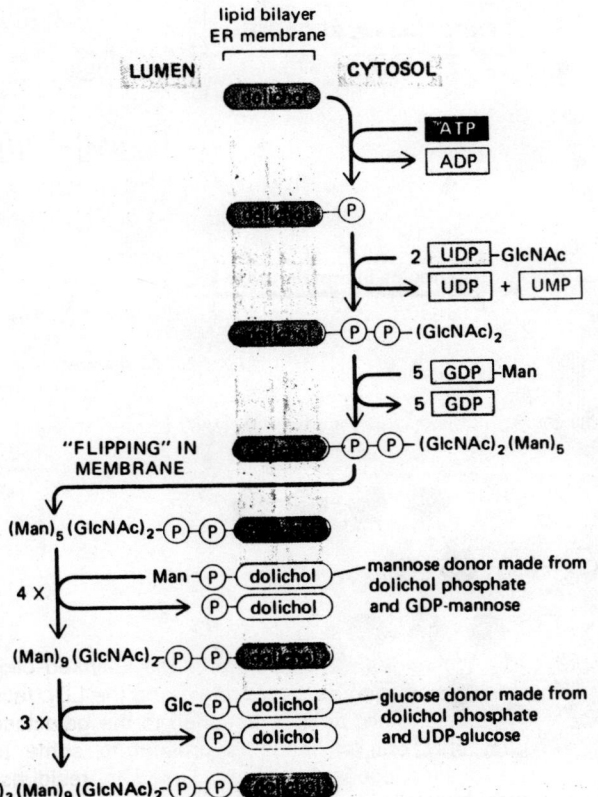

Fig. 7.51. Synthesis of the lipid-linked oligo-saccharide that is transferred to asparagine residues of nascent polypeptides on the luminal side of the ER membrane. The oligosaccharide is assembled sugar by sugar onto the carrier lipid dolichol, to which the first sugar is linked by a pyrophosphate bridge. The high-energy bond activates the oligosaccharide for its transfer from the lipid to an asparagine side chain. The synthesis of the oligosaccharide starts on the cytosolic side of the ER membrane and continues on the luminal face after the Man5-GlcNAc2 lipid intermediate is flipped across the bilayer. All of the glycosyl transfer reactions on the luminal side of the ER involve transfers from dolichol-P-glucose and dolichol-P-mannose. These activated, lipid-linked monosaccharides are synthesized from dolichol phosphate and UDP-glucose or GDP-mannose (as appropriate) on the cytosolic side of the ER and are then thought to be flipped across the ER membrane.

crosses the lipid bilayer of ER membrane 4-5 times. It is highly hydrophobic in nature. To initiate the synthesis of oligosaccharide core, first an ATP molecule reacts with dolichol at the cytosolic side of the ER membrane and transfers its phosphate group to dolichol, forming the lipid phosphate. The phosphorylated dolichol

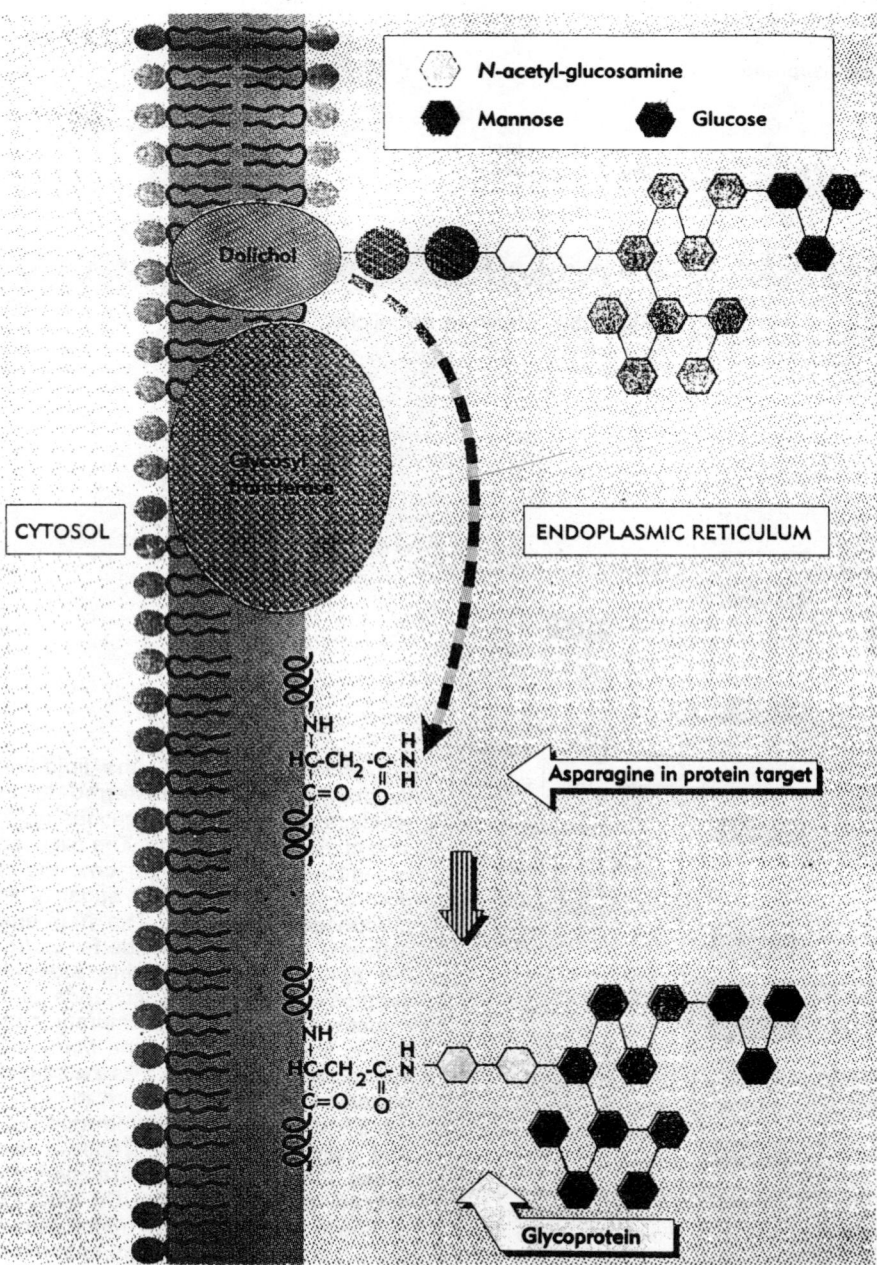

Fig. 7.52. Structure of core carbohydrates.

is the active form of dolichol which is now ready to receive the first sugar residue for the formation of the core carbohydrate moiety. The first sugar is always a GlcNAc, which is accepted as UDP-GlcNAc, UMP is given out and the sugar phosphate attaches itself to dolichol phosphate. The two phosphate groups (one from the dolichol phosphate and other from the sugar phosphate) form a pyrophosphate linkage between the sugar and the lipid. Further synthesis of the precursor takes place in a sequential manner and more sugar residues join this GlcNAc one by one. The addition of the sugars is on the cytosolic side of the membrane. These sugars are held together by glycosidic linkages. All these sugars are accepted as the nucleotide sugars, the nucleotide is released and sugar gets attached to the growing oligosaccharide chain. Another UDP-GlcNAc gets associated to dolichol-P-P-GlcNAc to form dolichol-P-P-(GlcNAc)$_2$, then 5 molecules of mannose get attached. Mannose is accepted as GDP-mannose. The dolichol-P-P-(GlcNAc)$_2$-(Man)$_5$ then flip-flops. The carbohydrate chain which was until now facing the cytosolic side, will now onward face the lumen side of the membrane. Further additions of the sugars take place on the lumen side of ER. For each addition the activated sugar is first accepted by a different dolichol molecule which carries it to the growing oligosaccharide chain and transfers it there. By a series of these transfers the complete core carbohydrate, which is the precursor molecule, is formed (Fig. 7.51). The core carbohydrate is madeup of 14 sugar residues, namely, 2 GlcNAc, 9 Man and 3 Glc residues in a highly defined sequence. As described earlier, the first GlcNAc is attached to lipid by a pyrophosphate bond and is joined to second GlcNAc which is joined to one Man. This mannose is joined to two mannoses forming a branch. Other mannoses are joined to these two mannoses. Glucose is attached to only one of the branch (Fig. 7.52). The whole carbohydrate molecule is present in the lumen of the ER. Once synthesized, the core oligosaccharide is transferred as a single unit to Asn in the target protein by the enzyme glycosyl transferase (Fig. 7.53). Glycosyl transferase is a membrane bound enzyme present in the ER. The attachment of carbohydrate to protein is through the free amino group of Asn. Further modification of core oligosaccharide takes place only after it has been attached to the target protein.

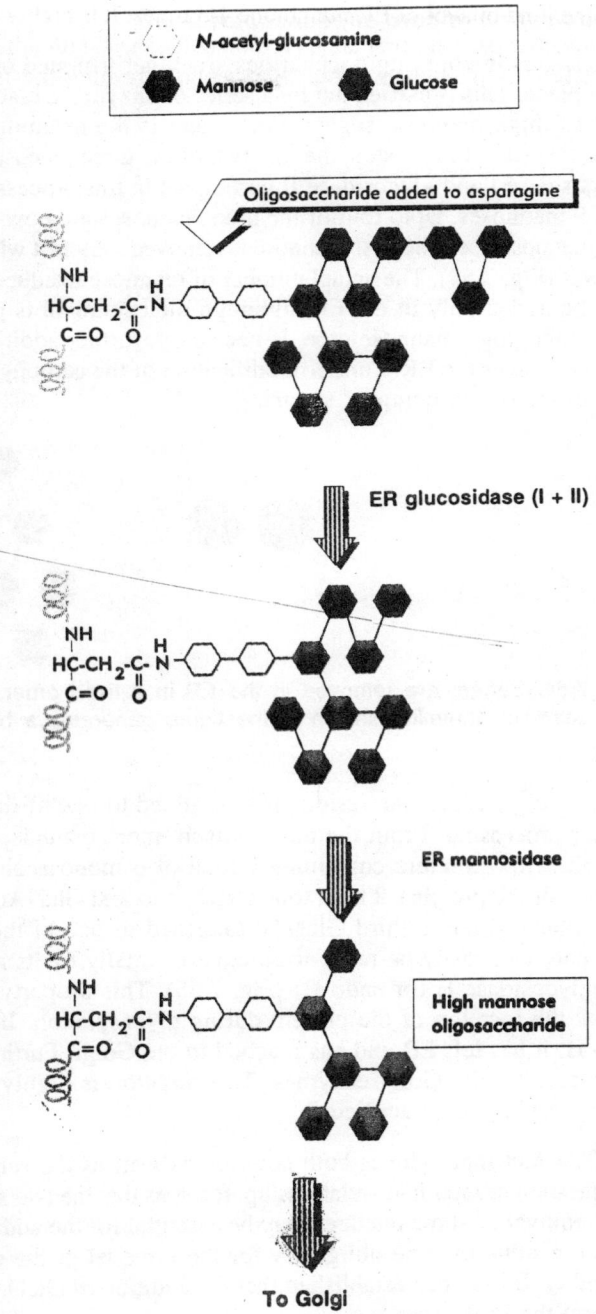

Fig. 7.53. An oligosaccharide is formed on dolichol and transferred by glycosyl transferase to asparagine of a target protein.

Modification of core oligosaccharide

The sugars in core oligosaccharides are either trimmed or other residues are added to it or both processes take place. This is carried out by a series of enzymatic reactions. The process is different for complex sugars and for high mannose sugars. First, there is the trimming of the sugars. The trimming in the ER is in a specific order. In first step, the removal of the three glucose residues takes place. Two different glucosidases, glucosidase I and glucosidase II participate in this process. The oligosaccharide at this stage has 2 GlcNAc and 9 mannoses. Upto four of the nine mannoses are now trimmed by the action of one of the ER enzymes, the mannosidase. The first mannose is removed very fast while the removal of subsequent residues is relatively slower (Fig. 7.54). The actual number of mannose residues varies from protein to protein. Mannose residues can be added only in the ER, although their removal is possible in Golgi also. The oligosaccharide is, at this stage, high mannose type. If necessary, further addition of mannose residues takes place and then the protein leaves the ER. Further modification of the carbohydrate moiety takes place only if the sugar is going to be one of the complex sugars.

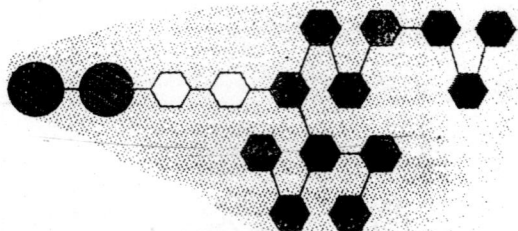

Fig. 7.54. Sugars are removed in the ER in a fixed order, initially comprising 3 glucose and 1-4 mannose residues. The trimming shown in the figure generates a high mannose oligosaccharide.

In Golgi, a GlcNAc residue is first added to one of the mannoses. The addition of this sugar triggers further processing. From the other branch, more mannoses are removed until a total of only 3 mannoses are left. This structure containing a total of 6 monosaccharides, 2 GlnNAc (one of which is attached to the Asn of the protein), 3 Man (one attached to 2nd GlcNAc and other two attached to this mannose forming two branches) and a third GlcNAc (attached to one of the mannose branch) is known as the inner core. This core can easily be recognized experimentally by its resistance to one of the glycosidic enzymes, the endoglycosidase H (or endo H) (Fig. 7.55). This property of resistance to endo H is used as a marker to follow the location of the protein during glycosylation. If the glycoprotein is resistant to degradation by endo H, it has left ER and has reached to the Golgi. Further addition of other residues takes place on this inner core by the Golgi enzymes. This addition is highly ordered. The residues which are added at this stage are Gal, sialic acid etc.

The fact that there is both addition as well as the removal of the sugar residues in the Golgi, raises the question of their inter-relationship. It seems that the two sets of reactions are corelated and inter-dependent. The removal of some residues may be essential for the addition of the other residues. Similarly the addition of one residue may be obligatory for the removal of the other residues, as is clear from the sequence of assembly. It has been established that the addition of GlcNAc is required for the removal of other mannoses to form the inner core.

Golgi has a very organised structure consisted of a series of stacks. Each stack is made of 4 or more (upto 8) cisternae. The Golgi apparatus is madeup of a number of compartments. These compartments are known as cis, medial, trans and trans-Golgi network (TGN), respectively. There is a type of polarity in all these compartments. The cis side of the Golgi faces the ER while the trans side faces the plasma membrane

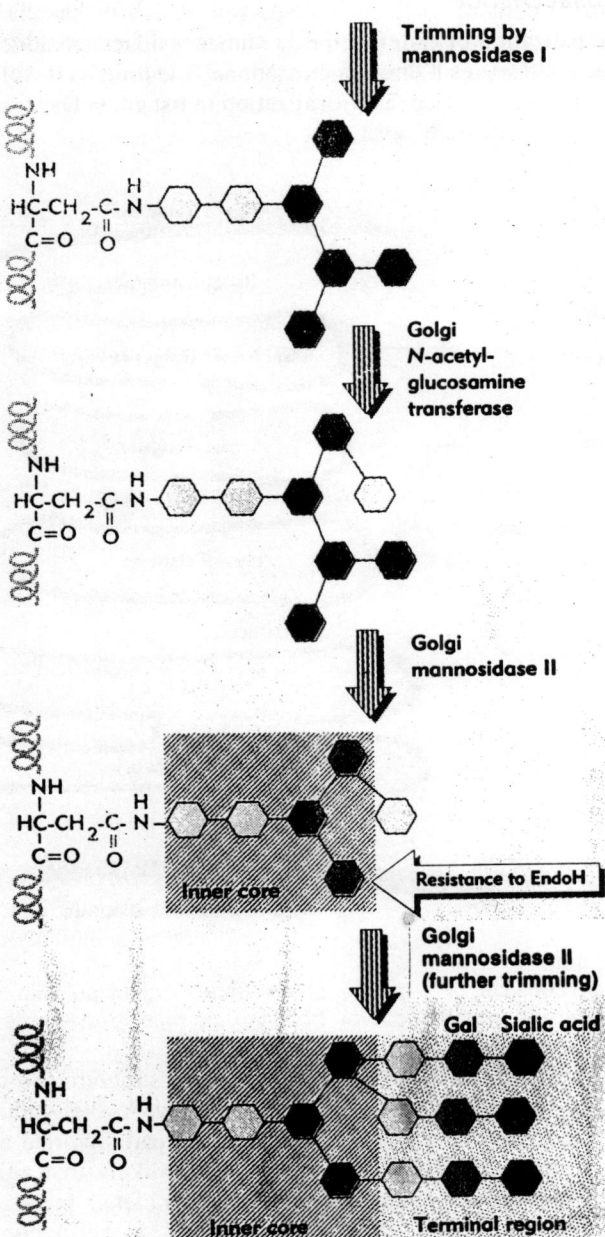

Fig. 7.55. Processing for a complex oligosaccharide occurs in the Golgi and trims the original preformed unit to the inner core consisting of 2 N-acetyl-glucosamine and 3 mannose residues. N-acetyl-glucosamine must be added before the final mannose residues can be removed. Other sugars can be added later in the order in which the transfer enzymes are encountered, to generate a terminal region containing N-acetyl-glucosamine, galactose, and sialic acid.

(Fig. 7.56). The molecular structure of the membrane changes across the folds of the Golgi apparatus. There is an increasing cholesterol content from cis to trans side which makes cis to be the heaviest and trans to be the lightest. The localization of different Golgi enzymes differs in different parts. The protein enters the Golgi from the cis face and leaves it through the trans face. During its travel inside the Golgi, the addition and removal of various sugars take place. The localization of the enzymes and the sequence of glycoprotein processing are in agreement with each other.

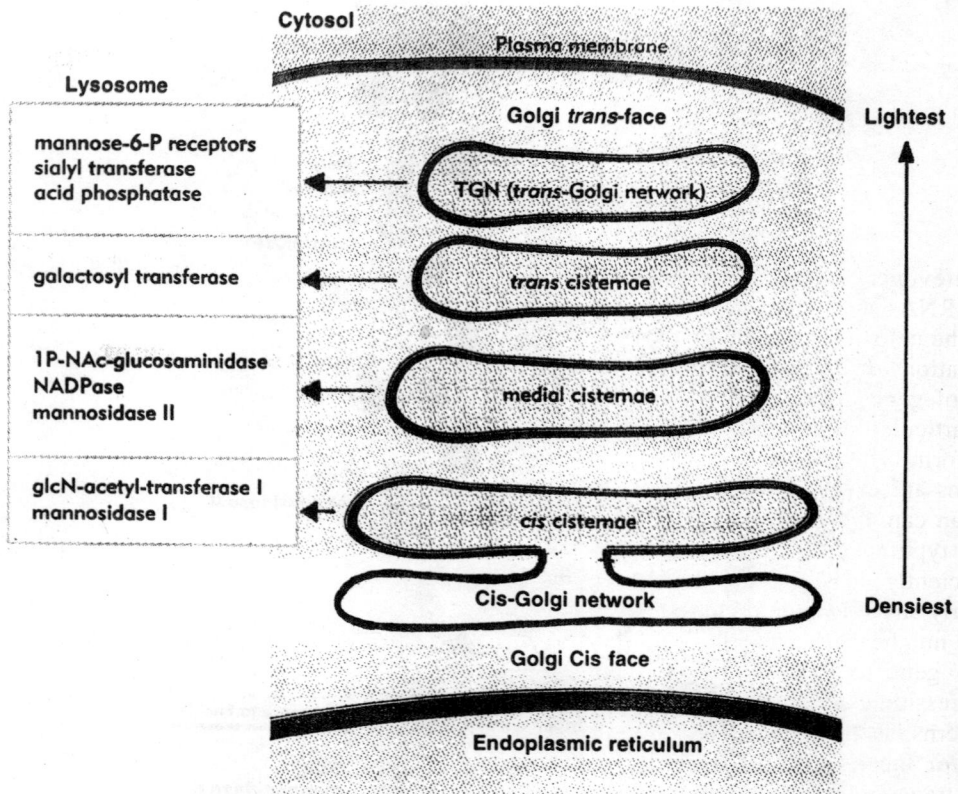

Fig. 7.56. A Golgi stack consists of a series of cisternae, organized with cis to trans polarity. Protein modifications occur in order as a protein moves from the cis face to the trans face.

It is not very clear as where the information for the sugar structure and their addition is present. It is very unlikely that it may be present with the carbohydrate moiety. As the synthesis of the core carbohydrates takes place on dolichol and then there is the transfer of this carbohydrate to the protein in an one step addition and all the proteins receive the same sugar, it is unlikely that either the dolichol or the core carbohydrate may be responsible for coding different sugar moieties present in different proteins. Early trimming for the formation of the inner core is also same in all the glycoproteins. It provides a strong circumstantial evidence that the information has to be present with the protein itself. However, the precise mechanism of the storage and transfer of the information is not understood.

8

Regulation of Gene Expression

In previous chapters we saw how the genetic information present in DNA can be expressed to form the RNAs and proteins. We also know that the genome of an organism is very well conserved and all the cells of an organism have the same genome. There are no cell to cell or individual to individual variations. It is therefore, logical to think that all the cells should have the same composition and same set of genes should be expressed in each one of the cells of any organism or all the individuals of a particular species. However, we know that it is not true. Different cells have different proteins and perform different function. This is because all genes are not expressed in all the cells, rather different genes are expressed in different organs and tissues. Many times, different cell types within the same organ can express different genes. Besides, the level of expression of different genes within the same cell type also varies. Sometimes this variation may be considerable. Some genes are expressed very efficiently and relatively large amounts of these proteins are made, while other genes are expressed poorly and very little proteins are formed. Further, there is also the developmental stage specific expression of a number of genes. All these specific and differential gene expression require very precise regulation. The gene expression involves both the transcription and the translation. The regulation of gene expression can, therefore, be either at the level of transcription or at the level of translation. The former governs the absolute amounts of translatable mRNA while in the later type of regulation, the translatability and/or the stability of mRNA is affected. In certain cases it may be at both the levels. However, the transcriptional regulation plays more important role than the translational regulation. There are a number of factors which affect the gene expression. These may be the 'cis' elements i.e. certain regulatory sequences present within the gene it self. The enhancers, activators and inhibitors are some of the examples of these elements. The regulation by 'trans' factors is more important. These include various protein molecules which bind to DNA and regulate its transcription. Some of these factors are tissue specific, others are dependent on the metabolic state and need of the cell, still others work in response to external signals such as the hormones and a number of other modulators of cellular functions. In general, the gene expression can be of two basic types, the constitutive expression and the regulated expression.

Constitutive Expression

The genes with this type of expression have their transcription taking place at a constant rate throughout the life of the cell. This rate does not vary with different stages of cell cycle. The efficiency of the promoter sequences is responsible for the relative rate of expression of the genes under this type of regulation. It has already been discussed that different promoters have different efficiency. For example, trp promoter of E. coli is more than three fold stronger than the tet promoter. The synthetic promoter, tac, which is the strongest bacterial promoter is more than 4 times stronger than the tet promoter and 3.5 times stronger than lac promoter (see Table 8.1).

Table 8.1. Strength of various E. coli promoters

Promoter	Strength (gal k activity)
tet	410 units
lac (UV5)	505 units
trp	1480 units
tac	1800 units

Regulated expression

In the genes with this type of expression, the rate of expression is the function of binding of specific regulatory factors to the promoter. These regulatory factors are usually protein in nature. Very few regulatory RNAs are known. These proteins (or the RNAs) are the product of regulatory genes. The regulatory proteins act in a 'trans' manner and play an important role in switching on, switching off and dimming a gene. A number of such control factors which affect the regulated expression of a gene are known. Different factors regulate different genes.

Dual control

Some of the genes are expressed in both constitutive as well as regulated manner. Through the constitutive expression of these genes, a certain level of protein is synthesized all the time, however, a regulatory factor changes the level of expression. How is it possible? One of the yeast genes, the HIS3 gene is a good example of genes with this type of regulation. In HIS3, there are two separate regulatory sites on the gene, each of which influences different TATA boxes of the promoter (Fig. 8.1). There are two transcription initiation sites located at the +1 and the +12 position, respectively. The first control site is dA/dT rich and governs the constitutive expression which is under the control of $TATA_c$. This uses the first transcription initiation site (at +1 position). The regulated expression, on the other hand, is controlled by a regulatory protein which is the product of the gene gnc4. The Gnc4 protein binds at two separate binding sites present in the HIS3 gene. These binding sites are made up of the repeats of a sequence TGACTC. The binding of Gnc4 to these site affects second TATA box ($TATA_r$) which controls the initiation from the +12 site. Thus a limited amount of HIS mRNA is always synthesized but Gnc4, in response to environmental factors, can stimulate its synthesis by several folds.

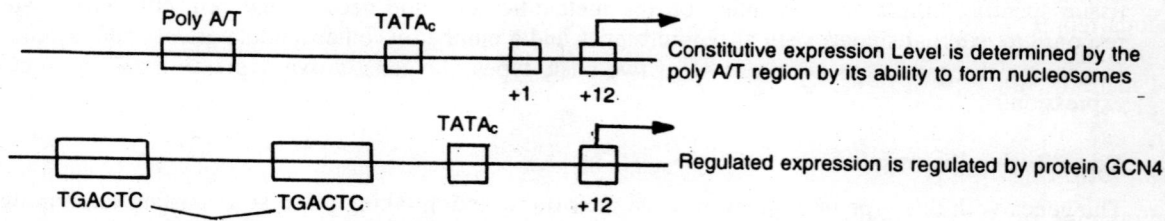

Fig. 8.1. Dual regulation of the expression of HIS3 gene.

DNA binding motiffs

Most of the 'trans' acting factors are protein in nature. Very few RNA molecules are known to have regulatory role. In order to exert their effect, these factors have to associate themselves with the target DNA molecule. The regulatory protein vary widely in their size, shape and confirmation. How does this interaction between the DNA and the proteins take place? Do the proteins bind to DNA? If yes, is it a covalent linkage. How this binding of proteins to DNA is achieved? How specific is the interaction? If only one of the two molecules (i.e. proteins and DNA) is responsible for the specific binding or both contribute to this specificity.

The analysis of a number of transcription factors have revealed that there are certain common structures present in all the DNA binding proteins. These structures allow the transcription factors (or other regulatory proteins) to bind to DNA. These specific domains of the DNA binding proteins are known as DNA binding motiffs. These motiffs are formed by a specific three dimensional folding of the proteins and facilitate the binding of the DNA–binding proteins to the target DNA. A number of such motiffs have been well characterized. The structure of some of the common and widely found motiffs has been discussed below.

Helix-turn-helix (HTH) motif

In this type of motif two alpha helices and a short region of the polypeptide present between these helices participate in binding to DNA. One of the two α-helices is known as the recognition helix which is involved in the identification of the target DNA sequences. Each of the two helices are usually 7-9 aminoacid long and are joined by a short stretch of polypeptide (upto 20 aminoacids long). This spacer polypeptide which lies between the two helices has a β-sheet type structure. The β-sheet turns itself in such a manner that the recognition helix interacts with DNA molecule and can bind to it, while the other alpha helix lies at an angle to it. The proteins with this type of motif are generally active in dimer form and always interact with the DNA at two sites. The distance between the two sites is exactly one turn of DNA helix (3.4 nm). Both recognition helices of the dimer bind to the DNA at the major grooves. Specific aminoacids in the α-helix can form hydrogen bonds with specific bases in DNA. Thus the binding site at the DNA have a twofold symmetry.

The activity of this type of proteins themselves is usually regulated by other small molecules. These control molecules can bind to the regulatory protein (with HTH modiff) in an allosteric manner and change its confirmation. As a result, the distance between two recognition helices can be changed which will, in turn, modulate their binding profile with target DNA. This binding of the regulatory protein to DNA regulates the transcription of the DNA and a gene can be turned on and off in response to environmental and metabolic status of the cell.

Helix-turn-helix was the first DNA binding motif recognized. Its identity was established in the lambda repressor molecules. Some other example of DNA-binding proteins having this type of motiffs are another lambda repressor, the cro-protein, many regulatory proteins present in bacteria, Drosophila and many of the eukaryotic transcription factors. The general structure of this type of motif is given in Fig. 8.2.

Helix-loop-helix (HLH) motif

The proteins with this type of motif contain two helices held together by a connecting loop. The helices are about 15 aminoacid each separated by the loop of 12-30 aminoacids. The total length of the motif is thus about 50-60 aa. Each of the helices is amphipathic in nature and has a hydrophobic region and a charged region. Very often the first helix is preceded by a basic region. Such proteins with basic

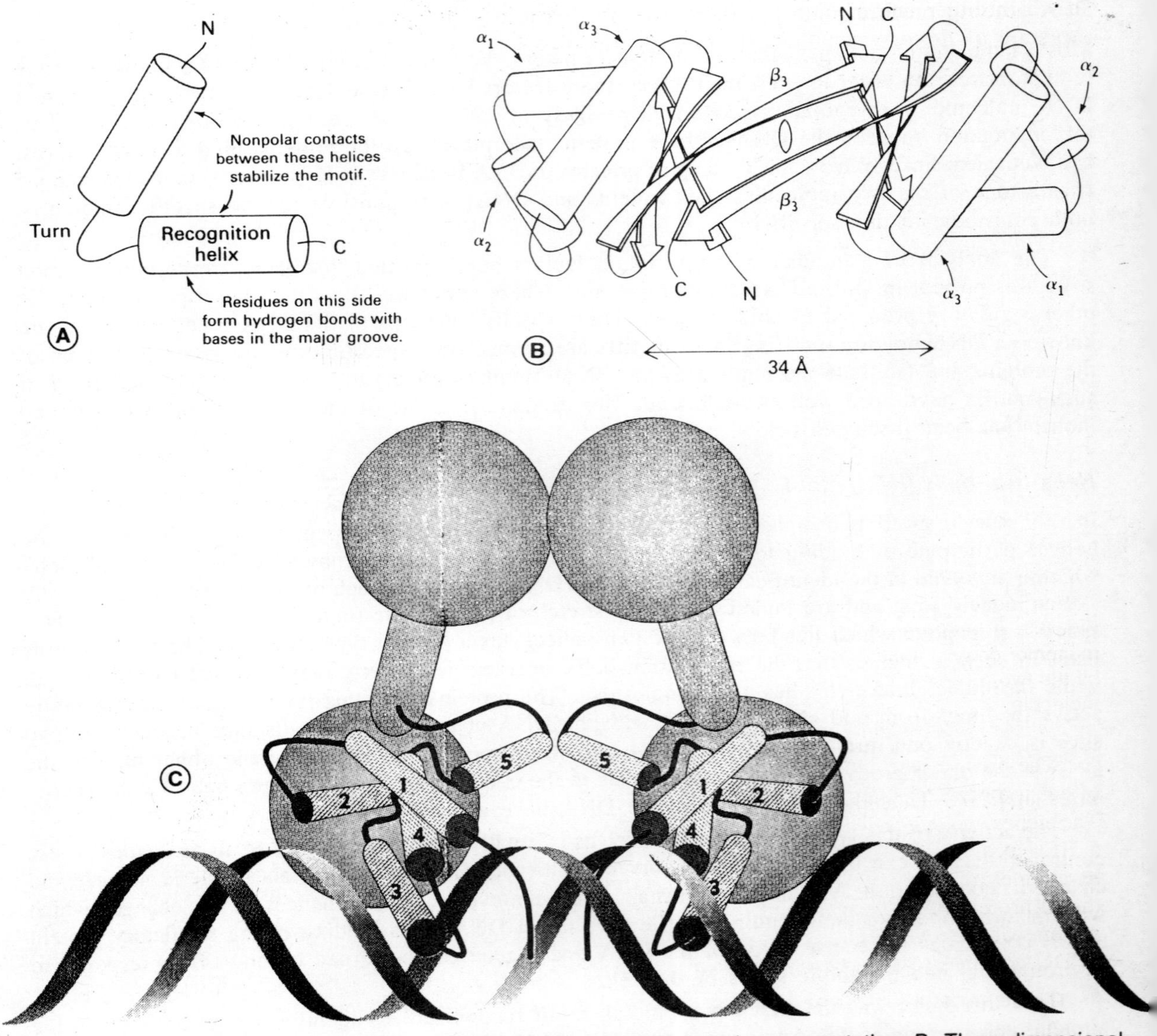

Fig. 8.2. Helix-turn-helix motif of DNA binding proteins. A. Diagramatic representation. B. Three-dimensional structure of cro protein, a dimer of identical subunits with HTH motif. C. Binding to the regulatory protein to DNA (λ repressor protein).

region are referred as bHLH proteins. These proteins are also active in the dimer form and very often the two monomers are held together in four bundles, each contributing two alpha helices which project from this. The dimers can be either homodimer or heterodimer. The dimer formation takes place by the interaction of hydrophobic residues on corresponding sites of the two subunit.

The basic region is often present in a stretch of about 15 aminoacids where ~6 aa are basic and are conserved. The basic region is usually essential for the binding of the protein to the DNA. A dimer in which either one or both monomers are non–basic usually does not efficiently bind to DNA. The structure of these type of motiffs is shown in Fig. 8.3.

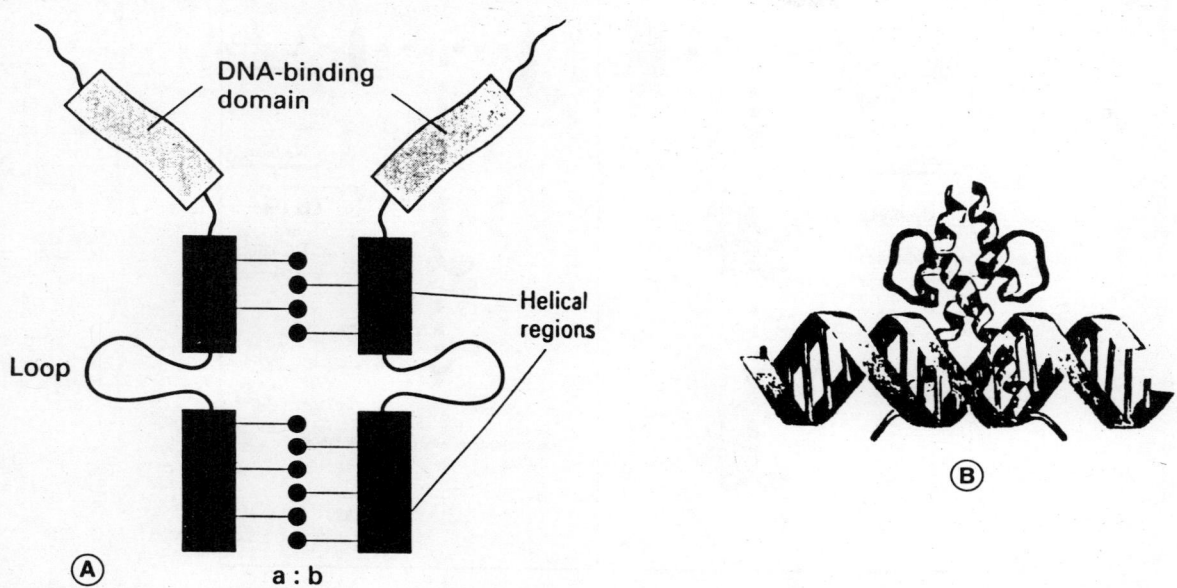

Fig. 8.3. A helix-loop helix forms a dimer. The two monomers are held together in a four-helix bundle, each monomer contributes two α helices connected by a flexible loop of protein. A specific DNA sequence is bound by the two α helices that project from the four helix bundle. A. Diagrammatic representation, B. Binding to DNA molecule.

The precise mechanism by which these motiffs bind to DNA is not very well understood. A number of eukaryotic genes which are expressed in developmentally related manner are regulated by HLH motif. The genes in myogenic cells are also regulated in this manner. For example, the over production of a HLH protein MyoD in certain precursor cells can initiate myogenesis. The trigger is switched on by a dimer of MyoD–E12 (both are bHLH proteins). Before the onset of myogenesis another HLH protein, the Id protein (without basic unit), binds to MyoD and/or to E12 and forms MyoD.Id/E12.Id complex. As one of the two proteins (Id protein) does not have the basic residues, the complex connot bind to DNA. This prevents myogenesis (Fig. 8.4).

These protein-protein interactions have established two general principals. First more than one proteins can associate together and this association may be responsible for the DNA binding characteristics of these proteins. Secondly, the association of two proteins with same type of structural motiffs (such as one basic and another non-basic, but both are HLH type motifs) may repress the activity of one of the proteins. The DNA binding of these proteins to the gene may either enhance or repress the transcription.

Zinc finger motif

These motiffs take their name from the shape of the protein which looks like a finger. In a typical finger a Zn^{++} radical is attached to four aminoacids located at such positions that a protuded structure is formed. The four aminoacid residues involved in Zn^{++} binding are usually 2 Cys and 2 His. However,

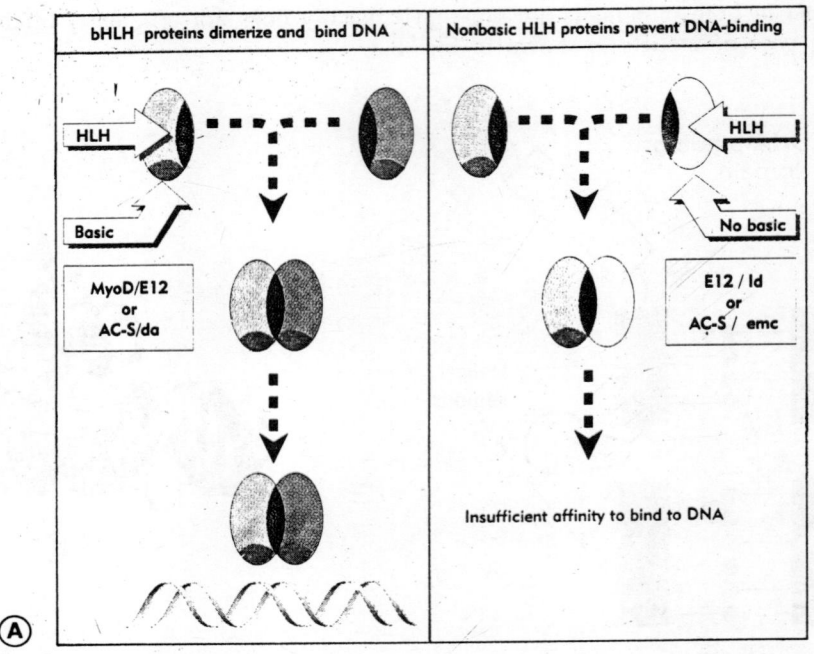

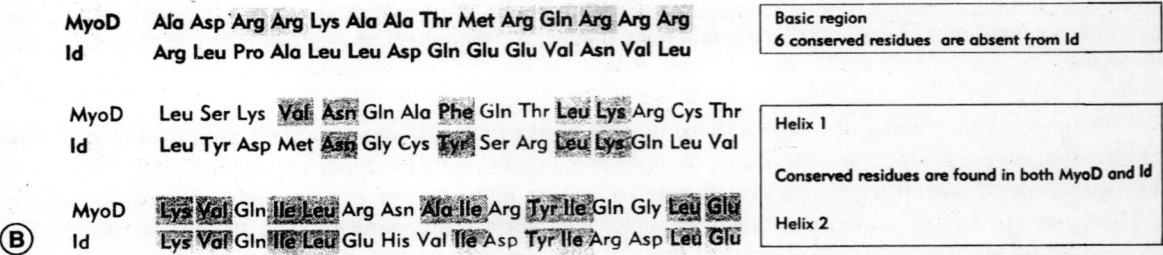

Fig. 8.4. A. An HLH dimer in which both subunits are of the bHLH type can bind DNA, but a dimer in which one subunit lacks the basic region cannot bind DNA. B. All HLH proteins have regions corresponding to helix 1 and helix 2, separated by a loop of 10-24 residues. Basic HLH proteins have a region with conserved positive charged immediately adjacent to helix 1.

occassionally 4 Cys may also be involved. Based on the aminoacids associated with Zn, the finger is known as Cys_2/His_2 or Cys_2/Cys_2 finger. The typical structure of a Cys_2/His_2 finger is Cys-X_{2-5}-Cys-X_3-Phe-X_5-Leu-X_2-His-X_3-His (Fig. 8.5). These residues are usually present repeatedly at regular interval and a finger protein contains a number of fingers. Usually a single finger is formed with 25-30 aminoacids and there are 5-8 aminoacids between two fingers. The proteins with this type of motif have any where between 2-9 fingers. However, if only one finger is present, it may not be a DNA binding protein but may bind to an RNA molecule. Very often half of a Zn^{++} finger may form an α-helix (usually the C-terminal part) while the N-terminal half may form a β-sheet. The α-helix can easily bind to the major groove of DNA. The α-helices of three fingers bind to a single major groove, each finger making two sequence specific contacts with the DNA.

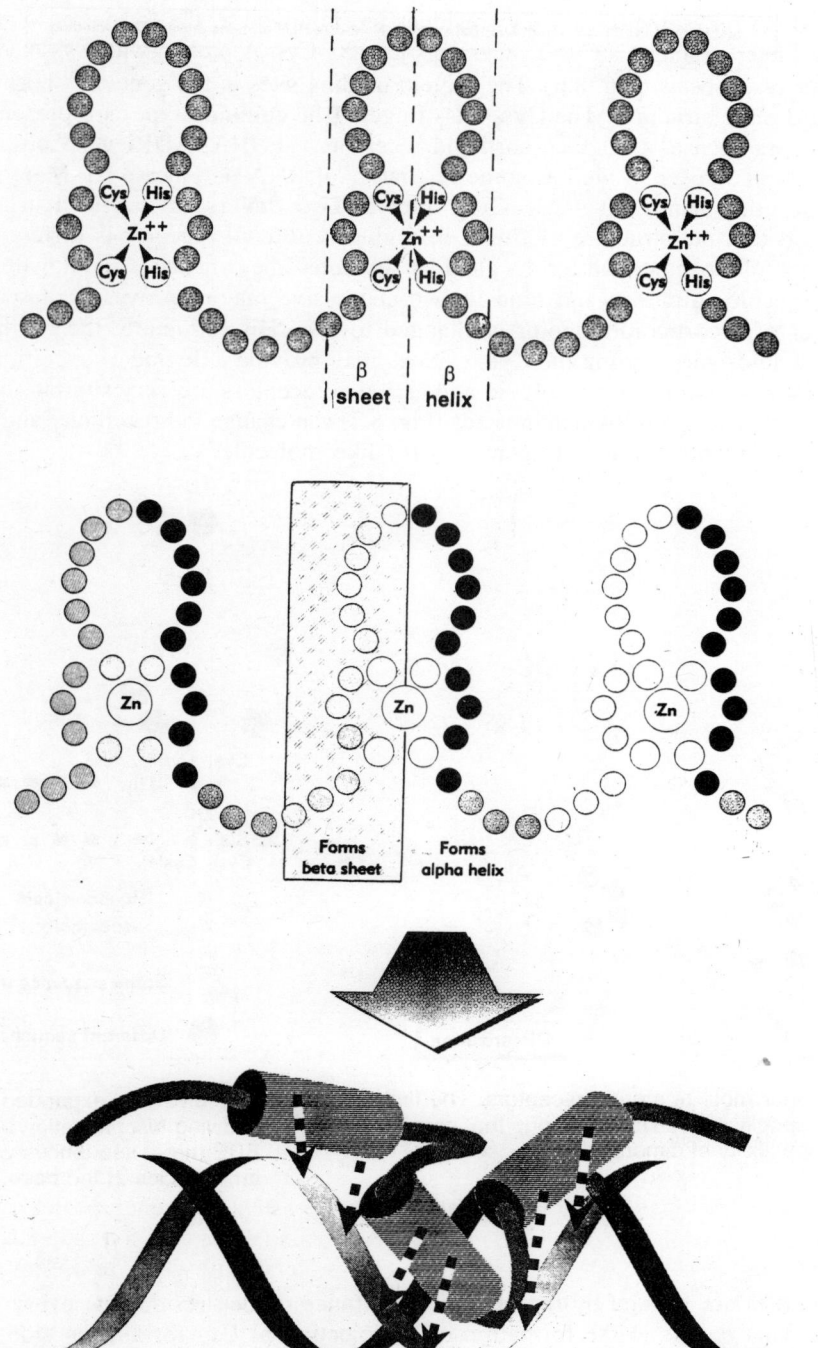

Fig. 8.5. Transcription factor SP1 has a series of three zinc fingers, each with a characteristic pattern of cysteine and histidine residues that constitute the zinc-binding site.

As discussed earlier, sometimes 4 Cys residues are involved in the formation of a finger. In such cases the typical finger structure is Cys-X_2-Cys-X_{1-3}-Cys-X_2-Cys. A protein with Cys_2/Cys_2 fingers usually have only one or two repeats (Fig. 8.6). The protein binding sites in the gene are short sequences which often have palindromic structure. The Cys_2/His_2 fingers (the common type) are present in a number of transcription factors such as the gluco-corticoid receptors, TF IIIA, ADRI gene product of yeast and gag gene products of viruses as well as some regulators of RNA polymerse III. Many steroid hormone receptors, on the other hand, have Cys_2/Cys_2 fingers. Two fingers are repeated in a typical protein. It has been found that the structure of finger in a gluco-corticoid receptor is different. The α-helices of both the fingers fold together and form a globular structure. The α-helices form a hydrophobic structure. Two protein molecules dimerise and bind to two successive major grooves. It has been seen that if Cys_2/Cys_2 finger of a corticoid receptor is changed to Cys_2/His_2 structure, the hormonal response is lost. Some aminoacids sorrounding the Cys residues may provide a degree of specificity. For example, the DNA binding motifs of gluco-corticoid and estrogen receptors are very similar and have a number of common residues. Change of two aminoacids (Fig. 8.7) can change the specificity and a gluco-corticoid receptor may be converted to an estrogen receptor like molecule.

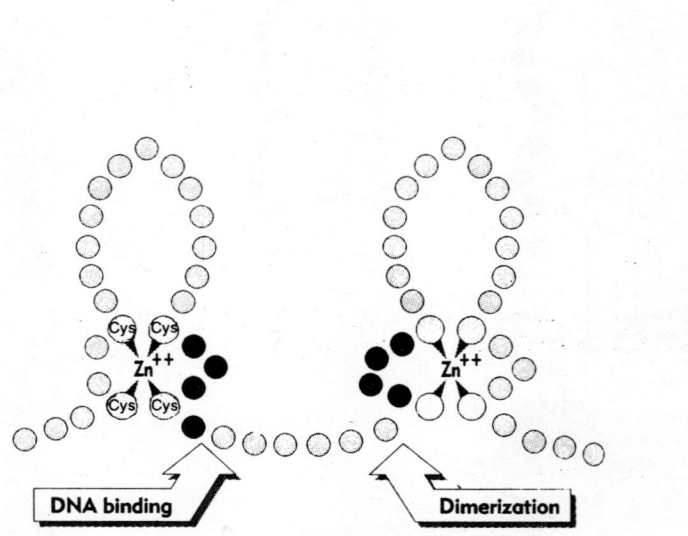

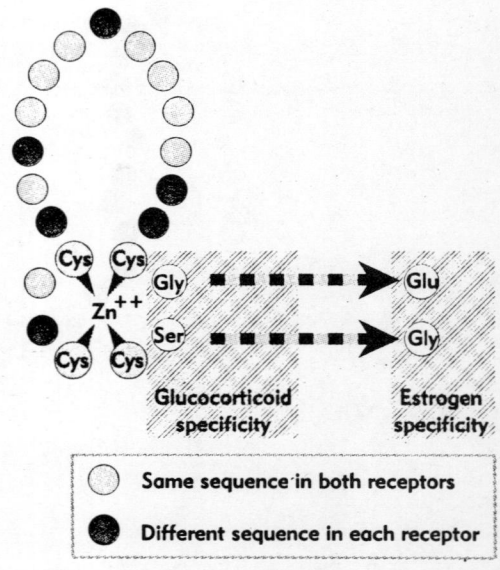

Fig. 8.6. Zn^{++} finger motif of steroid receptors. The first finger controls specificity of DNA-binding; the second finger controls specificity of dimerization.

Fig. 8.7. The expanded view of a finger showing discrimination between GRE and ERE target sequences which rests on two amino acids at the base of the finger.

Leucine Zipper

This type of motiffs are formed by the periodic occurance of Leu residues at every 7th position over 8 helical turns. This results in the formation of a projection of Leu residues at side chains at regular intervals. The leucine molecules are sorrounded by a region of basic aa. It has been found that the sequence of the basic region shows certain degree of conservation. A typical sequence is shown in Fig. 8.8. Two protein molecules with similar motiffs form a dimer where the leucine residues interlock with each other just like a zipper. The dimers may be either a homodimer or a hetrodimer. These zippers position the basic residues in such a manner that these can bind to the DNA and regulate its expression. Unlike other motiffs, in these motiffs, there is no direct binding of leucine zipper with the target DNA molecule but it folds the protein in such a way that the interaction of basic aa side chain with DNA can occur. These basic residues may form a scissor like structure where the DNA molecule is trapped between two arms (Fig. 8.9). The target DNA often has inverted repeats and the two arms of the scissor attach to these repeats. The CAAT Box enhancer binding proteins have this type of motif. Different proteins may have different number of repeats of these sequences. For example, SV40 enhancer binding protein has four repeats while Jun and Fos proteins (which are constituents of SV40 TF AP1) have five repeats. Some of the onco-proteins like C-myc and L-myc also have similar motiffs.

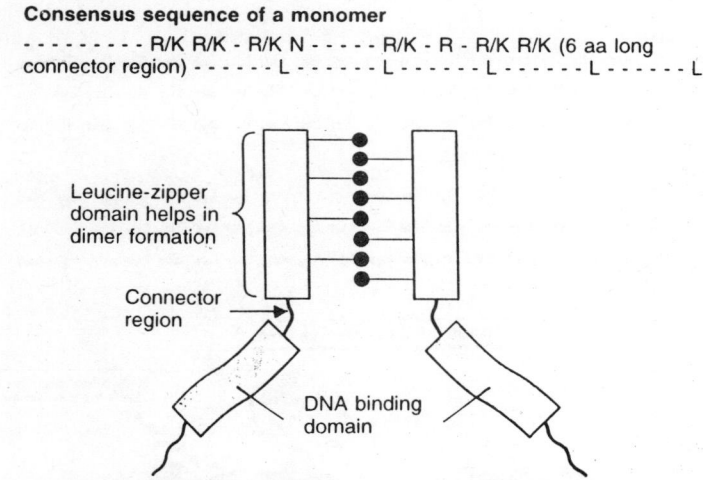

Fig. 8.8. Leucine Zipper motif of DNA binding proteins.

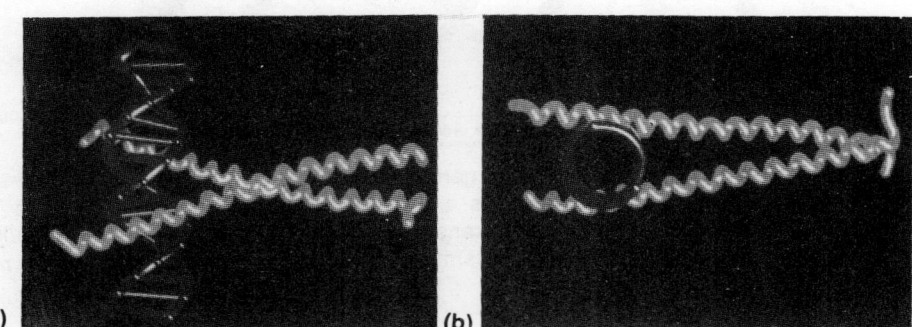

Fig. 8.9. The scissors-like structure of Leucine-zipper domain from (a) yeast Gcn4 with the two polypeptide backbones of the sub-unit C-termini of the dimeric protein and (b) The Gcn4-DNA complex viewed down the DNA axis. The dimerization domain in Gcn4 contains precisely spaced leucine residues. Some DNA-binding proteins with this same general motif contain other hydrophobic amino acids in these positions; hence, this structural motif is generally called a basic zipper.

Homeo domains: A sequence coding for 60 amino acids which was originally noticed in homeostatic loci of Drosophila, has been seen in many eukaryotic proteins. This sequence, referred as the homeo box, represents a DNA binding motif. Many transcription factors have this type of sequence. The domain has a homology with HTH type of motiffs. It contains three potential helices and a 17 aa long DNA recognition sequence which is responsible for the specificity of target site. The helices 1 and 2 interact the DNA on the outside of ds structure while helix 3 interacts with the major groove. The sequence of a highly conserved region of the homeo box has been shown in Fig. 8.10.

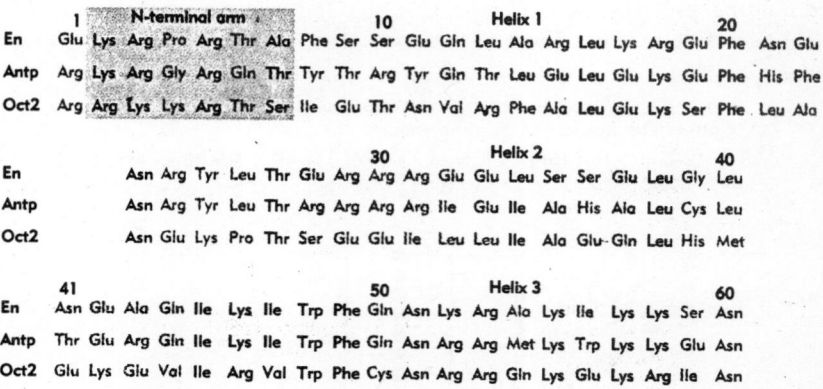

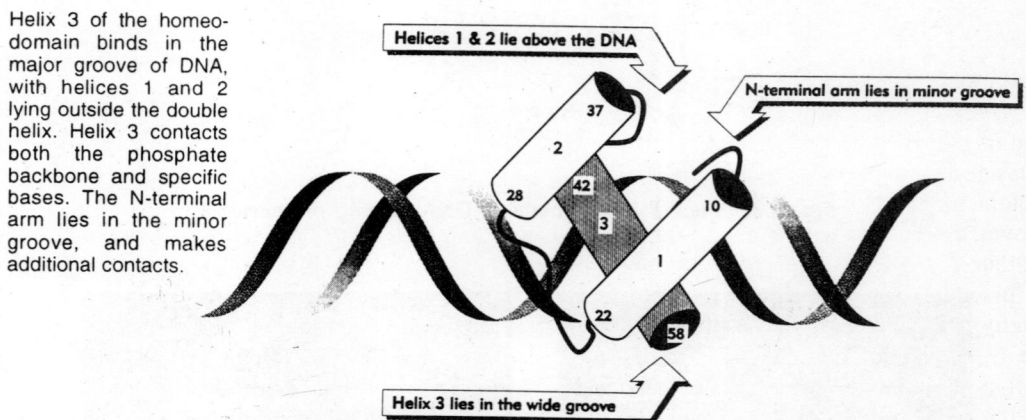

Helix 3 of the homeo-domain binds in the major groove of DNA, with helices 1 and 2 lying outside the double helix. Helix 3 contacts both the phosphate backbone and specific bases. The N-terminal arm lies in the minor groove, and makes additional contacts.

Fig. 8.10. The homeodomain of the Antennapedia gene represents the major group of genes containing homeoboxes in Drosophila; enlarged (en) represents another type of homeotic gene; and the mammalian factor Oct.-2 represents a distantly related group of transcription factors. The homeodomain is conventionally numbered from 1 to 60. It starts with the N-terminal arm, and the three helical regions occupy residues 10-22, 28-38 and 42-58.

Catabolic regulation of transcription in bacteria

Bacteria are very quick to adopt themselves with the changes in the environment. Their cell metabolism can be promptly changed to reflect these environmental changes. For example, it has been found that E. coli growing in presence of glucose as the primary carbon source, does not synthesize the enzymes involved in the catabolism of other sugars. This repression of the enzymes is referred as catabolic regulation of gene expression. It was observed that adenosine 3',5'-cyclic monophosphate (cAMP, structure is given in Fig. 8.11) plays an important role in such regulation. Glucose is known to lower the endogeneous levels of cAMP. The repression of catabolic enzymes is mediated through cAMP. Addition of exogeneous cAMP results in enhanced biosynthesis of these enzymes. In fact, cAMP acts as a hunger signal in both bacteria and in mammals. However, the mechanism of action of cAMP is different in both type of organisms (see later).

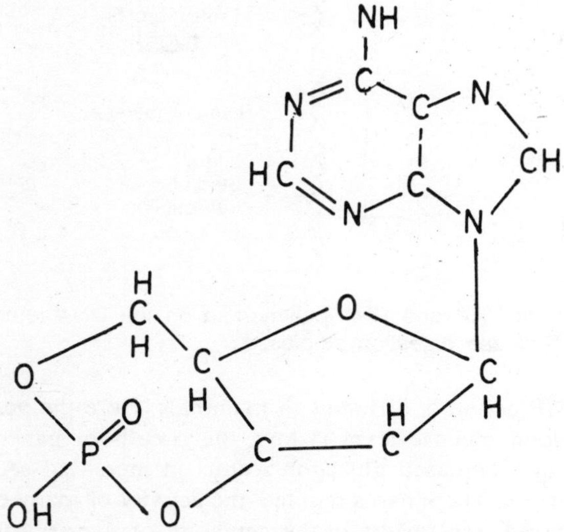

Fig. 8.11. Structure of adenosine 3',5'-cyclic monophosphate (cyclic AMP or cAMP).

The role of cAMP in induction of catabolic enzymes has been studied in great detail. During these studies it was found that cAMP can enhance the transcription of many inducible enzyme systems. A specific protein of 22KD has been identified in E.coli which binds to cAMP with high affinity. This protein, known as the catabolic gene activator protein (CAP) has two binding domains, one for the DNA and other for cAMP. Through its DNA binding domain, it can specifically bind to the target gene in the promoter region and can regulate its transcription. The site for CAP binding in the target DNA is usually present at the −87 to −48 region which is immediately upstream of the RNA polymerase binding site (−48 to +5) of the gene. The active form of CAP is a homodimer. The CAP is active only when it is associated with cAMP, free CAP is not active. It seems that binding of CAP-cAMP complex to the gene provides an extra site for the interaction with RNA polymerase, in other words an extra protein—protein interaction is possible. This protein-protein interaction between the RNA polymerase and the CAP-cAMP complex enhances the binding of the RNA polymerase to the promoter. This enhanced binding results in the enhancement of the transcription initiation and activation of gene expression (Fig. 8.12).

However, the CAP binding site is not always next to RNA polymerase binding site. It may be present within the promoter region as in case of gal operon (−50 to −23), when it is in close contact with RNA polymerase. In certain other cases, like in ara operon, it is further upstream (−107 to −78), and another protein binds between CAP and RNA polymerace. In general, CAP can activate transcription either by interacting with RNA polymerace directly or with DNA in such a way that the RNA polymerace binding is facilitated. Both these mechanism may work together.

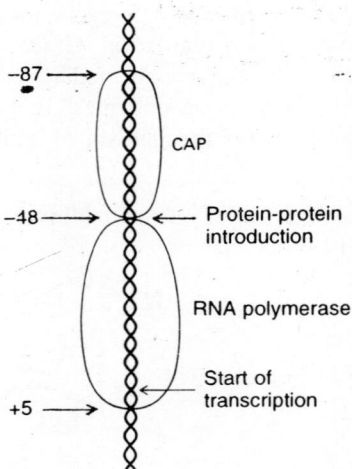

Fig. 8.12. Schematic diagram of CAP and RNA polymerase on the DNA template. The locations of these proteins were inferred from nuclease digestion studies.

The mechanism of cAMP action is different in mammals. Here the action of glucose is mediated through glucagon. When blood glucose level is low, the α-cells of pancreas are stimulated and the blood glucagon level goes up. Increased glucagon results in increased cAMP level which stimulates cAMP dependent protein kinases. The kinases regulate the activity of many enzymes by phosphorylation of the proteins. **The phosphorylation results in the acivation of liver phosphorylase and inhibition of glycogen synthetase.** This results in increased breakdown and decreased synthesis of glycogen. Thus, there is an increase in blood sugar levels. The entire cascade has been schematically represented in Fig. 8.13.

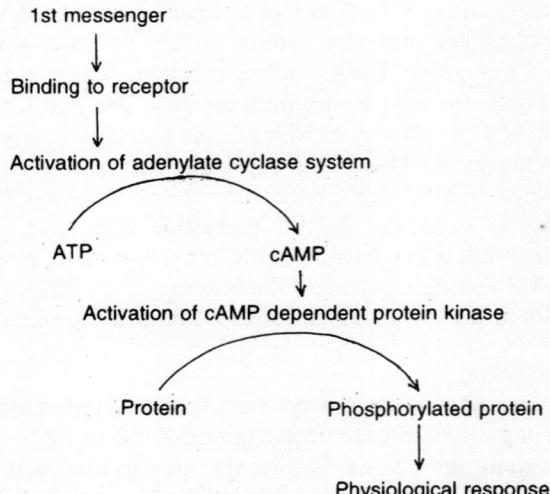

Fig. 8.13. The role of cAMP as second messenger in eliciting the response of various regulators through protein kinases.

The operon theory

During the studies on catabolic repression of a number of systems, many characteristic features of bacterial gene expression were discovered. Jacob and Monod studied the mechanism of these regulation in great detail and proposed a simple theory for the regulation of gene expression in bacteria. This theory, known as the operon theory, is based on the fact that the genes coding for the proteins having related functions are often clustered together. All the genes of such a cluster are transcribed as a single primary transcript in a polycistronic manner under the influence of a single strong promoter. These genes are thus regulated in a co-ordinated manner. This regulation is mediated through a regulatory element present at the begining of a polycistronic gene called the 'operator'. The operator can be defined as the naturally occuring regulatory element which modulates the function of a strong promoter. An operator is always present in close vicinity of the structural genes whose expression it regulates. The activity of the operator can be modulated by certain specific regulatory proteins. A regulatory protein is the product of a regulatory gene which is present either in a contiguous manner or at varying distance from the structural gene. The expression of the regulatory gene is under its own promoter and is independent of the operator region. The activity of this protein itself is modulated in response to cell metabolism. To regulate the gene expression, the protein binds to the operator. This binding modulates the promoter function. Entire gene system is known as the operon. The operon is thus made of three regions, the structural gene, the control region (operator and promoter) and the regulatory gene. The general structure of a typical operon is shown in Fig. 8.14. The regulation of the expression of the structural genes may be either positive or negative.

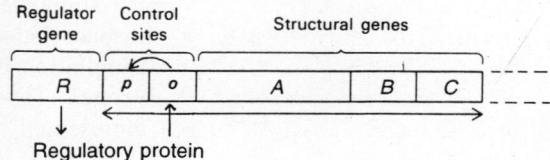

Fig. 8.14. General structure of a prokaryotic operon.

A number of different operons, each with different control mechanism, are present in bacteria. Following are some of the examples of regulation of such operons.

Lac operon

Lac operon is an example of negative regulation (repression) of the genes by a regulator (the repressor). It was the very first operon discovered and has been extensively studied. The operon is consisted of a multicistronic gene coding for three enzymes necessary for the utilization of lactose by the bacteria. The structural region is consisted of three genes, lac Z, lac Y and lac A, which code for β-galactosidase, permease and the trans-acetylase, respectively. The genes are under the control of a common promoter P whose function is controlled by the operator O. Upstream of P is the regulatory gene, lac I, coding for a lac repressor. The gene lac I is under its own promoter, independent of 'O'. Under normal conditions when glucose is present as the primary carbon source and there is no lactose in the system, efficient transcription of lac I gene takes place. This results in the synthesis of the lac repressor. The lac repressor is a DNA binding protein and is present in the cell in its biologically active form. The active form of the repressor is a homo-tetramer of a 37KD protein, which has very high specificity for the lac operon and binds with its operator. This binding is rapid and tight. The operator region has a 35 nucleotide segment which has a 28 base region with two fold dyad symmetry. The sequence of this region is shown in Fig. 8.15.

TGTGTG GAATTGTGAGCGGATAACAATTT CACACA

←—— 23 bp region protected ——→
by repressor

Fig. 8.15. The sequence of lac operator. The nucleotides with dyad symmetry have been underlined.

The protection experiments with DNase I digestion have revealed that the repressor binds to this region and protects 23 bases within this region. This binding of repressor down regulates the promoter activity and there is no transcription of the lac genes. As a result, none of the lactose metabolising enzymes are synthesized. However, when lactose is present in the system it acts as the inducer of transcription and the synthesis of all the three enzymes takes place. This has been diagrammatically represented in Fig. 8.16. The mechanism of induction is as following. The inducer binds with the repressor and inducer–repressor complex is formed. This inducer:repressor complex is biologically inactive and can not bind with the operator region. As a result, the transcription of structural genes take place and the enzymes are synthesized. The inducer can interact with the repressor which is already bound

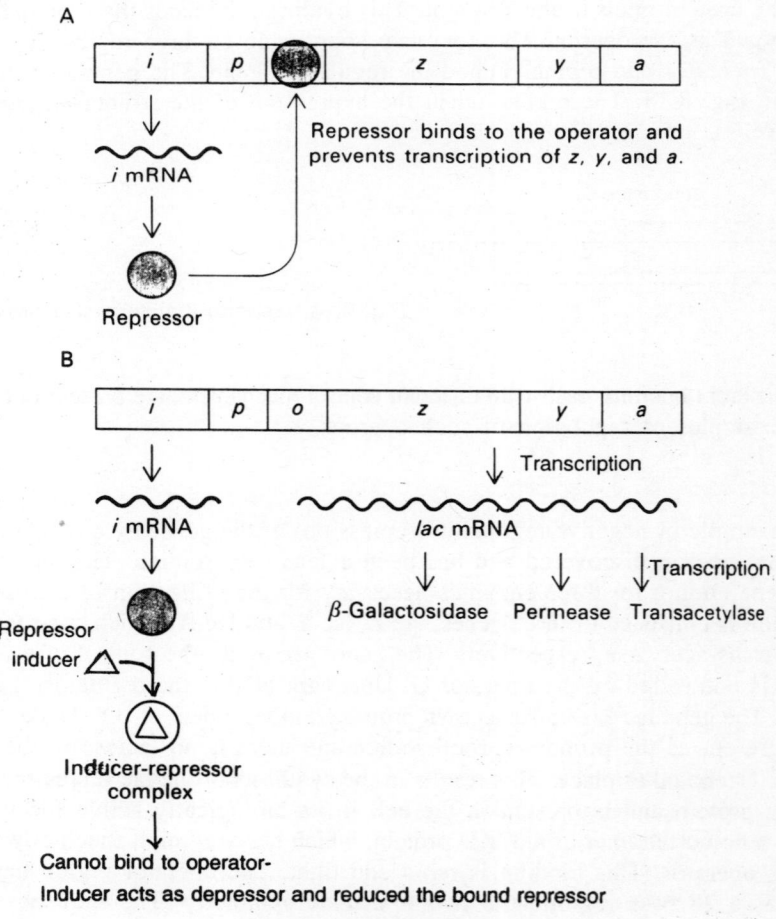

Fig. 8.16. The lac operon.

to operator region. This interaction will result in release of the bound repressor and activation of transcription of the genes. As the result of enhanced enzyme concentration, the lactose can be utilized by the cells. The induction can increase the enzyme level by as much as 1000 fold. An uninduced cell has an average of about 5 molecules of β-galactosidase/ cell, while induced culture can have upto 5000 molecules of the enzyme/ cell. If one follows the time kinetics of induction (Fig. 8.17) it shows that the increase in mRNA level starts within 2–3 min of induction. However, as the half life of mRNA is very short in bacteria, the levels go down to basal level immediately after the inducer is removed. Since the transcription–translation are coupled in bacteria, the enzyme concentration follows a similar profile for its enhancement (one or two miniute behind the RNA synthesis) but once synthesized, the concentration of enzyme remains elevated for relatively long time at the induced level (since the enzyme synthesized during the induction period does not breakdown immediately as the mRNA does). The role of inducer is, therefore, that of a derepressor for the transcription of structural gene.

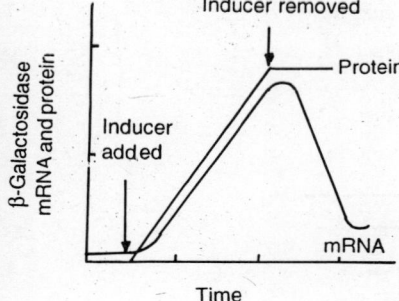

Fig. 8.17. The increase in the amount of β-galactosidase parallels the increase in the number of cells in a growing culture of *E. coli*. The slope of this plot indicates that 6.6% of the protein synthesized is β-galactosidase.

Lactose and one of its derivative, 1,6 allolactose, are the natural inducers of lac operon. However, there are certain analogs of inducers which bind with the repressor and de-repress the enzymes but are not recognized by the enzyme and are non-metabolizable. Certain other compounds can act as the substrate for the enzyme but cannot act as inducer as these are not recognized by the repressor. Such compounds are very useful in understanding the regulation of the system. Since the natural inducers get metabolized, these do not remain available in the system for long periods. It is, therefore, not possible to follow their effect. The non-metabolizable inducers, on the other hand, remain available continuously and their role can easily be studied. Isopropyl thiogalactoside (IPTG) is one of such inducers. (Fig. 8.18). It is not metabolized by the β-galactosidase but induces the synthesis of enzymes of the lac operon. It has therefore, been possible to study the mechanism of lac operon induction by using IPTG. As it can induce the enzymes without reacting with them, it shows that the regulation is entirely through the repressor and the amount of free enzyme does not play any role in downgrading its own synthesis by a feed back type mechanism.

As discussed, the lac repressor is active as a homo–tetramer and each of the 4 subunits has a site for inducer binding. The dissociation constant for the inducer is 10^{-6}. The repressor binds to the promoter at −3 to +21 region which partially overlaps with the RNA polymerase binding site (−48 to +5). The repressor binding thus interferes with the RNA polymerase binding and the polymerase can not bind when the repressor is bound to the gene. As a result, the repression of gene expression takes place. This is explained in Fig. 8.19.

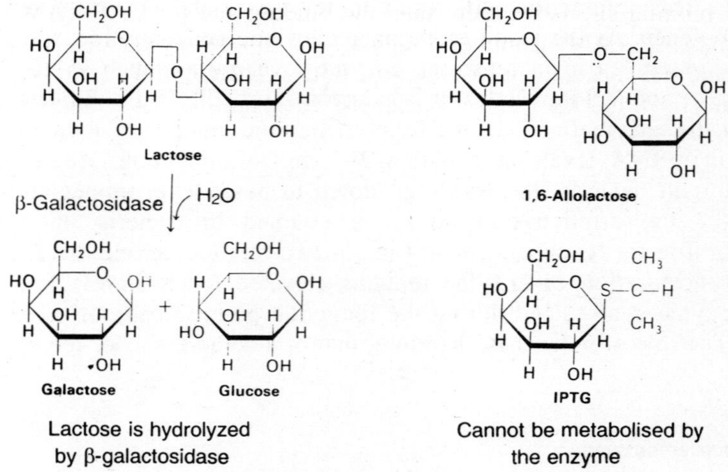

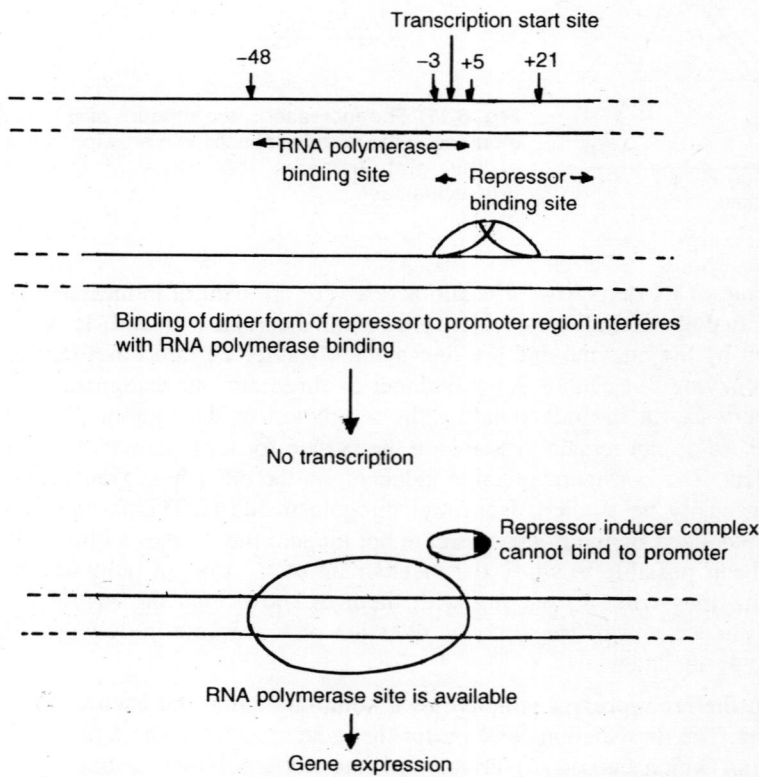

Fig. 8.18. Substrates for β-galactosidase.

Transcription start site

Binding of dimer form of repressor to promoter region interferes with RNA polymerase binding

No transcription

Repressor inducer complex cannot bind to promoter

RNA polymerase site is available

Gene expression

Fig. 8.19. The repressor binding site overlaps with RNA polymerase binding site.

The detailed analysis of induction of lac operon has shown that the level of enzymes can be elevated by cAMP. This effect is additive to the induction by IPTG. This can very well be explained by the fact that repressor binding site is different than the binding site for CAP–cAMP protein (as discussed in previous section, CAP–cAMP complex binds at −87 to −48 region, while the repressor binds at −3 to +21 region) and the mechanism of action of both is different. The enzyme levels can be further stimulated by about 50 fold in presence of cAMP. Thus the various scenerios can be present which have been discribed below.

1. When glucose is present, the cAMP levels are low, and if no lactose is present, the repressor gets associated to the operator region and no lac mRNA is transcribed.
2. If glucose is present (ie. cAMP is low) and lactose is also present, the induction takes place and the lac mRNA is transcribed.
3. If glucose is absent, the cAMP levels are high and if lactose is also present, then very high amounts of lac mRNAs are synthesized.

Trp Operon

The trp operon is another example of negative regulation. However, it works in a different manner than the lac operon. It is a polycistronic gene coding for a set of 5 enzymes involved in the synthesis of tryptophan. The genes are trpE, trpD, trpC, trpB and trpA, coding for anthranilase synthetase component I, anthranilase synthetase component II, N-(5'-phosphoribosyl)-anthranilate isomerase, tryptophan synthetase β-subunit and the tryptophan synthetase α-subunit, respectively. The pathway for tryptophan synthesis has been shown in Fig. 8.20.

The structural region of the operon is preceded by the control region which is consisted of the promoter and the operator. The operator is separated from the structural gene by a small segment of DNA, known as the leader segment. The leader segment plays an important role in an alternate mode of regulation of gene expression, known as the attenuation. The attenuation ensures that the bacteria responds very fast to aminoacid starvation and will be discussed separately at a later stage. The regulatory gene, trpR, is upstream of control region but is not contiguous with the operon. The trpR codes for the repressor which binds to the operator and regulates the promoter function. However, its mechanism of action is different than that of lac operon. The salient features of trp operon are shown in Fig. 8.21 and have been discribed below.

1. The trpR gene is autoregulated. Its product, the trp repressor, regulates its own synthesis by binding to a site within its own promoter region.
2. The repressor alone is biologically inactive and does not inhibit the function of the operator. Thus the synthesis of all the five enzymes goes on. However, when cellular concentration of tryptophan becomes high and free tryptophan is present, it binds to the trp repressor with high affinity and forms a repressor:trp complex. This causes a change in the repressor confirmation. The changed confirmation of repressor has active DNA binding motifs and the repressor-trp complex can bind to the 'O' region, resulting in the modulation of its function. As a result, the gene is switched off and the enzymes are not synthesized. Any variation in the concentration of tryptophan results in corresponding change in its synthesis. In a culture of bacteria, it is possible to manipulate the enzyme concentration by controling the availability of tryptophan in the medium. This scenerio is in contrast to that of the action of the inducer in lac operon. Tryptophan, thus, acts as a 'co-repressor' and activates the repressor molecule and inhibits the entire operon.
3. Certain compounds such as β indolyl acetic acid (IAA) and indole 3-propionic acid (IPA) can derepress the enzyme synthesis. These compounds are competitive inhibitors of the repressor binding to the 'O-P' region and can, therefore, inactivate the effect of the repressor in the same manner as caused by the low levels of tryptophan.

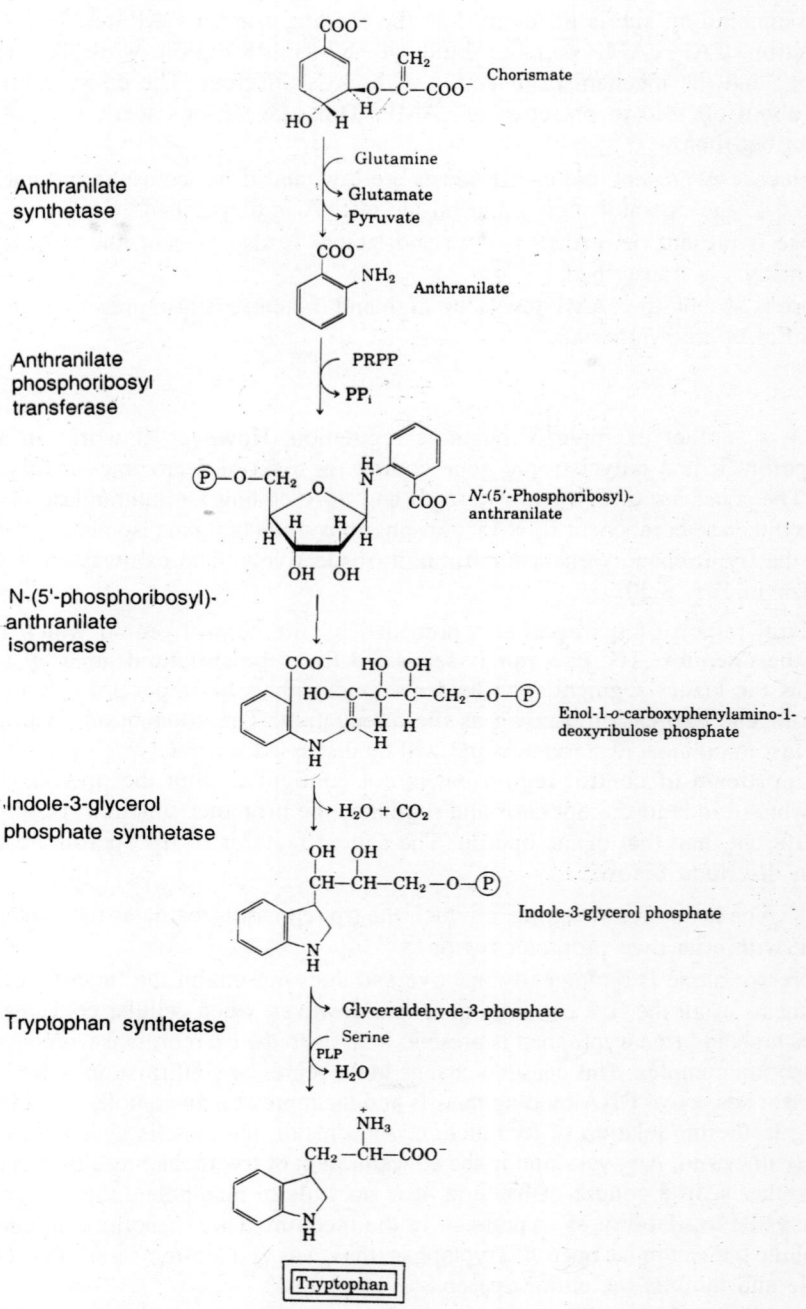

Fig. 8.20. Biosynthesis of tryptophan from chorismate. The pathway enzymes are : 1. anthranilate synthase, 2. anthranilate phosphoribosyl transferase, 3. N-(5'-phosphoribosyl)-anthranilate isomerase, 4. indole-3-glycerol phosphate synthase, and 5. tryptophan synthase. In E. coli, enzymes 1 and 2 are subunits of a single complex called anthranilate synthase.

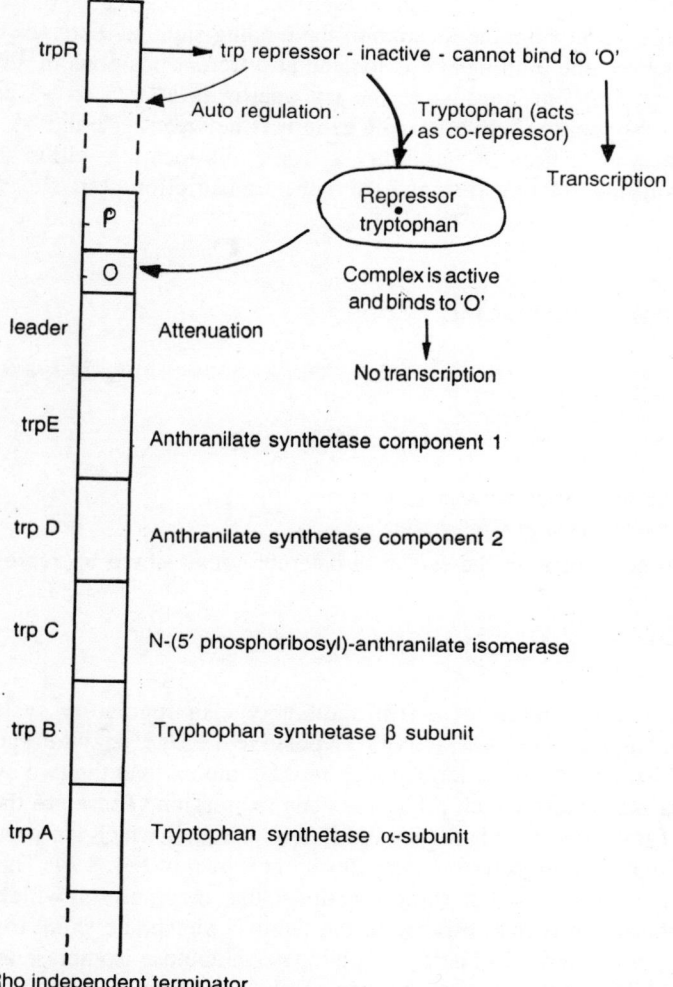

Fig. 8.21. The trp operon.

4. Besides the operon system, trp cascade is also regulated by another novel mechanism which is called 'attenuator' (see later). The combined function of the two systems helps in maintaining the optimal levels of tryptophan in the cell.

5. Besides acting at the operator region of the operon, the trp repressor also acts at another locus, the aroH gene. The aroH gene codes for one of the three enzymes involved in the synthesis of the common precursor for the bio-synthesis of different aromatic aminoacids. The action of trp repressor on aroH gene is same as its action on the trp operon.

Thus the trp repressor presents an important system where a single regulator molecule can bind to multiple loci and manipulate a number of gene clusters: How does it take place? Careful analysis of the sequences at the three loci show that there are common sequences in all the three loci which are recognized by the repressor and where the repressor binding takes place. The sites for repressor binding in all the three loci are given in Fig. 8.22. The binding sites are shown within the box and the transcription start site has been marked with an asterick. There is a degree of two fold dyad symmetry in these sequences. As is evident from the location of the binding site, the repressor binds to 21 nucleotides in each of the loci. However, the binding site is located at different positions in different gene in relation to the transcription start site. The binding at the trp operon is at −23 to −3 position, at aroH gene it is between −49 and −29 position while in trpR gene it is between −12 and +9 positions. This shows that the operator has a large degree of flexibility as for as its location within the gene is concerned. It may be present at varying relative distance from the transcription start site and still can modulate the gene expression.

trp AATC ATCGAACTAGTTAACTAGTAC GC*

aroH GCCG - AT - T - - - - - AG - - - - - - - G - ATNNNNNNNNNNNNNNNNNNNNNNNNNNNNNN*

trpR TGCT - - - - T - - - CT - * - - - G - - - - - AACC

- represents the same sequence as in trp operon
* represents the transcription initiation site

Fig. 8.22. The sequences of the region in different genes where trp repressor can bind.

Arabinose operon

The arabinose operon is an example of a still another type of regulatory system (Fig. 8.23). In this system, the regulation of the promoter activity is positive i.e. the enzyme synthesis is enhanced by the regulator. The mechanism of regulation is much more complex than the two systems discussed earlier and there are two separate factors which affect the gene expression. These are the arabinose and cAMP. The structural genes of this operon code for three different enzymes which are necessary for the utilization of arabinose as an alternate carbon source. This pathway is shown in Fig. 8.24. The cell converts arabinose to xylulose-5-phosphate by a series of three reactions, the enzymes for which are coded by the ara operon. Xylulose-5-phosphate is then utilised in the pentose phosphate shunt to produce energy. Three structural genes araB, araA and araD code for ribulokinase, arabinose isomerase and ribulose-5-phosphate epimerase respectively. The control region is made of two operators, O_1 and O_2. There is another locus, I, which also has the sites for the binding of the regulatory proteins. The regulatory protein, referred as the 'C protein' (C stands for control), is the product of the regulatory gene, araC. The gene araC is present at upstream of the control region. In fact, the I region has two independent sites for the binding of the C protein, referred as I_1 and I_2. Promoter P_{BAD} which controls the transcription of all the three structural genes is located near the I locus. Operator O_2 regulates the function of this promoter. As discussed, the regulatory part of the operon is consisted of gene araC, coding for protein C. The transcription of araC is controlled by the promoter P_c which is modulated by the operator O_1 and is located alongwith it. Promoter P_c transcribes the gene araC in leftward direction. On the other hand, promoter P_{BAD} transcribes the genes araB, araA and araD in rightward direction. The operon is under dual regulation. Both the C protein and the cAMP regulate it. The synthesis of C protein itself is auto-regulated. On one hand, it has a negative role for the autoregulation while on the other hand, it has both the positive and the negative roles for the regulation of the structural genes (see later).

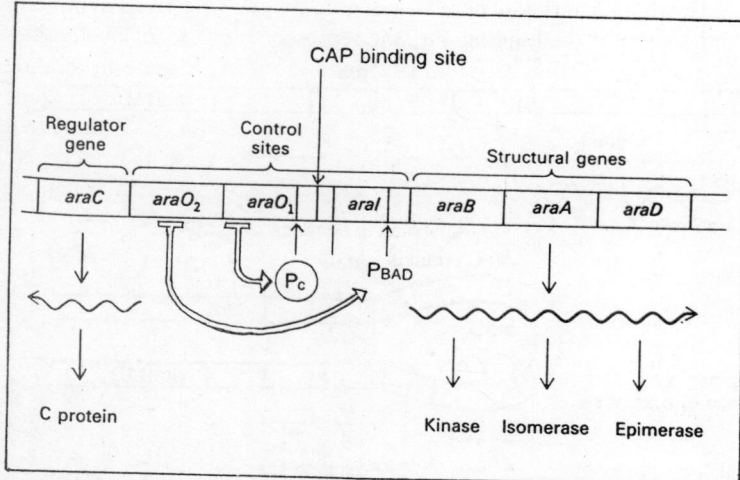

Fig. 8.23. The arabinose operon and its regulator genes.

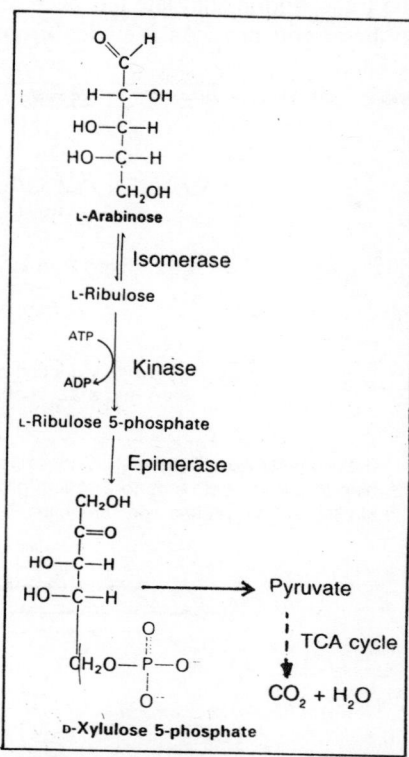

Fig. 8.24. The conversion of arabinose to xylulose 5-phosphate is catalyzed by the three enzymes encoded by the arabinose operon.

The regulatory mechanism can be summa-rised as following:

1. When the concentration of C protein is low and cAMP is also low, the synthesis of C protein takes place efficiently. However, as soon as free C protein concentration reaches beyond 40 molecules/cell (cAMP is still low), it binds with the opertator O_1 which negatively regulates the promoter P_c. This results in downgradation of C protein synthesis.

2. Once C protein has been synthesized and excess of C protein is present, a dimer from of the protein C binds with both the O_2 region and the site I_1 on the I locus. This two fold binding results in the stretching and bending of the DNA and a change in the configuration of the gene. A loop like structure is formed. This change in the configuration of gene brings the promoter P_{BAD} and operator O_2 in close proximity to each other. As a result, now the operator O_2 can modulate the promoter activity downward and the transcription of genes araB, araA and araD is repressed (Fig. 8.25A).

3. When arabinose is present, it binds with the C protein and arabinose:C protein complex is formed. This complex formation changes the confirmation of the C protein in such a way that it starts acting as an inducer in place of a repressor.

4. Arabinose-C protein complex does not have the DNA-binding sites available and can not remain bound to the operator O_2 and leaves this locus. As a result, the loop formation breaks. The O_2 and P_{BAD} move away from each other and the operator region can no longer repress the promoter activity (Fig. 8.25B).

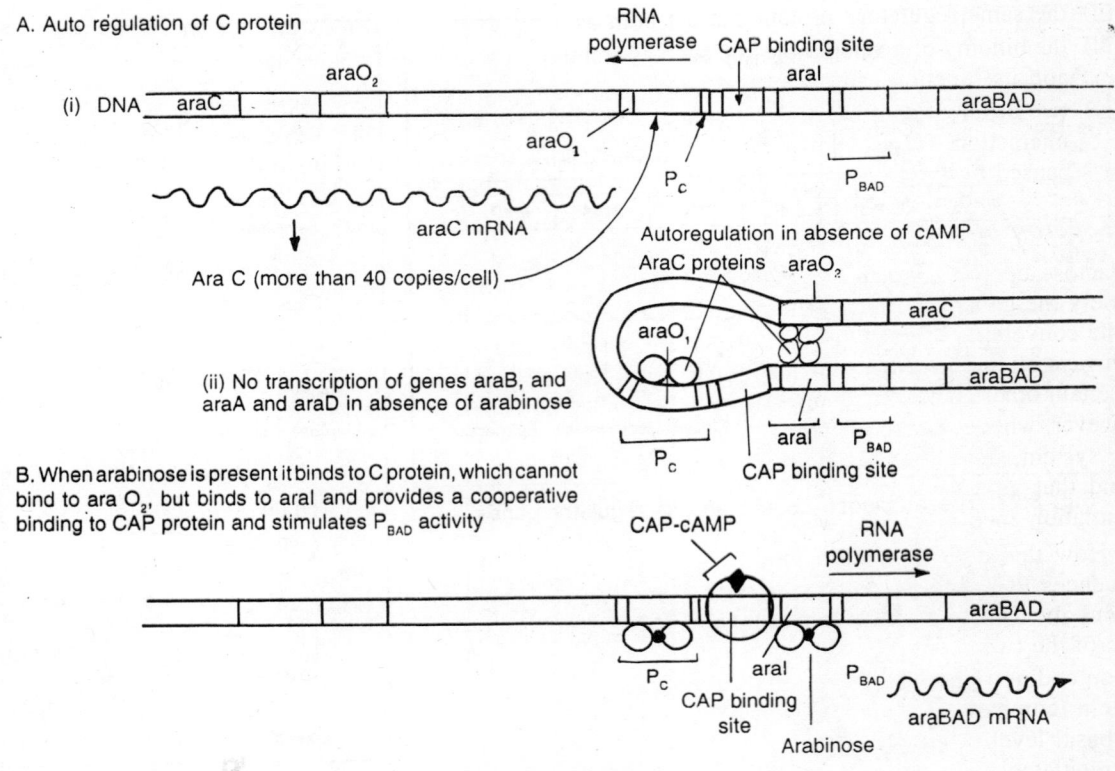

Fig. 8.25. Regulation of ara operon.

5. Arabinose-C protein complex binds to both the sites on I locus (I_1 and I_2) and also associates with the cAMP-CAP complex. The cAMP-CAP binds in between the two molecules of arabinose:C protein complex and gets sandwitched with it. The binding of these molecules at I site results in induced transcription of mRNAs for the structural genes which in turn enhances the synthesis of the enzyme complex.

6. The operator O_1 is still occupied by the C protein which downgrades the transcription of araC gene, thus the level of C protein remain low. As a result, the arabinose can be utilized effectively by the cells.

There are thus four different possible scenerios.

(a) The glucose is present and arabinose is absent, this will result in low cAMP levels and no synthesis of the enzymes will take place.

(b) Glucose is absent but arabinose is present which will result in high cAMP concentration. In this situation the structure of C protein is altered to its inducer confirmation. The inducer along with the CAP-cAMP complex enhances the enzyme synthesis and arabinose can be used.

(c) Both glucose and arabinose are present and

(d) both are absent. The picture is not very clear in both these cases. Probably low level of enzyme will be synthesized in (c) and no synthesis of the enzymes will take place in (d).

This system presents certain interesting facts. The salient features of this system are following:

(i) A regulatory protein can regulate the transcription of its own gene and thus can control its own concentration,

(ii) the same regulatory protein can act both as a repressor and also as an inducer,

(iii) the binding of a small molecule such as arabinose can drastically alter the confirmation of a protein and its function can be reversed and

(iv) two different control sites do not necessarily have to be contiguous with each other for their mutual interaction. These can be brought in close vicinity to each other by a change in the gene confirmation caused by the DNA-protein and/or protein-protein interactions.

Gal operon

Galactose operon presents yet another mode of gene regulation. The operon codes for three enzymes, namely the galactose kinase, the galactose transferase and the epimerase. These enzymes are involved in the conversion of galactose to glucose. As galactose is produced in the cell during various metabolic pathways of carbohydrate utilization and is also required for the cell wall synthesis and for the synthesis of certain other complex carbohydrates, the presence of a basal level of these enzymes is always required. However, when galactose becomes the primary carbon source, high level of these enzymes are required. The system, therefore, has both the constitutive and the regulated modes of expression. It has been found that galactose can stimulate the enzyme synthesis by 15 fold (compare with upto 1000 fold stimulation in lac operon) while glucose can repress it by 10-15 fold.

How this dual regulation functions? This is made possible by the presence of two pribnow box sequences PG1 and PG2 in the operon (Fig. 8.26). These sequences partially overlap each other and are involved in two fold regulation. There are also two separate transcription initiation sites, one for each of the two promoters. Thus the mRNAs produced by two promoters differ from each other in their 5'-non coding region. However, both the transcripts have the same coding region and code for the same protein (compare with the his3 gene). PG2 is responsible for the constitutive expression and maintains the basal level of enzymes. It can be downward regulated by cAMP. PG1 on the other hand, controls the regulated expression. It has much higher affinity for the RNA polymerase than PG2. Its activity can be stimulated both by galactose and also by cAMP. The concentration of cAMP itself is regulated by glucose. Thus cAMP affects both the sites in opposite manner. By the combination of two effects, the enzyme levels are maintained.

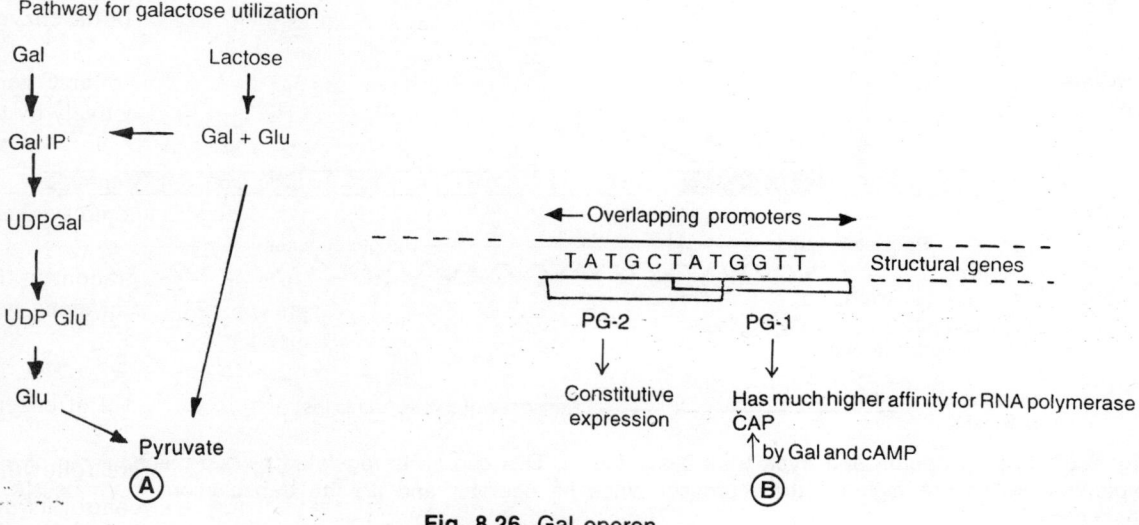

Fig. 8.26. Gal operon.

Attenuation

Attinuation is a very novel mode of regulation of gene expression. It was first discovered by Yonofsky in trp operon. While studying the effect of various growth conditions of bacterial culture, he noticed that E.coli can respond to the addition of tryptophan very quickly. The study showed that the time required for the transcription of the structural genes is about 4 min. However, the response time to the changes in tryptophan concentration is much less than that. How is it possible? The regulation by trp repressor can not explain it as trp repressor blocks the initiation of transcription. Even if initiation is totally shut off, there would be some preinitiated transcription complexes which will continue to elongate. Thus some amount of mRNAs should be formed. These mRNAs will be translated and keep the synthesis of the enzymes going on for some time. However, as the synthesis shuts off almost immediately, it is obvious that there has to be another mode of regulation working in this system.

It has already been discussed in the previous section that in the trp operon, the promoter/operator region is not contiguous with the structural gene. There is a small stretch of polynucleotide, referred as the leader, in between the two regions. This leader sequence is a 162 nucleotide long spacer region present in between the O region and the begining of the structural gene. Later on by mutation experiments, it was found that a mutation in the leader region can abolish the quick response. This mutation was later mapped between the nucleotide number 30-60 within the leader. This element was given the name attenuator. An attenuator can be described as an intrinsic terminator located at the begining of a transcription unit. It acts by the formation of a hairpin structure resulting in rho independent termination. The formation of the hairpin structure is dependent on the external signals. In trp operon, it was found that in presence of tryptophan a transcript of 130 nucleotides can be isolated in the wild type organisms. However, in those attenuator mutants which do not respond to tryptophan, a transcript of 7Kb is synthesized which has the mRNAs for all the five structural genes (Fig. 8.27). This observation confirmed the location of the attenuator element to be within the mutated sequences which are responsible for this regulation.

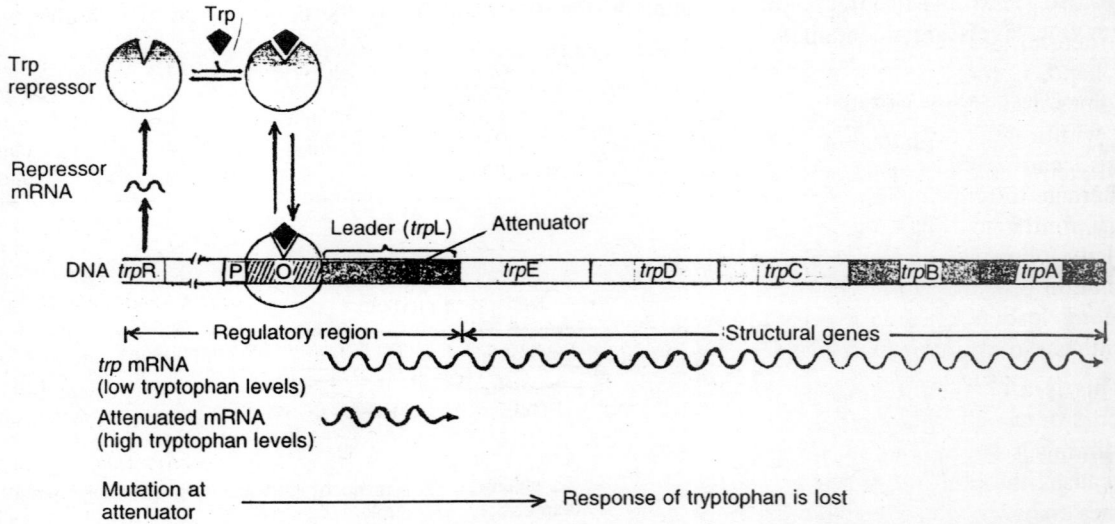

Fig. 8.27. The trp operon and tryptophan biosynthesis. This operon is regulated by two mechanisms. When tryptophan levels are high (1) the repressor binds its operator and (2) the transcription of trp mRNA is attenuated.

The sequence analysis of the leader region revealed that there is a putative ribosome binding site followed by an open reading frame which codes for a 14 aa long polypeptide, the 'leader peptide'. It further revealed that there are two tryptophan codons within this leader peptide. Furthermore, four regions with high degree of complementarity in the nucleotide sequence were also seen. These have been referred as sections 1, 2, 3 and 4, respectively, in Fig. 8.28 and have been highlighted.

AUG AAA GCA AUU UUC GUA CUG AAA GGU UGG UGG CGC ACU UCC **UGA AAC**
GGCAGUGUAUUCACCA **UGCGUA AAGCAAUCAG** AUACCCAGCCCGCC **UAAU** GAGCGGCU **UUUUUU**

Fig. 8.28. Sequence of attenuator region.

The region 2 is complementary to the regions 1 and 3 while the region 3 is complementary to the regions 2 and 4. Thus two alternate confirmations of the mRNA are possible. In first confirmation region 1 and 2 form a double stranded stem while 3 and 4 form another stem. In second confirmation, regions 2 and 3 form a double stranded stem while section 1 and 4 remain single stranded. These alternate confirmations of RNA are responsible for the functioning of the attenuator. The leader mRNA also has a G:C rich region within the regions 3 and 4, which is followed by a stretch of U residues. As discussed earlier, the transcription and translation are coupled in bacteria. When there is no trp in the growth medium, the trp-tRNA cannot be charged with the aminoacid and tryptonyl tRNA is not available in the cell. During protein synthesis when the ribosomes reach the trp codon, these have to pause due to the absence of tryptophanyl tRNA. As this trp codon rich portion of mRNA is within the region 1, the region 1 becomes embeded within the ribosome and is not available for base pairing with region 2. However, region 2 is free from the ribosome protection and is available for base pairing with region 3 as soon as it is synthesized by the growing transcription bubble. Region 4, when synthesized remains unpaired as region 3 has already formed the base pair with region 2. This confirmation of RNA (Fig. 8.29A) is entirely different from the structure of a terminator. Transcription, therefore, continues and the structural genes are transcribed to produce the 7Kb mRNA representing all the five genes. On the other hand, if enough trp is present in the system, there is no shortage of charged trp-tRNAs and the ribosomes donot pause at the trp codons. The translation continues and both, the region 1 and region 2 are within the ribosomes and not available for base pairing. Thus the pairing between region 2 and region 3 can not take place. Region 3 is now available for base pairing with region 4. As a result, the alternate loop formation takes place and RNA assumes an alternate confirmation (Fig. 8.29B), which is very similar to a rho-independent terminator. This terminator is formed due to the G:C rich dyad symmetry followed by a stretch of U which is very similar to the structure necessary for the rho-independent termination of trancription. The net result is the premature termination of the transcript, and only 140 base long leader mRNA is formed. This in turn blocks the synthesis of the enzymes necessary for biosynthesis of tryptophan and no tryptophan is synthesized.

This is a classical example how the alternate confirmation of same RNA can either terminate a transcript or can allow the transcription to continue. The system works on the precise timings of translation. This timing is maintained by a region of DNA preceding the attenuator which acts as a pause signal. This causes the pausing of RNA polymerase. Thus ribosomes get a chance to catch up and region 2 becomes embeded within the ribosomes and is not available for pairing with region 3 when it is synthesized. If translation is delayed, and region 1 is within ribosome but region 2 is free for the base pairing with region 3, attenuator will not work.

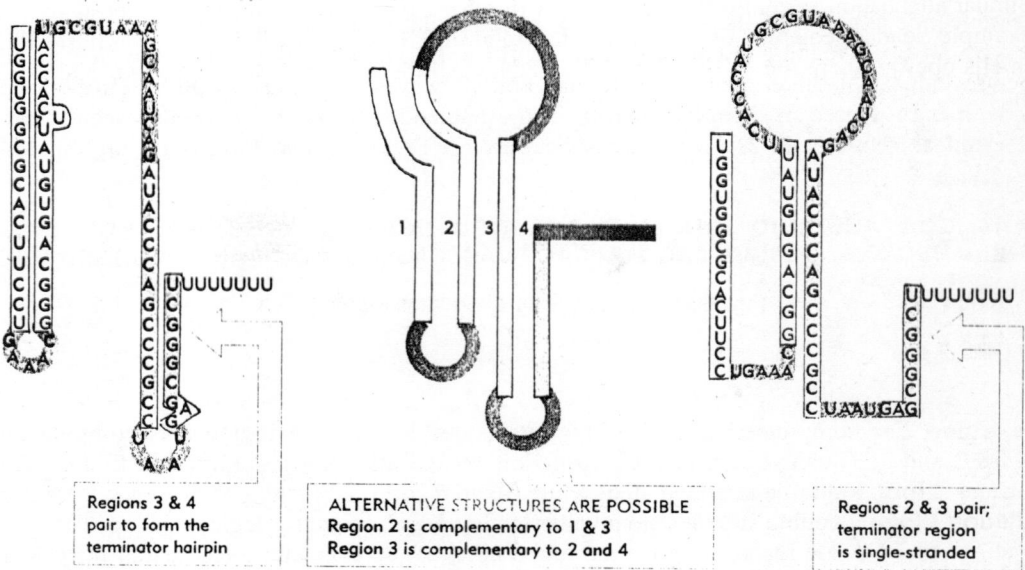

Fig. 8.29A. The trp leader region can exist in alternative base-paired conformations. The center shows the four regions that can base pair. Region 1 is complementary to region 2, which is complementary to region 3, which is complementary to region 4. On the left is the conformation produced when region 1 pairs with region 2, and region 3 pairs with region 4. On the right is the conformation when region 2 pairs with region 3, leaving regions 1 and 4 unpaired.

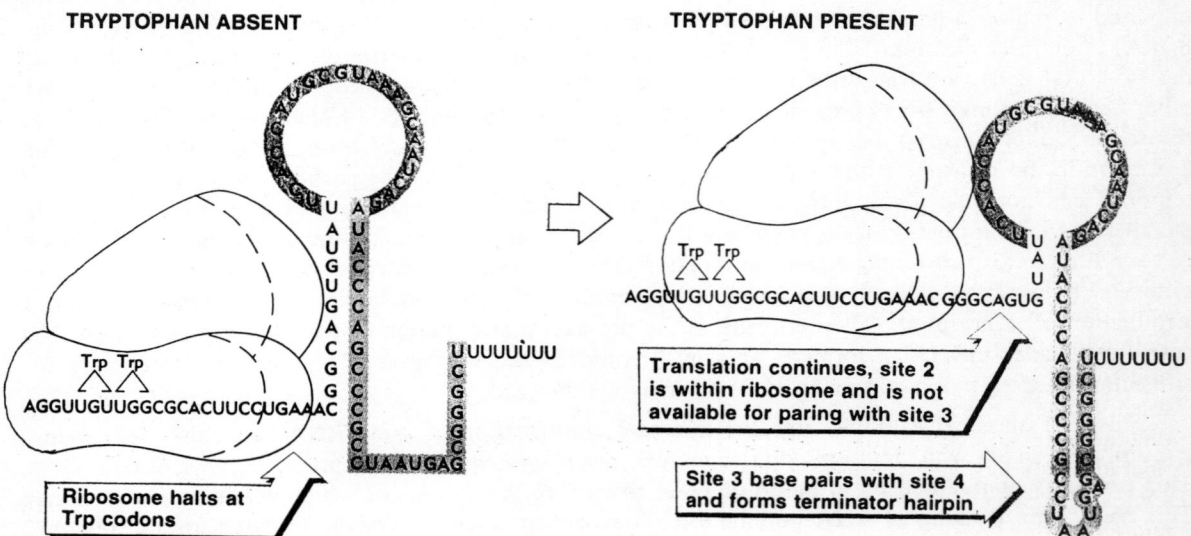

Fig. 8.29B. Attenuator depend on the location of the ribosome, which determines whether or not, the regions 3 and 4 can pair to form the terminator hairpin.

Similar attenuation system works in a number of other operons involved in the synthesis of aminoacids. For example, leader sequence of Thr operon has total of 9 Thr codons, in Phe operon has 7 Phe codons and in His operon, there are 5 His codons (Fig. 8.30). All these operons are regulated by the attenuation system.

Leader peptides

Thr operon   Met - Lys - Arg - Ile - Ser - Thr - Thr - Ile - Thr - Thr - Thr - Ile - Thr - Ile

Phe operon   Met - Lys - His - Ile - Pro - Phe - Phe - Phe - Ala - Phe - Phe - Phe - Thr - Phe - Pro - Stop

His operon   Met - Thr - Arg - Val - Gly - Phe - Lys - His - His - His - His - His - His - His - Pro - Asp

Fig. 8.30. Leader peptides of various operons with attenuators.

Regulation of lytic and lysogenic cascades in Lambda phage

Phages are the bacterial viruses which infect the host and replicate inside the host cells. They use the host cellular machinery for the replication of their genome. However, their genome codes for a number of regulatory proteins which are essential for their life cycle. Based on the mode of their life, the phages can be of two types. Many phages have only one type of life cycle. These multiply inside the bacteria resulting in high copy number of the particles. Once a threshold copy number of the phage has been attained, the bacterial death (the lysis) takes place and the phage particles are released in the media. These are now available for the infection of other bacterial cells. This is known as the lytic mode of life cycle. Many other phages, however, have two separate modes of life cycle. These either have the lytic cycle or a lysogenic cycle. In lysogenic cycle, the phage does not cause the death of the host. In this case, the viral genome gets integrated into the host genome, on the other hand, before the threshold level of phage copies have been formed. It then continues to grow with the host and forms multiple but non-infective copies of its genome. These DNA molecules, known as the virions, are naked and are not covered by the usual protein envalope and are often called the prophage. These do not kill the host and both, the host and the phage, are able to survive in a symbiotic manner. Lambda phage is the second type of phage and can undergo both lytic and lysogenic modes of life cycles.

The bacteriophage lambda is a relatively large phage, madeup of a double stranded linear genome of 48,514 base pairs. The DNA has 12 nt long single stranded region at the 5'–ends of both the strands which are complementary to each other. These cohessive ends are referred as the 'cos' sites (Fig. 8.31). Following the infection of the bacteria, the cos sites base pair with each other inside the host cells and form a circular DNA molecule. The replication of the phage genome takes place in its circular form. However, the progeny particles return back to linear form before these are packaged to form the phage particles. The genome contains a number of genes which are regulated by a series of promoter/ operator regions. The function of these sequences is regulated differently in the lytic and the lysogenic cycles. The selection of the mode of life cycle the phage will adopt primarily depends on the metabolic and environmental status of the cell. These factors regulate the expression of the genes which changes the phage behavior in response to environmental conditions.

Based on the timing of their expression, the phage genes can be divided into three sets. These are referred as the immediate early, the delayed early (or the intermediate) and the late genes. The immediate early and part of the intermediate genes are expressed in both the lytic and the lysogenic modes of life cycles. However, at later stages, the two cycles follow different pathways and the expression of different sets of genes takes place in the two modes. The general map of phage genome has been shown in Fig. 8.32. Two main genes, N and Cro are expressed in the early stage. Both of these genes code for the control proteins. Protein N is an anti-terminator which is essential for the expression of delayed early genes. Cro protein is an anti-repressor which is also important for switching the synthesis of early proteins off. The delayed early genes code for seven proteins responsible for recombination, two of which are essential for the integration of phage genome to the host genome. Besides, the intermediate genes include two genes which are responsible for the replication of phage genome and three regulatory genes. Two of the regulatory genes, the cII and cIII, code for an activator of integration and also participate in the repressor formation. The third gene codes for the Q protein which is an anti-terminator. Thus there are two anti-terminators, N and Q. However, these have different modes of action. Protein N binds to DNA at specific sites. These sites are known as nut (for N utilization) sites and are located just upstream of the terminators of early genes. The binding of N protein to nut sites modifies the confirmation of terminator. Three different host proteins also participate in this process. The modified form of terminator is biologically inactive and does not cause the termination of the transcript. It allows the RNA polymerase to proceed and transcribe the genes located beyond the terminator. The Q protein on the other hand, interacts with the RNA polymerase itself and modulates it, which results in prevention of termination. This interaction of RNA polymerase with Q protein takes place near the region of the late promoters which get activated and the transcription of late genes starts. The late genes include two genes necessary for lysis of the host. It also has the genes necessary for the packaging of viral genome. These include ten head genes and eleven tail genes. As the prophage formed during the lysogenic cycle is not envaloped and also the lysis of the host does not take place in lysogeny, the late genes are thus necessary only for the lytic cycle.

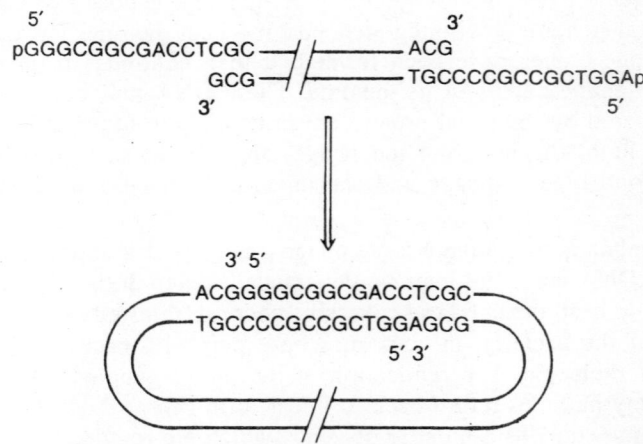

Fig. 8.31. Structures of cos region and the linear and circular forms of λ DNA.

Besides these genes, there is one more regulatory gene, cI. It codes for a regulatory protein, the lambda repressor. The repressor is a DNA binding protein. The DNA binding motif is of helix-turn-

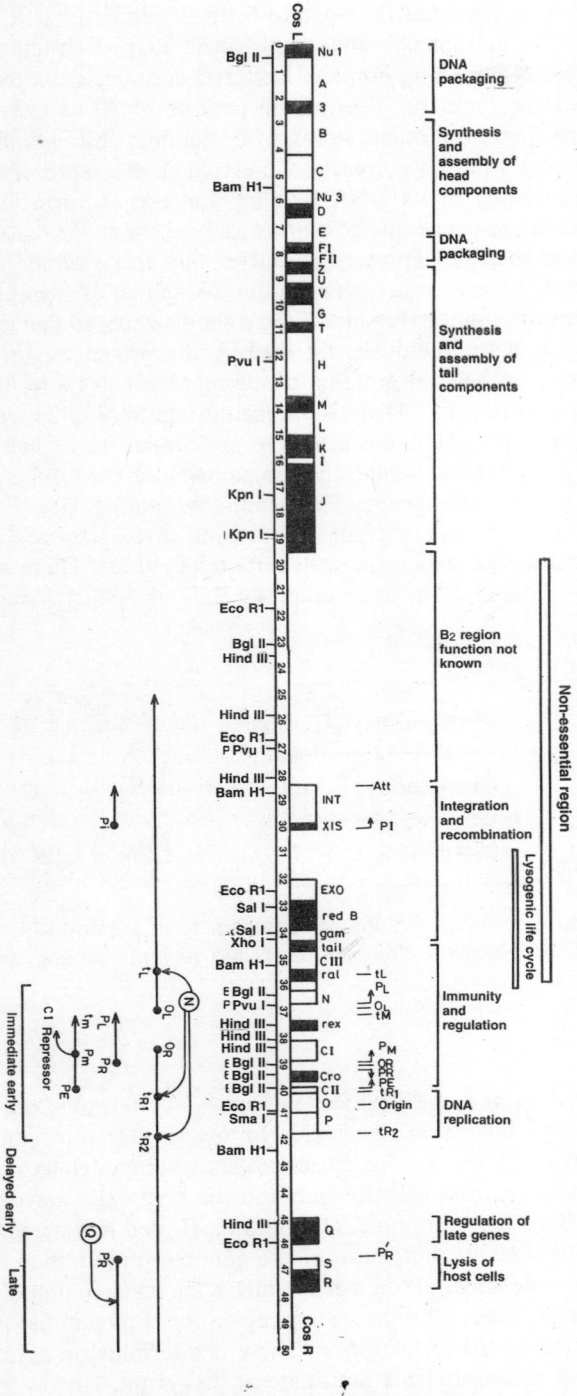

Fig. 8.32. The map of λ genome.

helix type. This type of DNA binding motif has already been discussed. In fact the lambda repressor was the first HTH motif to be discovered. The active form of repressor is a homodimer. Each subunit of the repressor dimer has 236 aminoacids and has a dumb shaped structure. First 92 aminoacids at the N-terminal end form the DNA binding domain. Last 105 aminoacids at the C-terminal end (number 132-236) form the dimer contact domain. The middle peptide of 39 aa (93-131) forms the connector region (Fig. 8.33). There are specific proteases present in the host cell, which can digest the connector region between the aa 111 and 113. This digestion inactivates the repressor. This inactivation of the repressor is caused by the inability of its DNA binding domains to form dimers without the help of C-terminal dimer formation domain (since this domain is cleaved off as the result of proteolytic digestion). It has already been discussed that the repressor is active only in its dimer form. The monomer form does not have biological activity. The contact between the C-terminal of two repressor molecules forming a dimer brings the N-terminals of both the subunits at the right distance, so that the protein-DNA interaction can take place. When the connector region is digested by the proteases, the repressor is broken into two pieces and there is change in the configuration of the repressor. As a result, the interaction between the repressor and DNA can not take place. There is a dynamic equilibrium between the repressor monomer and the dimer, and as we will see later, the effective concentration of active repressor plays a key role in determining whether the phage will enter in lytic pathway or the lysogenic pathway. The repressor binds to operator region for the early genes. The repressor binding site on the DNA includes a 17 bp region. Three separate repressor binding sites containing this 17 bp region are present in each of the operator region having conserved sequences with certain variations. These sites have different affinity for the repressor and are separated from each other by 3-7 bp A:T rich region.

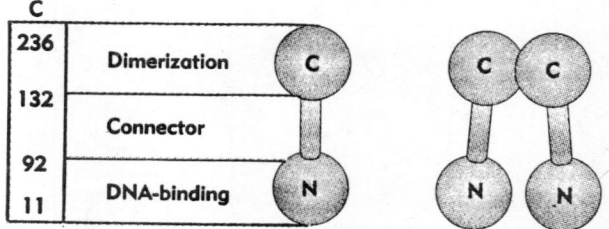

Fig. 8.33. The N-terminal and C-terminal regions of repressor form separate domains which are connected through the middle region. The C-terminal domains associate to form dimers; the N-terminal domains bind DNA.

The lytic cascade

Very simplified map of lambda genome is given in Fig. 8.34. It shows only the essential genes. As discussed earlier, the lytic and lysogenic life cycles follow similar route during the early period but diversify during the later part. However, for easier understanding, let us describe the two pathways separately. If the growth media is nutritionally rich and the host cells are rapidly growing, the phage follows the lytic life cycle. Two early promoters, P_L and P_R (L and R represent leftward and rightward, respectively) located on both sides of the centre of the genome initiate the early gene expression. The two promoters are in different orientation. Promoter P_L directs the transcription of the N gene. A terminator, t_L terminates the transcript immediately after the coding region for N protein has been transcribed. Similarly, the promoter P_R directs the rightward transcription. There is a terminator, t_{R1}, located immediately after the cro gene and majority of the transcripts terminate at this point. However, this terminator is leaky and a few transcripts pass beyond the terminator region and proceed upto the cII gene where another terminator t_{R2} is located. Once sufficient amounts of N protein has been synthesized, it binds to the nut sites present near all the three terminators (t_L, t_{R1} and t_{R2}) and inactivates them all. This inactivation of terminators allows the transcription of the delayed early genes. In the mean time, the expression of early genes has been switched off. Protein Cro is responsible for this function (switching the early genes off). Now the transcription of late genes takes place. It is directed by a late promoter, $P_{R'}$ located immediatly after the gene Q (which is the last rightward gene in delayed early region). The expression of these genes is constitutive. However, if enough amounts of protein Q are not present, the late transcript terminates at another terminator, t_{R3}, located near the promoter $P_{R'}$, forming a small transcript of only 194 bases. This transcript is referred as the the 6S RNA. In presence of protein Q, the terminator t_{R3} is inactivated and the transcription continues beyond it. This results in extension of the transcript and a large RNA is formed which is made up of the 6S RNA and also includes all the late genes. These sequences include the transcript of the genes responsible for the synthesis of proteins essential for the lysis of the host and packaging of the phage particles. The genes for head and tail proteins are normally at left hand side of the promoter. However, as the phage genome is present as a circular molecule at this time of the life, these genes are also expressed alongwith the lysis genes as a single transcript.

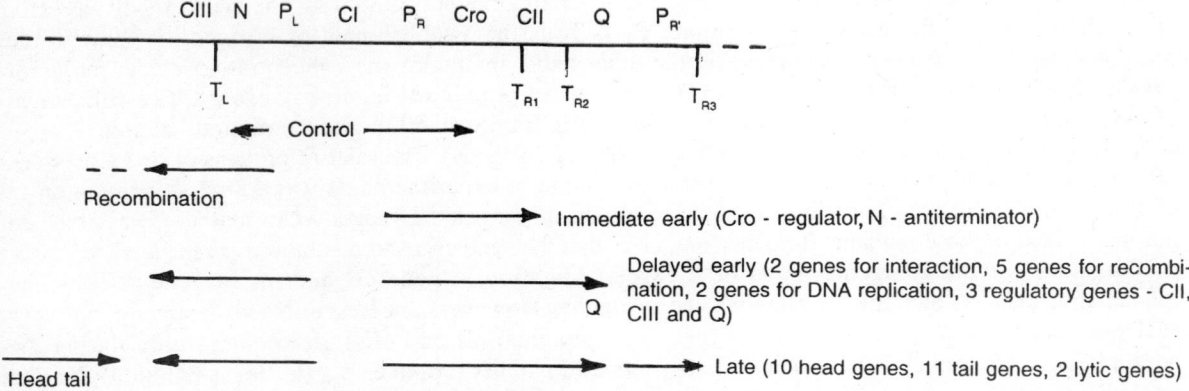

Fig. 8.34. Regulatory region of λ genome.

As discussed earlier, during this period the phage DNA is replicated as a circular molecule. The envalope proteins formed during the late phase cause the packaging of the DNA into phage particles. However, the circular DNA is converted into linear DNA before it is packaged. Once the host cell is lysed, the packaged phages are released into the media and are now available for infecting new host cells in the culture. The whole cycle is then repeated, fresh cells are lysed each time and more phage particles are formed which infect new cells and the cycle continues.

Lysogenic cascade

The early parts of both lytic and lysogenic cascades are same. Similar to the lytic cycle in lysogenic cascade also the early genes are expressed in the same manner. The proteins N and Cro are formed which allow the expression of delayed genes and products of genes cII and cIII are expressed. These play a crucial role in establishing the lysogeny (see later).

At this stage another promoter, P_{RM} (RM for repressor maintenance), starts the transcription of cI gene. The protein cII is essential for the activation of promoter P_{RM}. As has been discussed before, the gene cI codes for the lambda repressor. This repressor binds near the promoters P_R and P_L and causes their repression. As a result, the expression of all the genes except the cI gene, is stopped and the phage can not enter in the lytic mode. However, promoter P_{RM} itself is under the control of the repressor which acts as a positive regulator (i.e. enhances) for its activity. The presence of small amounts of repressor are obligatory for the activation of P_{RM}. This scenerio poses a problem for the initiation of the transcription of the repressor molecule. What is the source of this small amount of the repressor. Careful studies have shown that another promoter, P_{RE} (RE for repressor establishment), is present between the genes cro and cII (Fig. 8.35). This promoter is in leftward orientation. The promoter P_{RE} transcribes the cI gene. As their is no transcription terminator, it continues and along with cI, the transcript also includes the product of the cro gene but in reverse orientation (i.e. produces antisense RNA for cro). This results in the formation of sense:antisense ds RNA, resulting in unavailability of the Cro mRNA and blocking its translation. Thus there is repression of the synthesis of Cro protein while there is production of the repressor. The repression of the protein Cro ensures that the phage will go into lysogeny (role of Cro will be discussed later). The repressor gene has a very specific characteristic feature. It starts with the AUG codon without a typical ribosomal binding site. It is therefore, translated very poorly. Thus promoter P_{RE} provides only the small amounts of repressor protein. However, this quantity of repressor is sufficient to serve as the small amount essential for the synthesis of repressor under the control of the activity of promoter P_{RM}. Thus the establishment of lysogeny is through the promoter P_{RE} while the promoter P_{RM}, on the other hand, maintains the concentration of the repressor necessary for maintaining the lysogeny. The synthesis of protein cII is the key event for establishment of lysogeny. Protein cII, in turn, requires protein cIII for its stability and continuous action. Protein cIII acts through a host protein Hfl (for high frequency of lysogeny). The roles of proteins cI (the repressor), cII and cIII have been established by a series of mutation experiments. It was found that mutation in cI gene will abolish the capability of phage to undergo lysogeny. Lysogeny can neither be established nor maintained in these mutants. It is, therfore, clear that the synthesis and continuous presence of repressor is obligatory for the lysogenic mode of lifecycle. Mutation in gene cII and/ or in gene cIII, on the other hand, made it difficult to establish the lysogeny. However, once established, lysogeny can very easily be maintained. This showed that these two proteins (cII and cIII) are required only during the early phase of lysogenic cycle. Protein cII also activates another promoter P_{int} (int for integration), located immediately after the gene cIII. This transcribes the genes whose products are necessary for the integration of phage gene with the host genome (Fig. 8.36).

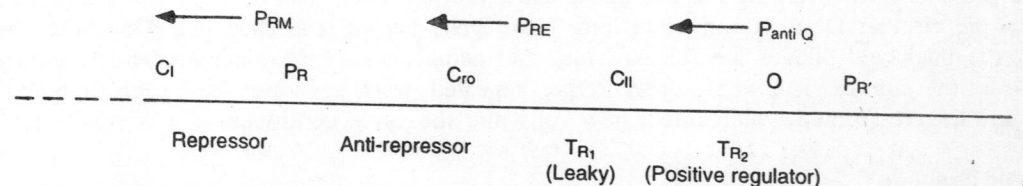

Fig. 8.36. The region of λ genome which is essential for lysogenic mode.

This dual control of the synthesis of repressor serves a very important function. It doesnot allow the synthesis of repressor until the early as well as some of the delayed genes have been expressed. Thus immediately after the infection, the phage expresses the early genes which are common between

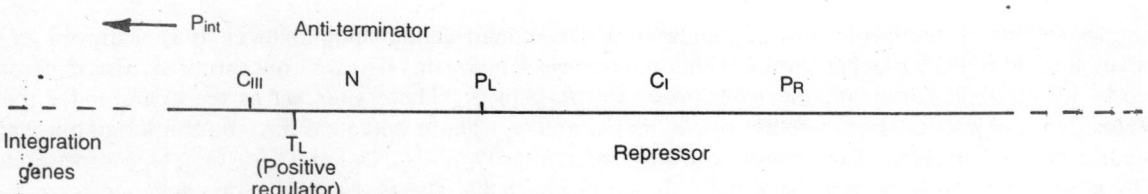

Fig. 8.35. Regulation of λ repressor synthesis.

the two modes for its life cycle. During this period it analyses the sorrounding environment and the growth conditions, and then decides which mode of life cycle it should adopt based on the metabolic status of the host cells. Only after the delayed genes have been expressed which amongst other functions, code for the proteins required for integration of the phage into host genome, the establishment of lysogeny takes place by the combined action of the proteins cII and cIII. As discussed above, protein cII is responsible for the establishment of lysogeny. However, small amounts of protein cII are formed during the immediate early gene expression also, since all the transcripts do not always terminate at the terminator t_{R1}. Some transcripts continue beyond this terminator and terminate at the alternate terminator t_{R2}, thus synthesizing small amounts of protein CII. If this amount of the protein is sufficient to start the synthesis of enough repressor molecules, the lytic functions will be stopped. On the other hand, the cell will not be able to sustain lysogeny yet as the proteins essential for integration of phage DNA into the host genome have not been synthesized so far. The possibility of this unacceptable situation is avoided by the fact that protein cIII is also needed for the activity of the protein cII. The protein cIII protects the cII protein from the proteolytic degradation. Though the presence of cIII protein does not necessarily mean that cII protein will not be broken, the cII is invariably degraded in absence of the protein cIII. Since cIII is synthesized only during the delayed early expression when the proteins for the integration are also being synthesized simultaneously, this ensures that the lysogeny will be established properly.

The protein cII has another function also. It activates another promoter, P_{antiQ}, which is located within the gene Q but is in a reverse orientation. Its activation, therefore, synthesizes an antisense RNA for a part of the Q mRNA. Thus the translation of Q mRNA and the synthesis of Q protein is strongly repressed. This results in the inactivation of the late promoters. The late genes are, therefore, not expressed and the lytic functions can not be carried out.

What are the signals which determine whether the phage will enter into the lytic or the lysogenic mode? A number of different factors are responsible for it, amongst them is the nutritional status of the host. It has been found that protein cII is very unstable. It can get hydrolysed very easily by a protease present in the host cells. If cells are growing very rapidly, large amounts of this protease are present which hydrolyses the cII protein, as a result, the repressor is not synthesised. The phage, therefore, undergoes the lytic cycle. It is beneficial for the phage as it can multiply and will have enough host cells to infect by its progeny. However, if the growth medium is not rich, the host cells grow slowly and relatively small amounts of this protease are formed. In such case, all of the cII protein is not hydrolysed and the repressor synthesis can easily be established. The phage, therefore, enters into lysogenic phase.

It should be clear from the above discussion that the amount of repressor is the key factor in the selection of the life cycle by the phage. If sufficient repressor is not present, the phage will go to lytic cycle and if too much repressor is present it will remain in lysogeny, without the possibility of returning to the lytic cycle even if the host becomes inhospitable at any future stage. It is therefore, important that the concentration of repressor is maintained at the optimal level. It is achieved by a novel auto-regulatory mechanism by which the repressor maintains its own concentration. The repressor works by binding to the sites near the promoters P_R and P_L. These sites act as the operator for their respective promoters. Thus there are operators O_R and O_L. These operators have not only one but three binding sites within each of the region which are referred as O_{R1}, O_{R2}, O_{R3} and O_{L1}, O_{L2}, O_{L3} respectively. The structure of these regions have been shown in Fig. 8.37. The first operator on each side is nearest to its promoter while the third one is the far most. These have different affinity for binding to the repressor. The mechanism of action of O_R operataors has been very well worked out and will be discussed in detail. The repressor has highest affinity for O_{R1}. As soon as small amount of repressor is formed through the action of the protein cII on promoter P_{RE}, it binds to O_{R1}. This binding of repressor to O_{R1} has a co-operative effect on the operator O_{R2} and increases its affinity for the repressor by many fold. As a result, when more molecules of the repressor are present, they will keep binding to O_{R2} unless it is fully saturated. The position of O_{R1} is such that on one hand it interferes with the binding of RNA polymerase to the promoter P_R and represses the transcription of early genes, on the other hand, it provides an extra site of interaction for the RNA polymerase which is initiating the transcription at the promoter P_{RM} and its activity is stimulated. The net result is that the repressor synthesis by the promoter P_{RM} is increased and the expression of all the other genes is switched off. However, when the repressor becomes in large excess and all the O_{R2} and also the O_{R1} sites have become saturated, the repressor binds to O_{R3}. Operator O_{R3} is located within the RNA polymerase binding site of the promoter P_{RM}. Therefore, the expression of the cI gene is blocked and the repressor synthesis is stopped. Binding of repressor to O_{R1} and O_{R2} does not have any co-operative effect on the O_{R3} site. Therefore, the O_{R3} gets saturated only after the O_{R1} and the O_{R2} sites are fully saturated. In this manner the repressor regulates its own synthesis and ensures that only appropriate concentration of repressor is maintained at any given time.

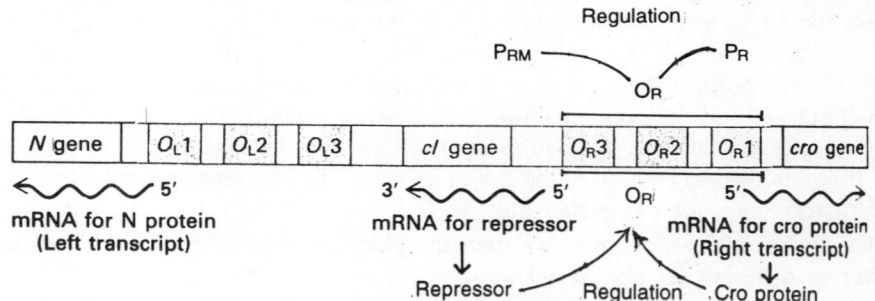

Fig. 8.37. Diagram of the O_L and O_R operator regions and the adjacent genes. O_{L1} and and O_{R1} have the highest affinity for the λ repressor. The repressor gene is cl. The left transcript starts with the N gene, whereas the right transcript starts with the cro gene.

Reversal to lytic phase

If the host becomes inhospitable, the phage goes back to the lytic mode and gets out of the host by lysing the bacteria. How does it do so? The key role is played by the Cro protein. The operators O_{R1}, O_{R2} and O_{R3} have the affinity for and may bind to the Cro protein also. Cro is a small protein of 9 KD which is active in its dimer form. It has similar DNA binding motiffs as the lambda repressor (the HTH type). However, the affinity of its binding to the operators O_{R1}, O_{R2} and O_{R3} is different than the affinity of the repressor binding to these operators. The Cro protein has highest affinity for O_{R3}. The affinity for O_{R1} and O_{R2} is much less. Also, the relative affinity of Cro for O_{R1} is about

10% of that of the affinity of the repressor for this site. Moreover, there is no co-operative effect of Cro which is bound to O_{R3} on its binding to O_{R1} or to O_{R2}. Thus even small amounts of the Cro protein can block the activity of the promoter P_{RM} and stop the repressor synthesis without blocking its own synthesis. It should be remembered that the site O_{R3} is not within the RNA polymerase binding region of the promoter P_R while the O_{R1} and O_{R2} are.

As discussed, the repressor is active only in its dimer form. When phage has to revert back to the lytic cycle, specific proteases digest the connector region of repressor (between aa 111-113, see earlier discussion) and the two domains of the repressor are separated. As a result, the dimer formation can not take place. There is a dynamic equilibrium between the monomer, the dimer and the bound form of the repressor. The inability of dimer formation results in release of the bound repressor so that equilibrium can be maintained. This releases the negative pressure on the promoter P_R and the Cro protein synthesis is established. This Cro protein, on the other hand, binds to O_{R3} and prevents the synthesis of fresh repressor. The collective result of these two activities is that the phage enters into lytic phase.

Any damage to the host cell DNA also activates the repressor hydrolysis and causes the reversal to the lytic cycle. For example, it can be mediated through another protein, RecA. RecA is normally responsible for the recombination events of host DNA. However, when bound to SS DNA, it possesses a protease activity. If there is damage to host DNA and SS DNA is formed, a protease activity is generated through RecA. This protease activity hydrolyses the repressor. Similarly, if there is extensive damage to the cells, it call the signal for a SOS response (Fig. 8.38). The SOS response is mediated through another protein, LexA. LexA also has protease activity and hydrolyses the repressor. This hydrolysis of the repressor, in both cases, leads to the reversal of the phage to the lytic mode of life cycle.

Balance between the lysogenic and the lytic cycles

Previous discussions have made it clear that the infection of host with the phage can lead either to the lytic or to lysogenic phases of life cycle. The critical point in determining the fate of the phage is whether the transcription through promoter P_{RE} will lead to the activation of the promoter P_{RM} or not. If promoter P_{RM} is activated, lysogeny will take over, otherwise the lytic cycle will continue. The relative concentrations of repressor and the Cro proteins are very important for this purpose. Protein cII plays a key role here in establishing the lysogeny. A number of factors, including the nutritional status of the cell, the sorrounding environment and the growth conditions of the host are very important.

REGULATION OF GENE EXPRESSION IN EUKARYOTES

A typical eukaryotic cell is much more complex than the prokaryotic cell. It has a large number of genes, many of these are under different regulatory mechanisms. The details of some of these mechanisms for regulation of gene expression are very well understood while certain other mechanisms are not fully understood. Efforts are being made to understand many more of these processes. Recent progress in genetics and recombinant DNA technology has made it possible to understand many of these mechanisms. However, many efforts have been made to understand and to explain various regulatory mechanisms and a number of different theories have been proposed from time to time to explain the regulation of gene expression. Back in 1969 R.J. Britten and E.H. Davidson proposed a model to explain the regulation of gene expression in higher animals involving complex circuits. This model became one of the most popular models at the time. Even though a lot is known about the regulation of gene expression today, the model is important and can explain the general mode of expression of many inducible eukaryotic gene under the control of exogeneous signals. It has been described below.

Britten-Davidson model of gene expression

The model proposes that many of the structural genes in the cell respond to different cell signals and are regulated in an integrated manner. The level of expression is controlled by certain regulatory genes which are present in a moderatory repeatitive manner. These genes have specific functions and are referred as the *sensor genes*. The sensor genes have sequence specific binding sites for and respond to a number of exogeneous cell signals such as the hormones and other messengers. These signals modulate the sensory genes, which in turn, regulate the transcription of the genes under their influence (the *integral genes*). The model has been represented in Fig. 8.39 in a simple diagramatic manner. The integral genes and the sensor genes are present adjacent to each other. The product of integral gene, which is an RNA molecule and is called as the *activator RNA*, then interacts with another gene, the receptor gene. The receptor gene is the last in the series of the regulatory genes. The interaction of activator RNA with regulatory genes is in a sequence specific manner. However, it was proposed that it will not make any difference if the product of the integrator gene was a protein in place of an RNA. A protein will also act in a similar manner. In other words, a regulatory protein can replace the activator RNA in this model. The interaction of activator RNA with receptor gene acts as a trigger for the transcription of the *producer gene*, which is the eukaryotic counterpart of the structural genes present in prokaryotic operon. These genes code for the proteins which regulate the cellular metabolism. Ultimately the transcription of producer genes and the production of essential proteins is modulated by the external signals.

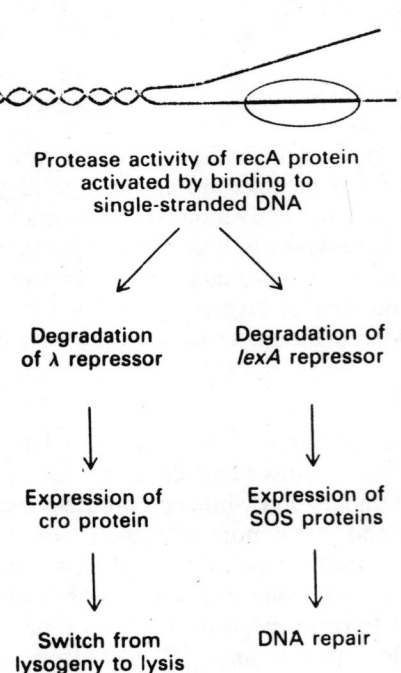

Fig. 8.38. Proteolysis of λ repressor by RecA protein bound to single-stranded DNA leads to the termination of lysogeny and the induction of the lytic pathway of this phage.

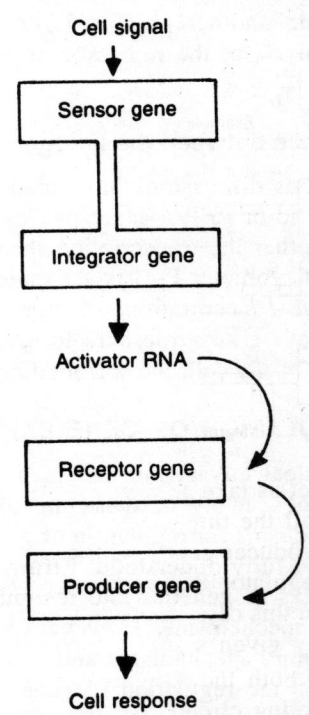

Fig. 8.39. Regulation of gene expression.

By using various possibilities one can devise a number of scenerios. For example, let us consider a case where there are three producer genes, P-1, P-2 and P-3; three receptor genes, namely, the R-1, R-2 and R-3. The receptor genes are redundant and are present in different combination with each of the three producer genes. Three different sensor genes S-1, S-2 and S-3 are present, each having its own integral gene, I-1; I-2 and I-3, respectively. Let us assume that P-1 is associated with all the three receptor genes R-1, R-2 and R-3, similarly P-2 is associated with R-1 and R-2 only while P-3 is associated with R-1 and R-3. Upon receiving the exogeneous regulatory signal, S-1 gets excited and activates I-1 which produces respective activator RNAs. This will activate the expression of all the three producer genes. Similarly, the excitation of S-2 will activate P-1 and P-2 while the excitation of S-3 will activate the transcription of P-1 and P-3. In other words, P-1 will be activated with any of the three signals, P-2 will be activated by S-1 and S-2 only while P-3 will be activated by S-1 and S-3. Thus the cellular response in relation with any given external signal will depend upon the presence of corresponding receptor gene which is associated with any producer gene (Fig. 8.40).

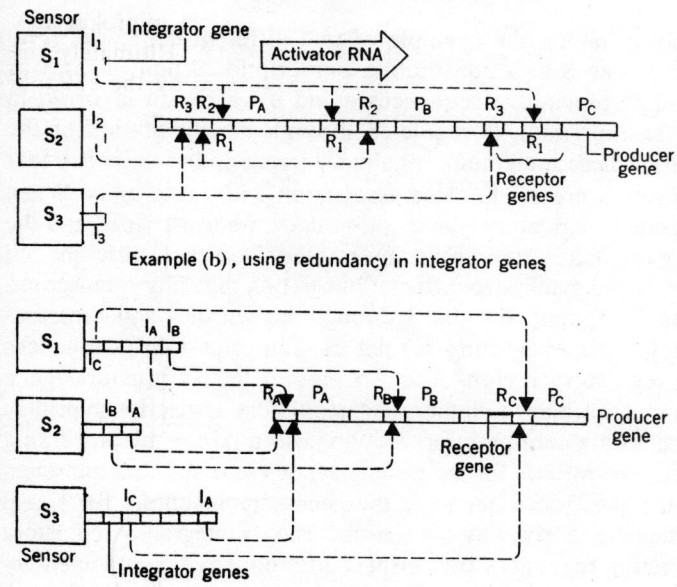

Fig. 8.40. The Britten and Davidson model of regulation of gene expression in eukaryotes. Two variations of integrated regulation are shown: (a) a system based on redundancy of "receptor" genes, and (b) a system based on redundancy of "integrator" genes. The three "sensor" genes (S_1, S_2, and S_3) respond to three different signals such as hormone-receptor complexes. The diagrams schematize the events proposed to occur after the sensor genes have triggered the transcription of their respective integrator genes (I_1, I_2, I_3 or I_A, I_B, I_C). The integrator gene products, "activator RNAs", diffuse from their sites of synthesis (integrator genes) to their sites of action (receptor genes). The binding of the various activator RNAs to the respective receptor genes somehow triggers the transcription of the contiguous producer genes (P_A, P_B, P_C). Depending on which integrator gene (or genes) is activated by its sensor gene (or genes), one, two, or all three of the producer genes (structural genes) may be turned on.

Let us take another case where the integrator genes are redundant. The sensor gene S-1 is associated with all the three integral genes I-1, I-2 and I-3 but have only one regulator gene, the R-1 and only one producer gene, the P-1. Similarly S-2 is associated with two integrals, the I-1 and I-2 but with only one regulator R-2 and one producer, P-2. Sensor S-3 on the other hand has I-1 and I-3 and R-3 and P-3. In this case, depending on which of the three (or how many of the three) integral genes are activated by any given signal, corresponding producer genes will be turned on.

If both the receptor genes and the integrating genes are redundant, then it is possible to devise integrating circuits for the gene expression. The model thus explains that the turning on or off of a gene depends on a complex circuit of a series of mutually dependent genes. The activation of one gene will modulate other genes under its influence, so for and so on. It is possible to explain tissue specific response of a particular signal by this model. However, testing the validity of these models are much more difficult than to devise these models. As the understanding of a number of processes progressed and new analytical methods were developed, it was observed that the primary transcript i.e hnRNA is much more complex than the mRNA. This led to the suggestion that considerable degree of regulation takes place during the post-transcriptional processing of RNA. Based on previous model and these observations, Davidson and Britten proposed another model referred as the Davidson-Britten model. This model has been described below.

The Davidson-Britten model of regulation of gene expression

The model proposes that most of the structural genes of an animal are present as *constitutive transcription units* and these are expressed in all the cells at a basal level. However, the post-transcriptional processing of these primary transcripts take place only in the cells which express the appropriate integral genes producing the *integral regulatory transcripts*. These transcripts are produced in a cell specific manner. The presence of an integral regulatory transcript is essential before a primary transcript of the structural gene can be processed to form respective mRNA.

This model can be understood very well by taking the example of two different cell types (Fig. 8.41). Both the cell types express a structural gene S as a constitutive transcriptional unit, using I as the initiation site. These transcripts have middle repeatitive sequences a and b which are involved in tissue specific expression. The tissue specific expression is regulated through the integration of the regulatory transcription units. The expression of these integrating regulatory transcription units is under the control of the sensors which are the sequences present in close association with these units. When sensors receive appropriate signals, the integrating regulatory transcription units are transcribed and the primary transcripts, referred as the integrating regulatory transcripts, are formed. However, different cell types have receptors for different types of signals and synthesize different integrating regulatory transcripts. For example, in the present case, the cell type 1 responds to signal 1 through the sensor 1 and expresses the integrating regulatory transcription unit 1. This integrating regulatory transcript 1 has sequences a' and b' which are complementary to the regulatory regions a and b present in the structural gene transcript. As a result, the structural gene transcript and the integrating regulatory transcript hybridize with each other and form a complex structure with a configuration which is essential for the processing of the primary transcript of the structural gene. The mRNA for the gene is synthesized and it is translated to form the protein. On the other hand, cell type 2 does not have the necessary receptors for signal 1. It has the receptors for another signal 2, which are received by the sensor 2 and its integrating regulatory transcription unit 2 is transcribed. This integrating regulatory transcript 2 does not have complementary sequences for a and b region of the structural gene, rather have different regulatory regions, c and d. The net result is that the primary transcript for structural gene can not hybridize with the integrating regulatory transcript 2 and the secondary structure essential for its processing is not formed. Thus no mature mRNA is formed and the translation does not take place. The net result is that the structural gene is not expressed in the cell type 2. However, the cell type two will express other specific genes by the same mechanism.

The integral regulatory transcripts have repetitive sequences which can interact with different structural gene transcripts in the same manner as the different receptor genes modulate the producer genes in the earlier model discussed previously. The major difference between two models is that the regulation at the transcriptional level can be explained by the earlier Bitten-Davidson model and the regulation taking place at post-transcriptional level can be understood by its modified version, the Davidson-Britten model of gene regulation.

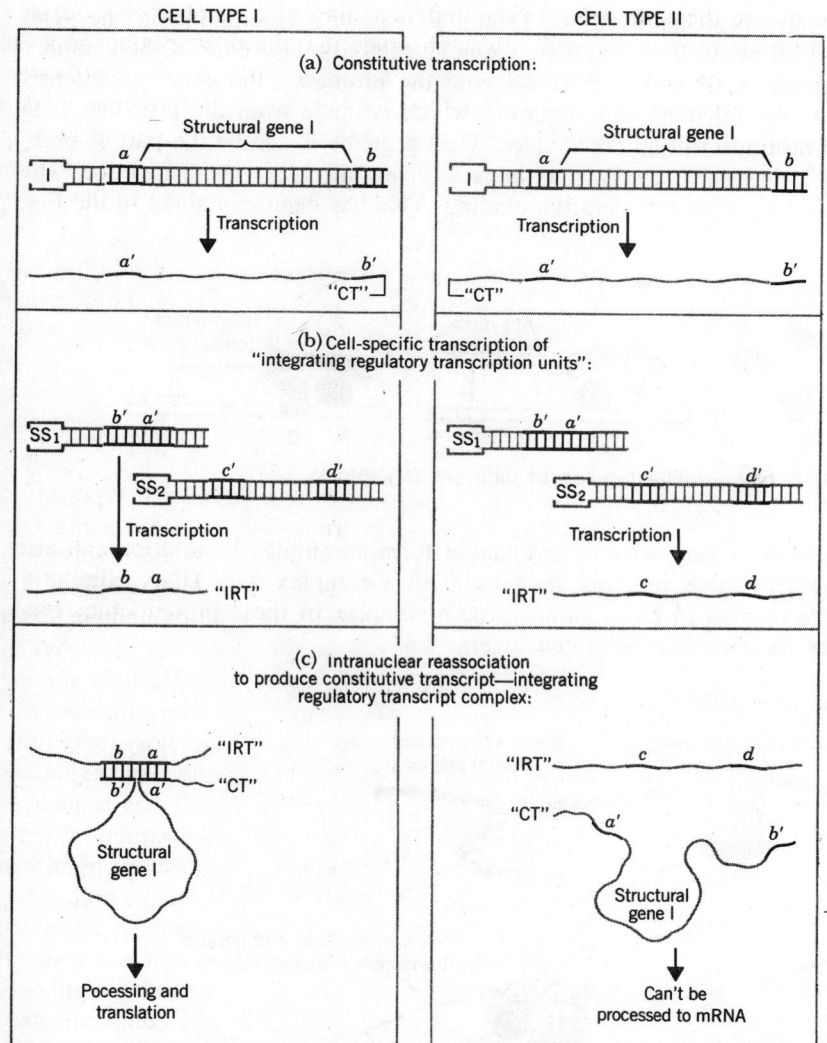

Fig. 8.41. The Davidson and Britten model for the regulation of gene expression at the RNA processing level in eukaryotes.

General mechanisms for regulation of gene expression

In the cell a number of regulatory factors, usually proteins, each with some effect on the gene expression are present. A number of modifications, processing and the mutual interaction of these factors may be essential for their effect. Some of the general mechanisms of these processes have been discussed below.

Co-operative binding of regulatory proteins

Sometimes more than one proteins form a complex and the complex is able to regulate the expression of a gene. In formation of these complexes, often a number of proteins participate. Some of these proteins may participate in the formation of more than one type of complexes, often with opposite activity. For example, four different proteins A, B, C, D and E may be participating in the gene regulation. None of these proteins all by itself can regulate the gene actaivity. However, if the complex 1 which is made up of the proteins A, B and C interacts with the promoter, the gene is switched on and its transcription starts. On the other hand, complex 2 which is made from the proteins A, D and E switches the gene off and no transcription takes place. Thus proteins A can be the part of both, the complex 1 and the complex 2. Note that the two complexes have entirely opposite function. The effect of these proteins is achieved by their co-operative binding. This has been explained in the Fig. 8.42.

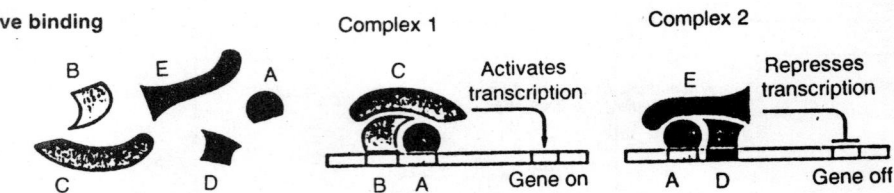

Fig. 8.42. Cooperative binding of different regulators.

Further, the proteins which interact very weakly and cannot form a complex in solution can also bind to each other if one or both of these proteins are present in a complex with DNA. Similarly, none of the proteins may be able to bind to DNA alone while a complex of these proteins may bind very strongly. These possibiities have been represented in. Fig. 8.43.

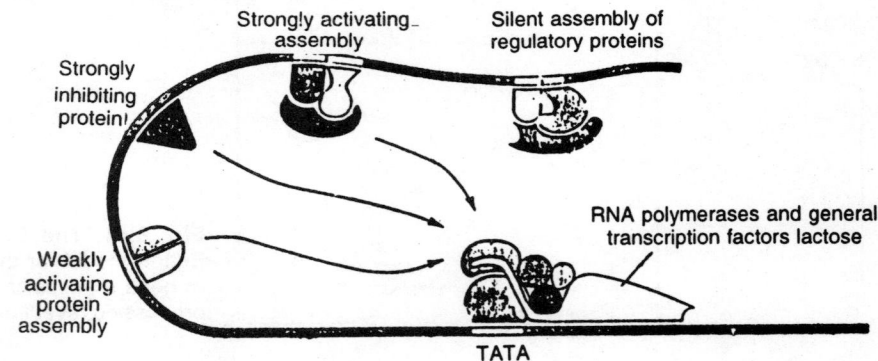

Fig. 8.43. Interaction of two proteins may result in stronger activity.

The complex regulatory modules are usually made of simple modules

A number of complex mammalian genes are regulated by a variety of different modules. The regulatory region of the genes may be very large, sometimes as big as 50 kb. This region has many binding sites where different regulatory proteins can bind. These proteins may be either a single protein or a module made up of many proteins. Each of these modules will have different effect on the promoter activity. Each of the module may have equal affinity for the interaction with the promoter region. Thus the level of expression will be governed by a very complex mechanism. The mechanism of the integration of various 'switches' is not always clear. This has been illustrated in Fig. 8.44. The promoter binds to the RNA polymerase and also to the general transcription factors and directs the transcription of the gene. However, the upstream regulatory region of the gene has a number of binding sites for different sets of regulatory proteins. Set A is strongly inhibitory, set B is weakly activating, set C is strongly activating while set D is a silencer which will totally shut off the gene. The topology of gene is such that each of these can interact with the promoter with equal affinity. The expression status of gene will depend on the integration of all these controls. A number of external factors may shift the balance to one or the other side.

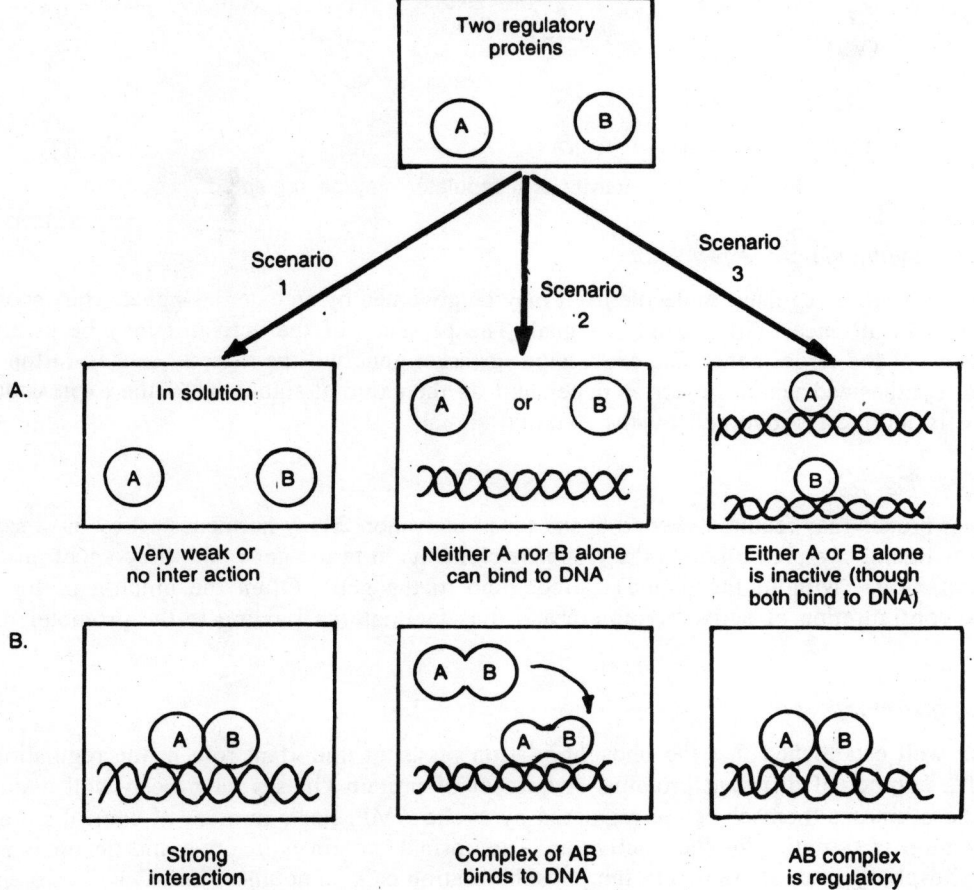

Fig. 8.44. Integration at a promoter. Multiple sets of gene regulatory proteins can work together to influence a promoter, as they do in the eve stripe 2 module. It is not yet understood to detail how the integration of multiple inputs is achieved.

The activity of the regulators may also be regulataed

Often a regulatory protein may be present in the cell which may be capable of regulating the gene expression under appropriate conditions. It may be present in an inactive form under normal conditions and may need some type of external signal for its activation. These signals may carry out one (or more) of the many functions. Some of these are enumerated below and have been represented in Fig. 8.45.

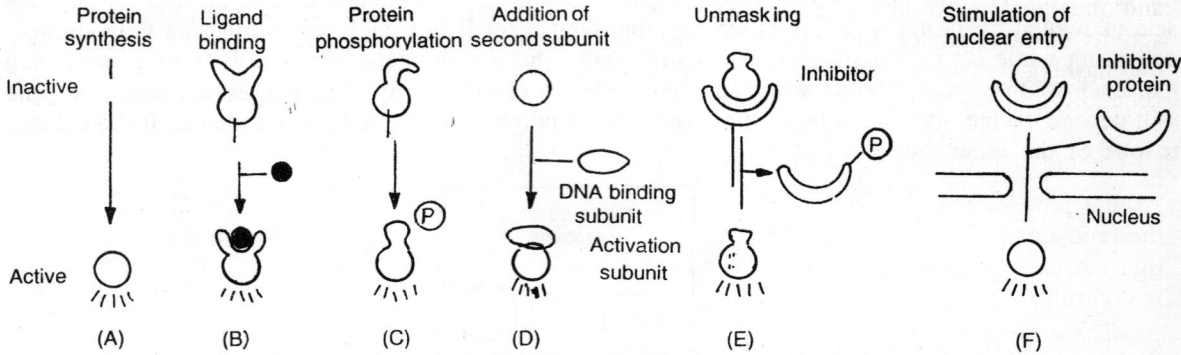

Fig. 8.45. The activity of a regulator may be regulated.

(a) Controlled synthesis of the regulator

The gene for a positive regulator molecule itself may be governed by an external signal. Thus no activator is synthesized in absence of the external signal. The presence of the activator may be essential for the expression of the target gene. The expression of target gene will be directly related to the amount of regulator synthesized which in turn is dependent on the external signal. Thus the expression of the target gene is indirectly governed by the external signal.

(b) Ligand binding

The regulator protein may require a second ligand for its activation. Many hormones act by this mechanism. The receptor-ligand complex binds to the response elements in target gene and affects its transcription. The receptor alone (without the ligand) cannot bind to the gene. Often the binding of ligand may change the configuration of activator protein and thus facilitate its binding to the promoter region of the gene.

(c) Protein phosphorylation

It has been well established that the phosphorylation plays an important role in the regulation of the activity of a number of different proteins. A number of protein kineses have been well documented. Many of these kineses themselves are regulated by cyclic AMP. For a number of control elements the phosphorylation is essential for their activities. The normal protein is inactive and becomes activated after it is phosphorylated, alternatively the phosphorylation can, sometimes, inactivate a protein which is otherwise active.

(d) Addition of another protein to the regulator protein may be essential

Some of the proteins may be active only when associated with another protein. The binding of second protein is regulated by the external signal. This protein-protein interaction regulates the activity of the control element and indirectly affects the expression of target gene.

(e) Derepression

The activity of a regulator may ordinarily be masked by the presence of another protein. This may take place either by changing the configuration of the regulator or just by covering the active site and thus making it unavailable. The removal of this masking protein may be essential for the activity of the regulator. Many times the phosphorylation of the masking protein may be required. Once the masking protein has dissociated, the regulator becomes activated and exerts its effect on the target gene.

(f) The nuclear transport of the regulator may be obligatory

As the proteins are synthesized in the cytoplasm while the transcription is a nuclear phenomenon, the regulator protein has to be transproted to the nucleus so that it may exert its effect. It is possible that the entry of the regulator to the nucleus can be regulated so that its effect on the target gene is controlled.

These are some of the commonly used processes for the regulation of the activity of a regulator protein. Many other less common processes may also be working in the cell.

Factors affecting the eukaryotic transcription

Living organisms have a remarkable property of adoptation according to change in the environment. This is achieved by changing the cell metabolism in response to external factors. Similar to prokaryates, eukaryotes can also change their cell metabolism in response to various factors. This is achieved by a change in the expression of a number of genes. A number of exogeneous factors affect the expression of the response genes. Some of these factors have been discussed below.

Response to Stress

A number of genes are present in almost all the animals which code for different proteins responsible for the adoptation to various types of stresses. Exposure to high temperature is one of such stresses. A number of specific proteins referred as the heat shock proteins are expressed as the result of exposure to high temperaure. HSP 70, a 70 KD protein is the most widely studied heat shock protein. This protein is one of the highly conserved proteins which has maintained its structure during the evolution and has very high degree of sequence homology amongst the different species. There is more than 50% homology between the HSP 70 of E. coli and its human counterpart. More than 85% homology is present between HSP 70 of human and Drosophila. The critical temperature for the expression of these proteins varies from organisms to organisms. For example, 30°C triggers its synthesis in drosophila while 40°C triggers its production in human. In bacteria, a specific σ factor is switched on as the result of heat shock. The normal σ factor which is the product of gene rpoD in E. coli, is 70 KD in size. The heat shock specific σ factor which is the product of gene rpoH is a 32 KD protein. This sigma factor recognizes the alternate promoter sequence (−35 region) CCCTTGAA-13-15bp-CCCGATNT (−10 region) in place of the consensus sequence of the promoter (−35 region) TTGACA-16-18bp-TATAAT (−10 region). In eukaryotes, on the other hand, the regulatory proteins bind to a upstream sequence at HSP genes and not to the promoter or the RNA polymerase. There is a heat shock binding factor (HSF, 110 KD) which is present in two metabolic forms, active and inactive, and regulates the expression of HSP. Exposure to high temperative activates HSF. Deletion studies have revealed that a 20 bp element present at a region of about 20 nucleotide upstream of TATA box is essential for this response. Within this element is the sequence which is recognized by this factor (HSF). This sequence is referred as the heat shock response element (HSRE or HRE) and has the following consensus sequence.

5' CNNGAANNTTCNNG 3'

The sequence analysis reveals that HSRE has a dyad symetry and the HSF acts as a transcription factor, which is essential for the transcription of HSP gene and synthesis of the HSP mRNA.

Similarly a set of specific proteins, the metallothioneins (MT), are synthesized in response to heavy metal exposure. Metallothioneins are low molecular weight proteins with an extra–ordinarily high Cys content. Exposure to Cd or Pb can increase the MT level by upto 50 fold in mouse. The MT gene has a regulatory region upstream of TATA box with following sequence:

5' CTNTGCPuCPyCGGCCC 3',

This sequence is known as the metal response element (MRE). The MRE seems to be the only requirement for responding to the heavy metals. It has been observed that MRE can confer metal inducibility to a gene which normally does not respond to the heavy metals. For example, by cloning the MRE upstream of the tk gene by genetic engineering procedures, it was found that the expression of the hybrid gene can be induced by heavy metals. It resulted in increased TK production when E. coli cells having the recombinant plasmids were grown in metal rich medium. In fact the expression of such chimeric genes is often amplified by exposure to heavy metals. In plant cells, MT is not present, however, an analogous protein, phytochelatin, is synthesized in plants in response to the metal stress. In plants a number of other proteins which are produced in response to salinity, alkaline soils and other stresses have been reported.

Hormone dependent genes

Hormones regulate the entire metabolism of the cells. A number of hormones, specially the gluco-corticoids and steroid hormones regulate the expression of a number of genes. The action of most of the hormones is usually mediated through the specific receptors. The hormones bind to specific receptors to form the receptor-hormone complexes. These complexes modulate the expression of the target genes. The receptors for a number of hormones such as the steroid hormones, corticoids, thyroid hormone as well as for certain vitamins and some other ligands have a general structure which has been shown in Fig. 8.46. These receptors have a variable region of 100-500 aa at the N-terminal end which gives the hormonal specificity to the receptor. This variable region is followed by a DNA binding motif of ~68 aa. The DNA binding domain is separated from the hormone binding domain by a spacer region of variable length. The hormone binding region is an epitope of 225-300 aa present at the C-terminal. The binding of hormone to its receptor modulates its DNA binding domain. The DNA binding domain of the receptors, can now bind to the target gene and modulate its expression. For example a DNA binding protein produced by adrenal glands in response to corticoid hormone increases the transcription of the MMTV genes.

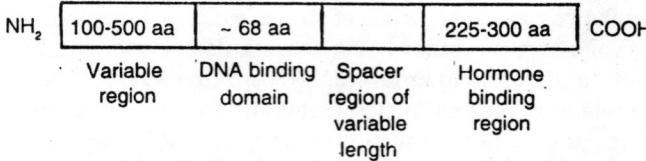

Fig. 8.46. General structure of a receptor.

It has been found that the receptor:hormone complex binds to the DNA through its DNA binding domain. The binding of this complex takes place within a 1.2 kb fragment of the target genes in MMTV. This region has hormone dependent transcription initiation sites. The sequences of different hormone response elements are given in Fig. 8.47.

Gluco-corticoid response element (GRE)	5' GGTACANNNTGTTCT 3'
Estrogen response element (ERE)	5' GGTCANNNTGA/TCC 3'
Thyroid hormone response element (TRE)	5' GTTCANNNNNNTGACC 3'

Fig. 8.47. Structures of hormone response elements.

Cell surface receptor-ligand interaction

A number of regulatory molecules, which affect the gene expression do not interact with the target genes at all. These regulators which are sometimes called as the first messenger, include a number of peptide hormones and many·other biomolecules. The first messenger has receptors at the cell surface to which it specifically binds, this binding stimulates (or inhibits) the synthesis of a small molecule (the second messenger). Some of these changes are the diacyl glycerol formation, changes in Ca^{++} ion concentration, formation of cAMP or other cyclic nucleotides (cGMP, for example) and other small regulatory molecules. The change in the concentration of the second messenger, on the other hand, triggers a cascade of cellular events which ultimately lead to various metabolic changes like the protein phosphorylation. These changes result in the regulation of a number of key events. These events may either result in immediate change in the gene expression or may result in a prompt change in the transcription by the involvement of DNA binding proteins (Fig. 8.48).

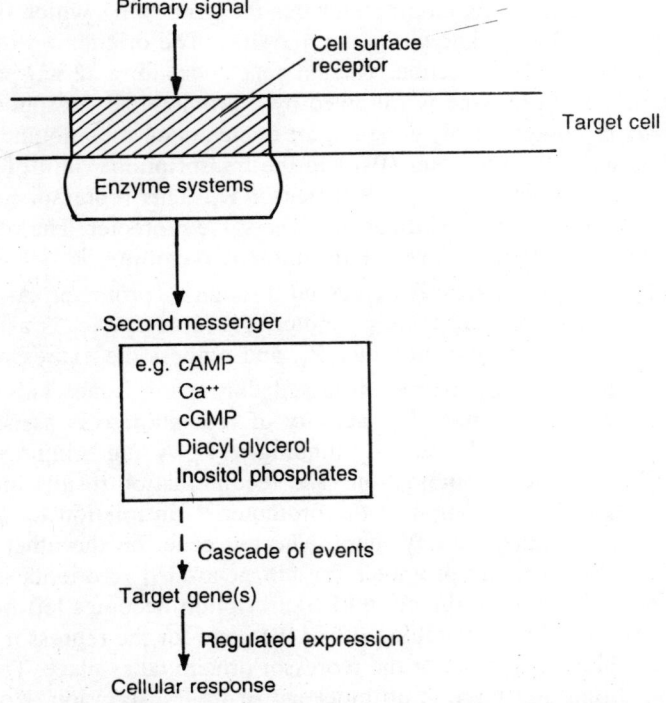

Fig. 8.48. The second messenger mediated cell responses.

Regulation of proto-ocncogenes

A number of genes are known to code for tumourogenic proteins. These genes, known as oncogenes, are often present in the cell in their precursor form, the proto-oncogenes. The proto-oncogenes are inactive and donot lead to malignancy. However, these can become tumourogenic as the result of a minor mutation and can cause cancers. A number of carcinogens lead to the activation of these genes resulting in their expression. On the other hand, the genes for a number of growth factors like PDGF and EGF may become hyperactive in response to the exposure to certain carcinogens. This hyperactivity will also ultimately lead to cancers.

Regulation of Gene Expression by genetic recombination

Many of the genes have either direct or inverted repeats in their sequence. These elements can undergo homologous recombination, as a result of this the internal arrangement of the gene will change. It is possible that this change will switch a particular gene either 'on' or 'off'. Phase veriation in Salmonella by gene inversion using a flipflop circuit is a good example of this type of regulation.

The movement of Salmonella inside the intestine of the host is achieved by the rotation of flagella present on its surface. This rotation of the flagella is essential for the survival of the organism. The flagella is primarily made of a protein flagellin which helps in its rotation. The flagellin is a 53 KD protein which is present in two molecular forms. The two forms of flagellin are related to each other and are coded by two separate genes H_1 and H_2 respectively. Both the genes are under the influence of separate promoters and are present at separate loci. The locus of gene H_2 is the regulatory site. This locus has a complex arrangement. The structural gene is preceded by a 1 kb regulatory region, which functions as the inversion module. This module includes the gene 'hin', which is flanked on both sides by a short inverted repeats of 14 bp, known as the hix sites. The orientation of the promoter and the gene hin transcribes it in right handed direction. The hin gene codes for a 22 KD protein, the recombinase, which is active as a dimer. The hin gene is followed by a promoter, P_2, responsible for regulating the H_2 gene expression. This promoter for H_2 gene is part of inversion module and the repeat at the right side (hix 2) is located between the promoter (P_2) and the transcriptional unit of H_2 gene. The H_2 gene is followed by another ORF which codes for a repressor R_1. This repressor gene is in a contiguous manner with the H_2 gene and is under the influence of the same promoter. The repressor acts on another gene H_1 which codes for the alternate form of the protein flagellin.

Under normal conditions, the H_2 gene is expressed through P_2 promoter. As both the repressor and the H_2 genes are under the influence of same promoter, the repressor R_1 is also expressed alongwith the H_2 gene. This repressor binds to the promoter P_1, and renders the expression of the gene H_1 off.

However, the recombinase is also being expressed during this time. This protein can cause the recombination between the two hix sites. The activity of recombinase is assisted by another protein Fis (factor for inversion stimulation). Fis acts by binding to DNA and bringing the two hix sites near to each other, thus facilitating the recombination. The recombination results into the inversion of the entire module. This results in re-orientation of the promoter P_2 in relation to the transcription unit of the gene H_2 which cannot be expressed any more. The hin gene, on the other hand, is also inverted along with the hix sites. However the promoter for hin gene also re-orients itself and the gene can continue to be transcribed. Though the direction of transcription becomes left handed in place of right handed. This inversion also results in switching off of the gene for the repressor R_1 alongwith the gene H_2. Thus no synthesis of either H_2 protein or the repressor protein takes place. The gene H_1 is expressed as the repressor is now absent and there is no blockage of its transcription. However, recombinase is still being produced. It will invert the entire module again and H_2 will again be expressed while the H_1 will be switched off. The process has been explained in Fig. 8.49.

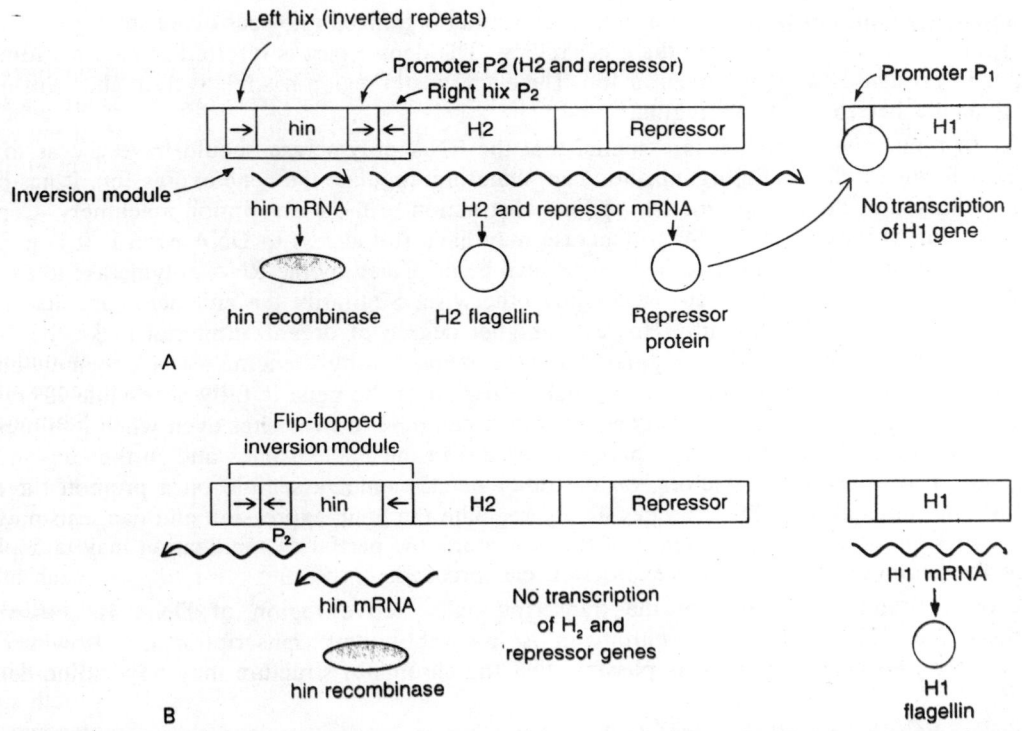

Fig. 8.49. Phase variation in Salmonella. Flagellins H1 and H2 are expressed in a mutually exclusive manner. (A) In phase 2, the HI gene is silenced by a repressor protein formed along with the H2 protein. (B) In phase I, inversion of a DNA segment catalyzed by a recombinase (Hin) encoded by it leads to the loss of the promoter for H2 and the repressor. H1 is then expressed. Further inversions switch the system back and forth between these phases.

The process continues and the Salmonella keeps on flip flopping between H_1 and H_2 forms of flagellins. This mechanism confuses the host immune system and helps the parasite to evade it. The regulation of these genes is absolute and even the background synthesis of the product of an 'off' gene does not take place. This is further ensured by the fact that upon inversion, the promoter for H_2 gene is physically about 1 kb away from the main body of the gene.

Similar mechanism also operates at a number of other systems. Some of these systems are as following.

(a) Host range variation of bacteriophage μ by inversion of the Gin/gix sites.

(b) Switching of the yeast mating types between a and α by recombination at HO endonuclease RAD 52 and other proteins/MAT locus resulting in non reciprocal gene conversion (see later).

(c) The antigenic variation of trypanosome at various non-reciprocal sites.

Regulation of gene expression by chromatin structure

As discussed earlier, the DNA of an average cell is present as a highly compact structure referred as the chromatin. The chromatin is nucleoprotein in nature, both DNA and protein contributing roughly equally. The proteins are either the histones or non-histone proteins. Certain amount of RNA may also be involved in the formation of the chromatin structure. The chromatin has three levels of organization. In first level, the DNA is wrapped arround the histones to form the nucleosomes, which are further organized into the 30 nm fibres. The 30 nm fibres are further organized into scaffolded structure. Certain parts of chromatin are more dense than the other region. The denser part is referred as heterochromatin while reletively less dense part is the euchromatin. The euchromatin region has relatively higher sensitivity to DNase than the heterochromatin region.

In order to transcribe a gene, it is essential that the RNA polymerase should have access to the DNA. Various levels of chromatin organization can, therefore, regulate the gene expression. It has been found that nucleosomes do not present any serious obstruction to the transcription machinery. Certain regulatory proteins as well as the RNA polymerase may have full access to DNA even if it is present as nucleosome (see later). It seems that the histones can be displaced by the RNA polymerase to expose the promoter region, if it is not already accessible otherwise. Similarily the enhancers are also fully active within the nucleosome structure. However, higher degree of organization can make the DNA unaccessible. The packaging can, thus, regulate the gene expression by silencing a DNA segment either in a reversible manner or irreversibily. The regulatory region of the gene is fully accessible if present in a nucleosome free region. Some of the gene activators can bind to their sites even when it is present within the nucleosome. This binding can partially destablize the nucleosomes and further unwinding can take place. The transcription factors, on the other hand, cannot assemble on a promoter if it is present within the nucleosome. This can negatively regulate the gene expression and can also prevent the leaky expression. However, in presence of the activators, the partial destabilization may take place and expose the promoter and the gene expression can proceed.

It has been found that generally the transcriptionally active region of DNA is present as euchromatin while DNA within heterochromatin is invariably inert transcriptionally. However, in response to certain specific signals, it is possible that the chromatin structure may have some degree of flexibility.

A few cases have been well understood where the chromatin structure switches a gene 'on' or 'off'. For example, the ADE 2 gene of yeast is expressed under normal organization of the genome. If one relocates this gene near the telomere of the chromosome, the gene becomes silent. Similar silencing of a number of other genes is seen if these are positioned within 10 kb of the telomere region. This phenomenon is referred as `silencing by positioning'.

The β-globin gene cluster is another example of this type of regulation. The entire cluster is consisted of a 50 kb region of the genome and contains 5 genes. The α and β genes are expressed in adults, the ε globin is expressed in embryonic yolk sac, γ-globin is present in yolk sac and in fetal liver while the δ and β-globins are present in the adult bone marrow. It has been found that the entire locus is DNase sensitive in the erythoid cells where it is expressed efficiently. On the other hand, it is DNase resistant in non-erythoid cells and is not expressed. This provides a strong case for the regulation of gene expression by chromatin orgenization. Further, the regulation of the entire globin cluster is by global chaperones in the chromatin structure. These chaperones are also responsible for the development stage specific expression of different genes of these clusters. These proteins interact at a specific region, the locus control region (LCR). If LCR is not present or if it is displaced, the genes cannot be expressed.

How does this work? There can be a number of different possible mechanisms. It is possible that the sequence specific DNA binding proteins may associate with various genes and cause the decondensation of the gene. Once, the gene is decondensed, there will be assembly of transcription factors and the RNA polymerase, resulting in the initiation of transcription. Thus the expression of the gene will be altered. This binding of the chaperones may also release the superhelical tension by gyration and may facilitate the expression. There may also be the nucleating effect due to the alteration of chromatin structure and/or the loss of protein coat from the gene, resulting in more efficient expression of the gene.

Role of sigma factor in regulation of gene expression

Sigma factor provides the specificity for the RNA polymerase and facilitates its binding to the promoter region. In absence of the sigma factor, the binding of RNA.polymerse to the DNA is non-specific and its binding to a region other than the promoter does not lead to successful transcription. The general sigma factor is a protein of ~70 KD in size and is the product of gene rpoD. However, under specific physiological, metabolic and environmental conditions inside and around the cell, such as in response to stress, specialised genes are expressed. During this period, the expression of the 'normal' genes is 'shut off' or is reduced to a very low level and the stress genes are switched on. This emergency response is achieved, amongst other mechanisms, by the synthesis of the specific sigma factors. In response to stress, the synthesis of stress specific sigma factors is enhanced. These factors, which recognize the promoters of the specific genes, bind to the core enzyme and the transcription of the stress genes is achieved. For example in E. coli a number of sigma factors have been recognized. Various sigma factors and their recognition sequence have been summmerised in Table 8.2.

Table 8.2. Various sigma factors of E.coli

Coding gene	Sigma factor: size, and specificity	Recognition sequence present on the promoter of target gene		
		−35 region	Spacer	−10 region
rpoD	General sigma factor, 70 KD	TTCACA	16-18nt	TATAAT
rpoH	Heat shock specific σ factor, 32KD	CCCTTGAA	13-15nt	CCCGATNT
rpoN	Nitrogen starvation specific σ factor, 54 KD	CTGGNA	6nt	TTGCA
fliA	Flagella specific σ factor, 28KD	CTAAA	15nt	GCCGATAA
	Consensus	TTGACA	16-19nt	TATAAT

Different sigma factors have different DNA binding domains which recognize a specific sequence present in (or near) the promoter region of their target gene. They regulate the gene expression by direct binding to DNA which results in correct positioning of the RNA polymerase. However, there are some common conserved regions among different sigma factors which may help in its association with the RNA polymerse. These specific sigma factors have one region for the association with RNA polymerase and another region which recognizes the specific gene sequences.

The expression of phage genes provides a good example of the role of sigma factors in regulation of gene expression. It has been found that there is a whole cascade of various sigma factors in the life cyeles of phages. The sequential expression of various genes of lambda phage is regulated by this cascade. Similarly the phage Spo1, which infects B. subtilis, depends on specific sigma factors for its life cycle. The genes of the phage are expressed in three groups, the early, the intermediate and the late genes. The expression of early genes is mediated through the sigma factors of the host. These early genes include amongst many genes coding for a number of other proteins, the genes which code for phage specific sigma factors also. The expression of intermediate and late genes is regulated by these phage specific sigma factors. Thus the late genes can not be expressed at a time earlier than when required (Fig. 8.50).

Similarily the sporulation of a number of bacteria is also governed by specific sigma factors. For example in B subtilis, there are at least 10 different sigma factors which are known. The general sigma factor σ 43 or σ A is needed for the vegetative growth of the bacteria. Other sigma factors are responsible for the sporulation (see later).

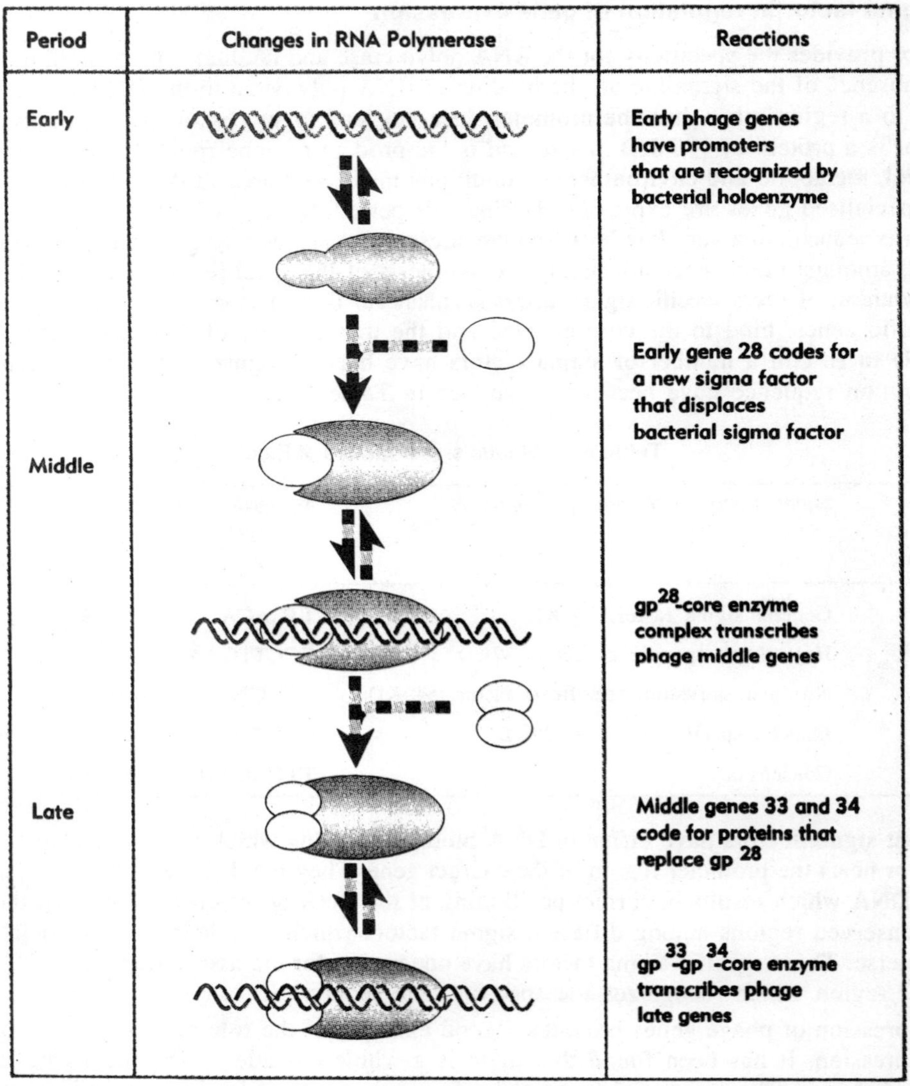

Period	Changes in RNA Polymerase	Reactions
Early		Early phage genes have promoters that are recognized by bacterial holoenzyme
Middle		Early gene 28 codes for a new sigma factor that displaces bacterial sigma factor
		gp^{28}-core enzyme complex transcribes phage middle genes
Late		Middle genes 33 and 34 code for proteins that replace gp^{28}
		gp^{33}-gp^{34}-core enzyme transcribes phage late genes

Fig. 8.50. Transcription of phage Spo1 genes is controlled by two successive substitutions of the sigma factor that change the initiation specificity.

Regulation of Sporulation

A number of micro-organisms have a novel mechanism to survive under adverse growth conditions. When the going gets tough and the organism finds that it cannot survive under these conditions, it secretes a tough coat around itself and enters into a metabolically inert phase, the spore. The spores are relatively inert phase of its life and these can remain as such for a very long time. Once the conditions become more favourable, the spores return back to the vegetative phase of life and restart the growth of the microorganism. The cycle has been explained in Fig. 8.51A.

Action	State of bacterium	Stage
Vegetative bacterium	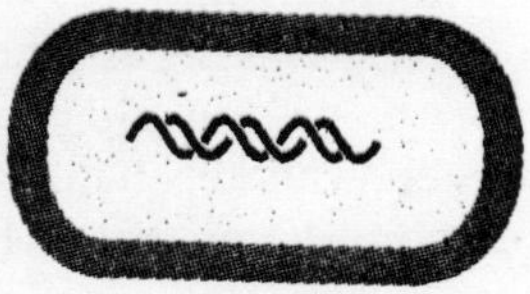	0
DNA replicates	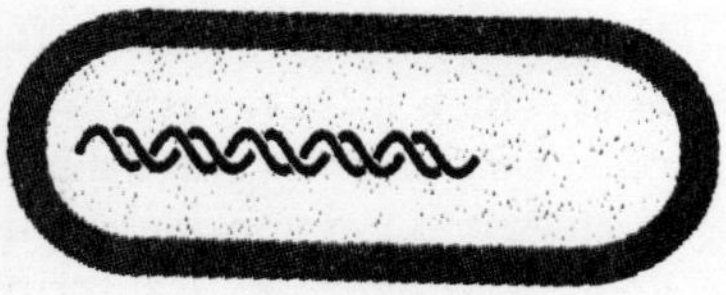	I
Septum forms	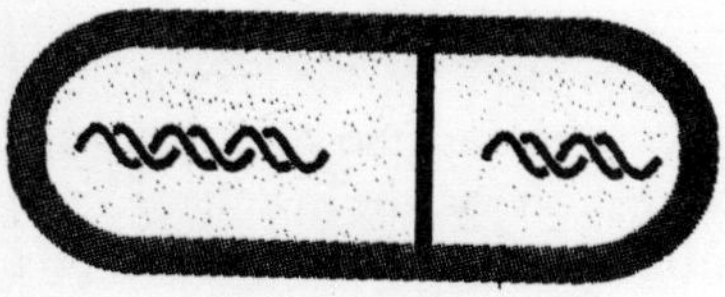	II
Spore is engulfed	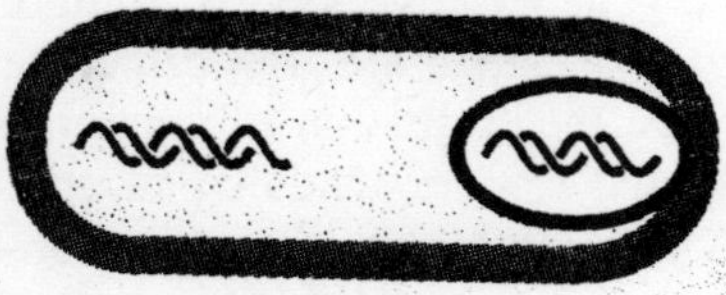	III
Spore coat forms	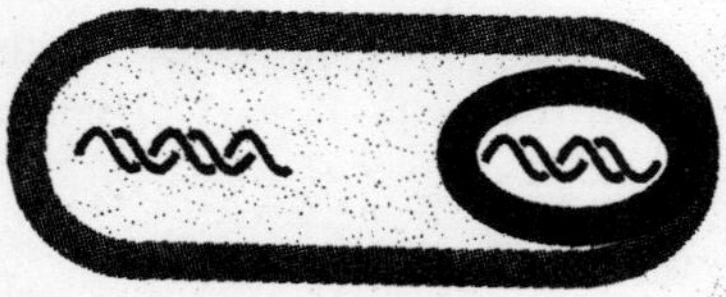	V
Mother cell is lysed	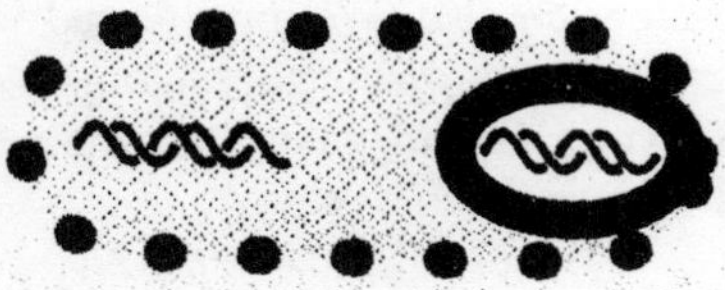	VI
Spore is released	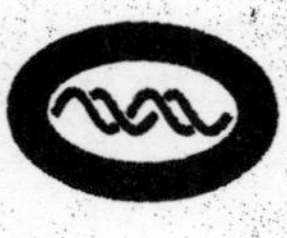	VII

Fig. 8.51A. Sporulation involves the differentiation of a vegetative bacterium into a mother cell that is lysed and a spore that is released.

The entire cycle of sporulation is achieved by a cascade of specific sigma factors. The phosphorylation relay plays an important role in this process. At the end of the log phase of the vegetative growth, when there is depletion of the nutrients, sporulation can occurs. The genome is replicated and the cell starts dividing. A septum is formed making two compartments within the cell. However, the two 'cells' do not separate from each other, rather the organism starts preparing for the formation of spores. There is the segregation of genes into the two compartments, the wall of the new 'cell' hardens and a spore coat is formed which is still present within the mother cell. This results in the formation of a 'protected cell' within the mother cell which is called the fore spore. Later this is followed by the lysis of the mother cell and the fore spore is released as a spore. During this stage upto 40% of entire RNA of the fore spore accounts for the sporulation specific mRNAs. These are translated and the factors necessary for the formation of spores are synthesized. The entire process of spore formation takes about 8 hrs.

To achieve this, a phosphorylation relay works which involves the products of a number of genes. The expression of these regulatory genes is controlled by a complex mechanism so that the spore formation does not take place unless essential. This relay results into the phosphorylation of a transcription factor SpoOA. The phosphorylated SpoOA is active and it facilitates the transcripition of a number of genes in both the mother cell and the fore spore. At this stage it uses the general sigma factor, σ 43, for the expression of genes. Amongst the genes being expressed, there is the expression of two sporulation specific sigma factor σ F in the fore spore and σ proE in the mother cell. The synthesis of σ proE is under the influence of a minor species of sigma factor, the σ H. The σ H does not contribute much during normal conditions but plays an important role as the result of the phosphorylation relay. The σ proE is biologically inactive. Under the influence of σ F a number of early sporulation genes are expressed and the σ proE of mother cell is converted into its active form, σ E. However, the amount of σ F is relatively small, therefore, the normal gene expression also continues. Further, the mother cell has an inhibitor of σ F, therefore, the sporulation genes are transcribed only in the fore spore. The synthesis of pro form of σ E takes place before the formation of septum but it becomes active only after the septum has formed. The σ E is essential for the synthesis of another sigma factor σ K (the pro form) in the mother cell. The gene for σ K is created by a recombination event and the σ K replaces the σ E. The early genes of the fore spores include a sigma factor σ G. The σ G is activited by σ K (pro form) of mother cell and the late genes of fore spore are transcribed. The transcription of late genes triggers the activation of the pro form of σ K to its active form, the σ K, which transcribes the late genes of the mother cell. This results into the lysis of mother cell and release of spore. This has been diagrammetically repressented in Fig. 8.51B.

Regulation by modulation of transcription termination

While most of the gene regulation in eukaryotes is at the level of initiation of transcription, sometimes the regulation may take place at the level of termination also. We have already seen this type of regulation in prokaryotes when the regulation of gene expression in bacteriophage λ was being discussed. Similar type of regulation is present in a number of eukaryotic viruses where the gene expression is in a sequential manner. A number of anti-terminators are known in such systems.

Differential splicing of mRNAs

This aspect has already been discussed in the earlier section. It is possible to produce more than one mRNA from a single primary transcript by alternate splicing. The pattern of splicing can be regulated. This in turn will govern the availability of one of these mRNAs and regulate the gene expression.

Overlapping transcription units

This is a special case when there are more than one transcription initiation signals present in a gene.

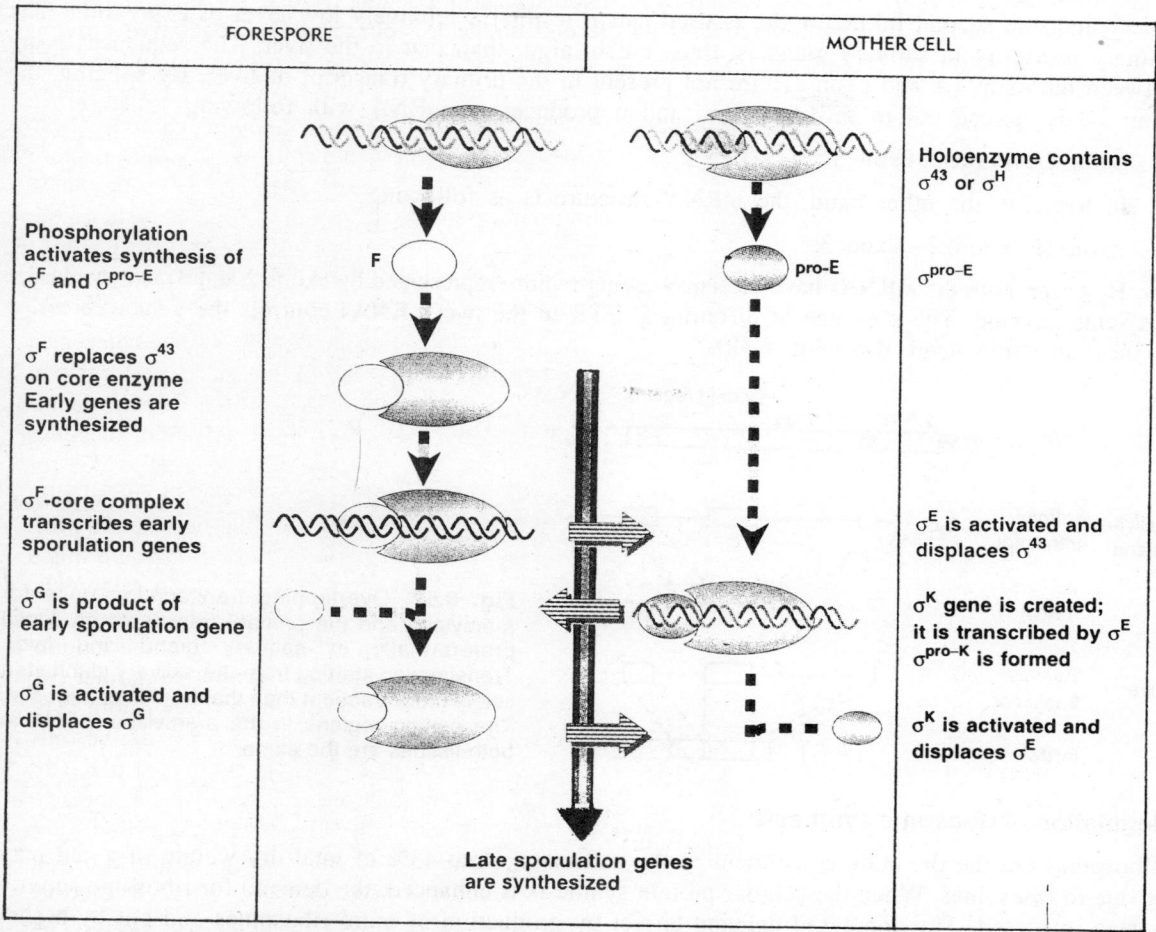

Fig. 8.51B. Sporulation involves successive changes in the sigma factors that control the initiation specificity of RNA polymerase. The cascades in the forespore and the mother cell are related by signals passed across the septum.

All of these signals can be functional and initiate the transcription. The RNA polymerase can select any one of these signals and initiate the transcription. However, these may have different control mechanisms which will result in varying rate of transcription and regulated expression of the gene. Furthermore, there can be more than one type of primary transcripts present, each arising from separate transcription start site and will vary in their 5'–end. The coding region and the 3'–UTR will be common and all the mRNA will code for the same protein. However, the 5'–UTR can regulate the translatability of mRNA. Thus the level of expression of the gene will be affected. The expression of α–amylase gene is a good example of such a case. It has been observed that there is 100 fold more enzyme in the saliva than in the liver. Even though in both the tissues the same gene is expressed. The analysis has revealed that the α–amylase gene has two transcription initiation sites, which are located 2.8 kb apart from each other. Each site is followed by a short exon which have the 5'UTR (Exon 1A and 1B respectively). The coding region of the gene is present in the two exons (Exon 2 and 3). In salivary gland the first initiation site is used resulting in high level expression of the gene. In liver, on the other hand, the second initiation site is used and it results in relatively low level of expression. The primary transcript in salivary gland is, thus, much larger than that in the liver. The sequences lying between the exon 1A and exon 1B are not present in the primary transcript of liver. By splicing, the exon 1B is spliced out in salivary gland and it produces an mRNA with following structure:

Exon 1A–exon 2–exon 3

In liver, on the other hand, the mRNA structure is as following:

Exon 1B–exon 2– exon 3.

However, both the mRNAs have the same coding region (represented by exons 2 and 3) and synthesize the same enzyme. The presence of different 5'-UTR in the two mRNAs controls the gene expression at the translation level also (Fig. 8.52).

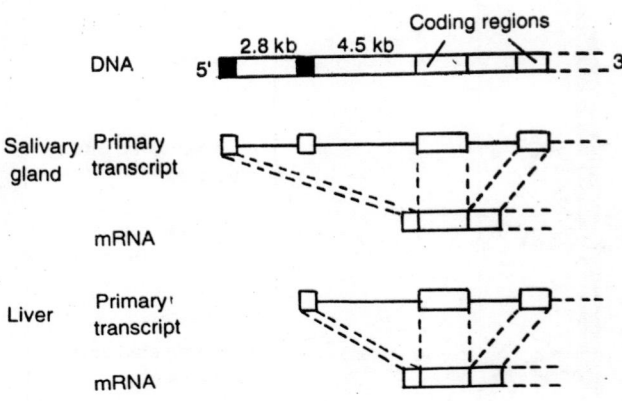

Fig. 8.52. Overlapping transcription units for a-amylase and the primary transcripts produced preferentially in salivary gland and liver. Transcription starting from the salivary gland start site is more frequent than that from liver start site. The coding regions in the a-amylase mRNA in both tissues are the same.

Regulation of ribosome synthesis

Ribosomes are the the main constituent of the cell mass. Upto 45% of total dry weight of a cell may be due to ribosomes. When the cellular protein synthesis is enhanced, the demand for ribosome activity is also increased. This increased demand is met by production of more ribosomes and not by higher activity of existing ribosomes. The ribosomes are nucleoprotein, their synthesis, therefore, requires the synthesis of r-proteins and rRNA. Both these arae regulated by different mechanisms.

Regulation of r-protein expression

The regulation of ribosomal proteins is by the translational feed back mechanism. In bacteria there are 52 genes for r-proteins which are arranged in 20 different operons. Few of these operons, specially the β-operon, Str-operon, α-operon, S_{10}-operon and the Spc-operon play an important role in the regulation of these proteins through a complex mechanism. The structure of these operons is given in Fig. 8.53. One of the proteins of each operon serves as the translational repressor. Often the protein coaded by the first structural gene of the operon acts as the repressor. For example, protein L10 in β-operon acts as the repressor, though the repressor does not necessarily have to be the first protein. For example in operon Str it is S-7, in operon α it is S-4, in operon S10 it is L-4 and in operon Spc it is S-8. However, in all of the operons, the protein which acts as repressor is always a protein which directly binds to the rRNA during the ribosomal assembly. It has already been discussed earlier that at the time of ribosomal assembly, some of the r-proteins directly bind to rRNA while other proteins bind to these proteins. Further, the repressor protein binds to the operon at a specific position. The site of binding has also been shown in Fig. 8.53 by an arrow. The binding of repressor to the operator region blocks the gene epression and proteins present at downstream position are not synthesized. However, the affinity of these proteins to rRNA is much higher than to the operator, as a result, the repressor protein will bind to its target gene only if no free rRNAs are available. Thus the amount of rRNA regulates the repressor activity of these proteins and the protein synthesis is inhibited only if it is not required for ribosome assembly.

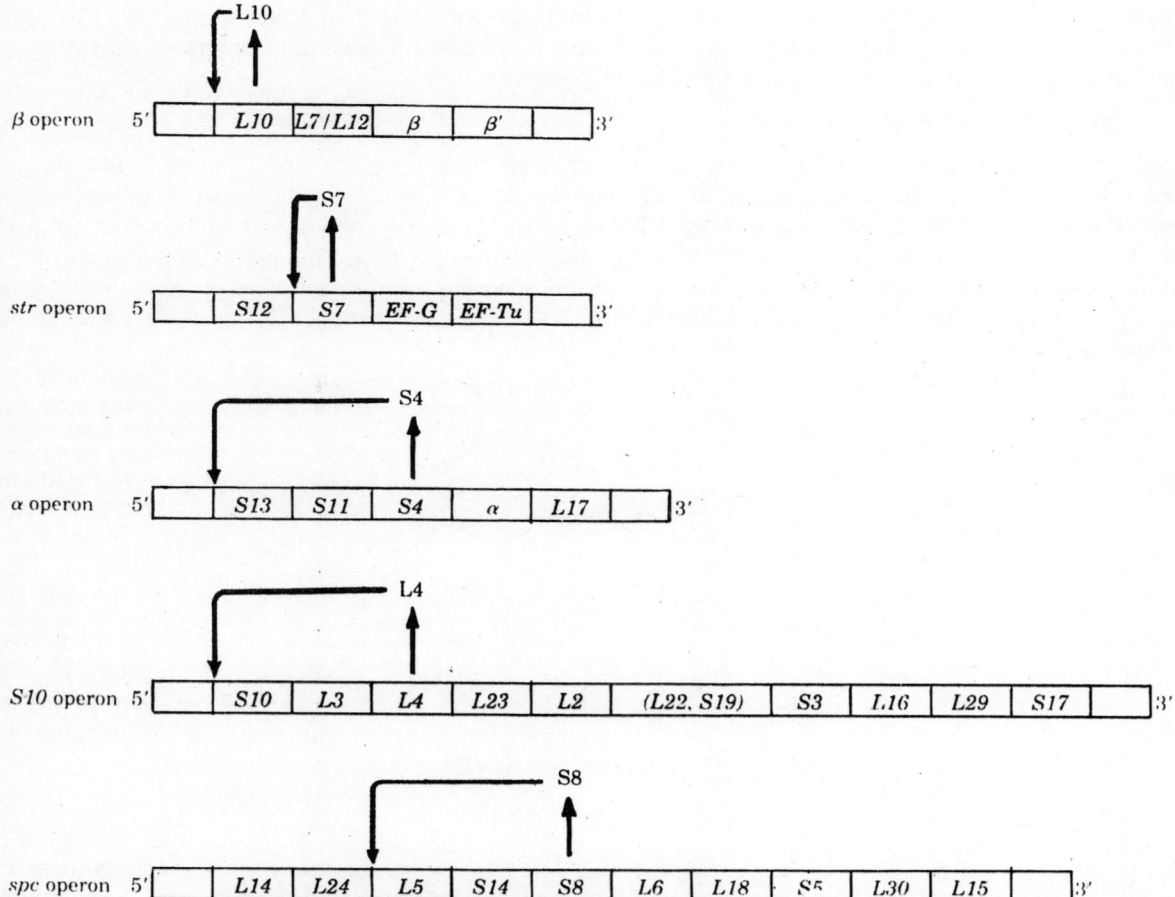

Fig. 8.53. Structure of some ribosomal protein operons in the mRNA transcripts. The r-protein acting as translation repressor has been shaded and its site of action is indicated by an arrow. Each translational repressor blocks the translation of all genes by binding to this one site on the mRNA. Genes that encode subunits of RNA polymerase are shaded yellow; genes that encode elongation factors are shaded blue.

Besides this control, cetain other mechanisms at the transcriptional as well as translational level may also regulate the r-protein synthesis.

Regulation of rRNA synthesis

The synthesis of rRNAs is regulated at the transcriptional level by the growth conditions and environment.

Especially the deficiency of nutritions play an important role in rRNA synthesis and formation of ribosomes. It may be pertinent to point out that the higher protein synthetic activity of a cell, resulting in higher demand for the ribosomes during enhanced activity of the cellular metabolism is met by increased number of ribosomes. There is no enhancement in the activity of the existing ribosomes. Similarly during reduced protein synthesis, the ribosome formation is also reduced. The unavailability of certain essential nutrients, specially the aa, causes a stringent response in the bacteria. In such cases the tRNAs cannot be charged and the A sites of ribosomes are occupied by the uncharged tRNA. This unusual phenomenon triggers a series of cellular response and an enzymatic factor, called the stringent factor comes and binds to these ribosomes. This causes the formation of an unusual nucleotide, the guanosine tetraphosphate (ppGpp) in the cells. Its synthesis takes place by following reaction.

$$GDP + ATP \longrightarrow ppGpp + AMP$$

The guanosine tetraphosphate has a very unusual structure. It has a pyrophosphate group attached to the 5'-position of G and another pyrophosphate attached at its 3' position (Fig. 8.54). This nucleotide was originally referred as the magic factor and is known to act as a cell signal in a manner similar to the cAMP. An increase in the concentration of ppGpp acts as the transcriptional inhibitor and results in the reduction in the synthesis of the rRNA. The precise mechanism of the action of ppGpp in regulation of rRNA transcription is not very clear. It should be noted that similar to cAMP, ppGpp is a starvation signal in E.coli.

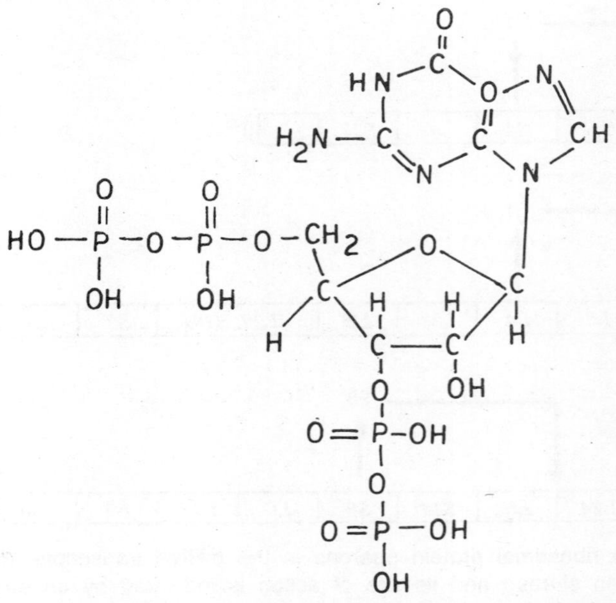

Fig. 8.54. Structure of guanosine tetraphosphate.

Regulation of gene expression in yeast

Yeast is the lowest eukaryote. It has a number of regulatory mechanisms which have certain degree of homology with various processes in bacteria. However, majority of the eukaryotic regulatory mechanisms have evolved in yeast and these cells follow many of the above mechanisms. We will discuss some of these in detail.

Regulation of expression of GAL genes

In yeast the GAL genes code for a series of galactose metabolizing enzymes. While small amounts of these enzymes are produced in a constitutive manner, these enzymes are inducible and their expression is enhanced if galactose is present as the carbon source in the growth medium. The pathway of galactose metabolism involves five enzymes which have a complex regulatory cascade for its control. The pathway has been shown in Fig. 8.55.

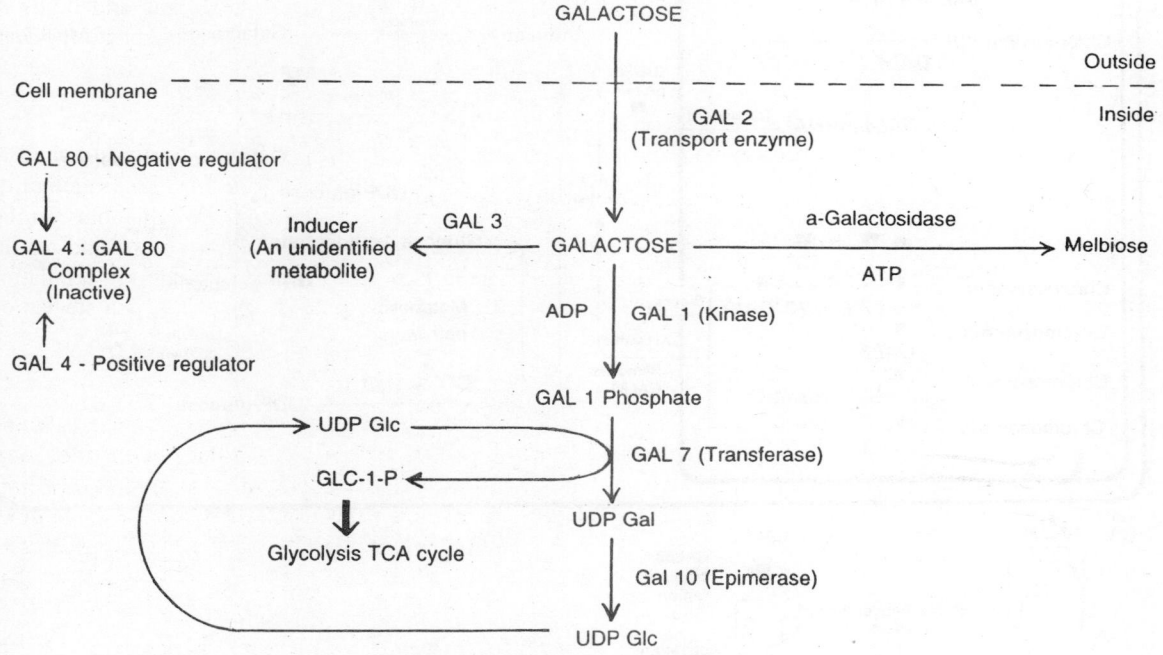

Fig. 8.55. Pathway of galactose metabolism.

The the genes for the five enzymes involved in the metabolism of galactose are present on different chromosomes. The genes for three of the enzymes, namely Gal1, Gal7 and Gal10 are present on chromosome II, Gal 2 is present on chromosome XII and the gene for α-galactosidase is present on chromosome U. The synthesis of the inducer is regulated by Gal3 which is present on chromosome IV. The activity of entire cascade of the expression of the enzymes is positively regulated by Gal 4, gene for which is present on the chromosome XVI. Gal 80 is involved in regulation of the activity of Gal 4. It can interact with Gal 4 and form a complex of Gal4:Gal80. This complex is inactive, thus Gal 80 acts as the negative regulator of the cascade. It is present on chromosome XIII. The inducer (coded by gene Gal 3) enhances the de novo formation of Gal 4 and also releases the Gal 4 which is present as the Gal4:Gal80 complex.

The mechanism of regulation of the cascade by Gal 4 and Gal 80 is quite complex (Fig. 8.56). Gal 4 contains three active centres. The first 147 aa at the N-terminal end constitute the DNA binding motif while the C-terminal of the protein is the site for Gal 80 binding. It has two acidic regions, one of which is essential for its activity as the activator of GAL genes. The three genes present on chromosome II (Gal 1, Gal 7 and Gal 10) have a common upstream activation sequence (UAS) and

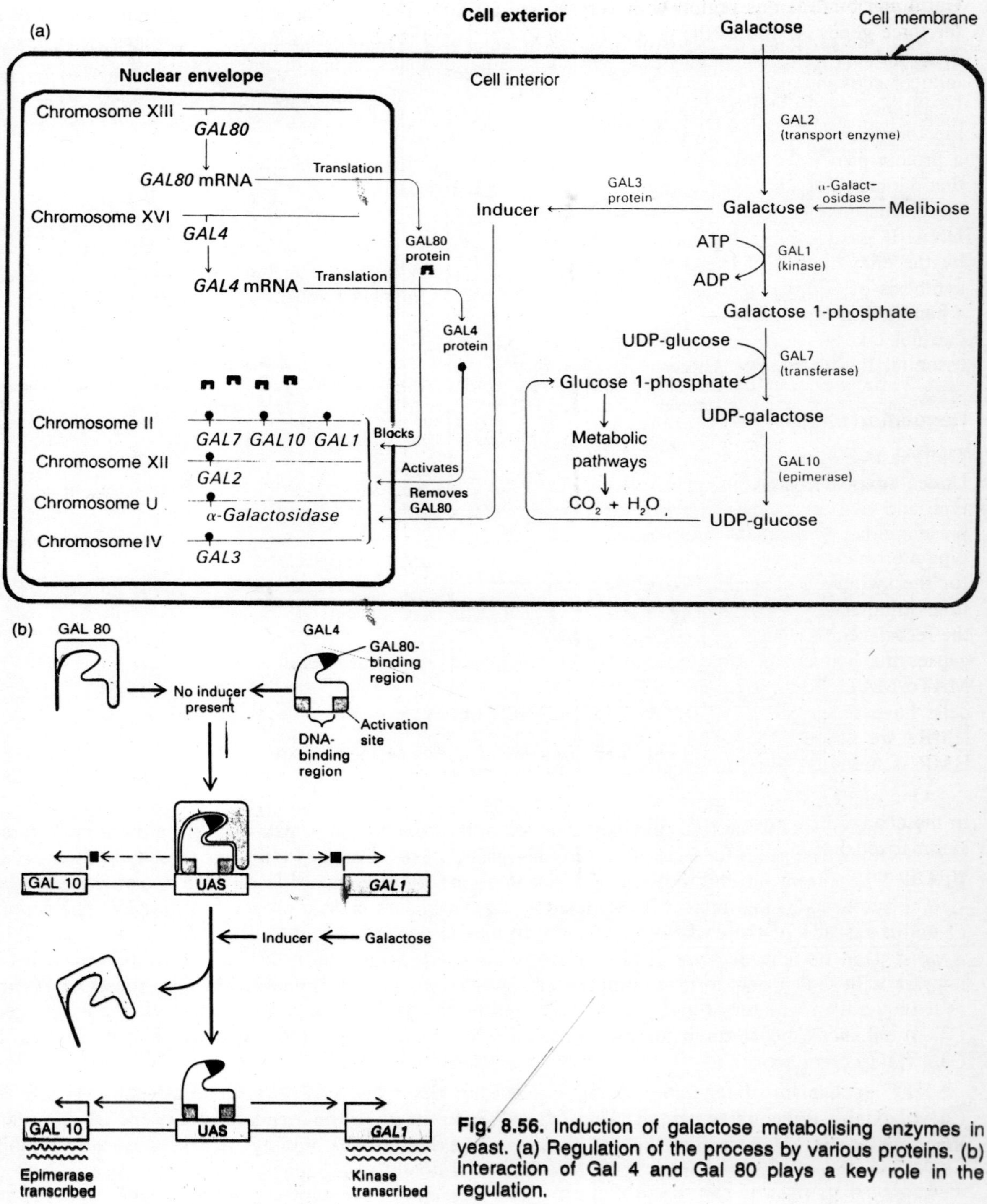

(a)

Cell exterior

Nuclear envelope

Cell interior

Galactose

Cell membrane

Chromosome XIII

GAL80

GAL80 mRNA — Translation

Chromosome XVI

GAL4

GAL4 mRNA — Translation

GAL80
protein

GAL4
protein

GAL2
(transport enzyme)

GAL3
protein

Inducer ← Galactose

α-Galact-
osidase

Melibiose

ATP

ADP

GAL1
(kinase)

Galactose 1-phosphate

Chromosome II

GAL7 GAL10 GAL1

Blocks

Chromosome XII

GAL2

Activates

Chromosome U

α-*Galactosidase*

Removes
GAL80

Chromosome IV

GAL3

UDP-glucose

GAL7
(transferase)

Glucose 1-phosphate

UDP-galactose

Metabolic
pathways

GAL10
(epimerase)

$CO_2 + H_2O$

UDP-glucose

(b)

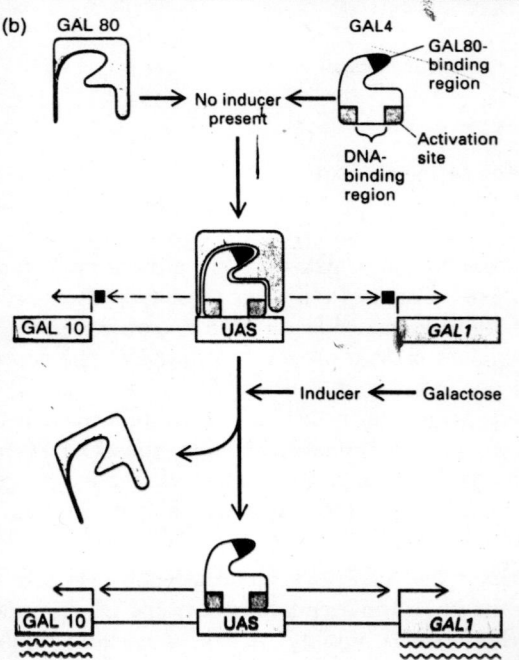

GAL 80

GAL4

GAL80-
binding
region

→ No inducer ←
present

Activation
site

DNA-
binding
region

GAL 10 — UAS — *GAL1*

Inducer ← Galactose

GAL 10 — UAS — *GAL1*

Epimerase
transcribed

Kinase
transcribed

Fig. 8.56. Induction of galactose metabolising enzymes in yeast. (a) Regulation of the process by various proteins. (b) Interaction of Gal 4 and Gal 80 plays a key role in the regulation.

Gal 4 can bind to this region with very strong affinity. This binding activates the transcription of all the three genes as well as the genes for Gal 2, Gal 3 and α-galactosidase. Gal 3 activates the formation of an inducer molecule produced as one of the intermediates during the metabolism of galactose. This inducer activates the Gal 4 synthesis. If galactose is not present, the inducer will not be synthesized. In absence of the inducer, there is reduced synthesis of Gal 4. Also the absence of inducer favours the formation of Gal 4:Gal 80 complex and the Gal 4 and Gal 80 interact with each other and form a protein-protein complex. As this complex is biologically inactive, the net result of this binding is that the enzymes for galactose metabolism are not synthesized. Gal 80, thus acts as a negative regulator. As discussed, the action of Gal 80 is through protein-protein interaction, it doesnot directly act on DNA. If galactose is added at this stage, small amounts of inducer are produced by its metabolism by the enzymes which were produced constitutely. As discussed, the inducer activates not only the synthesis of Gal 4 but also mediates the breakdown of Gal 4-Gal 80 complex. Thus pre-existing Gal 4 can be made available for the increased gene expression. Also the formation of Gal4-Gal 80 complex can not take place in presence of the inducer. Thus galactose can regulate the synthesis of enzyme essential for its metabolism by a cascade of events.

Regulation of yeast mating types

The yeast cells are present either as haploid or as diploids. The haploids are either a type or α type. Under adverse conditions, a mixed diploid a/α is formed which gives rise to four spores, two of a type and two of α type. The MAT gene which is primarily responsible for the diploid formation is present either as MATa or MATα. It is capable of converting either of the two mating types, the mating type a or mating type α by a series of complex mechanism. The MAT gene represents the active locus for the switching. The cells have the capability to switch frquently from one type to another (some times upto once in every generation). This change is brought by a dominant allele HO. However, if the recessive allele ho is present, the frequency of change becomes very low. The presence of HO allele causes the heploid cells to change the genotype, irrespective of the original genotype. The fact that MATα/MATa diploids are more stable, probably provides the reason for such switching. Thus all the cells have the potential to become either α type or a type and two extra loci, namely HMLα and HMRa are needed for such switching. As the name suggests, the HML is to the left of MAT while HMR is towards its right (Fig. 8.57). These represent the silent cassette for the switching.

One of the two silent cassettes have interaction with the active locus and replace it, which results in the change of mating type. A number of genes are involved in this process. These genes have been summarised in Table 8.3. There are common sequences between both the genotypes which flank the type specific region in the middle of both the active and the silent cassettes and are referred as the

Table 8.3. The genes which participate in mating type switching of yeast haploid cells

S.No.	Gene	Function
1.	MAT	Determination of mating type
2.	HM L/R	Storage of mating type information in silent cassettes
3.	SIR (1-4)	Repression of silent cassette expression
4.	HO	Endonuclease responsible for the initiation of switch type
5.	SIN (1-5)	Repression of the expression of HO
6.	SWI (1-5)	Essential for the expression of HO for switching initiation
7.	STE	Sites where mutations lead to sterility, mutants can not mate

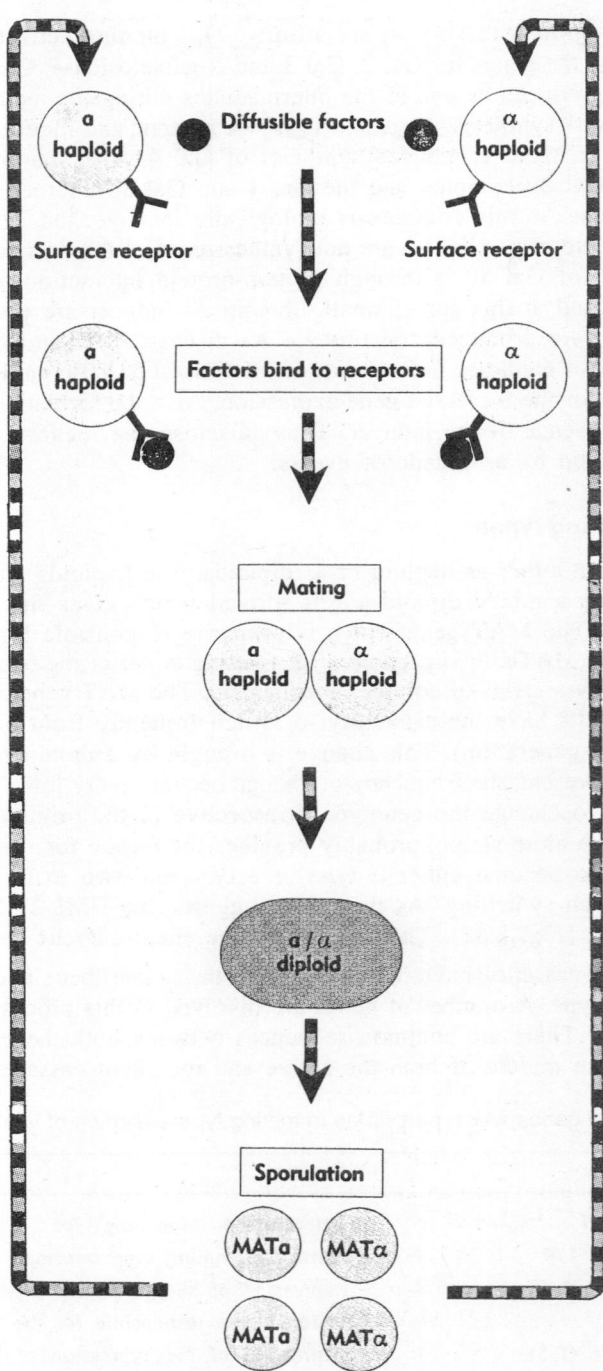

Fig. 8.57A. Overview of the yeast life cycle through mating of MATa and MATα haploids to give heterozygous diploids that sporulate to generate haploid spores.

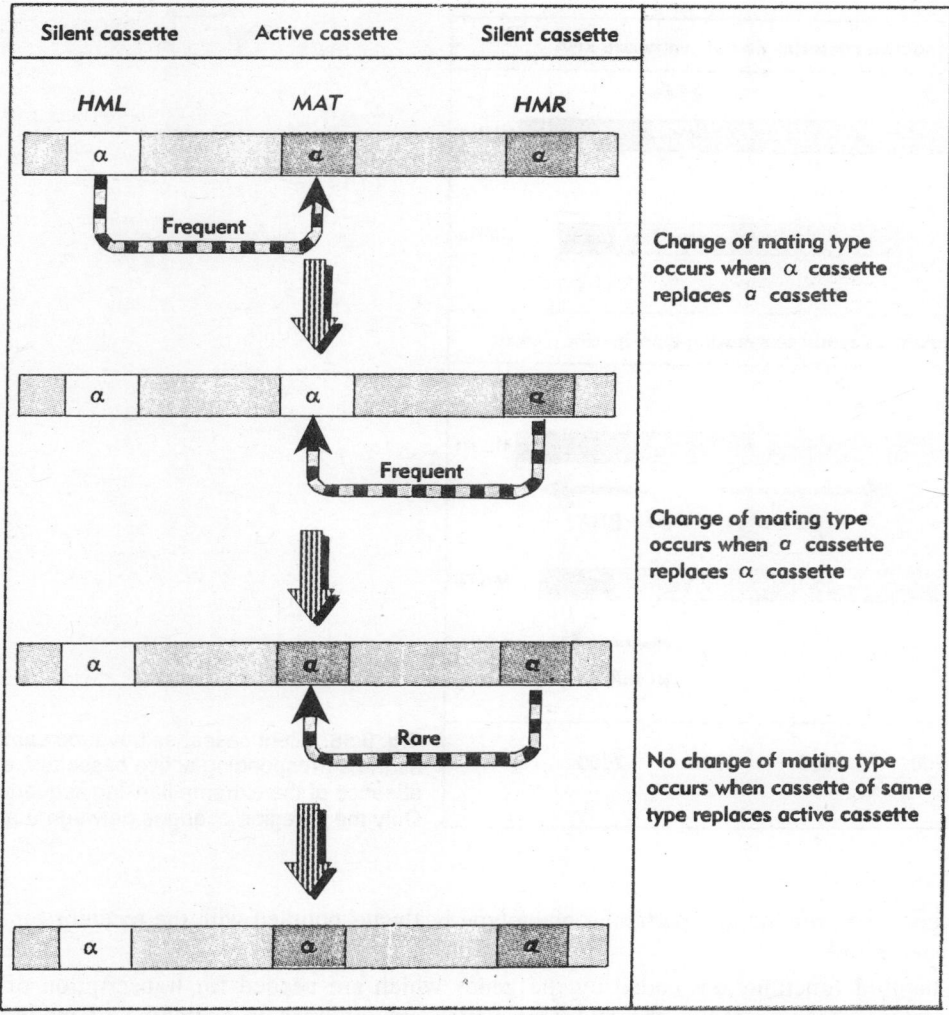

Fig. 8.57B. Changes of mating type occur when silent cassettes replace active cassettes of opposite genotype; when transpositions occur between cassettes of the same type, the mating type remains unaltered.

Yα and Yα. While the flanking sequences are identical, these are shorter in HMRa than in HMLα. However, the sequences in the silent regions are not transcribed while the active regions are transcribed and respective RNAs are synthesized (Fig. 8.58).

The a-specific genes are expressed constitutively in a-cells and remain repressed in α-cells. This group of genes include the a-factor structural gene, and STE2 (the gene for α-factor receptor). The a-type cells are thus ready to accept and respond to the pheromones produced by the cells of other mating type.

The α-functions, on the other hand, are expressed in α-cell type but are repressed in a-cells. These genes include the structural genes for the α-factor and the a-factor receptor gene, STE3. Thus the expression

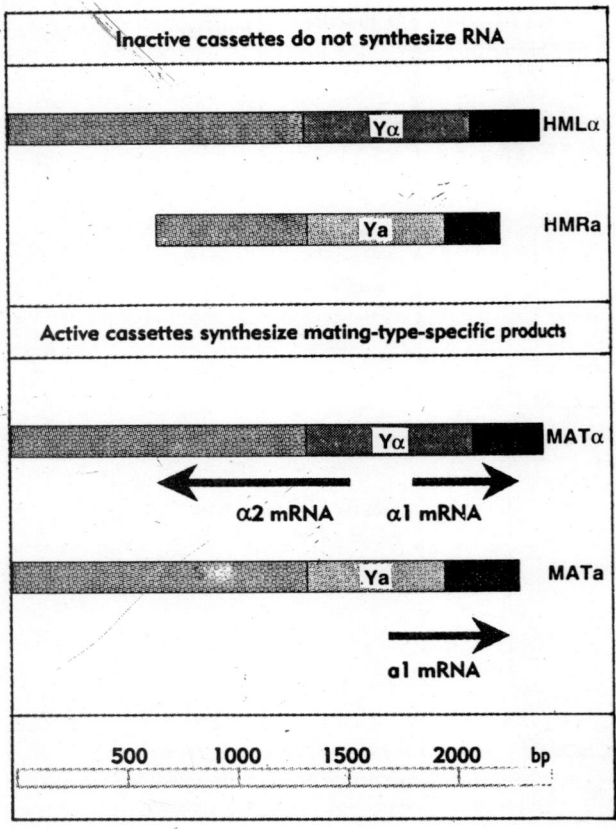

Fig. 8.58. Silent cassettes have the same sequences as the corresponding active cassettes, except for the absence of the extreme flanking sequences in HMRa. Only the Y region changes between a and a types.

of one type of pheromone in a particular phenotype is always coupled with the receptor for the opposite type of pheromone.

The haploid functions are coded by the genes which are needed for transcription of pheromone and pheromone receptor genes, the HO gene which are involved in switching of mating types, and the gene RME which codes for a repressor of sporulation. These are expressed constitutively in both types of haploid, but are repressed in α/a diploids. As a result, both the a-specific and the α-specific functions remain silent in the diploids.

The functions of the regulators and their targets, specially that of the MAT gene which is expressed in haploid and diploid yeast cells has been outlined in Fig. 8.59. The a and α-mating types are regulated by different mechanisms. In a-type haploids, a-mating functions are expressed constitutively. However, the functions of the product of MATa in the a-cell, if any, are not fully understood. It is probably required only to repress the haploid functions in the diploid cells.

In α-haploids, the α1 product turns on the α-specific genes whose products are needed for α-mating type. The α2 product represses the genes responsible for producing the a-mating type, by binding to an operator sequence located upstream of the target genes. In diploids, on the other hand, the a1 and α2 products cooperate to repress the haploid-specific genes. They combine to recognize an operator sequence different from the target for α2 alone.

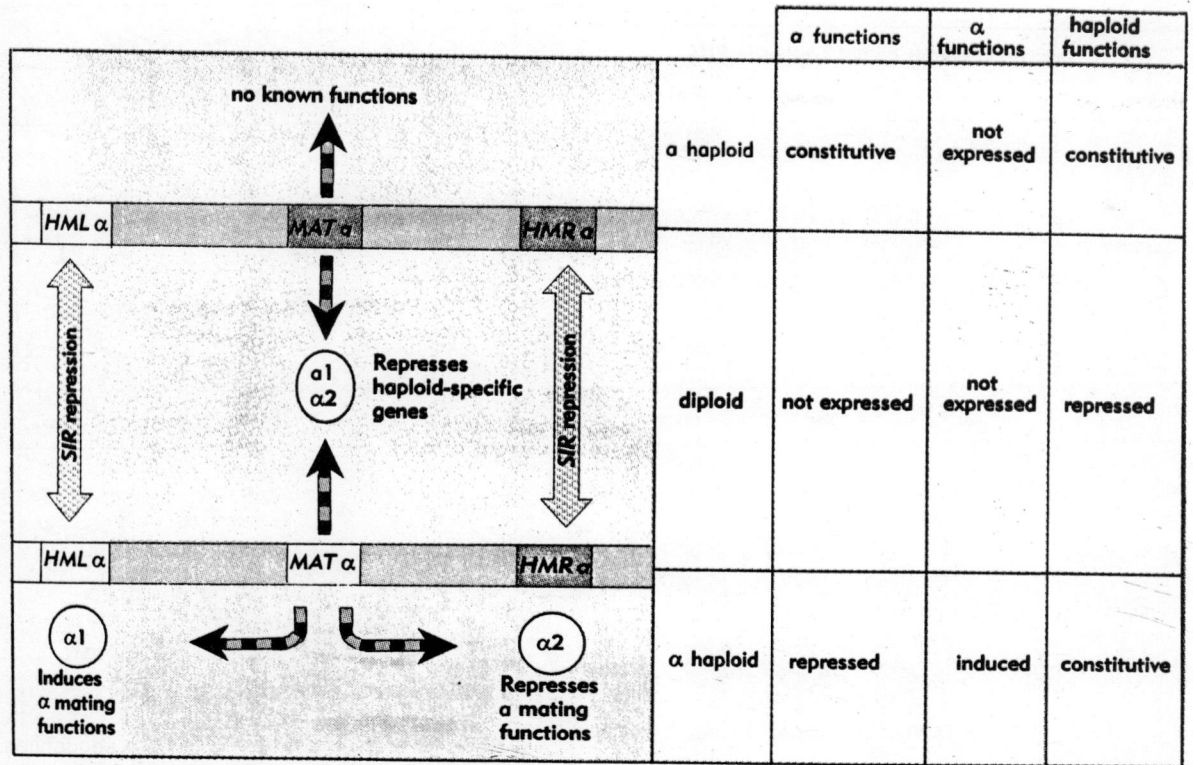

	a functions	α functions	haploid functions
a haploid	constitutive	not expressed	constitutive
diploid	not expressed	not expressed	repressed
α haploid	repressed	induced	constitutive

Fig. 8.59. In diploids the **a**1 and α2 functions cooperate to repress haploid-specific functions. In **a** haploids, mating functions are constitutive. In α haploids, the α2 function represses **a** mating functions, while α1 induces **a** mating functions.

The abilities of the α2, a1, and α1 proteins to regulate transcription primarily depends upon the protein–protein interactions between themselves and with other protein(s). A protein (which is not specific for mating type), PRTF is involved in a number of these interactions. It binds to a short consensus sequence called the P box (Fig. 8.60). The P–box sequences are found in a variety of locations and have diversified regulatory role. On one hand, the P box is essential for the activation of some of the genes, on the other hand, it is needed for the repression of certain other genes. Its effect depends on the presence of many other proteins that bind at the sites adjacent to the P box.

The genes that are a-specific may be activated by PRTF alone. This is adequate to ensure their expression in an α-haploid. These genes are repressed in an α-haploid by the combined action of the α2 protein and PRTF. The α2 protein contains two domains, the C-terminal domain binds to short palindromic elements present at the ends of an operator having a consensus sequence of 32 bp. However, binding of this fragment to DNA does not cause repression. The N-terminal domain is needed for the repression and is responsible for making the contact with PRTF. The binding site for PRTF is a P box in the center of the operator. In fact, α2 and PRTF bind to the operator cooperatively.

The expression of α-specific genes, on the other hand, requires the α1 activator which is a small protein of only 175 aminoacids. The sequences that confer α-specific transcription are located within

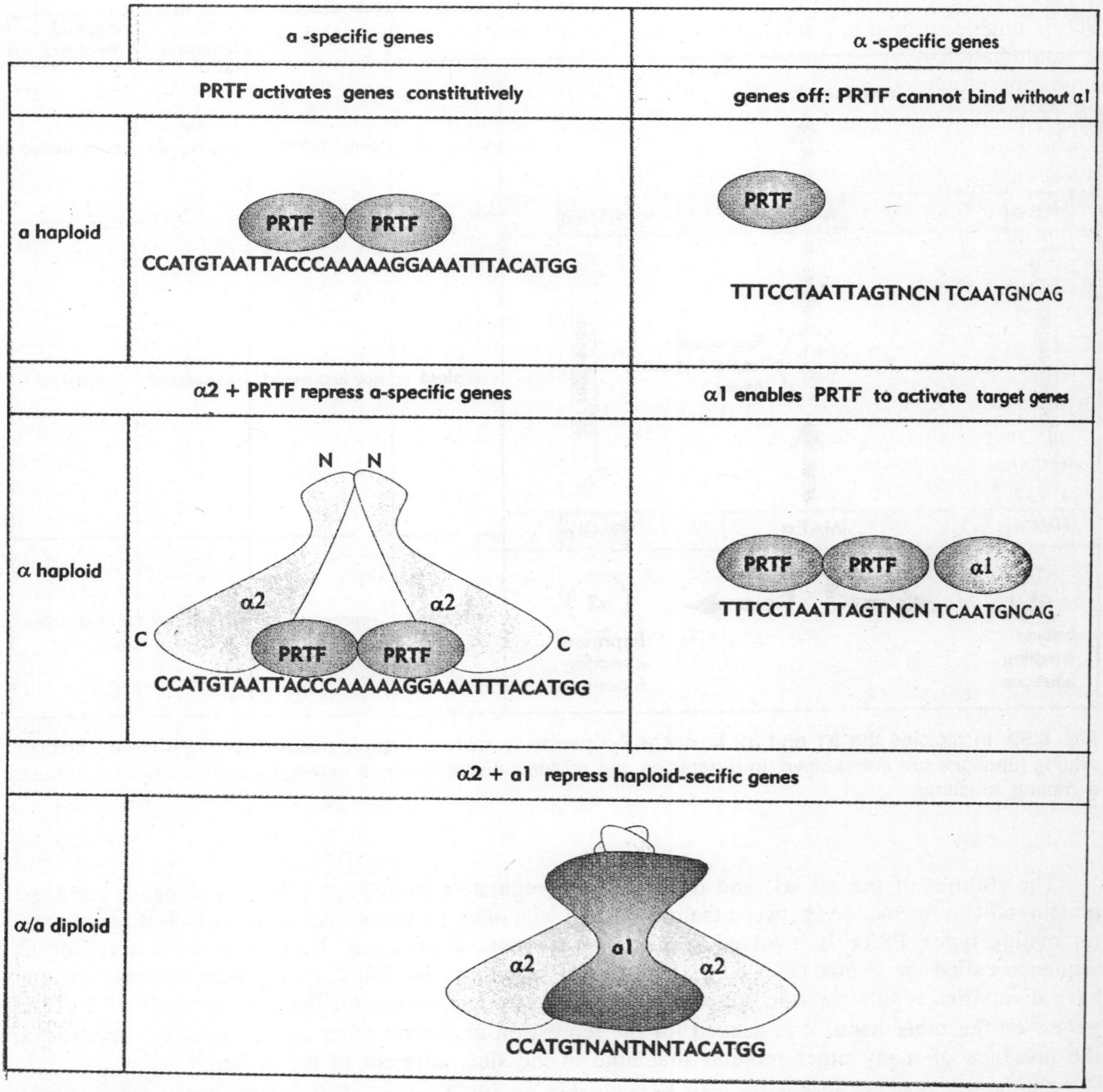

a -specific genes	α -specific genes
PRTF activates genes constitutively	genes off: PRTF cannot bind without α1

a haploid

PRTF PRTF
CCATGTAATTACCCAAAAAGGAAATTTACATGG

PRTF

TTTCCTAATTAGTNCN TCAATGNCAG

α2 + PRTF repress a-specific genes	α1 enables PRTF to activate target genes

α haploid

N N

α2 α2
C PRTF PRTF C
CCATGTAATTACCCAAAAAGGAAATTTACATGG

PRTF PRTF α1
TTTCCTAATTAGTNCN TCAATGNCAG

α2 + α1 repress haploid-secific genes

α/a diploid

α2 α1 α2
CCATGTNANTNNTACATGG

Fig. 8.60. Combinations of PRTF, a1, α1 and α2 activate or repress specific groups of genes to correspond with the mating type of the cell.

the UAS elements of the chromosome. The consensus sequence is 26 bp long and can be divided into two parts. The first 16 bp form the P box, to which PRTF binds while the adjacent 10 bp sequence forms the binding site for α1-factor. The α1-factor binds to this sequence only when PRTF is present at the P box. None of the proteins can bind to its target box alone, however, they can bind to DNA together. It may be due to a protein-protein interaction.

The α-specific genes are controlled by default in a-type haploids as in absence of the α1 protein, PRTF is unable to bind and to activate them. The α2 protein can also cooperate with the a1 protein. The combination of these proteins recognizes a different operator. The operator shares the outlying palindromic sequences with the sequence recognized by α2 alone, but is shorter because the sequence between them is different. The α2/a1 combination represses genes with this motif in the diploid cells.

The transcription of either MATa or MATα initiates within the Y region. However, only the MAT locus is expressed; yet the same Y region is present in the corresponding non-transcribed cassette (HML or HMR). This simply means that the regulation of expression can not be by direct recognition of some site(s) which may be overlapping with the promoter. A site outside the cassettes must distinguish the HML and HMR from the MAT gene. It has been found by deletion analysis that some sequences present at about the 1 kb upstream of both the HML and HMR are essential for the repression of their expression. These loci, called EL (near HML) and ER (near HMR), have two important properties. First, these act in a negative enhancers like manner and can function at a distance (up to 2.5 kb away from a promoter) in orientation independent manner. These are also referred as the silencers and secondly, these are associated with the ARS sequences, which probably function as origins of replication.

The search for the basis for the control of cassette activity by mutation in regulatory genes revealed that if a mutation permits the expression of an otherwise silent cassette at HML and HMR, both the a and α functions are produced, so that the cells behave like MATa/MATα diploids. Four complementation groups, called SIR (silent information regulator) have been identified. A mutation in any of these would lead to the expression of HML and HMR. The wild-type SIR loci maintain HML and HMR in the repressed state which are expressed as the result of a mutation in any one of these. Same regulatory events are involved in the repression of a silent cassette and in preventing it from being the recipient for its replacement by another cassette. An unidirectional transposition is initiated by the recipient MAT locus. The mutations identify a site at the right boundary of Y at MAT which is crucial for the switching event. Any deletion at the right end of Y do not have any effect until it crosses the boundary, when it abolishes the switching. Point mutations that abolish the switching occur near this boundary.

The Y-Z boundary is the site of the changes in DNA that marks the initiation of transposition events. In populations of cells undergoing the switching, about 1-3% of the DNA of the MAT locus has a double-stranded cut at this site which lies close to the boundary and coincides with the DNase hypersensitive site. It is possible that hypersensitive sites at the Y-Z1 boundary of MAT may become accessible as these lack a nucleosome and are recognized by an endonuclease which is coded by the HO locus. It is pertinent to assume that the hypersensitivity to DNase I in *in vitro* reflects a natural sensitivity to *HO* endonuclease *in vivo*. The *HO* endonuclease makes a doublestrand break immediately to the right of the Y boundary. Such cleavage generates the single-stranded ends of 4 bases (Fig. 8.61).

When the free end at the *MAT* gene invades either the *HML* or the *HMR* locus and pairs with the Z region, the Y region of *MAT* is degraded until a region which bears homology on the left side is exposed. At this point, *MAT* is paired either with *HML* or with *HMR* at both the left and the right side. The Y region of *HML* or *HMR* is copied to replace the region lost from *MAT* (which might extend beyond the limits of Y itself). The paired loci separate. The order of events could be different. Similar to the model involving a double-strand break for recombination, the process is initiated by *MAT*, the *locus that is to be replaced*. In this sense, the description of HML and HMR as donor loci refers to their ultimate role, but not to the mechanism of the process. The donor site remains unaffected, but a change in sequence occurs at the recipient site and the recipient locus suffers a substitution rather than the addition of material.

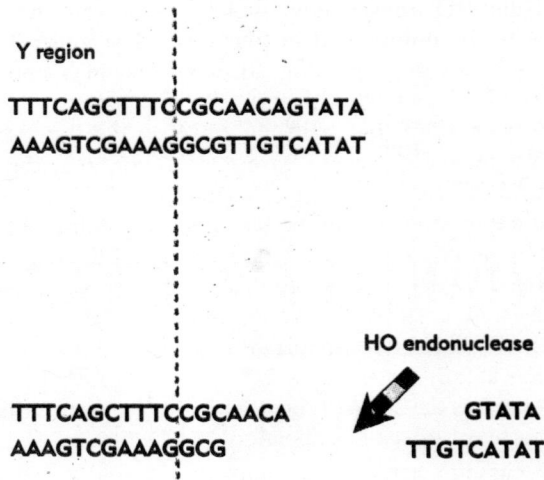

Y region

TTTCAGCTTTCCGCAACAGTATA
AAAGTCGAAAGGCGTTGTCATAT

HO endonuclease

TTTCAGCTTTCCGCAACA   GTATA
AAAGTCGAAAGGCG   TTGTCATAT

Fig. 8.61. HO endonuclease cleaves MAT just to the right of the Y region, generating sticky ends with a 4 base overhang.

Regulation of HO expression

The HO gene is regulated in an interesting manner. The transcription of HO responds to a number of controls. First the HO is under mating-type control, it is not synthesized in MATa/MATα diploids. Secondly, the HO is transcribed in mother cells but it is not expressed in the daughter cells. Thirdly, the HO transcription responds to the cell cycle also and the gene is expressed only at the end of the G_1 phase of the mother cell.

The timing of nuclease production explains the relationship between switching and the cell lineage. Switching is detected only in the products of a division; both daughter cells have the same mating type, switched from that of the parent. The restriction of HO expression to G_1 phase ensures that the mating type is switched before the MAT locus is replicated, with the result that both progeny have the new mating type (Fig. 8.62).

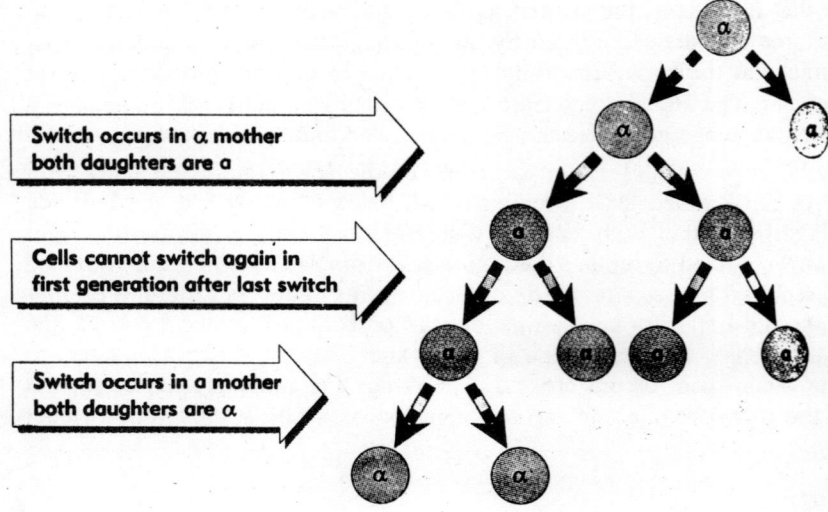

Switch occurs in α mother both daughters are a

Cells cannot switch again in first generation after last switch

Switch occurs in a mother both daughters are α

Fig. 8.62. Switching occurs only in mother cells; both daughter cells have the new mating type. A daughter cell must pass through an entire cycle before it becomes a mother cell that is able to switch again.

There are a few cis-acting sites that control the HO transcription which are present at a region of about 1500 bp upstream of the gene and have been summarized in Fig. 8.63. The general pattern of their control involves the repression responding to several regulatory circuits, that may prevent the transcription of HO.

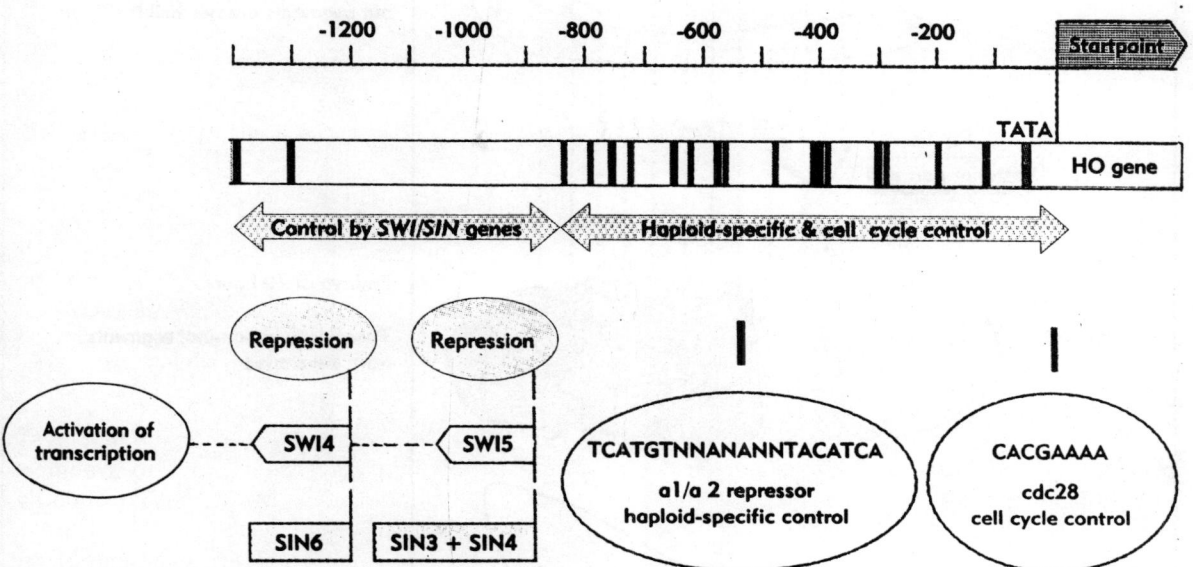

Fig. 8.63. The HO gene can be repressed by several control systems. Transcription occurs only when all repression is lifted.

In the diploids the transcription is prevented by the a1/α2 repressor. There are 10 binding sites for the repressor in the upstream region. These sites vary in their conformity to the consensus sequence; we do not know which and how many of them are required for haploid-specific repression. The cell-cycle control on the other hand, is conferred by 9 copies of an octanucleotide sequence that lie in the region between −150 and −900. A copy of the consensus sequence can confer cell-cycle control on a gene to which it is attached. A gene linked to this sequence is repressed except during a transient period toward the end of G_1 phase. Its activity depends on the function of the cell-cycle regulator CDC28, which executes the start stage of the cycle when the cell becomes committed for division. The interactions involving the SWI and SIN genes are involved in cell-cycle and mother-daughter control. The genes SWI1-5 are required for HO transcription.

Regulation of gene expression during development in Drosophila

The development of an organism starts with a single cell, the fertilized egg. However, during the development a sequential expression of a cascade of genes takes place which regulates the early development. This results in the differentiation of various cell types to form different organs. In fruitfly (D. melanogaster) the expression of such a cascade has been followed. An initial asymmetry in the fertilized egg gives rise to the four segments namely, the thorasic and abdominal segments, antenna and the wings. Fig. 8.64 shows the three basic stages of Drosophila development. The early embryogenesis is established by the maternal gene products and the anterior and posterior poles become well defined. This is followed by the creation of a number of parasegments, each representing a specific segment

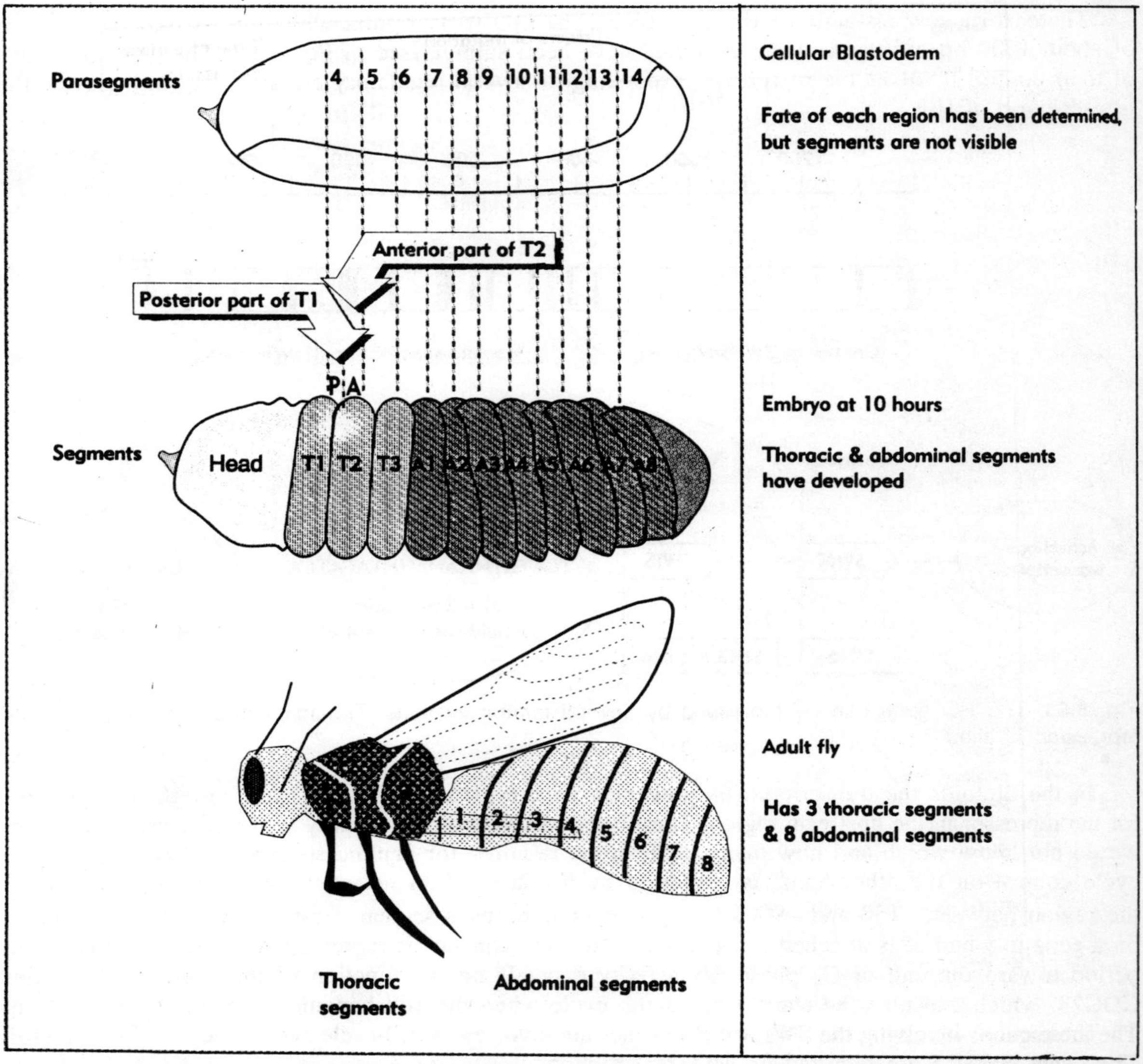

Fig. 8.64. Drosophila development proceeds through formation of compartments that form parasegments and segments.

of the adult fly. A number of segmentation genes (or the gap genes - a total of five in number) are responsible for this function. Any mutation in these genes (the gap mutants) results in the loss of adjacent segments. Similarly the eight pair-rule genes are responsible for the formation of a specific pattern of stripes in the larvae. The mutation here results in formation of fushi tarazu (ftz) type of larvae. The segment polarity genes (nine in number), on the other hand, ensure the correct development of anterior and posterior segments and the development of organs from these areas. Any mutation here will result in the replacement of segments by their mirror images. These possibilities have been shown in Fig. 8.65.

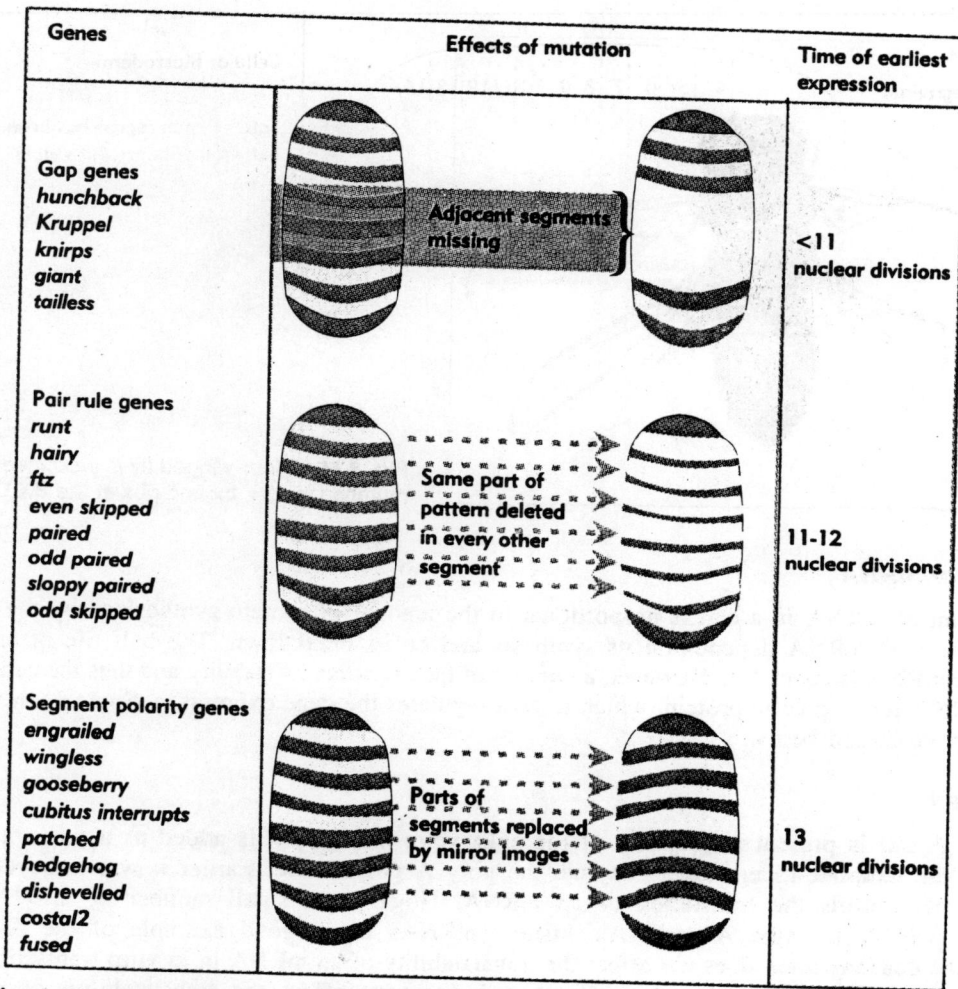

Genes	Effects of mutation	Time of earliest expression
Gap genes *hunchback* *Kruppel* *knirps* *giant* *tailless*	Adjacent segments missing	**<11** nuclear divisions
Pair rule genes *runt* *hairy* *ftz* *even skipped* *paired* *odd paired* *sloppy paired* *odd skipped*	Same part of pattern deleted in every other segment	**11-12** nuclear divisions
Segment polarity genes *engrailed* *wingless* *gooseberry* *cubitus interrupts* *patched* *hedgehog* *dishevelled* *costal2* *fused*	Parts of segments replaced by mirror images	**13** nuclear divisions

Fig. 8.65. Segmentation genes affect the number of segments and fall into three groups.

These genes are expressed in a precisely controlled sequential manner and mutation in these regulatory genes can cause the development of a leg in place of antenna or the formation of an extra pair of wings. For example a four winged fly can be produced by a triple mutation in the genes abx, bx and pbx (Fig. 8.66). All these genes are present in the BX–C locus. It should be pointed out that these complex loci involved in regulation are extremely large. Many of these are the homeotic genes having homeobox type of motif. The Drosophila homeobox genes have homology with Hox genes of mammals such as the mouse and human.

CYTOPLASMIC CONTROL OF GENE EXPRESSION

In cytoplasm the gene expression is regulated at the translational level. Following are some of the factors which affect translation.

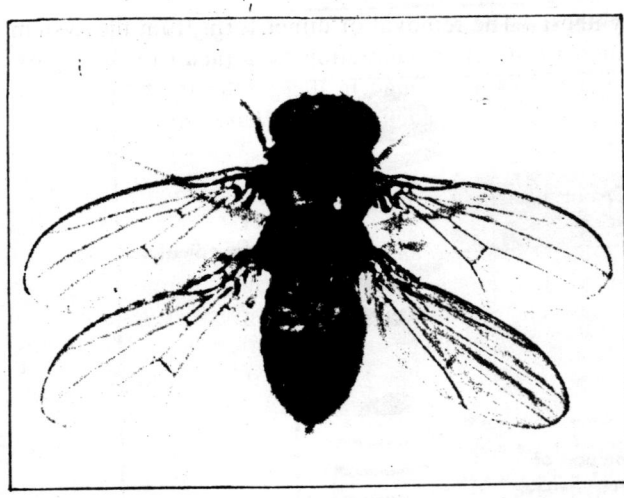

Fig. 8.66. A four-winged fly is produced by a triple mutation in abx, bx and pbx at the BX-C complex.

Stability of mRNA

The amount of mRNA in a cell is proportional to the amount of protein synthesized by the cell. The concentration of mRNA depends on its synthesis and on its breakdown. The half life of an average eukaryotic mRNA is about 18h. However, a number of factors affect its stability and thus the concentration of the mRNA for a specific protein, which in turn regulates the gene expression. Some of these factors have been described below.

Poly A tail

The poly A tail is present in majority of the eukaryotic mRNAs. It is added as a post-transcription event by the template-independent enzyme, the poly A polymerase. Earlier it was believed that the poly A tail controls the translation of an mRNA. However, a small number of mRNAs do not have the poly A tail (the A⁻ mRNAs, histone mRNAs are a good example of the A⁻ mRNAs). Further, the deadenylation does not affect the translatability of an mRNA in in vitro translation system. It is now well established that the poly A tail does not affect the translatability of mRNA as such. However, it plays an important role in the stability of the mRNA. The increased half life results in synthesis of multiple copies of the protein and thus play an indirect role in regulation of gene expressions.

Sequences at the 5' and 3' untranslated region of the mRNA

These apparently non-essential regions of mRNA may have many short sequences which play an important role in translation. For example, SD sequences in prokaryotes act by directing the binding of ribosomes. A number of other sequences act as 'cis' elements and also provide the site for the action of 'trans' acting regulatory factors.

Autoregulation

Certain proteins such as tubulin has two subunits α and β, which are post-translationally annealed to form a dimer. The dimers are then polymerized and are assembled in a precise manner to form the microtubules. Free dimers which have not polymerized, can interact with their own mRNAs and degrade it. Thus the protein is able to control their own synthesis. The removal of dimer form from the system increases the mRNA stability and there is a net increase in its concentration by a factor of 3-4 times. This regulation acts entirely at the level of translation and no change in the synthesis of mRNAs at the transcription level takes place. Certain hormones such as the gonadotropins also have similar regulatory mechanism along with the transcriptional regulation.

Hormonal regulation

Hormones are one of the most potent regulatory molecules known and affect both the transcription and the translation. Some of the examples of this class of hormones are steroid hormone, gluco-corticoid hormone etc. The hormone:receptor complex, on one hand stimulates the transcription of target genes by binding to upstream sequences, on the other hand, it also enhances the translation of the preformed mRNA and stimulates the protein synthesis.

Concentration of micronutrients

A number of micronutrients affect the expression of the enzymes involved in their metabolism. For example, the over-loading of cells with iron results in the increased synthesis of transferrin receptors as well as the higher ferritin content in the cell. These effects are blocked by cycloheximide suggesting that they are the translational effects.

Other factors affecting the rate of translation

There are many other factors which change the rate of translation. Some of these are the response to stress which produces specific proteins and shuts off the synthesis of some of the normal proteins. The mitotic cell division decreases the initiation of protein synthesis and results in decreased cellular proteins but increased specific factors. Similarily fertilization triggers the protein synthesis in the embryo. The unfertilized eggs of some of the eukaryotes, for example the frog oocytes, have large amounts of stored mRNAs which have been transcribed before the release of the eggs but are not translated until the fertilization has taken place. While the exact mechanism of this trigger is not very well understood, the 5'-untranslated region of the mRNAs modifies certain secondary structures. Sometimes the initiation factors are also modified. This type of mechanism takes place in stimulation of hemoglobin synthesis.

9

Protein Targetting

The proteins are synthesized in the cytoplasmic compartment of the cell on the ribosomes. Many of the proteins are released directly in the cytosolic pool and they manifest their biological activity there. However, a number of other proteins are localized in different subcellular compartments and some of these are also secreted out of the cell. A cellular machinery exists for the proper localisation of the proteins. The polysomes, which carryout the protein synthesis, can be classified into two broad classes based on their location. (1) The free polysomes and (2) the membrane bound polysomes. The free polysomes are present in the cytosolic fraction of the cell and the nascent polypeptide synthesized by these polysomes is released in the cytosol immediately after its translation. Majority of the proteins remain in the cytosol in a quasisoluble form. However, many other proteins are destined for other places within the cell. These proteins are taken to their final destination through a number of transport vesicles (see later). The final subcellular localization of the protein depends on a specific signal present in the protein. Common destinations for the proteins synthesised on free polysomes are the mitochondria, chloroplast, nucleus and the peroxisomes. If no specific signal is present, the protein remains in the cytosol in a soluble form by default.

The membrane bound polysomes, on the other hand, synthesize the proteins in association with the reticulo-endothelial system. The proteins which are synthesized by membrane bound polysomes contain a signal for the membrane insertion at the N-terminal end. This signal is known as the signal peptide or the leader sequence and is coded by the gene. The synthesis of these proteins is initiated on the free polysomes but soon after the signal peptide has been synthesized, it gets attached to the ER membrane. A specific nucleoprotein, the signal recognition particle (SRP) and the SRP-receptors which are present on the ER membrane, alongwith certain other factors are involved in this association. The signal peptide helps the protein to cross the membrane barrier and enter into the lumen of ER. Signal peptide itself is cleaved off during this process by a specific enzyme, the signal peptidase, and mature protein goes through the reticulo-endothelial system for the ultimate transportation to its final destination. Proteins are inserted in the ER membranes in a co-translational manner. The protein alongwith the signal peptide is known as the pro-protein and only after the signal peptide has been cleaved, the mature protein is formed. During the passing of the protein through the ER/Golgi complex, appropriate sugars are added (see earlier section for details of the glycosylation). There is a signal present at the N-terminal end of the protein, which codes for its final destination. As discussed earlier, the usual destinations for the proteins synthesized on the membrane bound polysomes are ER, lysosomes and the secretion out of the cell and in absence of a specific localization signal, a membrane bound protein is transported to the plasma membrane.

The synthesis and transportation of proteins is represented diagrammatically in Fig. 9.1. Various signals which code for ultimate transport of various proteins to their final destination are described in Table 9.1.

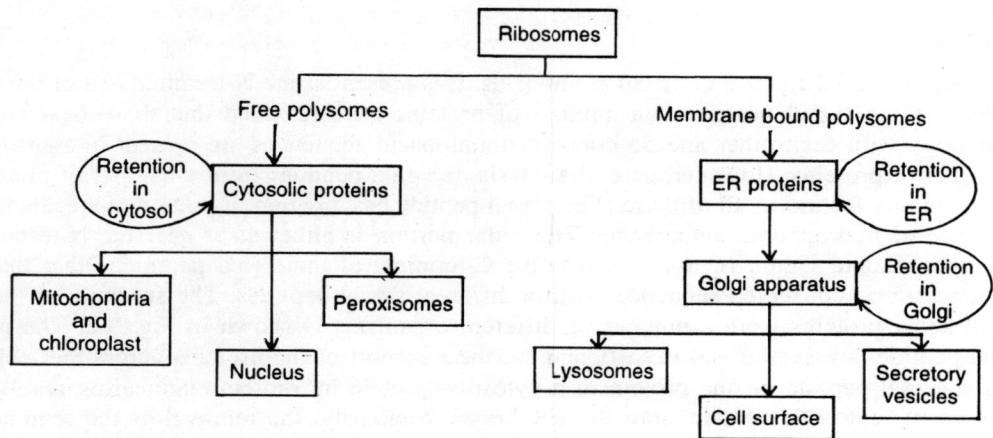

Fig. 9.1. Synthesis and transport of cellular proteins.

Table 9.1.

Destination	Signal location	Signal length	Nature of signal
A. Cytosolic proteins, synthesized on free polysomes			
Mitochondria	N-terminal	12-30 aa	Charged
Chloroplast	N-terminal	~25 aa	Charged
Nucleus	Internal Nuclear localisation signal	7-9 aa	Basic
Peroxisome	C-terminal	3 aa	Ser-Lys-Leu
B. Membrane proteins, synthesized on membrane-bound polysomes			
Insertion to membrane	N-terminal signal peptide	15-30 aa	Hydrophobic
ER	C-terminal	4 aa	Lys-Asp-Glu-Leu
Lysosomes	Carbohydrate moiety	1 sugar (modified)	Mannose-6-phosphate

Formation of the membrane bound polysomes

There is no intrinsic structural difference between the free polysomes and the membrane bound polysomes. The ribosomes are the same and the initiation of protein synthesis takes place in a similar manner. However, the membrane bound polysomes get associated co-translationally to the ER membrane. The experiments with isolated microsomes have shown that when the cell free protein synthesis is carried out in this system, the nascent polypeptide gets packaged with the membranes. However, if the pro-protein is incubated with the microsome, no such envaloping of the proteins takes place. This proves that the proteins are transported across the membrane in a co-translational manner. The membrane bound polysomes are associated with the sheets of ER and provide a characteristic roughness to the ER. These parts of ER are known as the rough ER. Other parts of ER to which polysomes are not attached, differ morphologically and these polysome-free ER membranes are known as the smooth ER. The components involved in the formation of membrane bound polysomes, insertion of protein and its crossing the membrane barrier and finally the removal of signal peptide include the signal peptide, the SRP, SRP-receptors and the signal peptidase. The mechanism of this process has been explained by G. Blobel who has put forward the signal hypothesis (see later).

Signal peptide

The signal peptide is a sequence of 15-30 aminoacids. It is present at the N-terminal end of the protein. The analysis of the signal peptide of a number of proteins have revealed that these bear very little or no homology with each other and no conserved aminoacid sequences are present in signal peptide from a number of proteins. However, careful analysis of signal peptides from a number of proteins has revealed a common feature in all of these. The signal peptide has a region of polar aminoacids followed by a sequence of hydrophobic aminoacids. The polar portion is either at or near the N-terminal end while the hydrophobic region is more towards the C-terminal of the signal peptide. Other than these regions, there are no conserved sequences within different signal peptides. The structure of the signal peptides of some proteins from a number of different organisms is shown in Fig. 9.2. The presence of a signal peptide is essential and is sufficient for the transport of the proteins across the membrane. Fusion of a signal peptide of one protein to a cytosolic protein by protein engineering results in the encapsulation of 'cytosolic protein' into the ER lumen. Similarly, the removal of the region having the codons for the signal peptide and inclusion of an arteficial initiation codon to the gene of a membrane protein results in the transformation of this protein into the cytosolic protein and its localization into the soluble fraction.

S.N.	Protein, source and nature	Size of signal peptide	Aminoacid sequence
1.	B-lactamase, pBR (secretory)	23 aa	MSIOHFRVALIPFFAAFCLPVFA H
2.	Maltose binding protein, E. coli (secretory)	28 aa	MKIKTGARILALSALTTMMFSASALA K
3.	OmpA protein, E. coli (membrane bound)	21 aa	MKKTAIAIAVALAGFATVAOA A
4.	Coat protein phage FD (membrane bound)	23 aa	MKKSLVLKASVAVATLVPMLSFA A
5.	B-lactamase, B. licheniformis (secretory)	34 aa	MLKKFSTLKLKKAAAVLLFSCVALAGCANNOTNA S
6.	Preproinsulin, Rat (secretory)	24 aa	MALWRMFLPLLALLVLWEPLPAEA F
7.	Growth hormone, Rat (secretory)	26 aa	MAADSOTPWLLTFSLLCLLWPOEAGA L
8.	Coat glycoprotein, vesicular stomatitis virus (membrane bound)	16 aa	MKCLLYLAFLFIHVNC K
9.	Lysozyme, chicken (secretory)	18 aa	MRSLLILVLCFLPLAALG K
10.	Igk light chain, Mouse (secretory)	22 aa	MDMRAPAGIFGFLLLLFPGTRC D

Fig. 9.2. Signal sequences of some prokaryotic and eukaryotic proteins.

Signal Recognition Particle

Signal recgnition particle is integral part of the cell membrane. It is a nucleoprotein of 11S in size and is rod-like in shape with dimensions of 5-6X22-25 nm. This has a single RNA of 7S size (305 bases, 100 KD) and 6 proteins. Of the 6 proteins, 5 are bound directly to RNA while the sixth protein (p54) is complexed with one of the five proteins (p19). The complex has a molecular weight of 240KD. It is possible to reconstitute the SRP in vitro by taking the 7S RNA from one membrane and the proteins from another. The RNA has a number of regions of base complementarity having high degree of secondary structure with a number of stems and loops. About 100 bases at the 5'-end and 40-45 bases at the 3'-end of RNA have structural similarity with the Alu class of RNA. This part is known as the Alu domain. The rest of the RNA is referred as the S domain. Four of the six proteins are associated with the S domain which is almost entirely covered with proteins. The Alu domain has only a dimer of two small proteins, the p9 and the p14. By reconstitution experiments it has been possible to assign various functions to different parts of SRP. The p9/p14 dimer is responsible for the temporary blockage of translation of the secretary protein. As will be discussed later, the association of SRP with signal peptide results in pausing of protein synthesis for a short while. Two major proteins (p68/p72) are associated with the midddle part of the 7S RNA and the dimer is responsible for the recognition of the SRP receptors and also for the translocation of the signal peptide across the membrane. Protein p19 is elongated in shape and is bound to the RNA at the two extremities. It is also complexed with the 6th protein (p54). The p54 is the only protein which is not bound to RNA and is responsible for the recognition of signal sequence. The detailed structure of SRP has been shown diagramatically in Fig. 9.3.

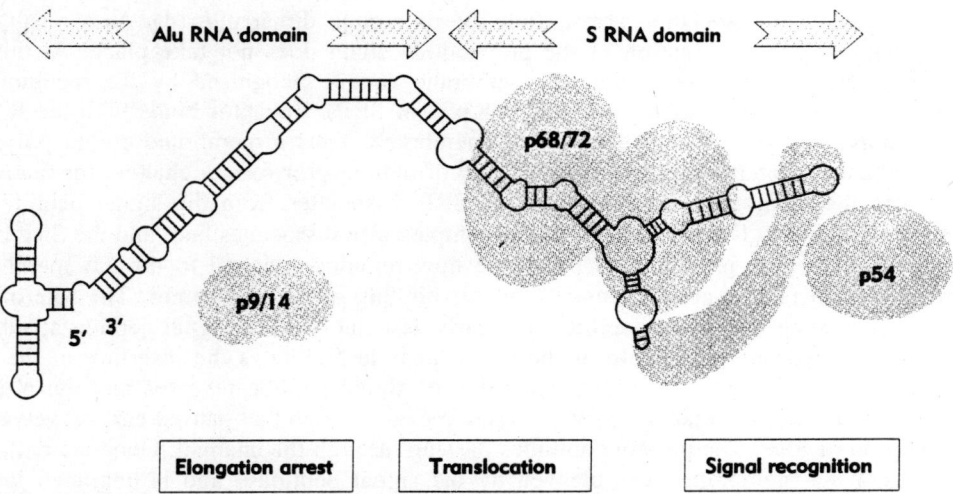

Fig. 9.3. Structure of SRP. The two domains of the 7S RNA of the SRP are defined by its relationship to the Alu sequence. Five of the six proteins bind directly to the 7S RNA. Each function of the SRP is associated with a particular protein(s).

SRP receptor

SRP-receptor is the integral part of the ER membrane. It is made of two proteins of 72 KD and 30 KD. Both proteins are associated with each other and are present as a dimer. The N-terminal of 72 KD protein is anchored to the ER in such a manner that most of the receptor protudes towards the cytosolic side of ER. The structure of receptor proteins is very similar to a number of nucleic acid binding proteins. This suggests that probably the binding of SRP to SRP receptor is through the RNA of SRP. However, the dimer of p68/p72 on SRP is responsible for the recognition of receptor by SRP.

Signal peptidase

Signal peptidase is a multimeric enzyme. It is a complex of six proteins. However, the enzymatic activity is associated with only one of these proteins. Other proteins are probably involved in providing the structural support to the enzyme. The enzyme is present at the lumen side of the membrane. Its location plays an important role in ensuring that the signal peptide is cleaved only after all of it has crossed the membrane and protein has become well anchored to the membrane. The enzyme is present in huge excess, almost in equimolar ratio to the membrane bound ribosomes in the cell. This means that the removal of signal peptide is very efficient and fast.

The signal hypothesis

The basic mechanism of the formation of membrane bound polysomes and the transfer of proteins from cytosol to the lumen of ER was first proposed by G. Blobel in 1975. This mechanism is referred as signal hypothesis. This explains the entire process in a very simple manner. The synthesis of a secretory protein is initiated just like any other protein on the polysomes. After about 50-75 aa have been incorporated and the entire signal peptide has emerged out of the ribosome (about 30-40 aminoacids of growing polypeptide remain within the ribosome during elongation), SRP recognizes the singnal peptide and gets associated with it (function of protein p54). This association of SRP with the growing polypeptide chain results in translation arrest (function of protein dimer p9/p14). As a result of this, the ribosome pauses and the elongation of the polypeptide chain does not take place. At this stage, the polysome-SRP complex moves to the ER membrane and is recognised by the receptor in the membrane (the function of dimer of the proteins p68/p72 of SRP). Receptor binds with the RNA part of SRP and the polysome gets associated with the membrane. Thus a membrane bound polysome is formed. Certain channel proteins present in the vicinity of the receptor form a channel for the insertion of the protein into the membrane. At this stage the SRP dissociates from the signal peptide (but is associated with the receptor). The SRP/SRP-receptor complex also dissociates later and the SRP becomes available for binding to next protein. The polysome now remains attached to the ER membrane. A number of other protein factors are responsible for this binding of the polysomes. The role of SRP is thus to bring the polysome to ER and facilitate the early association. The signal peptide attaches with the lipid bilayer. The hydrophobic nature of the signal peptide facilitates the insertion of the peptide into the lipid bilayer. At the time of insertion the end of signal peptide reverses and the N-terminal faces the cytosolic side. The elongation of the polypetide chain, which had paused earlier, gets resumed after the dissociation of SRP. The protein continues passing through the channel. Once the entire signal peptide has crossed the membrane, it is cleaved by the signal peptidase and is degraded later. The transfer of protein across the membrane continues. Once the stop codon is approached, the termination of protein synthesis occurs and the ribosome falls off the mRNA. However, the protein translocation continues until the entire molecule has crossed the membrane and all of the protein has reached the lumen of ER.

The pausing of elongation immediately after the signal peptide has emerged out of the ribosome and its resumption only after the nascent peptide has entered the membrane thus causing the co-translational translocation of the nascent polypeptide, plays an important role in maintaining the confirmation of the proteins. Many of the proteins are too large to be able to cross the membrane in their final confirmation. The co-translational translocation does not permit the protein to be exposed to the aqueous environment of the cytosol and thus maintains an alternate confirmation which helps the proteins to cross the membrane. This confirmation is maintained unless the protein leaves the membrane system when the final confirmation of the mature protein has been attained.

The entire process has been diagramatically shown in Fig. 9.4. It should be noted that although this hypothesis very well explains the translocation of the signal peptide across the membrane, a number of problems remain unanswered. The proteins are primarily hydrophilic in nature and a question, therefore, arises as how the protein is transferred across the hydrophilic environment of the membrane? It has been found that once the signal peptide has entered the lipid bilayer, some of the intrinsic proteins of the membrane form a channel around the protein. The nascent protein is thus not exposed to the hydrophobic environment and is rather sorrounded by a hydrophilic environment of the channel and passes through it (Fig. 9.5). The channel is very discretionary in its behaviour and does not allow any thing else but the protein to pass through it. No ions or other biomolecules can cross the channel

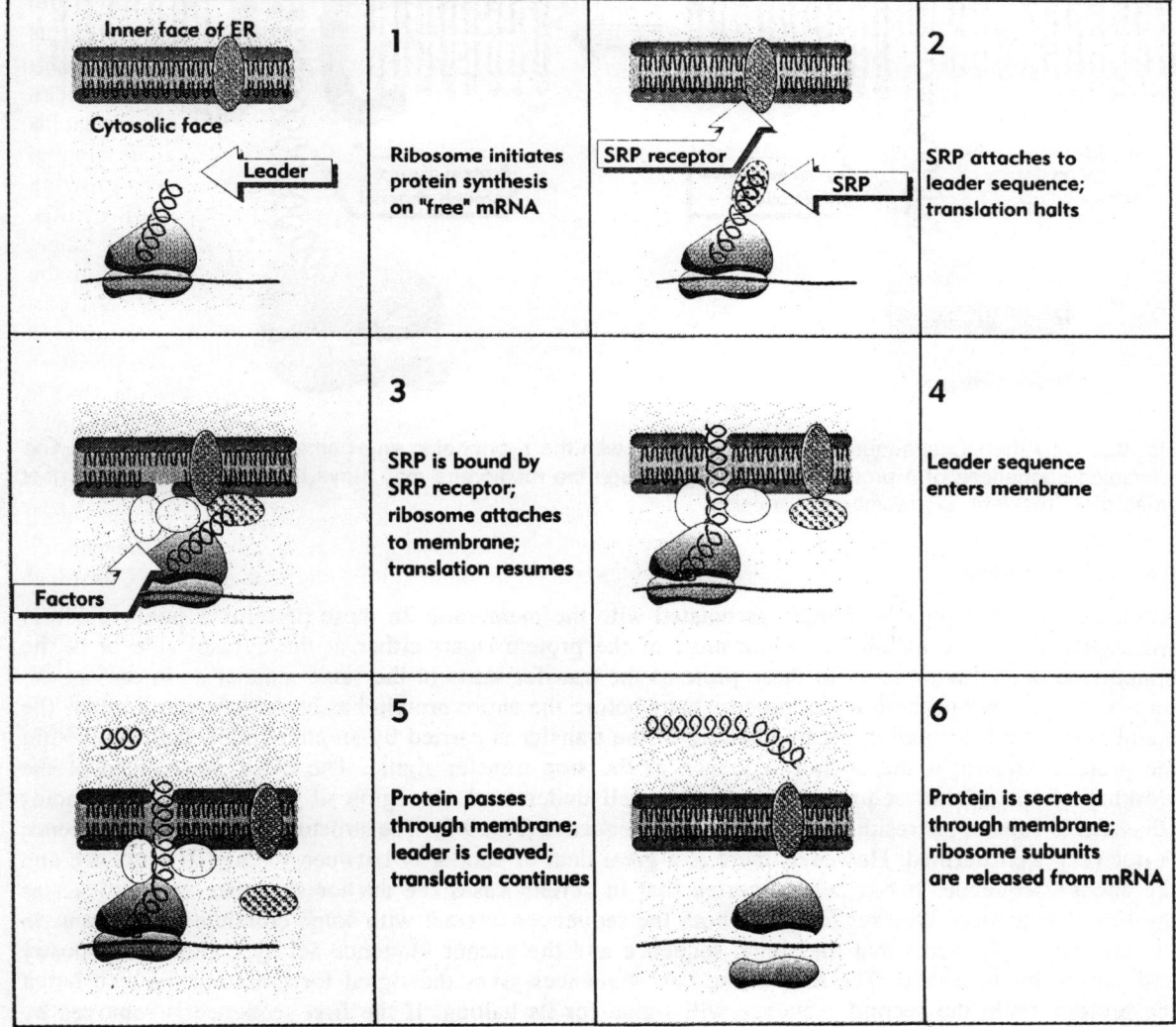

Fig. 9.4. The signal hypothesis. The ribosomes synthesizing secretory proteins are attached to the membrane via the leader sequence on the nascent polypeptide.

during the translocation. The presence of the signal peptide is essential and is also sufficient for this translocation. If the signal peptide is attached to another protein which was cytosolic otherwise, that protein will be transported across the membrane. Once protein synthesis is terminated and ribosome has dissociated, the channel closes and the memmbrane becomes intact.

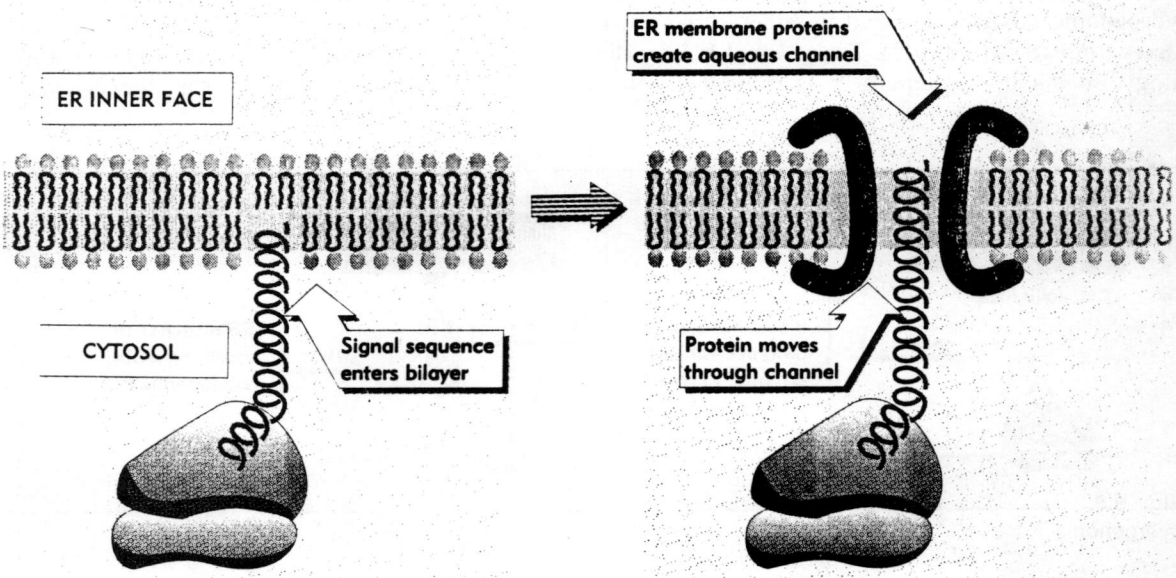

Fig. 9.5. Only the signal sequence interacts directly with the hypophobic environment of the lipid bilayer. The remaining sequences of a protein translocating through the membrane may move through an aqueous tunnel created by resident ER membrane proteins.

Resident Proteins

A number of other proteins remain associated with the membrane. In these proteins a small region is embedded inside the membrane while most of the protein floats either at the cytosol side or at the lumen side of the membrane. In these proteins the transfer starts in the same manner as in case of the secretory proteins but the transfer process halts before the entire protein has been transferred across the membrane. The information for this halting of the transfer is carried by another small sequence within the protein, known as the anchor sequence or the stop transfer signal. The exact mechanism of the working of the anchor sequence is not very well understood. A region of hydrophobic aminoacids adjacent to some ionic residues form the anchor sequence (Fig. 9.6). The structure of the anchor sequence is not very well defined. However, there is a great deal of similarity between the signal sequence and the anchor sequence. It has been reported that in certain cases the anchor sequence can also act as the signal sequence. This suggests that both the sequences interact with some common components in the membrane. It seems that the signal sequence and the anchor sequence act by a common pathway and can be interchanged. The first of the two sequences gives the signal for initiating the transfer of the protein while the second sequence will signal for its halting. If the first sequence is removed by protein engineering, the second region will function as the signal sequence. The whole scenerio can be compared with a push button type of electric switch; one push of the button allows the current to flow while the second push stops the current. If the current is already flowing then the first push will stop it.

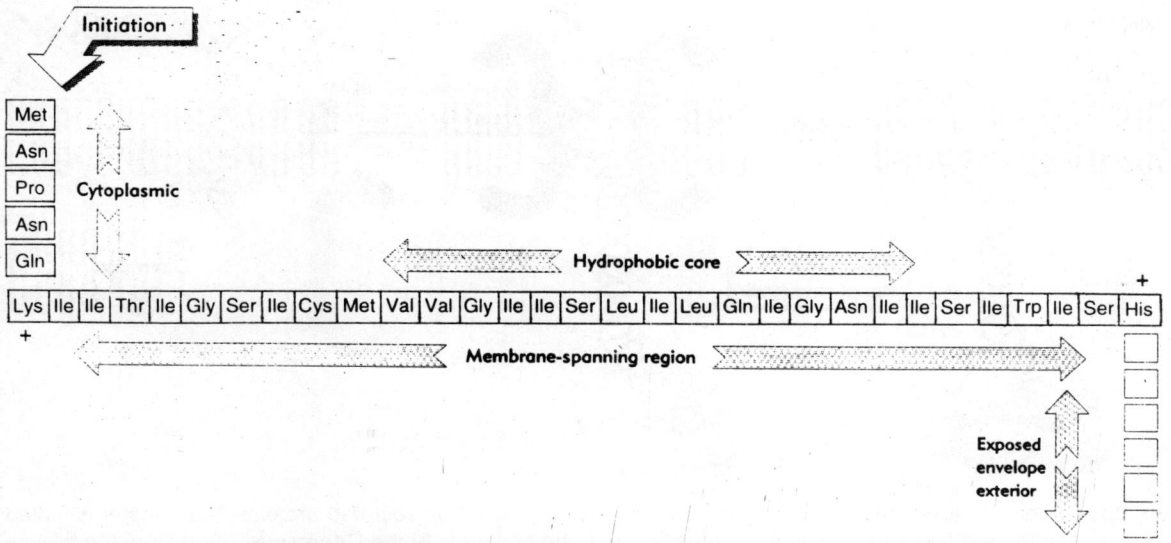

Fig. 9.6. The signal-anchor of influenza neuraminidase is located close to the N-terminus and has a hydrophobic core.

Based on the orientatation of the protein in relation to the membrane, there are two types of resident proteins. The type 1 proteins are anchored in the membranre by their C-terminal and have the N-treminal end floating in the lumen. Majority of the membrane associated proteins fall under this category. During transfer, the N-terminal signal sequence forms a hairpin like structure and gets anchored at the cytosolic side. The other end of the signal sequence keeps passing through the membrane and the channel is formed. Once entire signal sequence has crossed the membrane channel, it is cleaved. However, the protein keeps on passing and reaches on other side of the membrane. the anchor sequence is present on the C-terminal and stops the protein transfer. Thus the N-terminal is inside the lumen and protein is held by the membrane through its C-terminal (Fig. 9.7).

In the type 2 proteins, the orientation is reversed. The anchor sequence is present at or near the N-terminal. It is present in association with the signal peptide and is known as the combined signal-anchor sequence. This sequence is usually an internal sequence present near the N-terminal. There are 6-30 aminoacids present upstream of the combined signal-anchor sequence. The transfer of the nascent polypeptide starts in the same way as in case of type 1 proteins. However, as the signal sequence is located in an internal region, there will be some aminoacids which are already floating on the cytosolic side of the membrane before the signal peptide hits the membrane. At this stage, the hairpin structure is formed and the combined peptide enters the membrane. Once the sequence has entered, unlike the type 1 protein, it is not cleaved and remains associated with the protein. This sequence anchors the protein to the membrane. The transfer channel is formed and the transfer of the C-terminal of the protein continues. After whole protein is transferred, the C-terminal is at the lumen side of the membrane (Fig. 9.8).

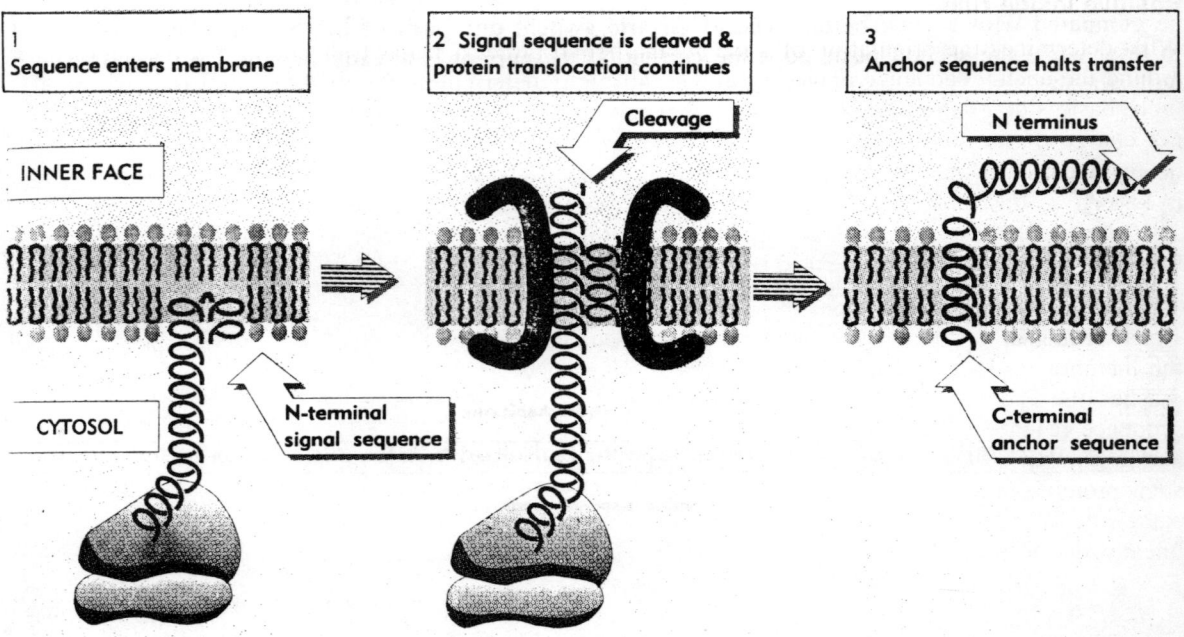

| 1 Sequence enters membrane | 2 Signal sequence is cleaved & protein translocation continues | 3 Anchor sequence halts transfer |

Fig. 9.7. Proteins that reside in membranes enter by the same route as secreted proteins, but transfer is halted when an anchor sequence passes into the membrane. If the anchor is at the C-terminus, the bulk of the protein passes through the membrane and is exposed on the far surface.

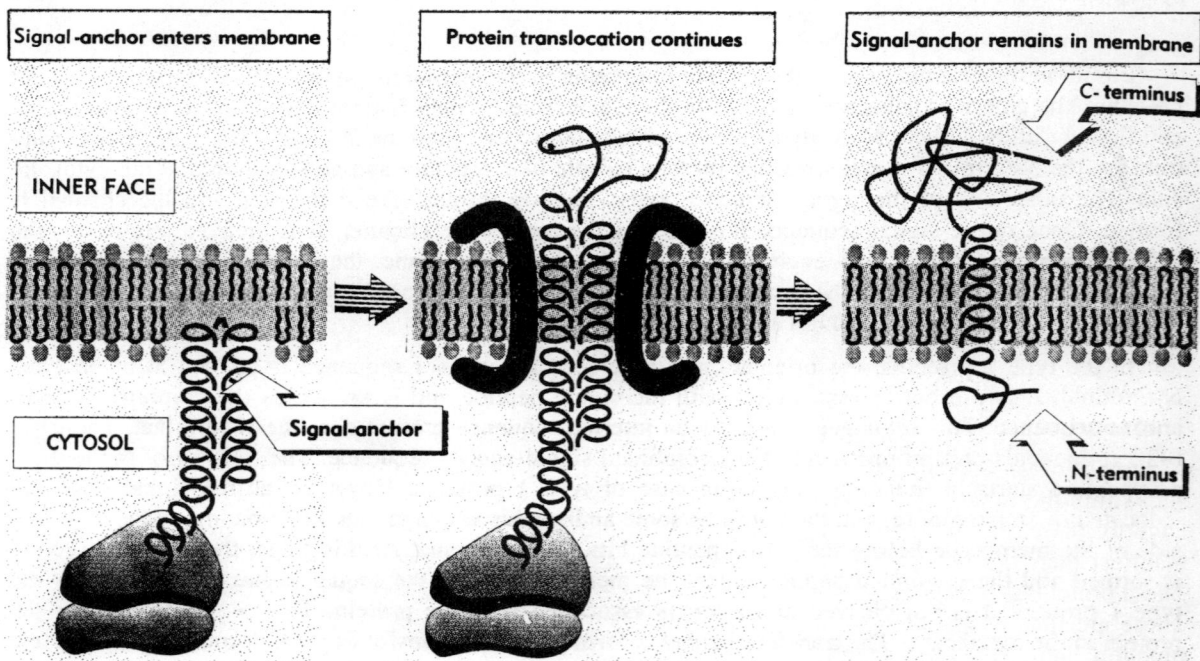

| Signal-anchor enters membrane | Protein translocation continues | Signal-anchor remains in membrane |

Fig. 9.8. A combined signal-anchor sequence causes a protein to reverse its orientation, so that the N-terminus remains on the inner face and the C-terminus is exposed on the outer face of the membrane.

Positive inside rule

What determines the orientation of a membrane bound protein? It has been found that the net charges around the anchor sequence play very important role in determining the orientation of the protein. The more basic side of the protein bearing higher net positive charge remains at the cytosolic side. If the net charge of the two sides are reversed by protein engineering, the orientation of the protein will be reversed. The end of the protein with higher positive charge always remains inside and this rule is known as the 'positive inside rule'.

Proteins with multiple anchoring regions

A number of proteins criss-cross the membrane a number of times. These proteins have more than one signal sequence and more than one anchor sequence. Once the signal sequence comes in contact with the membrane, the transfer of protein starts and continues until the anchor sequence is translated and reaches the channel. At this point the transfer of protein stops. However, when the second signal sequence reaches the channel, the transfer starts again. The entire process is repeated as many times as the number of signal sequences and the anchor sequences. The membrane embedding domains in such proteins may be either even or odd. Also either the N-terminal and the C-termnal may be on same side of the membrane or on different sides of the membrane. Any of the terminals may be present on any of the side. This has been shown in Fig. 9.9.

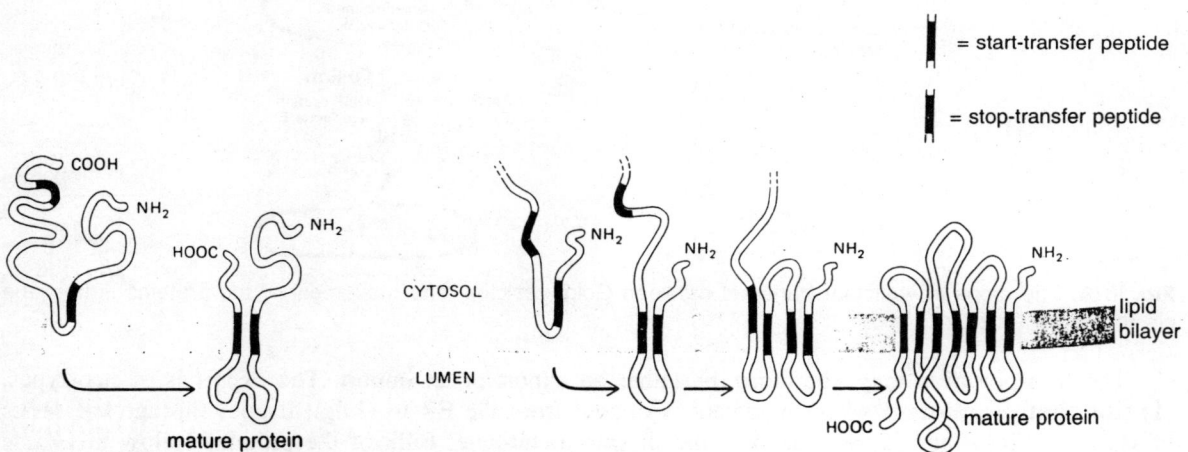

Fig. 9.9. The intrinsic membrane proteins have alternating start transfer and stop transfer sequences.

Transport vesicles

A number of proteins are transported from one site in the cell where these are synthesized, to another site within the same cell where these are finally localised and carry out their biological function. These have to, therefore, cross the cytoplasmic region for this translocation. Similarly, some of the proteins manifest their biological activity in a cell (or organ) other than the cell where these are synthesized. These proteins are secreted by the first cell and are carried to the other tissue where these are internalized. These are then transported to their subcellular location in the target cell and perform their biological function there. These transportations require a series of reactions involving a number of molecular interactions. In general, the transportation involves the formation of a transport vesicle which carries the protein of interest as its cargo. The vesicle then moves to the final destination where it docks and unloads the cargo. These vesicles are formed as a 'bud' protuding from the donor membrane and are coated with a number of proteins. The membrane and the lumen of the vesicle has the same structure as the membrane and the lumen of the donor site. After they have reached the target site, the coat proteins are shed off and the vesicle fuses with the target membrane. After fusion, the membrane and the lumen of the vesicle becomes the part of the target membrane (Fig. 9.10).

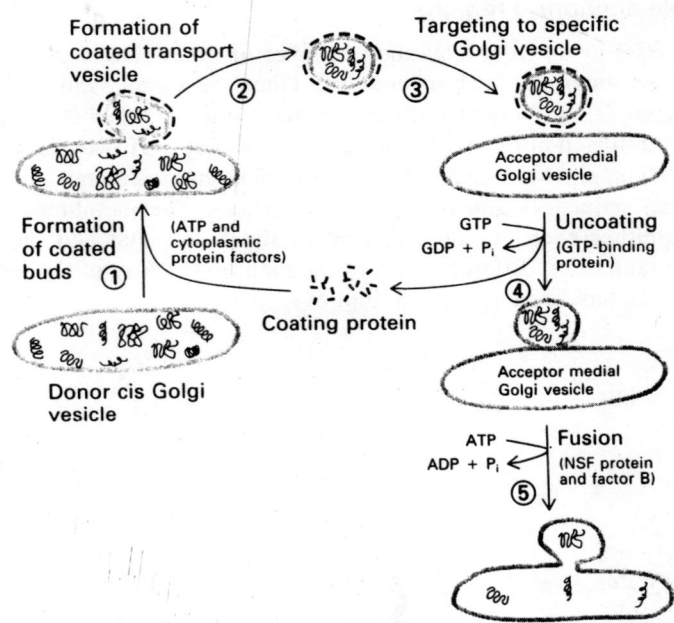

Fig. 9.10. The steps in vesicular transport between Golgi vesicles. The movement of the proteins is from the cis to medial Golgi.

The transportation may, therefore, be either an export or an import. The export is of two types. (1) Constitutive transport where a protein is carried from the ER to Golgi. It goes through the series of stacks in Golgi and is then taken to the plasma membrane. Bulk of the proteins follow this route which is also followed by a number of lipids. The vesicles carrying the proteins (or lipids) for constitutive export are known as transport vesicles. (2) Exocytosis, where the export is regulated by external signals such as a hormone. This is mediated through the vesicles, known as exocytic vesicle or secretory vesicles which are formed at the trans face of Golgi and act as the store house. They carry the protein to plasma membrane but do not fuse with the plasma membrane and unload the cargo. Only when an appropriate signal is received, the vesicles unload the cargo. The proteins which act at a tissue different than where they are synthesized, need to be taken in by the target cell. This is achieved by a process known as endocytosis. Once accepted by the target membrane, these proteins are transported within the cell by the endocytotic vesicles. The three vesicles involved in the three types of processes differ from each other in their structure.

As stated above, the vesicles have an outer coat sorrounding the vesicle membrane. This coat is made of a number of proteins. Some of the proteins are well characterized while certain other proteins have not been identified. The coat serves a number of useful purposes for the vesicles. First, it serves as a protective layer and guards the vesicles from the action of various cellular enzymes. The proteins also serve as an identification tag mark for the proper processing of the vesicle. The cellular transportation system determines the final destination of the vesicle by recognizing the information coded by the coat proteins. They also play an important role in the budding of the donor membrane and formation of the vesicle as well as in the triggering of the reaction leading to the final fusion of the vesicle with the target membrane. These may also exert a discretion in selecting the cargo which the vesicle will carry and transport with them. However, the mechanism of the role of the coat proteins in cargo selection is not very well understood.

The protein to be transported (the cargo) is incorporated inside the transport vesicle in the ER and is transported to the cis face of the Golgi. This transport is energy dependent and requires ATP. In Golgi, the protein is transported through the stacks towards the trans face by the transition vesicles. During this transition through Golgi stacks, the changes in glycosylation level of the protein also take place. At last, it is carried to their final destination through approprite vesicles. The final destination depends on specific localization signal present within the protein itself. If no signal for specific localization is present, the protein is destined to the plasma membrane by default.

Based on the nature of the coat proteins, the coated vesicles are of two types.

1. Clathrin coated vesicles; where the main protein of the coat is a heterodimer protein, clathrin. This forms the outer most layer of the coat. The endocytic vesicles and the exocytic vesicles are of this type. The two subunits of clathrin are a large H subunit which is 180KD in size and a much smaller L chain of 35 KD (it may vary between 30-40 KD). The coat is made of 3 H and 3 L subunits arranged in a polyhedral fashion. This structure is also referred as triskelion structure (Fig. 9.11). Clathrin is attached to the vesicle membrane by another protein referred as the adopter. The adopter is a heterotetramer of 4 subunits, each is known as the adoptin. The composition of adopter in exocytic and in endocytic vesicle is different. The adopter molecules involved in the formation of exocytic vesicle at the coated pits of Golgi apparatus are referred as the HA-1 adopters. These are made of one each of γ-adoptin, β-adoptin, p47 and p20. The adopters of endocytic vesicle at the plasma membrane are known as the HA-2 adopters and are made up of one each of α-adoptin, β-adoptin,

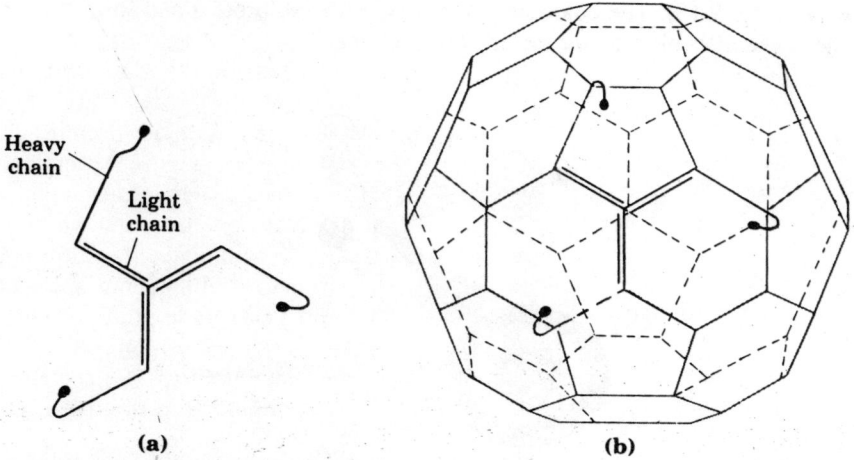

Fig. 9.11. The triskelion structure of a clathrin molecule. (a) A three legged trimer. (b) Assembly of triskelins to form polyhedral lattices.

p50 and p17. The β-adoptin subunit in both these adopters binds with the clathrin. Besides its binding to clathrin, the adopter also binds with the membrane of the vesicle through the cytoplasmic end of the membrane proteins. The structure of a clathrin coated vesicle has been shown in Fig. 9.12. The adopter molecules thus form the inner coat and act as the bridge between the clathrin portion of the coat and the membrane. These also provide specificity to the vesicle and play a role in selecting the cargo it would carry. During the fusion of the vesicle with the target membrane, the adopter and clathrin molecules are released and remain present in the cytoplasm in free form.

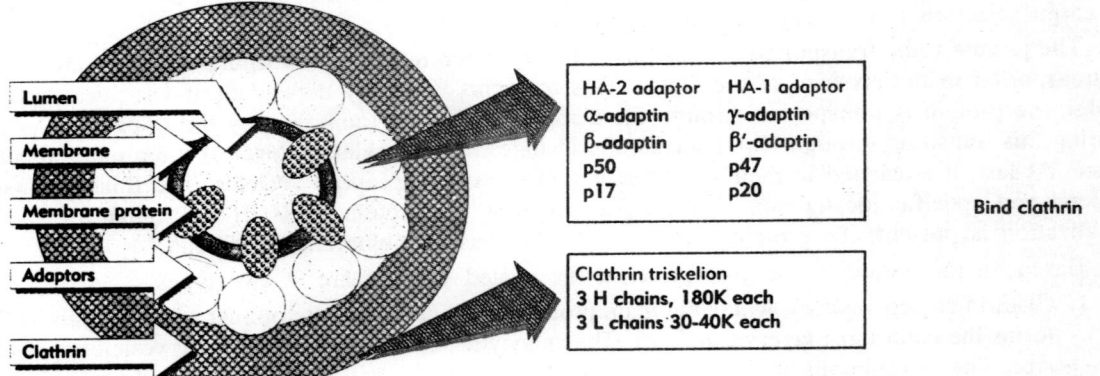

HA-2 adaptor	HA-1 adaptor
α-adaptin	γ-adaptin
β-adaptin	β′-adaptin
p50	p47
p17	p20

Bind clathrin

Clathrin triskelion
3 H chains, 180K each
3 L chains 30-40K each

Fig. 9.12. Clathrin-coated vesicles have a coat consisting of two layers: the outer layer is formed by clathrin, and the inner layer is formed by adaptors, which lie between clathrin and the integral membrane proteins.

2. Non-clathrin coated vesicles; as the name suggests, these vesicles donot contain clathrin in their coat. The nature of the proteins in their outer coat is relatively unknown. The transport vesicles and the transition vesicles belong to this type. Bulk of the proteins are transported through these vesicles. In this type of vesicles, the outer coat proteins are held together by seven types of major proteins known as COPs. These 7 types of COPs are α-COP, β-COP, β′-COP, γ-COP, δ-COP, p20 and p36. These COPs are present as a complex of very high molecular weight (~700 KD), which is known as coatomer (Fig. 9.13). The coatomers bind to membrane protein and form the inner coat. On the other side these also bind to the outer coat proteins.

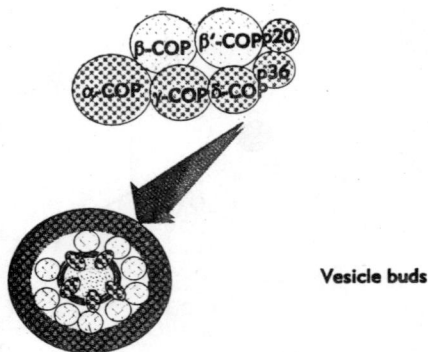

Vesicle buds

Fig. 9.13. The structure of a non-clathrin coated vesicle.

Formation of the coated vesicles

The vesicles are formed from the donor membranes in the form of a bud. The formation of a vesicle is shown in Fig. 9.14. The process is energy dependent and ATP is used. For vesicle formation the presence of lipid bilayer is necessary. Certain protein(s) binds to donor membrane by penetrating the lipid bilayer. This binding results in local destabilization and the membrane structure gets deformed. An extrusion of the membrane results which is referred as bud. This bud is surrounded by the coat proteins. The bud gets enlarged slowly and finally separates from the donor membrane in form of a vesicle. The protein which was originally bound to membrane and triggered the bud formation, also becomes the part of coat.

The formation of a non-clathrin coated vesicle has been well worked out. A GTP-binding protein, ARE (ADP-ribosylation factor) initiates the budding. ARF is N-myristylated and is capable of penetrating into the lipid bilayer of membrane through the fatty acid side chain. However, for its activity the ARF requires GTP. Either the free ARF or GDP-ARF complex is biologically inactive. The binding of GTP causes confirmational changes in ARF, as a result of which the myristylated residue becomes available for the penetration into membrane. Thus its activity and the binding and release are regulated by GTP hydrolysis. Once ARF has become bound to the membrane, the bud formation takes place and the coatomers (high molecular weight complex made of the COPs) surround the bud. Finally the outer coat proteins join and the vesicle is pinched off the donor membrane. ARF itself remains the part of the coat. There are 2-3 coatomers for each ARF molecule. The process has been shown in Fig. 9.15.

Fusion with target membrane

The vesicles carry their cargo proteins to the target membrane where the cargo is identified, sorted and the coat proteins of the vesicles are removed. The uncoated vesicles then fuse with the target membrane

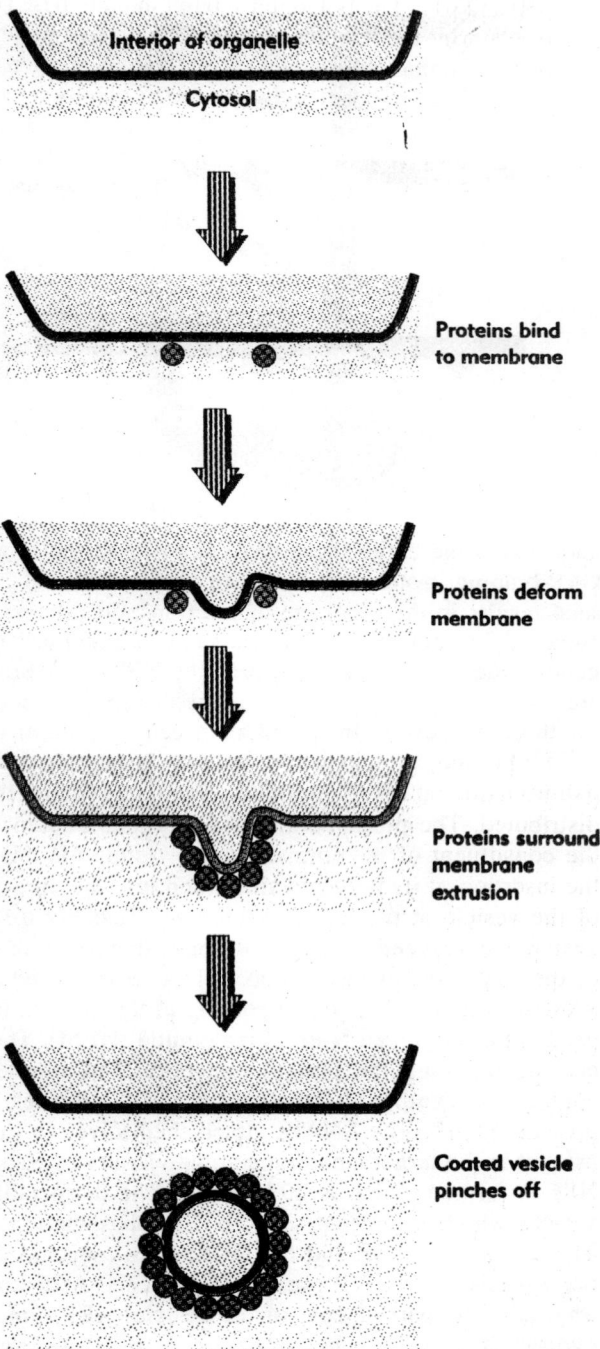

Fig. 9.14. Vesicle formation results when proteins bind to a membrane, deform it, and ultimately surround a membrane vesicle that is pinched off.

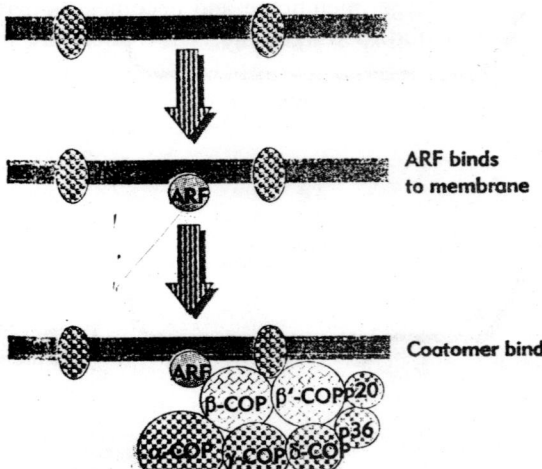

ARF binds
to membrane

Coatomer binds

Fig. 9.15. The budding of non-clathrin coated vesicle requires ARF and coatomers.

and unload the cargo these were carrying at the target. These processes are governed by a number of GTP-binding proteins. It has been established that in yeast cells the mutation in gene ypt1 or in gene sec4 results in the blockage of the transport process. The vesicles get accumulated either at the Golgi apparatus (in between various layers of stacks) or between the Golgi and the plasma membrane. These genes code for GTP-binding proteins YPT1 and SEC4. Similarly if non-hydrolysable analogs of GTP are incorporated in place of GTP, the transport is blocked. This confirms that GTP hydrolysis is required for these processes. In mammalian cells a protein Rab is present which carries this function. Rab is a GTP binding protein whose activity is regulated by GTP hydrolysis. The protein has prenylation or palmitylation at its C-terminal. There are more than 15 types of Rabs known which are widely distributed. The presence of Rabs has been documented in almost all the membranes. It is present as the constituent of membranes at the vesicle binding sites. Its attachment to the membrane is through the insertion of its fattyacid side chain into the lipid bilayer. Its function is to provide a site for docking of the vesicle at the target membrane. Probably different Rabs recognise different vesicles. Once the vesicle has reached its target, it docks there at a site provided by the Rab. At this stage the uncoating of the coat proteins have to take place. It is carried out by another protein, NSF. The NSF has soluble ATPase activity. The yeast homolog of this protein is SEC18. NSF is sensitive to one of the commonly used sulfa drugs, the N-ethyl maleimide (NEM). The drug acts against a number of viral diseases and acts by blocking the protein transport. This ultimately results in defective envalope formation and controls the synthesis of the progeny of the viruses. The NSF acts by forming a complex with another protein, SNAP. The SNAPs attach themselves to the membrane through specific receptors which are present in the target membrane at the vicinity of Rab protein. Thus a large complex of receptor-SNAPs-NSF is formed which is 20S in size. The dissociation of this complex results in the uncoating of the vesicle which is present on Rab. The dissociation of this complex involves the hydrolysis of ATP. The dissociated NSF and the SNAPs are recycled. The dissociation of 20S complex seems to trigger the hydrolysis of GTP present in the GTP-ARF complex. It may be recalled that this complex was originally the part of coat of the vesicle. ARF remains associated with GDP, which is formed by the hydrolysis of GTP. The formation of GDP-ARF complex changes the confirmation of ARF which ultimately results in uncoating of the vesicle. The GDP-ARF complex is later recycled through its interaction with another molecule of GTP and regeneration of the GTP-ARF.

Once the vesicle has been uncoated, it fuses with the target membrane and becomes its part. The protein which was being carried by the vesicle is unloaded at the target site. The vesicle are formed at the ER and the Golgi and as the integral part of their structure, the vesicles carry a small portion of the ER/Golgi membrane including some of the membrane proteins with them. When the vesicle fuses with the target membrane, this portion of ER/Golgi membrane becomes part of the target site. Thus, there is a constant flow of membrane structure from the reticuloendothelial system to the plasma membrane. This should normally result in the depletion of ER/Golgi system and enlargement of the plasma membrane. However, this is not what actually happens and both the systems maintain their size. Therefore, a reverse transport of membrane structure has to take place. The mechanism of such a reverse flow is not very well understood. It seems that this type of reverse flow takes place in the form of tubules which have high surface to volume ratio and thus can carry large portion of membrane components in a relatively small volume. It is in contrast to the transport vesicles, which are round in shape and have low surface to volume ratio, thus carrying relatively small amounts of membrane structures but have large capacity to carry the cargo. Fig. 9.16 represents these processes.

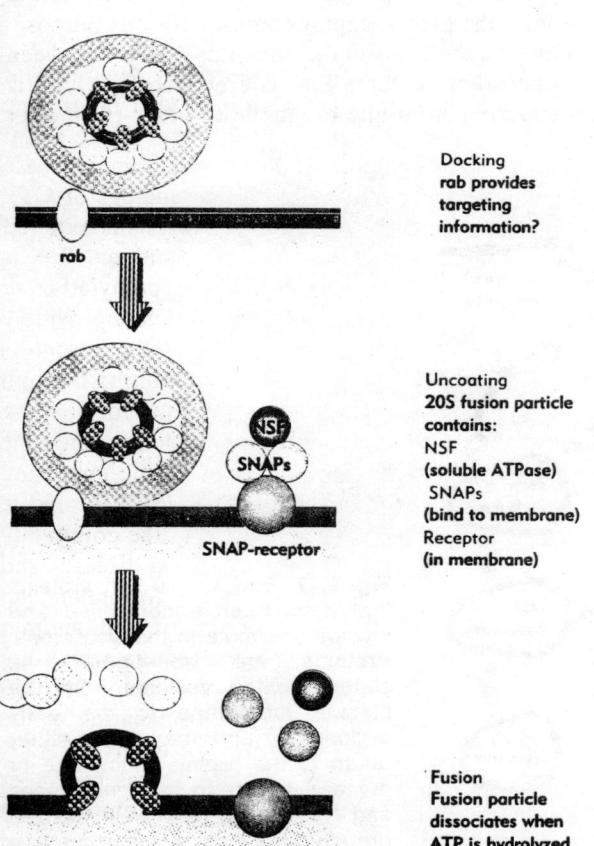

Docking
rab provides targeting information?

Uncoating
20S fusion particle contains:
NSF
(soluble ATPase)
SNAPs
(bind to membrane)
Receptor
(in membrane)

Fusion
Fusion particle dissociates when ATP is hydrolyzed

Fig. 9.16. Different proteins are required for vesicle targetting, uncoating, and membrane fusion.

Transport of proteins to their final destination

Once the cargo protein has reached to the Golgi and has become matured, it is then transported to its final destination. The final localization of the protein depends on the signal carried by the protein. The recognition of the signal and sorting of the proteins for further transport takes place only after the protein has become matured. Thus, different signals are processed at different location within the Golgi network. Some of the commonly present signals have already been shown in Table 9.1.

It should be noted that if a protein is to be localised in the ER, it has to first go through the entire Golgi network where it becomes mature. Only then it is exported from the Golgi at the trans-cisternae and is taken to the ER through a vesicle. It does not go back to ER through the Golgi stacks.

Localization into lysosomes

As discussed earlier, further transport of the cargo protein is dependent on the signal carried by it. Lysosomes are one of the organelles which accept the proteins from Golgi for their final distribution to a member of other places. Besides, majority of the cellular import of the proteins from other cells is also handled by lysosomes. The imported cargo is endocytosised inside the cell and is brought to the endosomes by the endocytic vesicles. The endocytic vesicles are clathrin-containing coated vesicles. The endosomes are the intermediate stop for ultimate destination of the proteins to the lysosomes. There are two types of endosomes, the early endosomes and the late endosomes. Endo-somes act as the location for sorting of the import proteins. The early endosomes are located just below the plasma membrane. The proteins take approximately 1 min to reach the early endosome. These have an acidic environment inside the lumen (pH less than 6). The acidic pH helps in changing the structure of the imported proteins. For example, if a receptor-ligand complex is received, it is dissociated and the two components are separated. The proteins are sorted here. If necessary, a protein may be returned back to the plasma membrane. For example, in case of receptor-ligand complex cited above the dissociated receptor may return back to the original membrane. If it goes back to membrane, the site of its fusion is either the original site at the parent membrane or somewhere near it. Alternatively, it may be transported to the lysosomes and get degraded. The proteins which are destined to lysosome, are then transferred to the late endosomes. Late endosomes are located near the nucleus. Late endosomes also have a similar structure as the early endosomes and also same environment as the early endosomes. Once a protein is accepted by the late endosome, it can not go back to either plasma membrane or to any other site. It is now destined to go to lysosome. The internal proteins being transported from the Golgi to lysosome are also accepted by late endosomes. These proteins require the M6P receptor complex for this purpose. The proteins are ultimately transferred from late endosomes to the lysosomes. The inter-transfer between endosome-lysosome is in two ways. Either the early endosome matures into late endosome which is further matured into the lysosome or the protein is transferred from one organelle to other for further processing (Fig. 9.17).

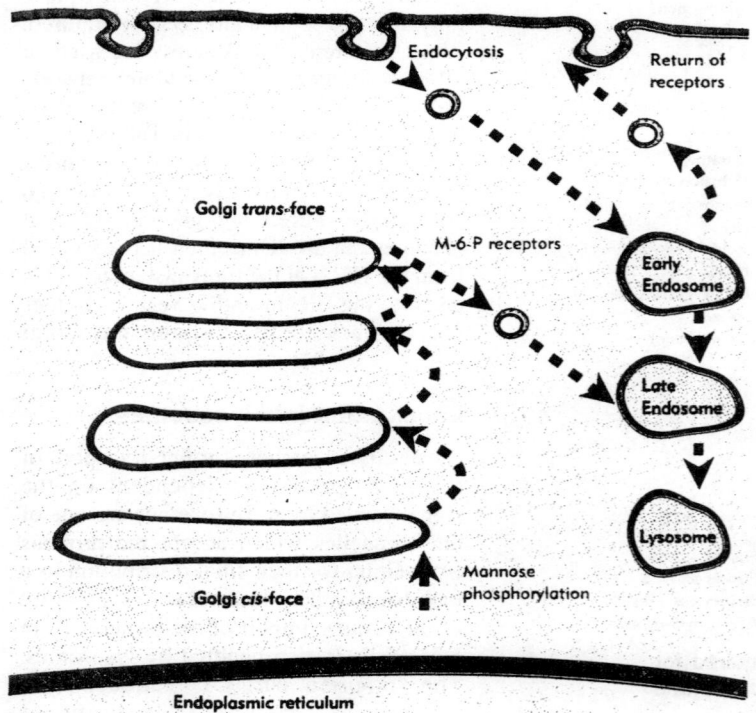

Fig. 9.17. Endosomes sort proteins that have been endocytosed and provide one route to the lysosomes. Proteins are transported via clathrin-coated vesicles from the plasma membrane to the early endosome, and may then either return to the plasma membrane or proceed further to late endosomes and lysosomes. Newly synthesized proteins may be directed to late endosomes (and then to lysosomes) from the Golgi stacks. The common signal in lysosomal targeting is the recognition of mannose-6-phosphate by a specific receptor.

Multiple signals

Normally a protein has only a single signal for its destination and is transported to the location coded by this signal. However, by protein engineering it is possible to attach multiple signals to a single protein. These engineered proteins have been used for the study of mechanism of localization. For example, a hybrid protein can be synthesized which has the signals for localisation to ER as well as to the lysosome. This has been achieved by attaching a C-terminal ER localisation signal to a lysosome-bound protein. When its fate is followed, it has been found that it reaches to ER and not to lysosome. This can be explained by the fact that phosphorylation of mannose to M6P, which is the signal for lysosome localization, takes place in TGN. The maturation of ER proteins on the other hand, is completed much earlier in the Golgi apparatus (at the trans cisternae), the protein is thus, transported to ER even before the phosphorylation of mannose has taken place.

Direction of the protein transport

The proteins are received by the ER, transferred to Golgi system where these go through the Golgi stack system and are finally dispatched to their final destination. The transport is only in this direction and this undirectional movement is referred as the anterograde transport. There is no reverse flow until the anterograde transport is blocked by some arteficial means. A lot of information has been obtained in this regard by the use of Brefeldin A (BFA), a drug which blocks the forward transport of proteins. BFA blocks the formation of ARF-GTP complex from ARF-GDP which results in the accumulation of inactive ARF. Thus the binding of β-COP to form the coatomers is blocked. As a result, the budding at the site of origin of vesicles can not take place and the vesicles are not formed. The proteins are, therefore, accumulated between the cisternae of the Golgi. The formation of tubules between different layers of cisternae takes place which results in their joining into ER. The proteins then go back to ER from Golgi. This reverse flow of proteins is referred as retrograde transport.

Transport to Nucleus

Nucleus is the store house of the genetic information in any eukaryotic cell. A number of proteins participate in its function as well as in chromatin formation. However, the nucleus does not carry out the protein synthesis. All the nuclear proteins are synthesized at and transported from the cytosol to the nucleus. Further, all nuclear proteins are synthesized on free polysomes. These proteins carry an internal signal (see Table 9.2) which directs them to nucleus. The entry to nucleus is by a different mode than the normal membrane transport discussed above. The nuclear membrane has a number of small pores which permit the passage of the proteins in a very selective manner. The precise mechanism of the nuclear transport is poorly understood. The diagrammatic representation of the nuclear structure is given in Fig 9.18. The nucleus is enveloped by double membrane layers, the outer and the inner nuclear membranes. There is perinuclear space between the two membranes. The outer nuclear membrane is in fact, a specialized extension of the ER membrane. The perinuclear space is connected to the ER lumen. The nuclear lamina is within this membrane system. There are a number of small pores in the membrane which make it perforated and form the channels between cytoplasmic compartment and the lumen of the nucleus. A typical mammalian nucleus has 3,000-4,000 pores. The pores are embedded in a large disc like structure known as the nuclear pore complex. The complex has a diameter of about 100 nm. It is sorrounded by octagonally arranged protein particles referred as granules. The molecular weight of a complex is 50,000-100,000 KD. There is a channel at the centre of the complex which contains an aqueous environment. Sometimes the pore seems to be clogged by the large molecules (such as the ribosomes which are assembled in nucleus and are then transported to the cytoplasm where they carry out their biological function) being transported. This looks like another granule and is referred as the central granule. The structure of a nuclear pore is shown in Fig. 9.19. The opening of this channel

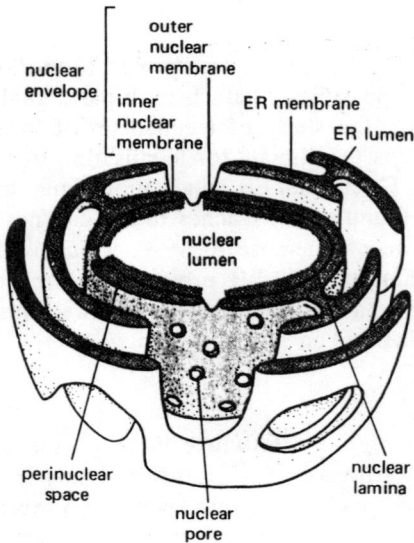

Fig. 9.18. A three-dimensional sketch of the double-membrane envelope that surrounds the nucleus. The nuclear envelope is penetrated by nuclear pores and is continuous with the endoplasmic reticulum.

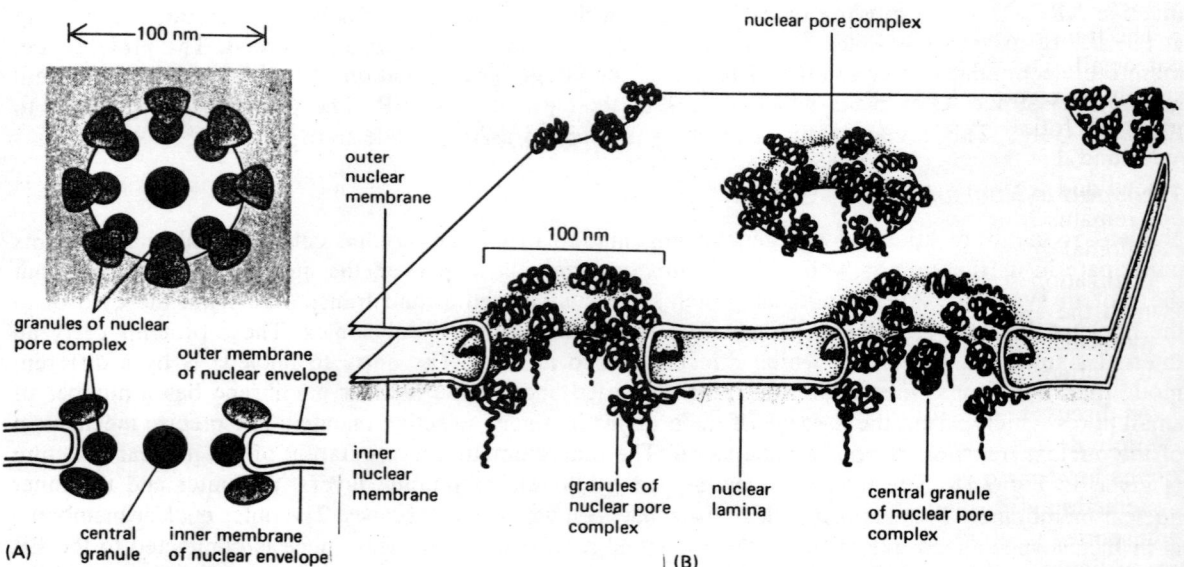

Fig. 9.19. The arrangement of the nuclear pore complexes in the nuclear envelope. (A) A top view and a central vertical section. The 'central granule" is seen in some pores but not others; these granules may be part of the pore, or they may be large complexes caught in transit through it. (B) Three-dimensional sketch of a small region of the nuclear envelope.

is about 9 nm and the water soluble molecules can shuttle through this channel by passive transport. A small protein of about 17KD can equilibrate between the nuclear and the cytosolic compartments in 1-2 min while a protein of 44KD will take about 30 min for equilibration. However, this is too slow to account for the requirement of nuclear proteins of a cell. Further, the globular proteins, more than 60KD in size, can not enter the channel. Thus passive diffusion can not explain the process of transport of larger molecules. For example, during the active DNA synthesis, a cell may require upto 300,000-400,000 histone molecules per min, which means that about 100 histone molecules enter each pore per minute. The transport is, therefore, the active transport which is energy dependent and requires ATP.

Table 9.2. Nuclear proteins have an internal signal which is not cleared after transport into nucleus. Length of the signal - 7-9 aa.

Nature of signal - basic

Examples :

SV4O 'T' antigen	-Pro-Lys-Lys-Lys-Arg-Lys-Val- (aminoacids 126-132)
Influenza virus nucleoprotein	-Ala-Ala-Phe-Glu-Asp-Leu-Arg-Val-Len-Ser- (Aminoacids 336-345)
Adeno virus Ela protein	-Lys-Arg-Pro-Arg-Pro (C-terminal aminoacids)
Yeast Mat α2 protein	-Lys-Ile-Pro-Ile-Lys- (aminoacids 3-7)
Yeast ribosomal protein L3	-Pro-Arg-Lys-Arg (aminoacids 18-21)

The transport of nucleoplasmin, one of the most abundant nuclear proteins, has been followed in great detail. The protein can be cleaved into two fragments by limited proteolytic digestions. These fragments are referred as the head and the tail. The nuclear localization signal is present in the tail region. By following the transport of nucleoplasmin with double labelled head and tail pieces, it has been found that the complete nucleoplasmin is easily taken in through the nuclear pore. However, when the head and the tail are separately incubated with nuclei, only the tail enteres the nucleus. The head piece remains in the cytosolic compartment. On the other hand, if the tail pieces are conjugated with the colloidal gold, the gold particles are taken in by the nucleus (Fig. 9.20). This clearly suggests that the localization signal alone is sufficient for the nuclear transport. The nature or the size of the cargo to which the signal is attached is not important for the purpose of transport. The signal will direct any molecule which is attached to it, to the nucleus. This observation is same as for the N–terminal signal peptides which is the only requirement for the transport of a membrane bound protein.

As discussed, the size of the nuclear channel is only 9 nm, it is, therefore, surprising how the larger protein molecules are transported to the nucleus. There are evidences to suggest that the large nuclear proteins have specific receptors at the pore margin. Once a large protein reaches to the nuclear pore, its interaction with the receptors transmits a signal to the pore ordering it to get enlarged and the protein is transported through enlarged pore by active transportation. The octagonal arrangement of the granules form a diaphragm like structure which functions in the same manner as the diaphragm guarding the aperture of the lens in a camera works and controls the opening.

Unlike the 'signal peptide', the nuclear localization signal is not cleaved after the protein has been transported to the nucleus. This process is very important functionally. During the mitosis, nucleus is disassembled and the nuclear proteins get mixed with the cytoplasmic proteins. However, these are not degraded and are reimported into the nucleus after the nuclear reassembly. During the reassembly, first the chromosomes are envaloped within a membrane which does not permit any other molecule except the chromosomes to get encapsulated within it. These chromosomes then complex together to form the nuclear core and the 'old' nuclear proteins are re-transported to this structure as the nuclear localisation

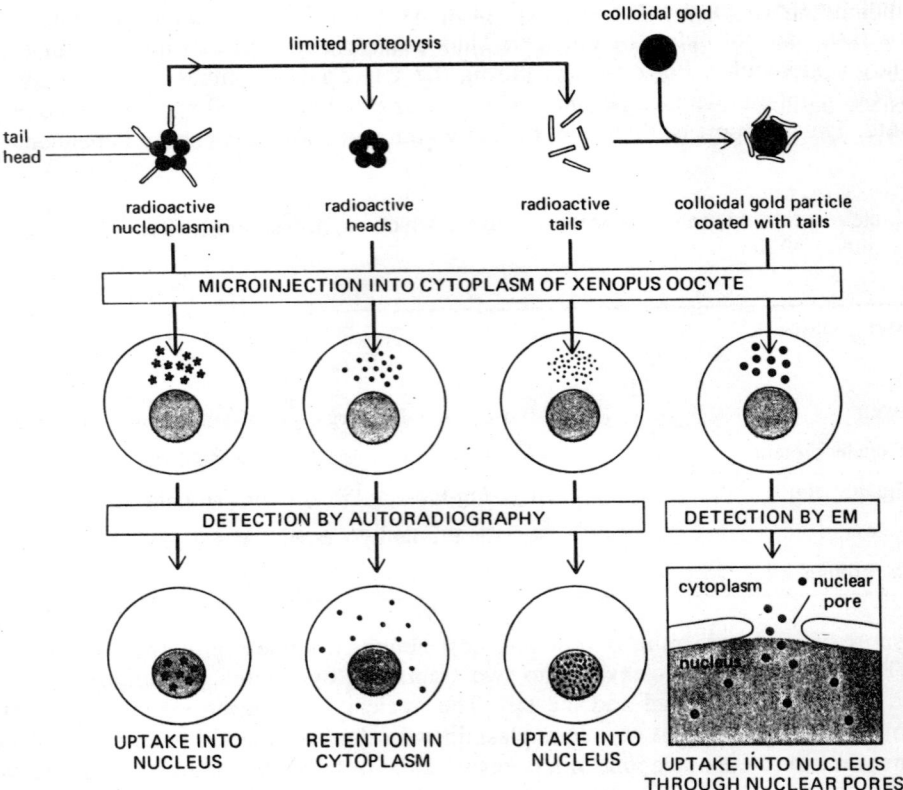

Fig. 9.20. The uptake of selected proteins into nuclei via nuclear pores. Nucleoplasmin is a large pentameric nuclear protein with distinct head and tail domains. The heads can be cleaved from the tails by limited proteolysis. When injected into the cytoplasm of a frog oocyte, intact nucleoplasmin molecules rapidly accumulate in the nucleus even though they are too large to diffuse passively through the small channel in the centre of a nuclear pore complex. The signal for this nuclear import apparently resides in the tail domains, since injected tails are taken up by the nucleus but heads are not. The role of nuclear pores in this signal-directed import is demonstrated by electron microscopy using nucleoplasmin tails coupled to spheres of colloidal gold, which are easily visualized because of their high electron density. The attached nucleoplasmin tails direct the entry of the gold particles via nuclear pores.

signals are still intact. Has the nuclear localisation signal been cleaved during the transport, the re-entry of these proteins would not have been possible. The cell in that case, would have been forced to resynthesize all the nuclear proteins. This would have created a number of procedural problems as the process of transcription would have been difficult in absence of the formation of complete nucleus.

These pores also permit the export of RNA and the ribosomes and other molecules from the nucleus to the cytoplasm. However, there are separate receptors for the export of these molecules.

Transport to peroxisomes

Peroxisomes or the microbodies are very heterogeneous orgenelles. These can be defined as a collection of organelles with a constant membrane and variable content within the membrane structure. Except for their membrane structure, different peroxisomes differ widely from one another. These play an important role in the oxygen metabolism. Unlike many of the other organelles such as the nucleus, mitochondria and the chloroplast, the peroxisomes donot have their own genome. All their proteins are synthesized in the cytoplasm and these have to be imported. The peroxisomal proteins are synthesized on free polysomes. These orgenelles have only a single membrane which envelopes their content. The membrane surface contains specific protein(s) which serve as the receptor and can recognize the translocation signals present on the protein being transported. Atleast one such receptor protein has been characterized which is specific to the peroxisome. These receptor protein(s) are present on the cytosolic side of the peroxisome and recognize a C-terminal tripeptide of the transported protein. These proteins are taken inside the peroxisomes through active transport.

Catalase is one of the major enzymes present in the peroxisome which has been extensively studied. The active enzyme is a homo-tetramer and contains heme as its prosthetic group. It is synthesized in the cytosol and is imported inside the organelle as the monomer without heme. The assembly of the enzyme takes place inside the peroxisome where heme is added. There is no cleavable signal peptide in these proteins.

Transport in bacteria

The transport of proteins in bacteria is predominantly export. Commonly the proteins are transported across the inner membrane to the periplasm of the cell. However, some proteins can cross the outer membrane also and these are secreted out of the cell into the culture medium. The basic process is very similar to the eukaryotic transport. Both co-translational as well as the post-translational transport take place in bacteria. However, the co-translational transport is more common. The export requires a N-terminal leader sequence which has a hydrophilic terminus followed by a hydrophobic core. The structure of this signal peptide is very similar to the eukaryotic signal peptide. The export apparatus of bacteria can recognize the eukaryotic leader sequences also and some of the eukaryotic secretory proteins can be actively transported by the bacteria during their expression in bacteria by genetic engineering experiments.

The export apparatus of the bacteria has strong resemblance with its eukaryotic counterpart. It has been shown in Fig. 9.21. A number of proteins, which are the product of sec (for secretory) genes, participate in this process. First a protein, SecB, binds to the nascent pro-protein at its N-terminal sequence (similar to the SRP binding) and brings it to the membrane. SecB acts as a chaperone and retards the folding of the protein. However, it cannot reverse the foldings which have already taken place before its binding and does not act as an unfolding agent. This is very important as the folded protein may be too big to be transported. SecB has high affinity for the signal sequence and also for another protein SecA. There are separate binding sites for the signal peptide and the SecA protein. The Sec A is a large peripheral membrane protein which has affinity for acidic lipids and also for another protein, SecY. SecY is an integral protein of the bacterial membrane. SecY along with yet another integral membrane protein, the SecE, forms the channel along the membrane. SecY is much larger, having ten trans-membrane segments. SecE on the other hand, has only three trans-membrane segments. Both the SecE and the SecY together constitute the enzyme translocase which is needed for the purpose of transport. SecA recognizes both the SecB (which is bound to N-terminal signal of the pro-protein) and the pro-protein. Thus, both, the sequence of the N-terminal peptide and that of the mature protein are very important for the transport in bacteria. This is in contrast to the eukaryotic system where only the signal peptide is important and sequences of the mature protein do not play any role. SecA also has an ATPase activity which is regulated by the binding of SecA with both, the SecY and also with the pro-protein. Once SecB has brought the protein near the membrane, SecA binds to the protein and

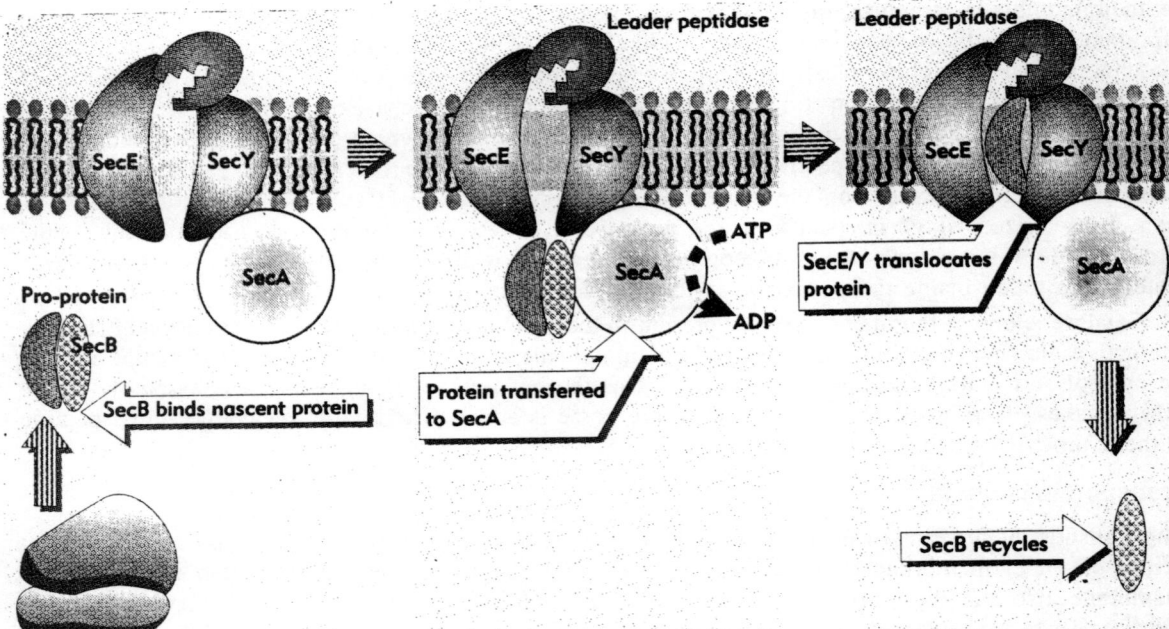

Fig. 9.21. Protein translocation in bacteria requires SecB to function as a chaperone and bind the nascent protein; then SecB transfers the protein to SecA, which is a peripheral membrane protein associated with the integral membrane proteins SecE/Y. Translocation requires hydrolysis of ATP and a protonmotive force. Leader peptidase is an integral membrane protein that cleaves the leader sequence.

forms a complex. This complex, then associates with ATP and its entry through the transport channel is initiated. Now ATP is hydrolysed and ~20 aminoacids are transported across the membrane. This forms a structure which is somewhat similar to the membrane bound polysomes of the eukaryotic system. The transport of the precursor takes place by the repetition of this process and is also facilitated by the electron potential across the membrane. Finally, the precursor is released in the periplasm. Another membrane bound protein has the leader peptidase function and can cleave the signal peptide to form the mature protein.

The presence of a SRP like nucleoprotein has also been reported in bacteria. It has a 4.5S RNA and a single 48KD protein. This particle is involved in the secretion of certain proteins through the outer membrane.

10

Structure and Genesis of Mitochondrial and Chloroplast Genome

In eukaryotes, the nucleus is the primary organelle for storing the genetic information of the cell. Here, this information is transcribed to form the RNA which is modified and is later transported to the cytoplasm. The mRNA is translated in the cytoplasm and the proteins are synthesized. However, certain organelles other than nucleus also contain their own genome. These organelles are the mitochondria and the chloroplast. Though the genome of these organelles is very small and codes for only a fraction of the information which is necessary for the biological function of these organelles. Thus a dual system of genetic information works in these organelles, one set is coded by the organelle itself while the other set is coded by the nucleus. It has been found that majority of the RNA present within the organelles and needed for their function, is coded by the organelle genome while majority of the proteins are coded by the nuclear genome. There is a co-ordination between the contributions made by the two genomes, however, an absolute coupling between the two systems is not present. The precise mechanism by which the expression of two genomes is co-ordinated is not very clear. The organelle genomes differ from the nuclear genome in their sensitivity to a number of metabolic inhibitors. It is therefore, possible to study the organelle genomes as isolated entity in an in vitro system. For example, the nuclear transcription is inhibited by α-aminitin while the transcription of the mitochondrial genome is not sensitive to it but is sensitive to the acridines and the ethidium salts. Similarly, the translation of the nucleus coded mRNAs is blocked by cycloheximide while the mitochondrial translation is not affected by it but is sensitive to certain other antibiotics such as chloramphenicol, erythromycin and tetracycline. As discussed above, majority of the organelle proteins are synthesized in the cytoplasm and are transported to the organelles. However, this is only one way traffic and none of the cytoplasmic proteins are synthesized in the mitochondria. There is no transport of biomacromolecules from organelles to cytoplasm. These characteristics of organelle genome have been illustrated in Fig. 10.1.

The size of organelle genome shows a wide variation. In general, the animal organelles have relatively small genome than the genome of plant organelles. Further, there is a great deal of variation from species to species. Also sizes of some of the genomes have been shown in Table 10.1.

Replication of organelle genome

There is no de novo genesis of the organelles. For the formation of new organelles, the genome of the organelle is replicated resulting in doubling of its mass. The replication of DNA takes place throughout the cell cycle and is not restricted only to the S phase as is the case in replication of the nuclear genome. After the DNA replication, the two DNA molecules move apart and the formation

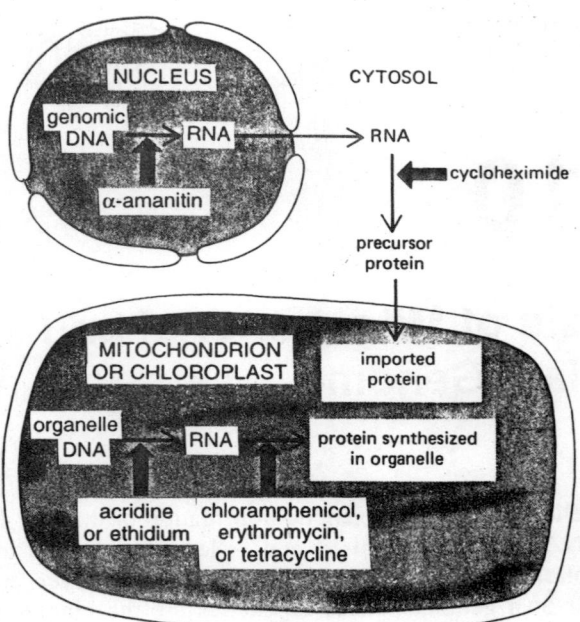

Fig. 10.1. An overview of the biosynthesis of mitochondrial and chloroplast proteins. The site of action of an inhibitor that is specific for either organelle or cytosolic protein synthesis has been shown by arrows.

Table 10.1. Organelle genome : Size and variation

DNA	*Size*
Chloroplast DNA of higher plants	120-200 kb
Chloroplast DNA of green algae	150-200 kb
Mitochondrial DNA of animals	15-20 kb
Mitochondrial DNA of plants	150-2500 kb
Mitochondrial DNA of fungi	15-80 kb
Mitochondrial DNA of algae	15-18 kb
Mitochondrial DNA of protozoa	20-40 kb
Examples :	
Chloroplast DNA of chlamydomonas	180 kb
Chloroplast DNA of liverwort	121 kb
Chloroplast DNA of Zea mays	140 kb
Mitochondrial DNA of yeast	78 kb
Mitochondrial DNA of Aspigillus	32 kb
Mitochondrial DNA of Neurospora	60 kb
Mitochondrial DNA of Trypanosoma	22 kb
Mitochondrial DNA of Paramecium	40 kb
Mitochondrial DNA of human	16.5 kb
Mitochondrial DNA of Drosophilla	18.4 kb
Mitochondrial DNA of Xenopus	184 kb

of a septum starts which divides the mitochondria (or chloroplast) into two unequal compartments. Both the compartments are then separated and two organelles are formed (Fig. 10.2). For the DNA replication, the individual molecules of DNA are selected in a random manner and there is no preferential order for the replication of any individual molecule. However, the entire mitochondrial DNA is doubled during each cell cycle and the number of DNA molecules within an organelle is always kept constant. The entire process of the mitochondrial genesis is carefully controlled, however, the regulatory mechanisms are not well understood. It may be worth mentioning that multiple copies of the DNA are present in any organelle and it is possible that two organelles can fuse together by the reversal of the divisionary process and form a organelle with higher copy number of DNA molecules in it. Further, the cells have the capability to enhance the copy number of organelles in it if so required. For example, in the muscles of athletes, who perform lot of physical exercise and have much higher demand for the energy, the number of mitochondria per cell is much higher. Probably this is what is meant by the stamina building.

The transfer of organelle genome is in random manner and it does not follow the typical Mendelian laws and is non-Mendelian in nature. It has been found that if two strains of yeast differing in mitochondrial genome are mated, the number of offsprings inheriting the desired characters are not what would have been expected according to Mendel's theory. This has been very clearly shown in case of mating between petite yeast (having defective oxidative phosphorylation) with wild type yeast or mating of the chloramphenicol resistant and wild type strains of yeast. In majority of the cases the inheritance is uniparental. In higher eukaryotes it is maternal. The sperms have almost no cytoplasm and donot contribute to organelle genome. However, in lower eukaryotes such as in yeast, it is biparental.

Another important character of organelle genome is its deviation from the universal genetic code. So far we have maintained that the genetic code is universal and all the known organism follow the same code. However, this statement is true only for the nuclear genome. In the organelle genome, some of the codons are translated differently. Not only this, certain variations are seen between organisms to organism also. These variations have been shown in Table 10.2.

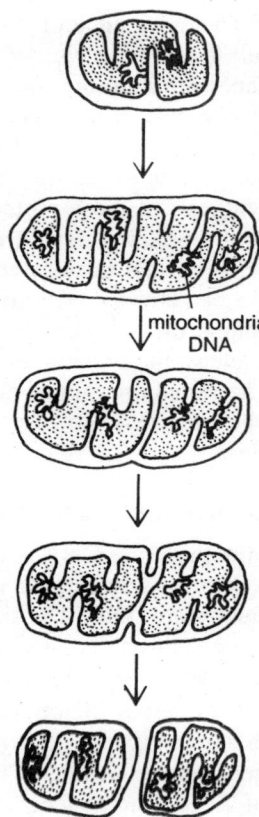

mitochondrial DNA

Fig. 10.2. Diagram of a dividing mitochondrion. The pathway shown has been postulated from static view of dividing mitochondria.

Table 10.2. The organelle genetic code : There are some differences between the 'Universal Code' as followed by chromosomal genome and the code followed by organelles, specially by mitochondria. The codes which have different meanings between two genomes have been enumerated.

Codon	Universal Code Chromosomal	Mammalian mitochondria	Drosophila mitochondria	Yeast mitochondria	Plant mitochondria
TGA	Stop	Trp	Trp	Trp	Stop
ATA	Ile	Met	Met	Met	Ile
CTA	Leu	Leu	Leu	Thr	Leu
AGA	Arg	Stop	Ser	Arg	Arg
AGG	Arg	Stop	Ser	Arg	Arg

The presence of double sets of genome raises a question about the logic and the necessity for the cell to maintain two separate sets of genome, as it is very expensive for the cell. As much as 90 nuclear genes are required just for maintaining the organelle genome. This puts enormous amount of taxation on the cell. It has been found that many of the organelle proteins are too hydrophobic in nature and it was earlier believed that the aqueous environment of the cytoplasm may not be able to synthesise these proteins. It, therefore, becomes obligatory for the cell to maintain a separate mechanism for the synthesis of these proteins. However, it is now well established that a number of hydrophobic proteins or the proteins having highly hydrophobic structural epitopes are synthesized in cytoplasm. It is now believed that during the course of evolution these organelles have been formed by the engulfment of the bacteria by primitive eukaryotic cells (the endosymbiont hypothesis, see later). While during the course of evolution, majority of the genes got transferred from the prokaryotic part of this cell to its nucleus, the process, however, reached to a dead end after some time and no further transfer took place. The remaining genes maintained their independent entity and have given rise to the present day cells. The precise reason for this freeze in the transfer of genome from one compartment to another is not clear.

Mitochondrial genome

Mitochondrial DNA is circular in all the known species except in Chlamydomonas and in Paramaecium where it is linear. In its structure, it has more similarities with prokaryotic genome than with the eukaryotic DNA. The size and the complexiety of mitochondrial DNA varies substantially from organism to organisms. For example, the human mitochondrial DNA is about 16.6 Kb in size while in yeast it is about 84 Kb and in certain plants it may be upto 250Kb or even larger.

In certain plants such as in *Brassica campestris* (the Chinese cabbage), mitochondria with more than one type of DNA may be present. However, the careful analysis of the *B. compestris* mitochondrial genome has revealed that its DNA is 218 Kb in size which has two copies of a repeated element of 2 Kb. The genetic recombination of these repeat units can give rise to two fragments of this DNA, one is 135 Kb and other is 83 Kb (Fig. 10.3). Thus a mitochondria may have DNAs of three different sizes, 218 Kb, 135 Kb and 83 Kb.

Recombination in plant mtDNA

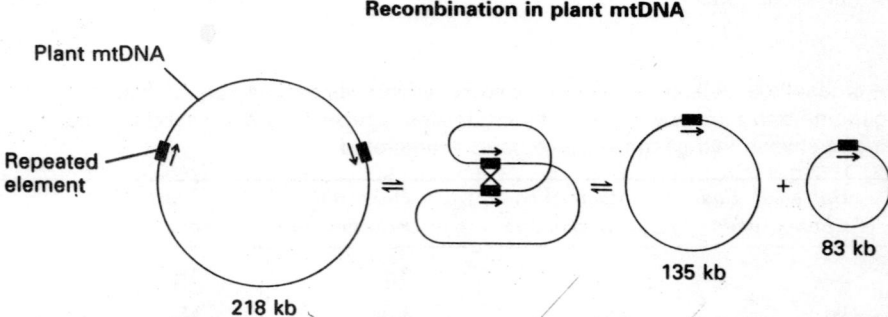

Fig. 10.3. Many plant mitochondria contain multiple but related DNA species. Bruma campestris (Chinese cabbage) mitochondria contains three different DNA molecules. The 218 kb DNA (the largest DNA species) contains two repeated 2 kb domains. Recombination between these two sequences generates the small DNAs (135 kb and 83 kb).

Similarly the number of DNA molecules per organelle and the number of mitochondria per cell also vary considerably. In general, the mitochondrial DNA accounts for only a small amount of total genome (0.5% in human, ~1% in other mammals). However, in yeast it may constitute upto 18% of the total DNA. In certain specialised cells it may account for most of the cellular DNA. For example in the frog eggs, where the number of mitochondria per cell can be upto 10,000,000, the mitochondrial DNA accounts for almost 99% of the total DNA. These data have been summarised in Table 10.3.

Table 10.3. Mitochondrial genome of different organisms

Organism	Tissue	DNA molecules per mitochondria	Average no. of mitochondria per cell	Mitochondrial genome as fraction of total DNA of the cell
Human	Liver	2-3	750	0.5%
Rat	Liver	5-10	1000	1%
Mouse	L-cells	5-10	100	< 1%
Yeast	Vegetative	2-50	1-50	Upto 15%
Frog	Eggs	5-10	10^7	99%

The location of the mitochondrial genome is in the matrix of the mitochondria. Ocassionally it may be present in the inner membrane or may be present in association with the mitochondrial ribosomes. As discussed earlier, the mitochondrial genome codes only for a small part of its protein requirement. Almost 95% of the mitochondrial proteins are coded by nuclear genome. These proteins are synthesized in cytoplasm and later transported to mitochondria. Rest of the proteins (about 5%) are coded by its own genome and synthesized inside the mitochondria by its own ribosomes. However, mitochondrial genome codes for almost all of the mitochondrial RNAs including the rRNAs, tRNAs and some of the mRNAs. Only mitochondrial RNA which is coded by nuclear genome is a small RNA of 135 bases which is involved in the metabolism of the RNA primer essential for the replication of mitochondrial genome.

The mitochondria have their own protein synthesizing machinery. However, there are certain characteristic differences between the cytoplasmic ribosomes and the mitochondrial ribosomes. Mitochondrial ribosomes are smaller in size, have different RNA/protein ratio and have different sensitivity for certain antibiotics such as cycloheximide. Further, the size and the composition of mitochondrial ribosomes also vary between organism to organism. Table 10.4 summarises the mitochondrial genes and their products in different organisms. Similarly the structural data of mitochondrial ribosomes have been summarised in Table 10.5.

In human mitochondria, almost all of the DNA comparises of the coding region, either for RNA or for proteins. There are no introns in human mitochondrial genome. In fact many of the genes run into each other and have very little or no regulatory sequences. Some of the genes donot even have the complete stop codon, TAA, at the end of the coding region. It is coded only by one or two nucleotides and the addition of A residues to form the poly (A) tail accounts for the completion of the stop codon. However, in yeast and also in plants, which have much larger mitochondrial genome, lot of 'junk DNA' is present. In fact in plants which probably have largest mitochondrial genome, majority of the DNA is junk. Besides, introns are also present in certain genes of these organism. Many times a particular gene may have introns in one strain of a given species and may not have intron in another strain of the same species. In other words the introns are, often, 'optional'. Further, these introns may move in and out of a gene in the same manner as the transposable elements of the nuclear

Table 10.4A. Mitochondrial RNAs and proteins synthesized in mitochondria

	Animals	*Fungi*	*Plants*
Genome size	14-18 kb	19-108 kb	150-2500 kb
Ribosomal RNAs	2	2	3
No. of tRNAs 22	23-25	~30	
No. of r-proteins	~75	~75	–
r-protein (var.-1)	–	+	?
Cytoctrome coxidase subunits	+	+	+
CoQ cytochrome	+	+	+
C-reductase Apocytochrome b	+	+	+
Fo ATPase subunits			
6	+	+	+
8	+	+	+
9	+	±	+
F_1 ATPase α subunit	–	–	+
No. of subunits in NADH–CoQ reductase	7	0-6	6?

Table 10.4B. Mitochondrial proteins—synthesized in cytosol and transported to mitochondria (usually in precursor form)

Mitochondrial location	*Protein*
Matrix	F_1 AtPase α (except in plants), β, γ & δ (fungi) subunits
	Carbamoyl phosphate synthetase (mammals only)
	Magnese—SOD
	RNA polymerase
	Ribosomal proteins
	Citrate synthetase
	Ornithine aminotransferace (mammal)
	Ornithine trans carbamoylase (mammal)
	Alcohol dehydrogenase (yeast)
Inner membrane	Cytochrome C_1
	ADP-ATP carrier
	Cytochrome C oxidase subunits
	Proteolipids of Fo ATPase complex
	Cytochrome b.C.$_1$ complex subunits
	Uncoupling proteins
Intermembrane space	Cytochrome C
	Cytochrome C pzoxidace
	Cytochrome b$_2$
Outer membrane	Porin

Table 10.5. The mitochondrial ribosomes and protein synthesis

1. Size of ribosomes	From 60S (mammals) to 70S (plants)
2. Ribosomal RNAs	Synthesized in mitochondria
Small subunits	12S in animals
	15S in yeast
	18S in plants
Large subunits	16S in animals
	21S in yeast
	26S in plants
5S RNA	Present only in plants
3. Ribosomal proteins	Upto 75 proteins - all (except one or two) are synthesized in cytosol and transported to mitochondria
4. tRNAs	22 tRNAs in animals
	25 tRNAs in yeast
	~30 tRNAs in plants
5. Amino acyl tRNA synthelice	20, synthesized in cytoplasm
6. Sensitivity to antibiotics	Mitochondrial protein synthesis is not inhibited by cycloheximide but is inhibited by chloramphenicol, erythromycin and tetracyclin
7. Genetic code	Certain variations from the nuclear code e.g.:
	UGA codes for Trp in animals and fungi
	AUA codes for Met in animals and fungi
	CUA codes for Thr in yeast
	AGA and AGG code for termination in mammals

genome. Many times the relative position of an intron is at a common place within a gene in a wide variety of organisms, suggesting that these may have derived from a common ancestral gene. The presence of such introns is common between yeast, aspergillus and neurospora species.

Other special features of mitochondrial genome are the presence of only 22 tRNAs (as against 40 different tRNAs in cytoplasm). To accomodate 61 codons with only 20 tRNAs, often the anticodon recognizes only two of the three nucleotides of a codon. In other words, the occurance of bobbling is much more in mitochondria than in cytoplasm. Mitochondrial DNA polymerase has much less fidility than the nuclear DNA polymerase and as a result the rate of substitution is much higher during mitochondrial DNA replication.

Human mitochondria

Human mitochondrial genome is 16,569 bp in length. It is one of the smallest mitochondrial genome of all the species. It is circular molecule and both the strands code for the gene products. Each of the two strands are transcribed by a single promoter. When the mitochondrial DNA is denatured, the two strands are separated and are centrifuged through the cesium chloride gradients, both strands show slightly different buoyant densities. This is because of the characteristically different base composition of the two strands. One of the strands which is heavier, is referred as the 'H' strand while the other is known as the 'L' strand. The H strand codes for 2 rRNAs, most of the tRNAs and about 10 mRNAs. The L strand codes for 8 tRNAs and 1 small A+ mRNA. Almost 90% of the L strand doesnot code for any product and is not transcribed. Mitochondrial mRNAs have poly A tail but donot have a cap at their 5'-end. The map of human mitochondrial DNA has been shown in Fig. 10.4. Its transcriptional pattern is shown in Fig. 10.5. The H strand has 2 transcription initiation sites, both under the same promoter. The primary transcript initiating from the first site (transcript I) starts at a point immediately upstream of tRNA$_{Phe}$ and produces a small transcript coding for both 12S and 16S rRNAs (small and large ribosomal RNAs respectively, compare with the sizes for cytoplasmic rRNAs - 18S and 28S) and two tRNAs namely, tRNA$_{Phe}$ and tRNA$_{Val}$ The frequency of its initiation is about 10 times higher than the frequency of initiation for transcript II. The second transcript starts at 5'end of 12S rRNA and produces 12 tRNAs and most of the mRNAs. The L strand has a single transcript which is processed to produce 8 tRNAs and a single mRNA.

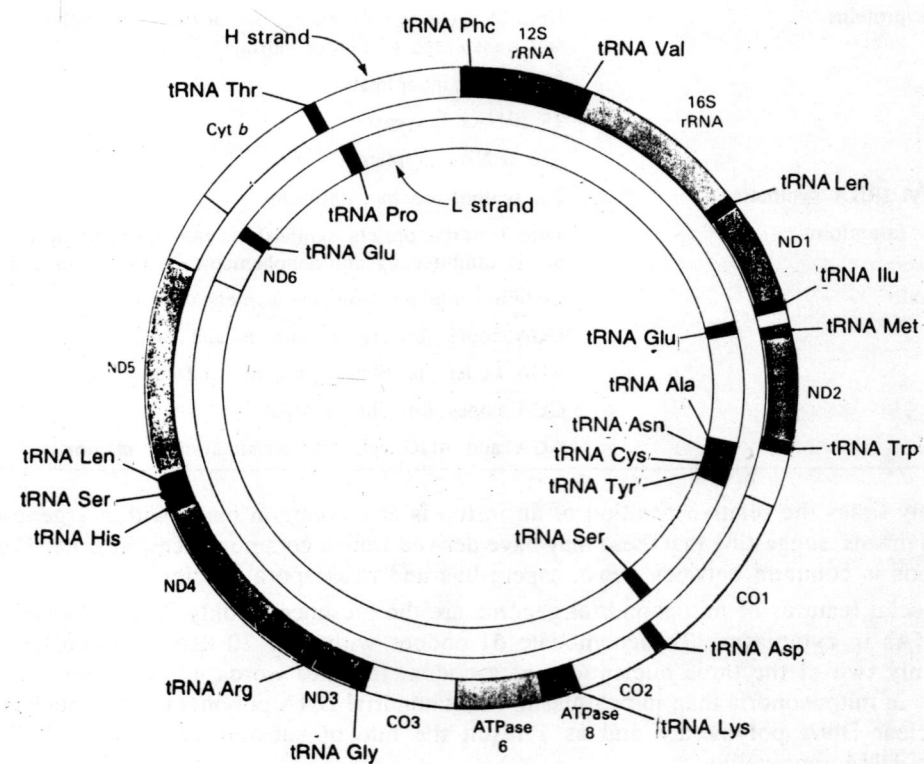

Fig. 10.4. Map of the 16,559-bp human mitochondrial genome. ND1-ND6 represent the genes for various subunits of NADH-CoQ reductase complex, CO represents gene for CytC oxidase.

Yeast mitochondria

Yeast mitochondrial genome, on the other hand, is about five times larger than the human mitochondrial DNA (84Kb). Its genomic map has been shown in Fig. 10.6. However, it codes for almost same number of genes as the human mitochondrial genome. Thus a large amount of the DNA is 'junk'. Besides,

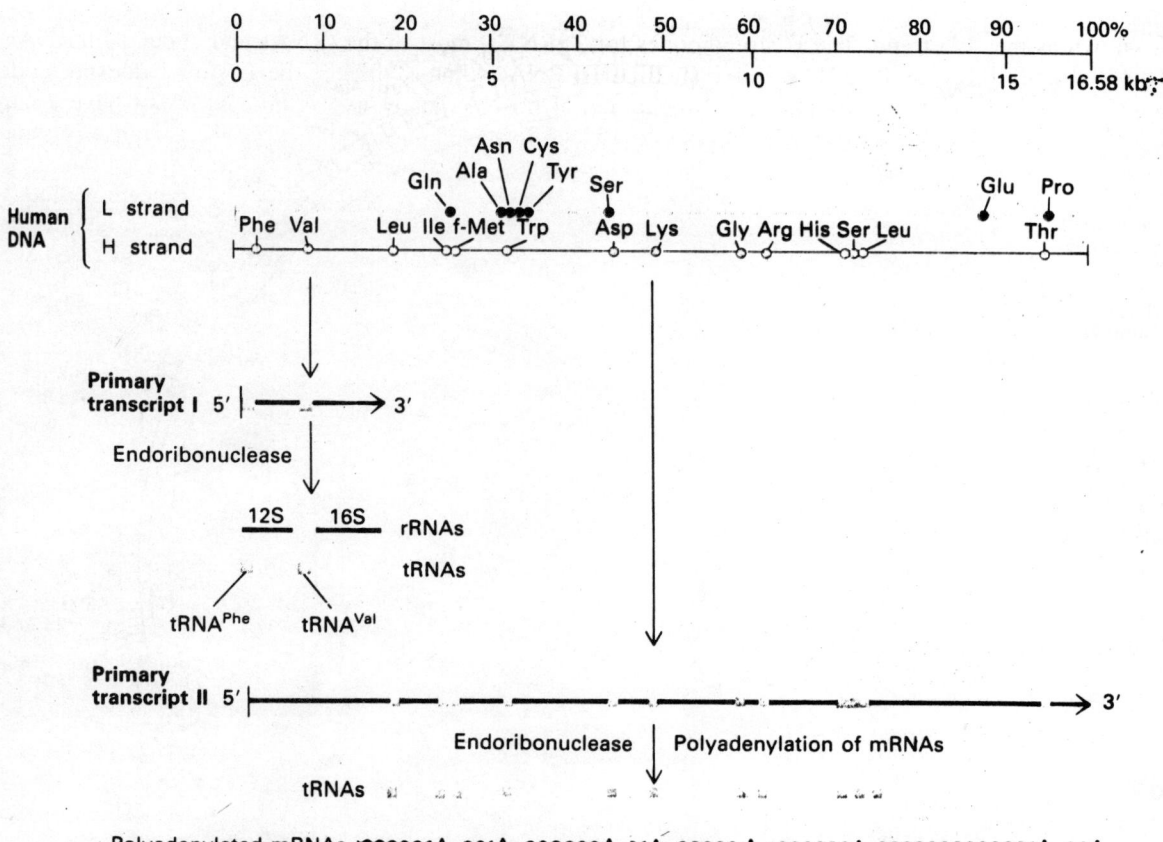

Fig. 10.5. Transcription map of human mtDNA, deduced from the DNA sequence and RNA-DNA hybridization studies, the light (L) DNA strand encodes only eight tRNAs; this strand is transcribed right to left. The heavy (H) DNA strand encodes the 12S and 16S RNAs, 14 tRNAs, and 11 predominant species of polyadenylated mRNAs. The mRNAs encode all mitochondrial proteins. Transcription of the H strand starts at two sites. Primary transcript I initiates just up stream of the tRNA^{Phe} gene and terminates just after the 16S rRNA; it is processed by endoribonucleases to yield one molecule each of tRNA^{Phe}, tRNA^{Val}, and 12S and 16S rRNA. Primary transcript II initiates near the 5' end of the 12S rRNA and apparently continues completely around the circular mtDNA; it is processed to yield the other tRNAs and mRNAs, which are subsequently polyadenylated (A$_n$). Some of the cleavages of this transcript begin while the chain is nascent.

a number of yeast mitochondrial genes also have introns. These introns are of type I and type II. Recall the discussion on splicing; the type I and type II introns were originally discovered in mitochondrial DNA of fungi.

The introns of the gene for cytochrome b in yeast have a very speciical characteristic which is specific for it and no counterpart of such introns is present in any of the higher eukaryotes. The gene for cyt b has already been discussed earlier (Fig. 6.32) and is again shown as Fig. 10.7 here. There are two types of genes present for cyt b, both differing only in the introns and code for the same protein. Many strains have the 'long' gene which is 6.4 kb in size and has 6 exons and 5 introns.

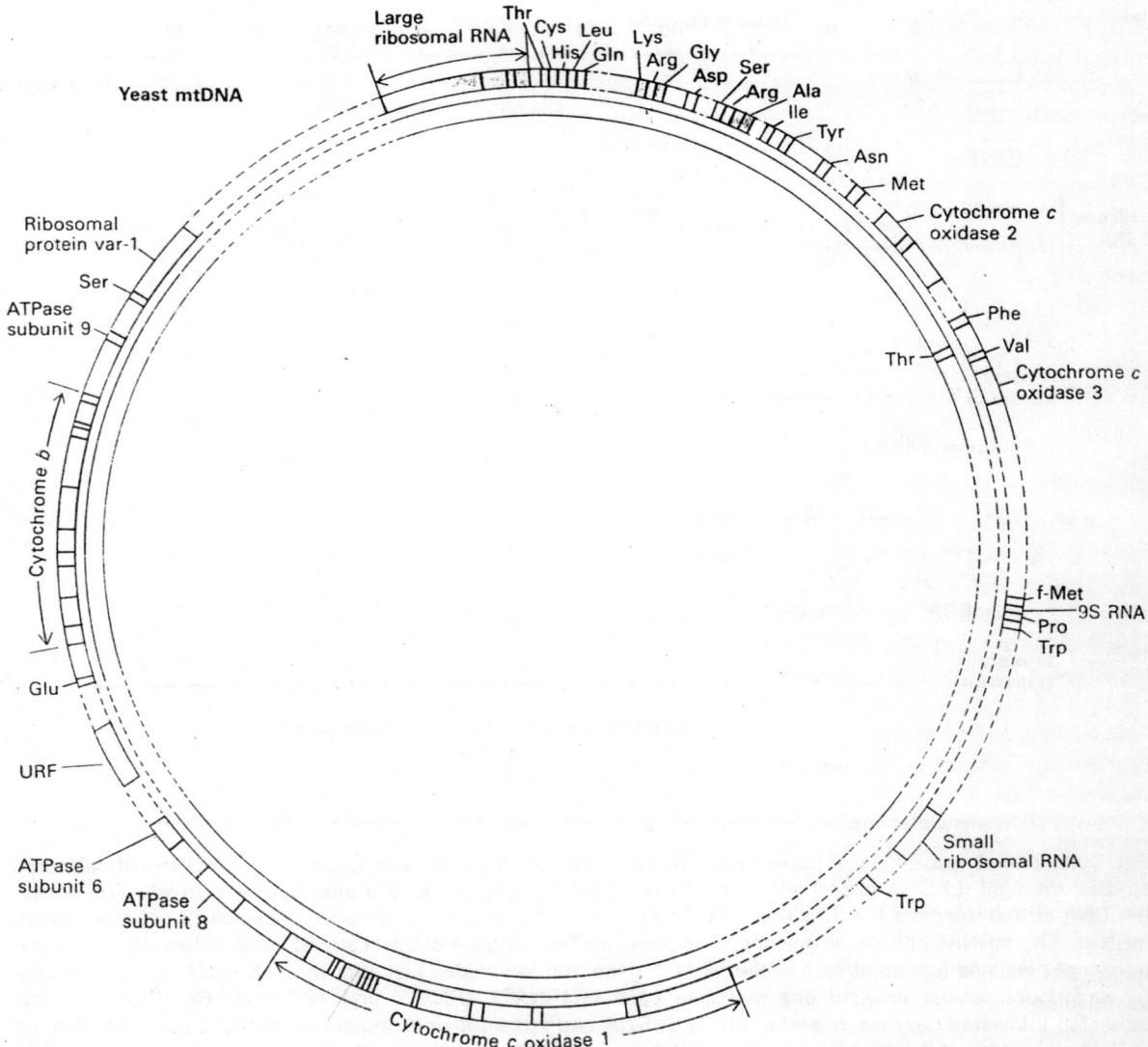

Fig. 10.6. The organization of yeast mtDNA. Yeast mtDNA is five times larger than human mtDNA. Proteins and RNAs encoded by each of the two strands are shown separately. Transcription of H strand of each mtDNA is clockwise and of the L strand is counterclockwise.

Certain other strains have a 'short' gene of 3.3 Kb in which first four exons of the long gene have fused together to form a single large exon. This has occured due to the loss of first three introns. Rest of the gene structure remains the same. The splicing of short gene follows the usual splicing pathway and the mature mRNA is produced. However, in the long gene the splicing pattern is unique. After the primary transcript is formed, intron 1 is removed in the first step, in a self catalysed manner. A

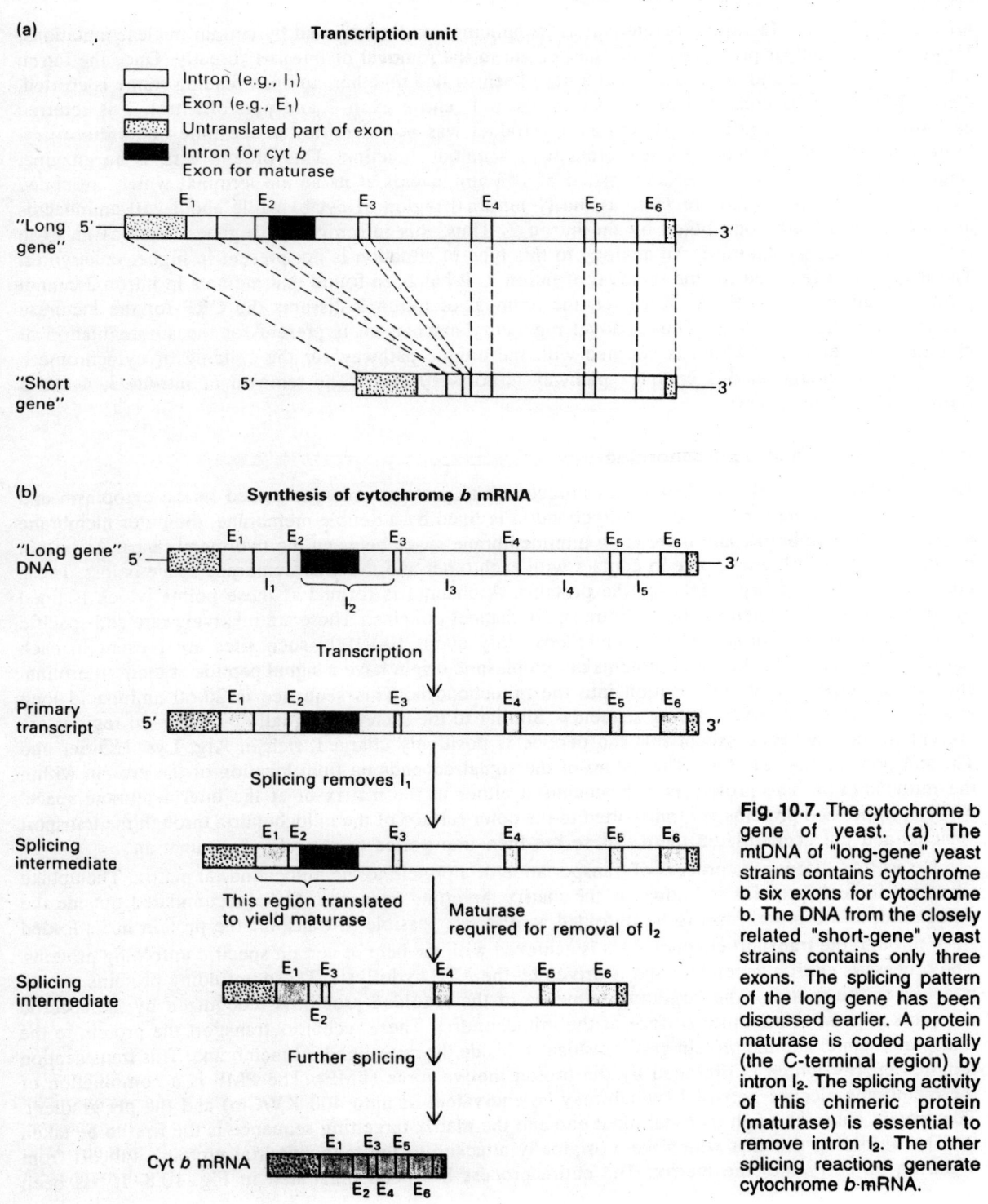

Fig. 10.7. The cytochrome b gene of yeast. (a) The mtDNA of "long-gene" yeast strains contains cytochrome b six exons for cytochrome b. The DNA from the closely related "short-gene" yeast strains contains only three exons. The splicing pattern of the long gene has been discussed earlier. A protein maturase is coded partially (the C-terminal region) by intron I_2. The splicing activity of this chimeric protein (maturase) is essential to remove intron I_2. The other splicing reactions generate cytochrome b·mRNA.

nuclear protein may facilitate its removal as its splicing can be inhibited by certain nuclear mutations. However, this nuclear protein does not participate in the removal of intron 1 directly. Once the intron 1 has been removed and the exons 1 and 2 have been ligated together, an open reading frame is created. This ORF, which is consisted of the part of exon 1, entire exon 2 and part of intron 2 is referred as 'unidentified reading frame' (URF) as its product was not identified at the time of its discovery. Now we know that it codes for a protein with a unique function. This protein acts as an enzyme, referred as maturase. Maturase is consisted of 143 aminoacids at its amino terminal which are coded by the exons 1 and 2 (and are same as the N–terminal region of cyt b) while about 250 aminoacids at its C–terminal are contributed by the intron 2. Thus, this intron of cyt b gene serves as an exon for the synthesis of maturase. An analogy to this type of situation is not present in higher eukaryotes. The maturase is required for the removal of intron 2. It has been found that mutants in intron 2 cannot produce mature cyt b mRNA. However, the removal of intron 2 disrupts the ORF for the maturase and its synthesis is blocked. Thus a novel regulatory mechanism is present for the autoregulation of maturase concentration which is coupled with the unique pathway for the splicing of cytochrome b gene. The advantage of this complex pathway is not very clear. The removal of introns 3, 4 and 5 follows the normal course.

Import of proteins into mitochondria

As discussed earlier, almost 95% of all mitochondrial proteins are synthesized in the cytoplasm and are imported into the mitochondria. Mitochondria is lined by a double membrane, the outer membrane and the inner membrane, and there is an intermembrane space between the two membranes. At certain points the two membranes come in contact with each other and the intermembrane space is lost. These points serve as the entry points for the proteins. A channel is formed at these points which is lined by specific intrinsic proteins called the 'transport channel proteins'. These are relatively rare and specific sites present in the mitochondrial membranes, only about 100-1000 such sites are present in each mitochondria. The mitochondrial proteins of cytoplasmic origin have a signal peptide at their N-terminal end which helps in their localisation into the mitochondria. This sequence is 20-60 aminoacid long and is referred as uptake targetting sequence. Similar to the secretory signal, no conserved regions are present in this sequence except that the peptide is positively charged, rich in Arg, Lys, HO-Ser and Thr and poor in Asp and Glu. The nature of the signal depends on final location of the protein within the mitochondria. The protein may be localised either in the matrix or at the intermembrane space. Newly synthesized proteins are transported to the outer surface of the mitochondria through the transport vesicles and get accumulated there. These are then transported to their final destination.

Let us first discuss the process of transportation of a protein to the mitochondrial matrix. The uptake sequence in such proteins is known as the matrix targetting sequence. Once accumulated outside the mitochondria, the protein has to be unfolded as it is not possible to transport the protein in its folded form through the transport channel. This is achieved with the help of certain specific unfolding proteins. The process is energy dependent and is driven by the ATP hydrolysis. These unfolding proteins remain attached to the protein. The targetting sequence of the unfolded protein is recognized by the specific receptors present at the outer surface of the mitochondria. These receptors transport the protein to the transport channel and the protein gets translocated inside the mitochondrial membrane. This translocation requires energy which is provided by the proton motive force (PMF). The PMF is a combination of the membrane electric potential (which may be equivalent of upto 400 KV/Cm) and the pH gradient. The protein enters through its N-terminal end and the matrix targetting sequence is the first to be taken in. The unfolding proteins which were originally attached to the mitochondrial proteins, fall off from it during its entry into the matrix. The entire process has been illustrated in Fig. 10.8. It has been

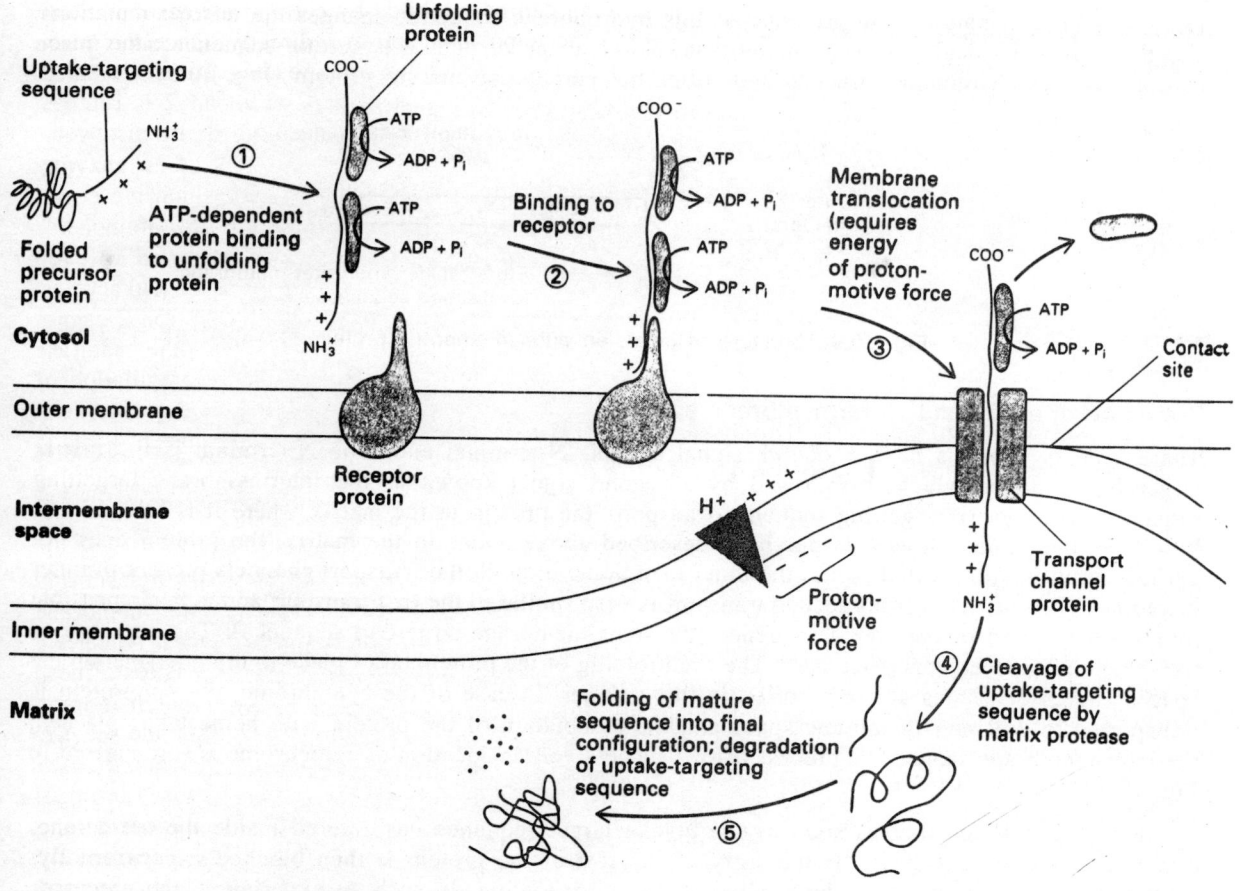

Fig. 10.8. The transport of a protein to the matrix of mitochondria.

found that the matrix targetting sequence is the only region of the protein which is required for its transport into the matrix. The sequence of the mature protein does not play any role in the transport. If the matrix targetting sequence of one protein is attached to a non-mitochondrial protein, the later protein would be transported into the mitochondria. By genetic engineering technology, a chimeric protein has been constructed in which the matrix targetting sequence of alcohol dehydrogenase, a mitochondrial protein, has been fused to DHFR, a cytosolic protein. It has been abserved that this recombinant protein is transported into the matrix of mitochondria. Once the protein has entered inside the matrix, the N-terminal uptake sequence is cleaved by specific proteases present in the matrix. These proteases which are specific for matrix targetting sequence, have two subunits and also have different metals as their prosthetic group. Once localised in its final destination, the protein is then folded into its mature form. Many times the proteins may require some chaperones for their final folding in the matrix. One of the heat shock proteins, the HSP60, may play the role of such chaperone.

Only a few proteins are present at the mitochondrial membranes. Porin is one such protein which is present in the outer membrane. In porin the matrix targetting sequence is present which is very short. It is followed by another region of signal known as the stop transfer sequence. The stop transfer sequence is hydrophobic in nature. The presence of this hydrophobic sequence changes the transport pathway and the protein is localized in the membrane. No cleavage of uptake targetting sequence takes place in this case which remains attached and forms the part of the mature protein (Fig. 10.9).

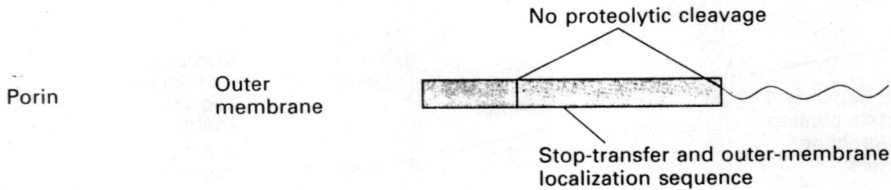

Fig. 10.9. Structure of porin, an outer membrane protein.

Transport of a protein to intermembrane space

These type of proteins have a double signal at their N-terminal end. The N-terminal is the matrix targetting sequence which is followed by a second signal known as the intermembrane targetting sequence. The matrix targetting sequence transports the protein to the matrix where it is cleaved off. It follows the same pathway as has been described above. Once in the matrix, the protein does not get folded but is transported across the inner membrane through the transport channels present in inner membrane. The process of this second transport is very similar to the first transport and is made possible by the second part of the signal sequence (the trans-membrane targetting sequence). The cleavage of the second sequence takes place here. The final folding of the protein takes place in the inter-membrane space. The cytochromes are transported in this manner. In case of the cytochrome, the apoprotein is transported to the inter-membrane space and the association of the protein with heme takes place in the inter-membrane space. The process of two successive translocation of cytochrome is summarised in Fig. 10.10.

It has been found that as soon as the uptake target sequence has entered inside the membrane, it is immediately cleaved off. If the entry of the rest of the protein is then blocked experimentally, the protein can be detected at the surface of the mitochondria. In such an experiment, the precursor of ATPase, one of the matrix proteins, was first incubated with the antibodies specific for its C–terminal domains. The antibodies attached themselves to the C–terminal while the N–terminal uptake specific sequence remained free. When this protein was incubated with mitochondria, its translocation was initiated and part of the protein was imported inside. The signal sequence was cleaved off (summarised in Fig. 10.11). However, the association of antibodies prevented the entry of the C–terminal and the protein remained at the surface of the mitochondrial membrane. This could easily be visualized by incubating the entire system either with a labelled second antibody or with IgG binding proteins such as the protein A. These antibodies which are attached to the protein, can easily be labelled with gold particles and visualised under electron microscope.

Chloroplast Genome

The chloroplast genome is similar to mitochondrial genome except that it is relatively larger and codes for many more proteins than the mitochondrial genome. The size of chloroplast DNA varies between 121-155 Kb. In fact the bacterial RNA polymerase can easily transcribe the chloroplast genome, suggesting that it has strong similarities with the bacterial DNA. There are much less variations in complexiety of the chloroplast genome of different plants than the variations in the size of mitochondrial genome. The average size of chloroplast DNA from a number of plants is shown in Table 10.6.

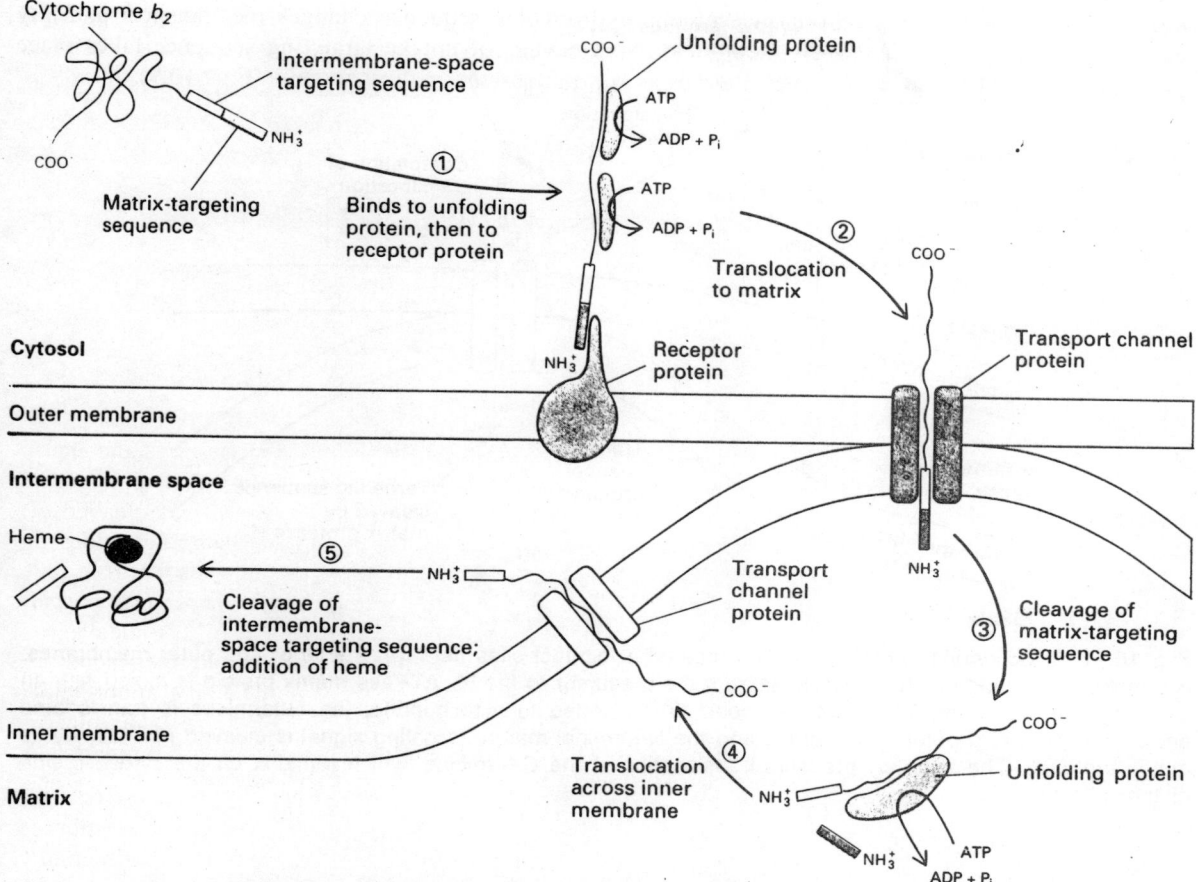

Fig. 10.10. Two successive translocations are required to target proteins such as cytochrome c_1 and cytochrome b_2 to the intermembrane space. The precursors of cytochrome c_1 and cytochrome b_2 have two uptake-targeting sequences at N-termini. The first, a matrix-targeting sequence is involved to target the protein to the mitochondrial matrix, exactly as if it were a typical mitochondrial matrix protein. This segment of the sequence is cleaved by the matrix protease (step 3). The second, an intermembrane-space targetin sequence, targets the protein to the inner membrane, presumably by binding to a receptor, and directs the translocation of the protein to the intermembrane space (step 4). There, the sequence is cleaved by a specific protease; heme is added, and the cytochrome folds into its mature configuration (step 5).

Table 10.6. Size of chloroplast genome

Plant	Genome size
Higher plants	120-200 kb
Chlamydomonas	180 kb
Euglene	135 kb
Liverwort	121 kb
Tobacco	156 kb
Zea mays	140 kb

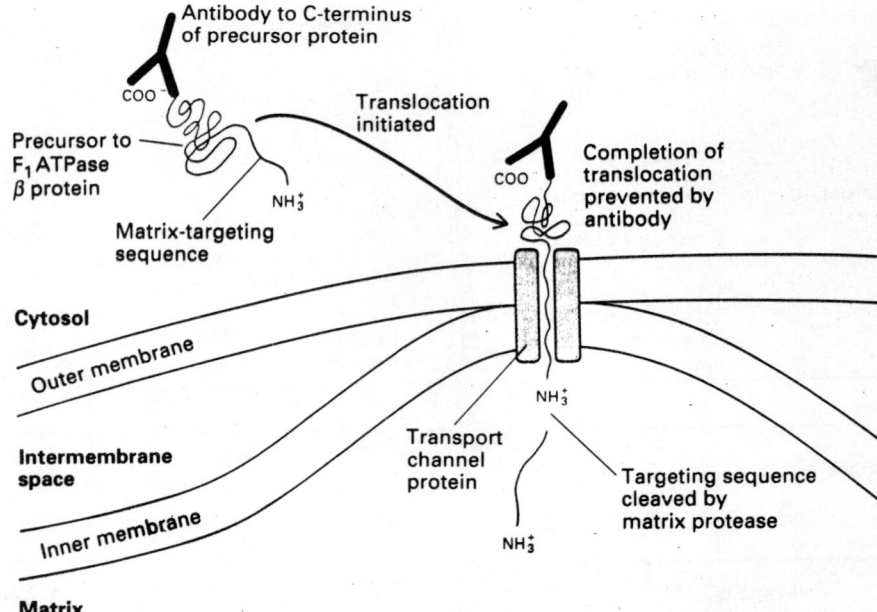

Fig. 10.11. Mitochondrial proteins are translocated at contact sites between the inner and outer membranes. A translocation intermediate is accumulated if the precursor to the F1 ATPase matrix protein is mixed with an antibody specific for its C-terminal segment. When added to mitochondria, the N-terminus is translocated across the inner and outer membranes, and the N-terminal mature targeting signal is cleaved normally by its matrix protease. The antibody prevents translocation of the C-terminus, which remains on the cytosolic side of the mitochondria.

The chloroplast DNA is circular in nature. The DNA has two regions of inverted repeats (IR) which devide the single copy region into two unequal parts these are referred as short single copy (SSC) and long single copy (LSC) region (Fig. 10.12). The comparision of the sizes of SSC, LSC and IR show that the variation between the sizes of chloroplast genome of different organisms is primarily in the IR region. The LSC and SSC regions are relatively constant (Table 10.7).

Table 10.7. The variation in size of chloroplast DNA of various plant species is primarily in inverted repeat region. The sizes of the chloroplast genome of two of the most characterized plants are given below

	Liverwort	Tobacco	
Single copy regions			
SSC	19.8 kb	18.5 kb	
LSC	81.0 kb	86.7 kb	
	100.8 kb	105.2 kb	
2 IRs, each of	10.1 kb	25.3 kb	× 2
	(i.e. 20.2 kb)	(i.e. 50.6 kb)	
Total genome	121.0 kb	155.8 kb	

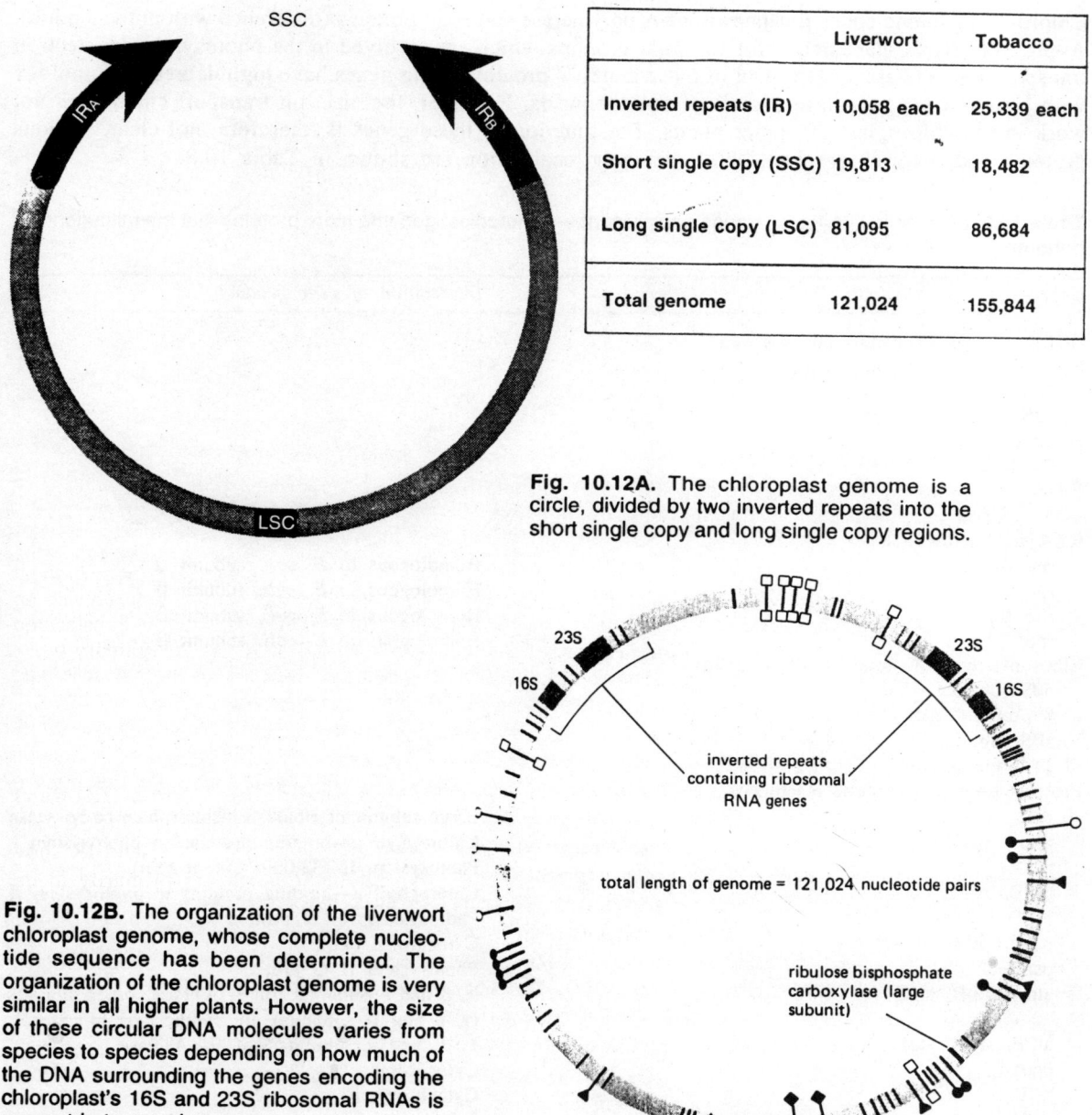

	Liverwort	Tobacco
Inverted repeats (IR)	10,058 each	25,339 each
Short single copy (SSC)	19,813	18,482
Long single copy (LSC)	81,095	86,684
Total genome	121,024	155,844

Fig. 10.12A. The chloroplast genome is a circle, divided by two inverted repeats into the short single copy and long single copy regions.

Fig. 10.12B. The organization of the liverwort chloroplast genome, whose complete nucleotide sequence has been determined. The organization of the chloroplast genome is very similar in all higher plants. However, the size of these circular DNA molecules varies from species to species depending on how much of the DNA surrounding the genes encoding the chloroplast's 16S and 23S ribosomal RNAs is present in two copies.

Chloroplast genome codes for about 120 genes, out of which about 20 genes have introns in them. A substantial amount of DNA is 'junk', not coding for any genes. The introns of the genes are spliced off either by self splicing mechanism or by the RNA mediated catalysis. The IR region codes for rRNAs and a few other genes which are present in duplicate. Majority of the genes are present in the LSC region. There are about 60 genes which are related to DNA replication, transcription and translation.

Chloroplast genome codes for its own RNA polymerase and the r-proteins (difference with mitochondria). Approximately 20 genes code for essential proteins which are involved in the photosynthesis, electron transport and ATPase system. Out of these genes, 7 protein coding genes have high degree of homology with NADH-CoQ reductase system of motochondria. However, the electron transport chain does not work in the chloroplast of higher plants. The function of these genes is, therefore, not clear. Various proteins coded by chloroplast DNA and their localization are shown in Table 10.8.

Table 10.8. Chloroplast genome : genes and proteins— Chloroplast genome more proteins that the mitochondrial genome

Genes	Description of gene product
rRNAs (2 sets of genes, one each in inverted repeats IR_A and IR_B)	
16S RNA	
23S RNA	
4.55 RNA	
5S RNA	
tRNA	
37 tRNAs	
RNA polymerase	
rpo A	Homologous to *E. coli*, subunit α
rpo B	Homologous to *E. coli*, subunit β
rpo C1	Homologous to *E. coli*, subunit β'
rpo C2	Homologous to *E. coli*, subunit β'
Ribosomal protein—total of 19 r-proteins	
50S subunit:	
8 proteins (rpl)	
30S subunit:	
11 proteins (rps)	
Proteins for photosynthetic machinery	
rbcL	Large subunit of ribulose bisphosphate carboxylase
psaA, psaB	Chlorophyll a—binding proteins in photosystem I
psbA	Photosystem II (32,000-MW protein)
psbB, psbC	Chlorophyll a—binding proteins in photosystem II
psbD	Photosystem II D2 protein
psbE, psbF	Cytochrome b_{559}
psbG	Photosystem II G protein
atpA, atpB, atpE	α, β and ϵ Subunits of F_1 ATPase, other subunits (γ, δ and II subunits) are synthesized in cytosol
atPF, atpH, atpI	1, 3, and 4 subunits of F_0 ATPase
petA	Cytochrome f
petB	Cytochrome b_6
petD	Subunit 4 of cytochrome b_6/f complex
ndh1, ndh2, ndh3,	Homologous to the subunits of
ndh4, ndh4L,	human mitochondrial
ndh5, ndh6	NADH-CoQ reductase complex
frxA, frxB, frxC	Homologous to a 4-Fe-type ferredoxin
Others	29 unidentified open reading frames (URF)
Total no. of genes	~ 110

Rest of the proteins, including the 3 subunits of light harvesting system are synthesized in cytoplasm

The chloroplast ribosomes are similar in size as the bacterial ribosomes (50S and 30S, respectively, note that mitochondrial ribosomes are much smaller in size). These defer from mitochondrial ribosome in the fact that the large subunit also contains two small RNA molecules of 4.5S and 5S alongwith the 23S RNA. There are 37 tRNAs present in chloroplast (compared to only 20-22 tRNAs in mitochondria). The RNA polymerase of chloroplast has 4 subunits which are very similar to α, β and β' subunits of bacterial RNA polymerase.

Even though the chloroplast DNA codes for many of its proteins, a large number of these proteins are coded by the nuclear DNA and are transported to the chloroplast. The mechanism of import of these proteins is very similar to that of mitochondrial proteins. The site of import is relatively rare site where the inner and the outer membranes are fused together. The transport channel is lined by a protein/ group of proteins which serve as the receptor as well as the channel protein. This multifunctional protein is known as the receptor-transport protein. A stromal import sequence, usually approximately 30 amino acids in length, is present on the N-terminal end of the protein and is recognized by this receptor. The protein is internalised in a receptor mediated manner. The signal is cleaved by specific proteases present in the lumen and the mature protein is folded in its final form. For the proteins which have to be localized in the thylakoid vesicle (such as the plastocyanin) or at the inter-membrane space, a second signal, the thylakoid uptake targetting sequence (or the intermembrane targetting sequence, as the case may be), is present following the stromal import sequence. The process is similar to mitochondria (Fig. 10.13).

The thylakoid uptake targetting sequence is a 25 aa long peptide which is very hydrophobic and is cleaved by a specific endoprotease present in the thylakoid vesicle.

Differentiation of chloroplast

Chloroplast and other similar organelles are differentiated from a common precursor, the proplastid. A proplastid can differentiate into 5 different plastids, namely the chloroplast, etioplast, amyloplast, elioplast and the chromoplast. Some of these plastids can interconvert to each other. For example, etioplast can convert to chloroplast and chloroplast can convert to chromoplast (Fig. 10.14). Etioplast is an intermediate formed during the final differentiation to chloroplast and is present only in the embryonic tissues or in the leaves stored in dark. Chloroplast is the only plastid which has internal thylakoid membrane. Light plays an important role in the formation of these plastids. All the plant tissues have a light sensitive regulatory protein known as the phytochrome. The light absorbing pigment of phytochrome is a tetrapyrrole which is linked to the protein. The pigment can have two forms, P_r and P_{fr} (the r and fr in subscript denote red and far red, respectively). The P_r form has an absorption maxima at 660 nm. When exposed to light, it absorbs red light and converts to the P_{fr} form. A number of physiological responses are mediated through this form. The P_{fr} has an absorption maxima at 730 nm. It quickly converts to P_r form when exposed to infra red light. In dark P_{fr} converts to P_r, but the conversion is slow (Fig. 10.15). A number of physiological processes are regulated by these phytochromes. For example, for the germination of lettuce seeds it is essential that these are pre-exposed to light.

The genesis of organelles

The fact that the organelles have very high degree of homology with prokaryotic cells, raises a very important question related to the genesis of these organelles. How and why are the two genome at different (and for away from each other) stages of evolution are similar in their structure. A theory referred as the endosymbiont hypothesis has been proposed to explain the evolution of both the

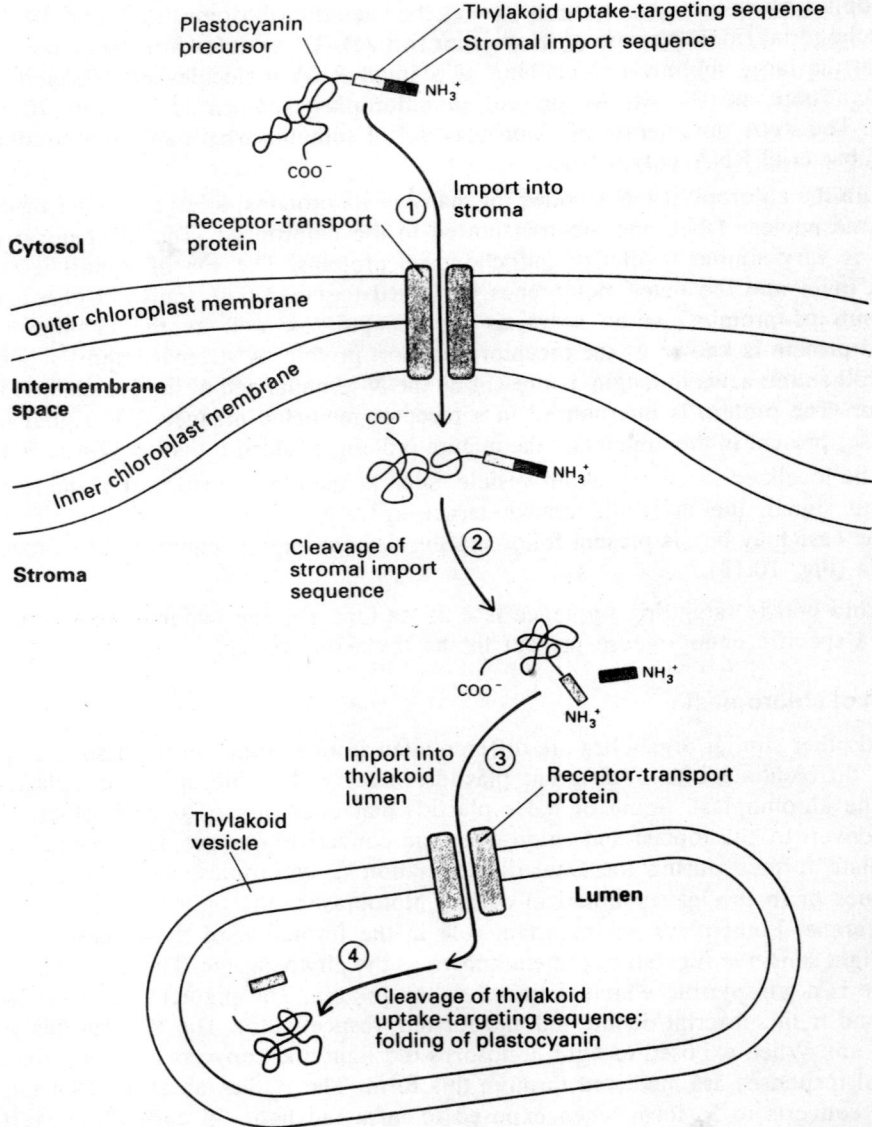

Fig. 10.13. The successive action of two uptake-targeting sequence direct plastocyanin to the thylakoid lumen. The plastocyanin precursor is synthesized at the cytosol; the 66 amino acids at N-terminus are not found in the mature protein in the thylakoid lumen. First 30 N-terminal residues import into the chloroplast stroma. As with import into the mitochondria, translocation from the cytosol to the stroma is mediated by a receptor-transport protein localized to the points of contact at the outer and inner chloroplast membranes. The stromal import sequence is removed by a stromal signal protease. The thylakoid uptake-targeting sequence of ~25 residues is very hydrophobic; it causes the stromal protein to be imported into the thylakoid lumen and presumably binds to a distinct import receptor-transport protein on the thylakoid membrane. This sequence is removed in the thylakoid lumen by a separate endoprotease.

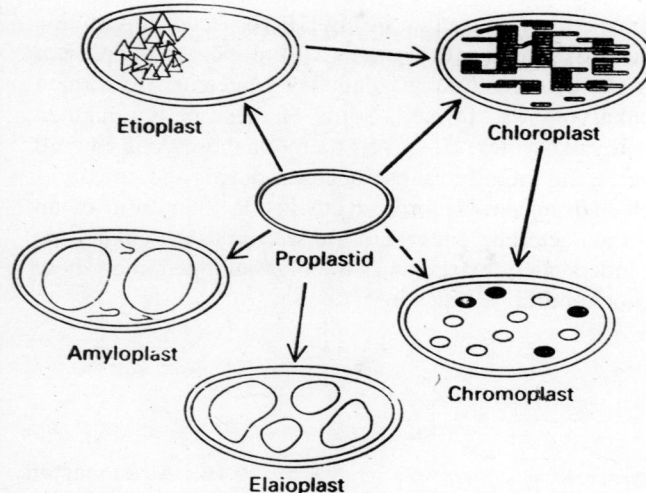

Fig. 10.14. Proplastids can differentiate into many organelles depending on the plant tissue in which they are found and/or on exposure to light. The etioplast is an intermediate in the conversion of a proplastid to a chloroplast. Thus the choroplast contains internal thylakoid membranes.

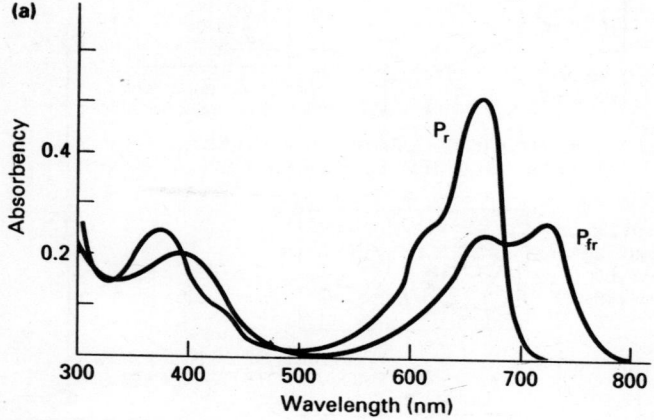

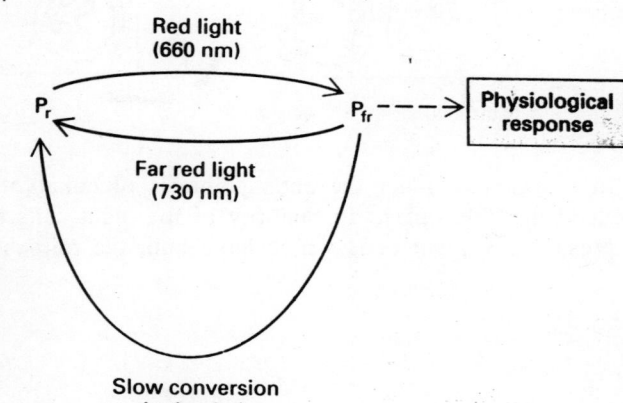

Fig. 10.15. (a) Light absorbency by the two interconvertible forms of phytochrome. The P_r form maximally absorbs light of 660 nm; the P_{fr} form maximally absorbs light of 730 nm. (b) Absorption of a quantum of red light by one molecule of the P_r form converts it to P_{fr}. P_{fr} can be reconverted to P_r by absorption of a quantum of far red light.

mitochondria and the chloroplast. This is diagrammatically represented in Fig. 10.16. According to this theory, the life orginated in the form of an anaerobic prokaryotic cell. From this primitive cell the present day aerobic prokaryotes have evolved. Through an alternate evolutionary pathway a nucleus was formed in the anaerobic prokaryotes and an anaerobic eukaryote was formed. Some of these cells remained unchanged and can be seen as present day anaerobic eukaryotes. However, many of these cells entered in a symbiotic arrangement with the aerobic bacteria and engulfed these bacteria during the course of time. Thus an eukaryotic cell was evolved which had an aerobic prokaryote inside it in form of an endosymbiont. During the course of time, some of the bacterial genes were transferred to the eukaryotic nucleus while certain other genes maintained their independent existance as the organelle genome. These are the present day aerobic eukaryote having mitochondria.

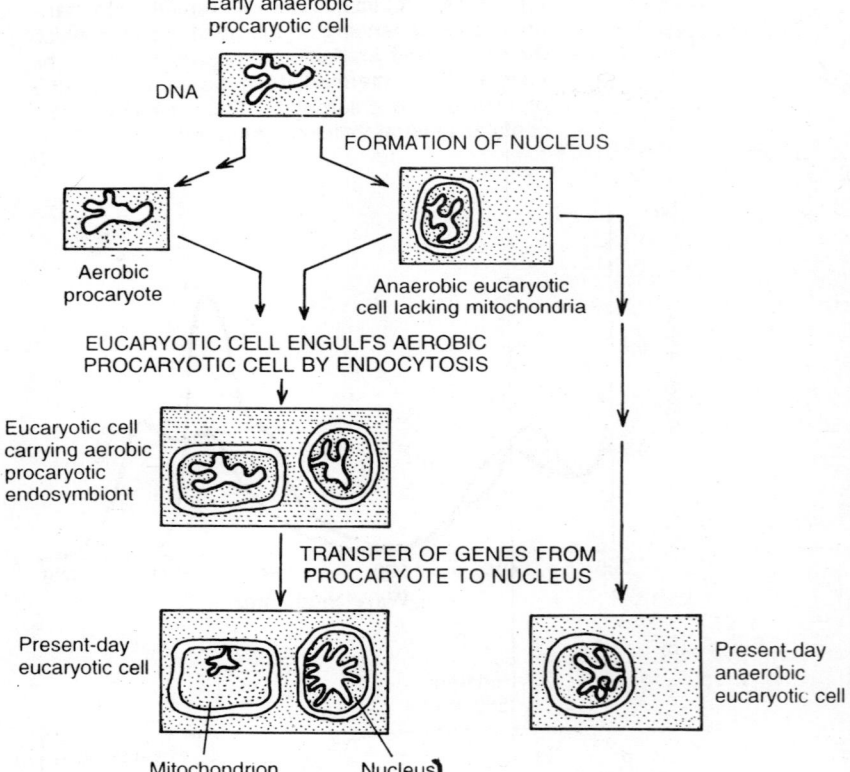

Fig. 10.16. A suggested evolutionary pathway for the origin of mitochondria. Although a single origin for all mitochondria is sometimes postulated, separate endosymbiotic events may have led to the mitochondria found in such distantly related eukaryotes as trypanosomes and euglenoids. Microsporidia are present-day anaerobic single-celled eucaryotes (protozoa) without mitochondria that live in the gut of many animals. Because they have an rRNA sequence that suggests a great deal of evolutionary distance from all other known eucaryotes, it has been postulated that their ancestors were also anaerobic and resembled the eucaryote that first engulfed the precursors of mitochondria.

In a similar manner the endosymbiosis of eukaryotic cells with photosynthesizing prokaryotes produced the chloroplast. In majority of the plant cells both types of endosymbiosis took place and the present day plant cells which have both the mitochondria and the chloroplast have evolved.

11

Mutation and the DNA Damage and Repair System

Mutation

The cell is continuously exposed to a number of environmental and biological factors which can cause damage to its genome. In fact a number of changes, both major and minor, in the basic structure of DNA keep taking place throughout the life of the cell. However, majority of the damages are repaired by the celluler machinery. Only a small proportion of these damages remain unrepaired and some of these changes are inherited to the next generation. Sudden inheritable changes in genetic material of an organism as well as the process by which these changes take place are known as the mutation. Following the occurance of a mutation in the genome, the cell or the organism is known as the mutant. A mutant can be recognized from the normal organism (the wild type) by the exhibition of some novel characters or phenotype in the mutant.

Mutation is the ultimate source of all genetic variations and is the raw material for evolution. Had there been no mutation, all the genes would have been present in only one form and there would have been no evolution and no adoptation to the environment. On the other hand, too frequent mutations will disturb the entire process of the transfer of genetic information from one generation to another and will be biologically unacceptable.

The mutation may result in one of the following changes:

(i) Change in chromosome number

In this type of mutations, an entire chromosome may either be lost or get duplicated resulting in an aneuploidy. If a chromosome is gained, it will result in the formation of one chromosome which will have three homologues and will be referred as the trisomic. The loss of one chromosome will result in one chromosome having only a single homologue and the organism can be referred as a monosomic organism. Sometimes it may be the loss or gain of a complete pair of chromosomes resulting in the formation of euploidy.

(ii) Chromosome Abberation

Chromosome abberations are extensive damage in the DNA which may be due to breakage of chromosomes or due to transposition of the transposons. Such mutations result in major changes in genetic information and are caused due to some unusual events such as in the survivors of atomic bombs exploded in Japan during the second world war.

(iii) Changes in individual genes

Most of the mutations result in the changes in individual genes. These changes can either be a single base change or relatively longer changes. In case of the change in a single base, the mutation is referred as the point mutation. The point mutation can be a replacement change where a base is changed for another base. The replacement changes can be of two types, the transition and the transversion. In transition a purine is replaced by another purine (G for A or A for G) or a pyrimidine is replaced by another pyrimidine (T for C or C for T). In transversion a purine is replaced by a pyrimidine and vice versa (i.e. A for T, A for C, C for A, C for G, G for C, G for T, T for G or T for A). The possible changes are shown in Fig. 11.1. In the replacement type of mutations only one of the codons will be changed and it will either have no effect on protein (i.e. another codon for the same amino acid may be created resulting in a silent mutation) or it will change only one amino acid of the protein. One aminoacid change may not affect the biological function or may change the entire function of the protein as is the case in sickle cell anaemia.

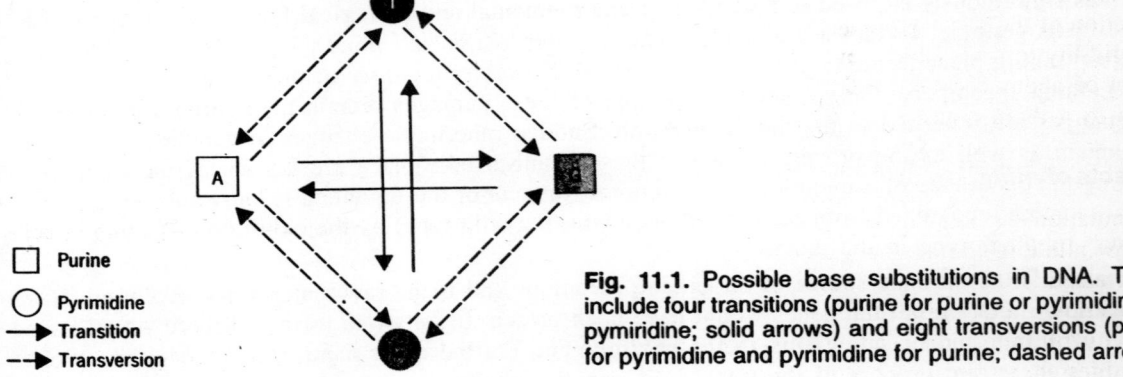

☐ Purine
◯ Pyrimidine
→ Transition
--→ Transversion

Fig. 11.1. Possible base substitutions in DNA. These include four transitions (purine for purine or pyrimidine for pymiridine; solid arrows) and eight transversions (purine for pyrimidine and pyrimidine for purine; dashed arrows).

Another possible point mutation is the addition or deletion of a base. In both these cases the reading frame will be shifted and the gene product will be totally different than the normal gene product. All the codons after the mutation will, therefore, be changed.

Based on the reason behind the occurance of mutation, these may be of two types:

(a) Spontaneous mutations

In this type of mutation, there is no apparent reason for the change(s) in the DNA. These take place spontaneously without any known cause. The deamination of bases, specially of cytosine and the spontaneous depurination (which is very slow) are good example of this type of mutation.

(b) Induced mutation

In this type of mutation, the changes in DNA are caused by certain physical or chemical agents. These agents are known as the mutagens. Exposure to a mutagen results in the mutation. Some of the known mutagens are the ionizing radiations such as the X-rays, γ-rays, cosmic rays and the UV light (specially of very low wave length). The radiations with UV light of the wave length of less than 100 nm are very strong mutagens. Other mutagens include the chemicals which react with nucleic acids (see later) and the nucleotide analogs which can be incorporated in place of a normal nucleotide. These analogs can form a mis-base pairing with a wrong nucleotide and a mutation will take place during the next cycle of DNA replication.

The mutagens which change certain genes resulting in the transformation of a normal cell into malignant cell (the proto—oncogenes) and onset of cancers are known as carcinogens.

Based on the location of the change in the DNA chain, the mutation can be either random or site specific. In random mutations, the changes occur at any location within the genome. Most of the environmentally induced mutations are random. Similarly most of the spontaneous mutations are also random. On the other hand, by using a specific mutagen under well defined specific conditions, it is possible to modify the DNA precisely at a specific place, usually at a pre—determined place. Such mutations are referred as the site directed mutations.

Intrinsic error frequency

It is the frequency of incorporation of a wrong base during the replication of DNA. As discussed, the fidility of DNA structure during the replication is primarily maintained by the template directed base pairing. This is followed by the correction of any mistake which may have occured, by the proof reading function of the DNA polymerase and finally the methylation directed mismatch repair process increases the fidility to a very high level. These processes together bring the degree of mistakes to an acceptable level of about 1 mistake/10^8-10^{10} bases incorporated. If there is a higher frequency of errors, it will lead to a disruption in the transfer of genetic information from generation to generation.

Effects of mutation

A mutation can lead to the expression of new characters. It is usually achieved by the creation of a new allele in the genome. If the changes are at multiple alleles, an entirely new form of DNA may be created. If the changes are very small which can be detected only by specialized techniques, then it is known as the formation of an isoallele. Occasionally a mutation can lead to total loss of the activity of an essential gene. This may eventually lead to the death of the organism. Such mutations are referred as the lethal mutations.

Reversion of mutation

If a mutant is again mutated at the same site in such a manner that its phenotype returns back to the wild type, the second mutation will be the reversion of the first mutation or a back mutation. The back mutation can be of two types:

(a) True back mutation, where the second mutation is at the same genetic site where the first mutation had taken place and the phenotype as well as the genotype of the organism revert back to wild type.

(b) Supression mutation: In such mutation, the second mutation is at a site other than the site of the first mutation. However, the second mutation nullifies the effect of the first mutation and the phenotype of the organism is back to the wild type. But the genotype of the revertant will show the mutations at two separate locations.

Conditional Mutation

Sometimes the mutation is in such a genetic locus that under one set of canditions the organism grows normally while under a different set of conditions, either the growth is not normal or the organism does not grow at all. Such mutations are known as the conditional mutations. The conditions which premit the normal growth are known as the permissive conditions and the other conditions are referred as the non-permissive or the restrictive conditions. If under restrictive conditions the organism is unable to grow at all, the mutation becomes a conditional lethal mutation. Based on the conditions required for the growth, the mutation may be an axotropic where the growth media and the metabolic conditions are responsible for the expression of mutation. For example, certain mutants can easily grow in presence of glucose but replacement of glucose with any other sugar will cause the growth to stop. It may be temperature sensitive (both cold or heat sensitive) or may be supressor sensitive where the organism is viable in presence of a supressor but in the absence of supressor the mutation is lethal. The supressor contains a gene which either complements or corrects the defect in the mutant, either recessive or dominant.

Radiation Induced mutations

A number of radiations specially the electromagnetic waves with 100 nm or smaller wave length cause ionization. The example are the X-rays, γ-rays and the cosmic rays. The effect of these rays was investigated as early as in 1927, when H.J. Muller found that excessive exposure to X-rays increased the incidence of sex linked recessive lethal mutation in Drosophila. It was found that there is a direct relationship between the radiation dose and the incidence of mutation. For example, at an exposure of 5000 r about 15% occurance of mutation was observed. The rate was found to be about 3% for each 1000 r exposure (Fig. 11.2).

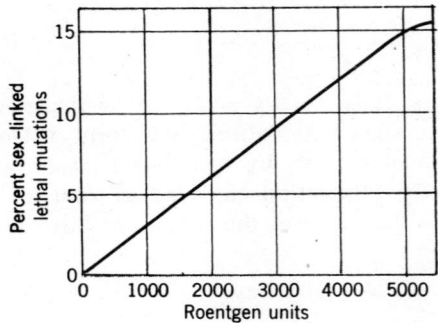

Fig. 11.2. Relationship between the frequency of sex-linked lethal mutations and ionizing irradiation dosage.

However, it was found that some mutations can take place even at very low exposure dose occuring for long time or at high dose for relatively short time. Thus, there is no safe level of radiation and even a very small dose may be unsafe. In rats, it has been found that the chances of mutation are much less if a chronic irradiation with low dose is given than if same dose is given in one hit.

The environmental conditions also affect the effect of ionization. For example, at low oxygen tension the incidence of mutation is low. Similarly, if high oxygen tension is present at the time of irradiation, the incidence of mutation will be higher even if the animal is kept at low oxygen tension later on. The ionic radiation causes all sort of mutations. There are incidences of chromosome abberation of all types, for example, there can be deletion, duplication, inversion and transversion.

The state of cellular metabolism and the phase of cell cycle also play a role on the effect of ionizing radiations. For example, A.H. Sporrow has reported that in response to irradiation of the plant Trillium, the mutations were 60 times more prevelent at the metaphose than at the interphase of the cell cycle.

Effect of UV

UV is relatively weak mutagen. The normal levels of UV in the sun light are not strong enough to cause mutation. Any damage to DNA is repaired readily by the cell. However, UV is absorbed by both the purine and the pyrimidine bases and these are converted into an excitable state when these are more reacative. The UV of 254 nm or lower wave length is most damaging. It can cause the formation of pyrimidine dimers and pyrimidine hydrates. The relationship between the UV dose and the mutation rate is highly variable.

Chemically induced mutations

A number of chemicals are mutagenic in nature. Some of these chemicals are commonly used by human beings, while the others are not that common. The saliant features of these are enumerated below. In general, the chemicals can be grouped in two classes.

(a) Chemicals which can cause mutation to both the replicating and the non-replicating DNA. Some of the examples of this class of chemicals are nitrous acid (HNO_2), alkylating agents, etc

(b) Certain other chemicals are mutagenic only to the replicating DNA, such as acridine dyes and the base analogs.

The mechanism of action of some of these chemicals will be described briefly.

Nitrous acid

It causes the oxidative deamination of bases in DNA. As a result, A is converted to hypoxanthine which can base pair with C during replication and convert an A : T pair to a G : C pair. Similarly C is converted to U which can base pair with A, converting a C : G pair to an A:T pair. The G, on the other hand, is converted to xanthine which can also base pair with C. This change, therefore, does not cause a mutation. As the effect of HNO_2 is to convert an A : T to G : C and a G : C to A:T, it can also be used to revert a mutant back to the wild type.

Alkylating agents and hydroxylating agents

These chemicals transfer a CH_3 or C_2H_5 group to the bases. For example, mustard gas [Di (2-chloro ethyl) sulphide] and EMS (ethyl methane sulphonate) carry out the ethylation at the N7 and O6 positions. These modified bases form a base pair with a wrong base. For example, 7-ethyl G base pairs with T, converting a G : C pair to an A : T pair. NTG (N-methyl-N'-nitro, N-nitroso guanidine), is one of the most potent alkaylating agents. It causes a number of multiple and closely related mutations in DNA. Ethylene sulphonate (EES) is another example of these type of chemicals. The NH_2OH is a hydroxylating agent, specific for G : C base pair converting it to an A : T pair. These chemicals, besides causing a base change, can also cause the cross-linking and may occasionally result in chromosomal breakage and abberations. They can also activate the repair mechanism of the cell.

Acridines

Acridine dyes cause the frame shift mutations. These dyes, such as proflavin, acridine orange, ICR 170 and ICR 190 interchelate between the stacked base pairs in the DNA and get sandwitched between two bases. This results in an increased rigidity of the DNA and change in its confirmation. This confirmational change causes the addition and deletion of one or more bases during replication and results in the frame shift mutation.

Base analogs

A number of modified bases can be incorporated in place of a normal base during the DNA replication as the DNA polymerase cannot differentiate between the normal base and its analog. However, often the analog forms a base pair with an alternate base and results in a replacement change during the next cycle of replication. For example 5-bromo-deoxyuridine (Brdu) is a thymidine analog and can convert a G : C pair to an A : T pair when it is present in enol form and converts an A : T pair to a G : C pair in its keto form (Fig. 11.3). Similar mutation can be caused by 2-amino purine. These chemicals can also be used for reverting a mutation. Other base analogs are N^4-hydroxy CTP which is copied either as a G or an A and results into the replacement of G to A or C to T in 30% of the molecules.

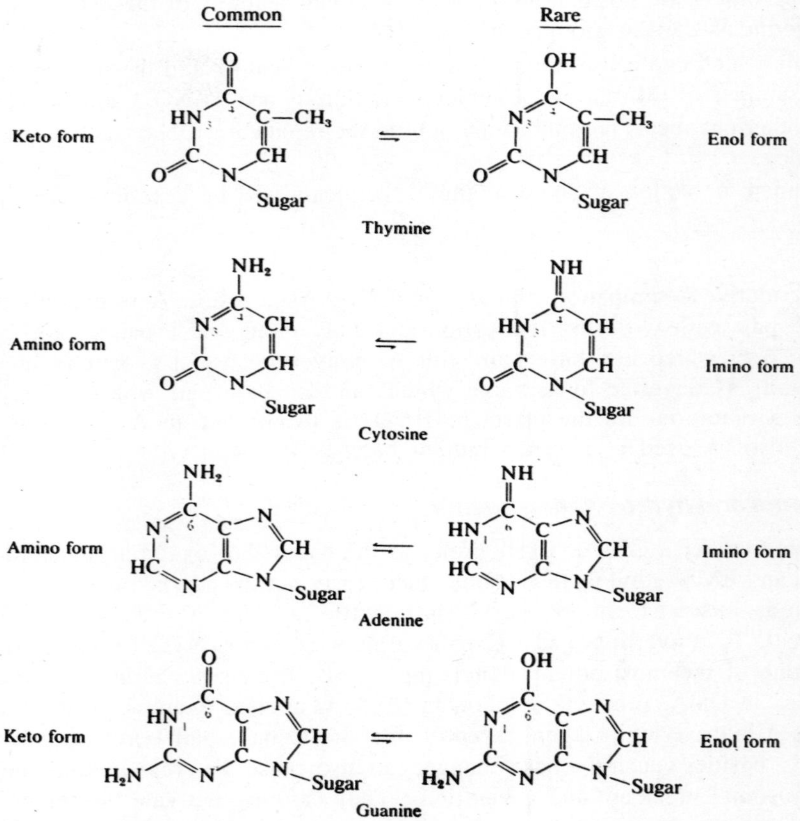

Fig. 11.3. Tautomeric forms of the four common bases in DNA. The shifts of hydrogen atoms between the number 3 and number 4 positions of the pyrimidines and between the number I and number 6 positions of the purines results in change in the base-pairing potential of the bases.

Beneficial mutation

Most of the spontaneous mutations are harmful to the organism as these usually render an organism less efficient. However, the entire process of evolution has been possible only because of the slow mutations. Many mutations allow an organism to be more suitable to survive in an unfriendly environment. These mutations permit the development of new characters, while also give the adoptability to the sorrounding.

The induced mutations can be used for providing new characters. The applications of such mutations have been more in plant sciences. It has been possible to provide an organism with useful characters, such as pest resistance, stress resistance or the high yielding varieties etc. For example, it has been possible to develop the variety of Pennicilium which has higher yields of penicillin. Such over producers have been very valuable commercially.

Mutagenicity of a substance

In recent years the use of chemicals has greatly increased and human are exposed to various chemicals. It is therefore, essential to assess these chemicals for their safety. B. Ames developed a simple test for assessing the mutagenicity of a substance. In this test a specially constructed strain of Salmonella typhimurium, having auxotrophic mutation is used. A limited number of these bacteria are plated in an agar plate having trace amounts of the necessary growth factor. The concentration of growth factor is just sufficient enough for supporting only a few cell divisions. Thus while the survival and very slow growth of bacteria is maintained, no visible colonies are formed. The compound to be tested for mutagenicity is then applied at the centre of the plate in a small disc of filter paper. If the compound is a mutagen, it should cause a mutation which in all probability would be at a locus that will allow the growth of the bacteria under restrictive conditions. Normally the selection pressure will ensure that the mutagen would reverse mutate the mutant and the mutant should be able to grow. By counting the number of colonies, it is possible to estimate the mutagenicity of the compound.

The practical details of Ame's test are shown in Fig. 11.4. A tester strain of S. typhimurium which requires histidine for its growth, is plated on agar plates with only traces of histidine. Various concentrations of different test compounds are applied at the centre of the plate in a filter disc. Higher the mutagenicity of a compound, more colonies will be formed even at low concentration of the compound.

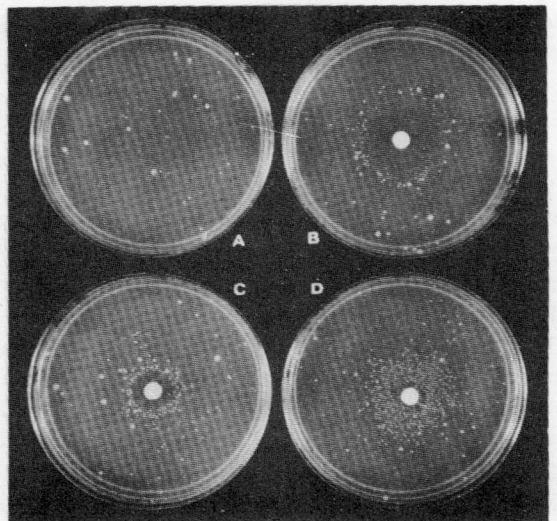

Fig. 11.4. Ame's test for mutagenicity using Salmonella mutants. Each petri dish contains a layer of agar medium containing only a trace of histidine and a known number of "testing strain" cells, which are carrying a frameshift mutation that results in histidine auxotrophy. Plates C and D also contain the rat-liver microsomal activation system. The potential mutagens are applied to filter paper disks, which are placed in the centre of plates B, C and D. (A) Control plate with no addition, showing the background level of spontaneous reversion to prototrophy. (B) Plate to which the carcinogen furylfuramide (a food additive) has been added. (C) Plate to which the carcinogen aflotoxin B (a fungal toxin) has been added. (D) Plate to which the carcinogen 2-aminofluorene has been added.

Over the years a corelation between the mutagenicity and carcinogenecity has been seen in more than 90% of the tested substances. Many times a compound itself may not be mutagenic, but it may get metabolised by the cell to produce an intermediary metabolite which is mutagenic. As a result, the compound acts as a potent mutagen.

Somatic and Germinal Mutations

Mutation can take place in any cell as well as at any stage of the cell cycle. A mutation in a somatic cell will be perpetuated only in its descendant cells and not in the whole organism. As animal cells donot have totipotency, these changes will be restricted only to the original organism and will not be passed on to next generation. However, these are inherited by the daughter cells of the originally mutated cell. Thus the term 'inherited' in the original definition of the mutation does not necessary means the next generation of the organism but means only the daughter cells (next generation of the cell). However, in plants it is possible to obtain the plants with mutation by vegetative propagation as the plant cells are totipotent.

On the other hand, if a dominant mutation occurs in the germ cells, their effect will be immediately visible in the next progeny. The recessive mutation, may not produce phenotypic changes in progeny. However, these gametes will carry a mutated allele.

Mutagenesis

Many times during the genetic engineering experiments one has to modulate a region of the gene of interest in order to be able to manipulate it in a desired manner. For any such manipulation, it is necessary that the desired gene should be fully characterized. Its restriction map should be known. The sequence of the entire gene or atleast that of the target region should be known. While the details of these processes are beyond the scope of this topic it may be pertinent to breifly discuss some of these processes.

Most common method of creating a mutation is to expose the culture of the bacteria to a mutagen. The HNO_2 is one of the most commonly used chemicals for this purpose. Following the exposure to the mutagen, the bacteria are allowed to grow under a number of different conditions and the mutants with desired phenotypic characters are isolated. The genotype of these bacteria is then characterized so that the gene responsible for the changed characters can be scored. However, such mutations are random and the mutants are recognized by phenotypic changes in desired characters.

Site directed mutagenesis

Often the aim of the experiment is to carry out the mutation at a desired site. This can be achieved by a number of different methods. One of the ways is to delete an entire restriction fragment of the gene while other is to mutate a single (or only a few) base. The second type of mutation is known as the point mutation.

For deletion of a restriction fragment, the restriction degestion with appropriate enzymes is carried out and the DNA minus the fragment to be deleted is ligated. Alternatively, an exonuclese can be used to cleave the bases from the end of a DNA. The kinetics of the digestion is carefully scored so that only the desired number of bases are deleted. Very often a combination of endo– and exonucleases is used. The endonuclease creates a cut at desired position while the exonuclease will remove the bases from the ends. A number of sequence specific nucleases have been identified and are aften used for this purpose.

For insertional mutation, the use of a transposon is a natural method. An modification of this method is to clone a DNA fragment by genetic engineering route. In fact, the entire gene cloning can be visualized as a specialized form of mutation in the vector DNA.

For the addition or deletion of a few bases, one can use the restriction digestion followed by filling (or digestion, as the case may be) of the sticky ends and ligating the blunt ends (Fig. 11.5).

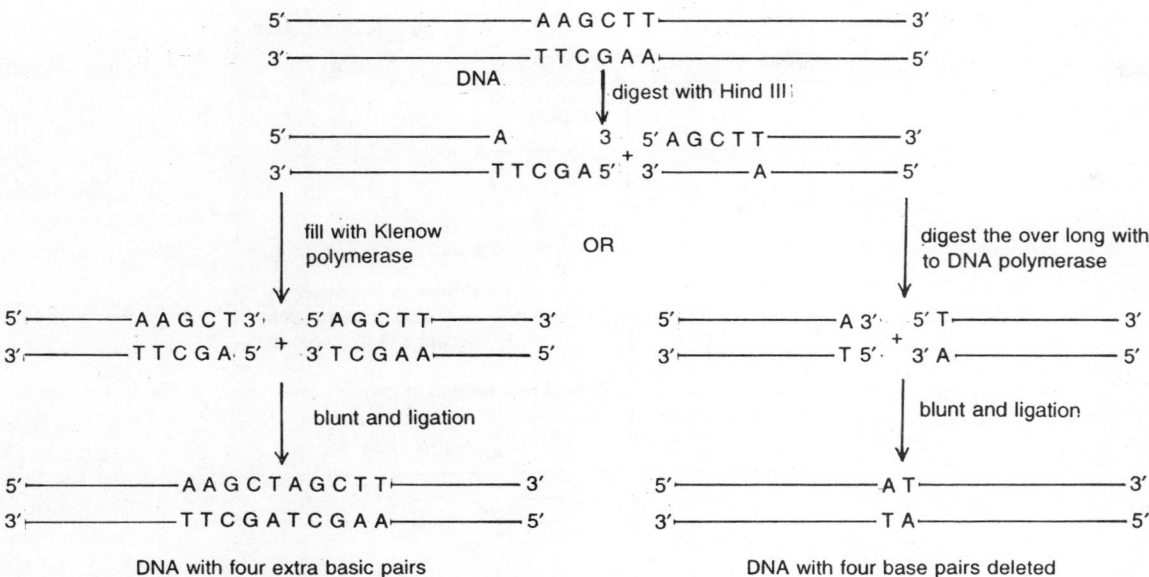

Fig. 11.5. Addition or deletion of bases by restriction digestion.

Site directed point mutation

Very often the aim of the mutagenesis is to change only a single base at a specified locus. It can be achieved by a number of ways. Bisulphite can be conviniently used for this purpose. In a single stranded DNA, bisulphite changes the C to uracil which will later be copied as an 'A'. For this purpose a number of strategies have been deviced. A DNA can be cleaved with a restriction enzyme in presence of ethidium bromide when only one of the two strands will be cleaved and a nick will be created. A region of SS DNA can be generated through the nick and a mutation with bisulphite can be created. The DNA is then filled with pol I when the C (which has become converted to an U by the bisulphite treatment) is copied as A. M 13, one of the coliophages, can be used for generating the SS DNA. This can then be mutated. Other chemicals used for mutation are formic acid (converts an A or a G to any of the four bases), hydrazine (C or T are mutated to any of the four bases) and KMnO$_4$ (acts on T and converts it to any of the four bases). However, often a very specific method of mutagenesis is used which uses a synthetic oligonucleotide. The details of this method are discussed below.

Oligonucleotide directed site mutagenesis

This is a very powerful technique for creating a mutation at a specific site in a fool proof manner. The DNA to be mutated, is isolated in a single stranded form. Bacteriophage M 13 provides a convinient method for generating the SS DNA. A oligonucleotide is synthesized against the region which has to be mutated. This oligonucleotide (primer) is complementary to the target region except for the base which is to be mutated. Desired change is included in the oligonucleotide sequence. The mutated primer is allowed to anneal with the target DNA. It forms base pairing with the target gene alongwith the mismatch which is looped out. The length of the primer and the annealing conditions are carefully monitored so that a mismatched primer can get annealed with the gene in a stable manner. The primer is now enzymatically extended, using the DNA polymerase. A copy of the template is thus obtained which will contain the desired mutation (Fig. 11.6). This mutated strand can now be used as the template to get the ds DNA which will have the desired mutation.

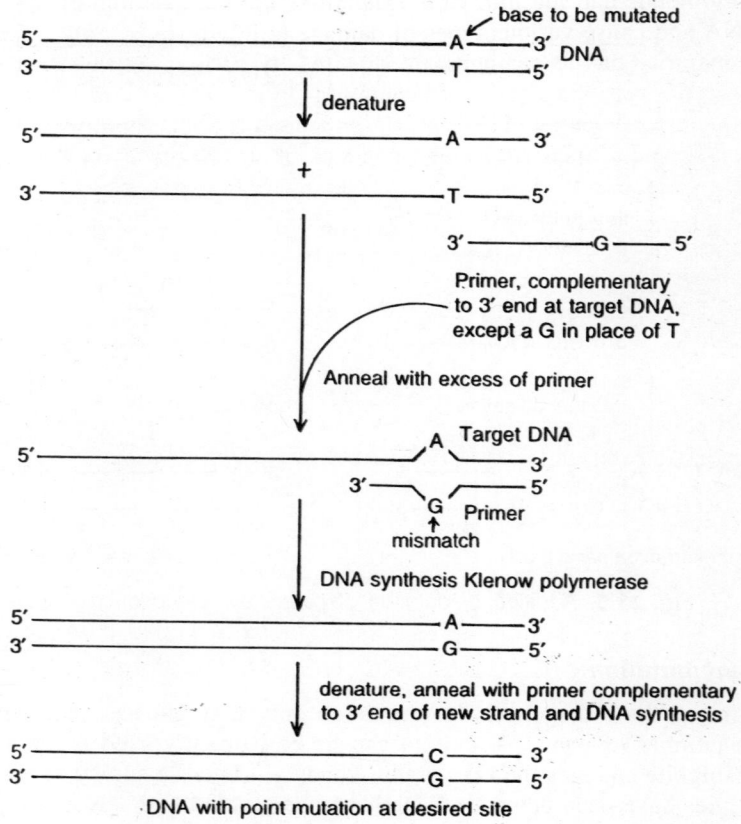

Fig. 11.6. Oligonucleotide directed site mutagenesis.

As a modification of this method, it is possible to automatise the process through PCR when the mutated DNA can be suitably amplified. By using modification of the process it is also possible either to delete or add a single nucleotide in the gene at the desired place.

The point to remember is that the length of the primer should be carefully calculated. Usually a formula is used where an 'n' nucleotide long primer is used if the length of the entire genome is 4^n. For example, for E. coli a 9 base long primer should be sufficient. However, 2 extra nucleotides are added to the length of primer for each of the mismatches. Further the mismatch should be as much far away from the 3'-end of the primer as possible. In general practice, a 15–20 nucleotide long primer is usually used.

DNA DAMAGE AND REPAIR

The DNA of the cell is continuously exposed to a number of harmful biological, chemical and physical agents. Some of these agents, specially the chemical agents, are produced inside the cell during the course of normal metabolic processes. Of course, these harmful chemicals are removed from the cell by the detoxification processes. However, the DNA may be exposed to these harmful agents, atleast for short period of time. Other agents are present in the environment and different cells of the body get varying degree of exposure to these agents. Highly reactive oxygen radicals are the example of first type while many metals and the ultraviolet radiations are the example of the second type. These agents affect the DNA and cause various types of damage to it. However, only a few of these damages are permanent and majority of the damages are repaired by various mechanisms present in the cell. Any damage which is not repaired, leads to a mutation. In one of the rare inherited genetic diseases of human, the person is deficient in DNA repair enzymes. In this condition, referred as 'Bloom's Syndrome', there is a dramatic increase in the incidence of various cancers. The damage to DNA can either be a single base change or the damage to an extended region which results in structural distortion and affects the function of the genome.

Types of DNA damage

The common damage to DNA is caused by any of the following processes.

1. Deamination

Deamination is a spontaneous process. As a result of deamination, the cytidine residue is converted to uracil and adenine is converted to hypoxanthine. Similarly guanine is converted to xanthine and 5-methyl cytosine is converted to thymine (Fig. 11.7). It has been estimated that in human, the spontaneous deamination will result in change of approximately 100 bases/genome/day. It should be pertinent to point out here that the products of G and A deamination, xanthine and hypoxanthine respectively, are not the constituents of nucleic acids. The 5 methyl cytosine which is not present in DNA normally, is a precursor for T formation. However, the product of C deamination U, is a normal constituent of RNA. Probably this is the reason why nature does not have U in DNA. Had U been the normal constituent of DNA, the formation of U by deamination of C may not have been recognized as a damage and as a result, the rate of spontaneous mutation would have been extraordinarily high.

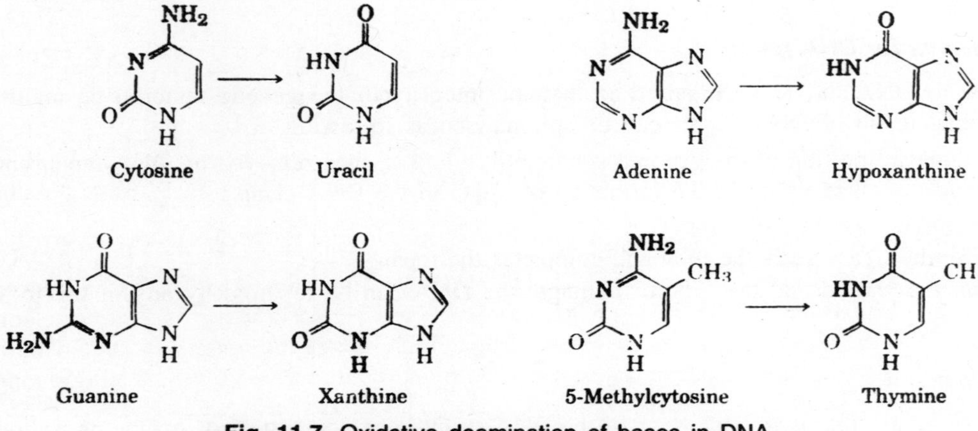

Fig. 11.7. Oxidative deamination of bases in DNA.

2. Depurination

Under different environmental conditions, there is loss of the bases, specially that of the purines, from DNA. Should a sugar become debasic, it is prone to break down and results in DNA damage. It has been estimated that due to fluctuations in environmental temperature, an average of about 5000 purines are lost from human genome every day from an eukaryotic cell.

3. Thymine dimer formation

Ultraviolet light is highly damaging. The body is consistantly exposed to UV of solar radiation. The UV causes the formation of thymine dimers by following reaction (Fig. 11.8). Similar dimer formation can take place by oxidative damage also. Cytosine, on the other hand, forms cytosine hydrate by reacting with atmospheric water in presence of UV.

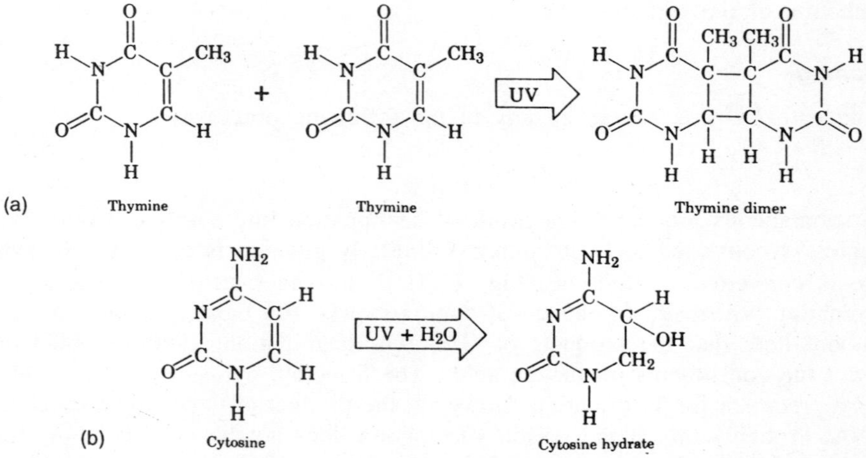

Fig. 11.8. Pyrimidine photoproducts of UV irradiation. (a) Crosslinking of adjacent thymine molecules to form thymine dimers, which block replication. (b) Hydrolysis of cytosine to a hydrate form that may cause mispairing of bases during replication.

Basic pathways for DNA repair

Any damage to DNA has to be repaired so that the integrity of the genetic material be maintained. The basic mechanism of DNA repair can be summarised as following.

  (i) The damaged portion of the genome is recognized and is, then removed by DNA repair enzymes (the nucleases), resulting in the formation of a gap in the DNA chain.
 (ii) DNA polymerase fills this gap.
(iii) Finally, the ligase seals the nick and completes the repair.

  Based on the extend and the type of damage, the DNA can be repaired by any of the following pathways.

A. Direct repair

In this type of repair, the basic back bone of the DNA structure is not disturbed. All the phosphodiester bonds remain intact. The damaged base is recognized and is replaced by the repair enzymes. Following are some of the cases where the DNA is repaired by the direct repair mechanism.

(a) Repair of pyrimidine dimers by photolyasis

In an energy dependent process assisted by flavin nucleotides, the pyrimidine dimers are converted to individual pyrimidines. The energy is provided by light and the enzyme is the photolyase. In E. coli, the photolyase is a 54 KD protein. The reaction is shown in Fig. 11.9.

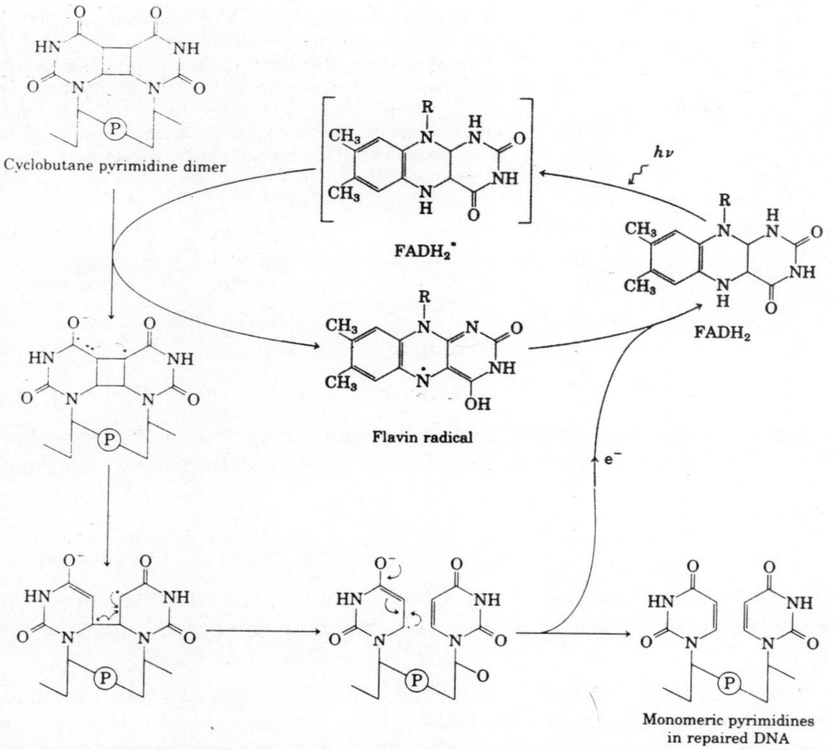

Fig. 11.9. Repair of pyrimidine dimers with photolyase. Shown here is a simplified representation of a pyrimidine dimer. Energy derived from absorbed light is used to reverse the photoreaction that had caused the lesion. The two chromophores in E. coli photolyase, 5,10-methyenyltetrahydrofolate and FADH$_2$, complement each other in terms of the light wavelengths at which they absorb efficiently. Most of the photoreactivating light energy is absorbed by the folate and transferred to FADH$_2$; some of it is absorbed directly by FADH$_2$. The excited form of FADH$_2$ transfers an electron to the pyrimidine dimer, regenerating FADH$_2$. The pyrimidine dimer species containing a free radical is unstable and breaks down to form the monomeric pyrimidines.

(b) Repair of O⁶-methylguanine

Guanine can be methylated at the O^6 position to form 6-methyl guanine. The configiration of O^6 methyl guanine allows its base pairing with thymine (in place of cytosine). As a result, a T can be incorporated in place of C during the replication, should the O^{6}mG remain unrepaired. The O^{6}mG is converted back to G by the activity of an enzyme O^6 methyl guanine DNA methyl transferse by following reaction (Fig. 11.10).

The mechanism of the action of the enzyme is complex. The enzyme has a Cys residue which is capable of accepting the methyl group. Once methylated, the enzyme becomes inactive. A fresh molecule of enzyme is required for the transfer of every methyl group. Thus the enzyme itself participates in the reaction and acts as a methyl group acceptor. As an enzyme itself does not participate in a normal reaction, the protein methyl transferase is not an enzyme in true sense.

The fact that an entire protein molecule is required for the repair of a single damaged base and the protein is not recycled but has to be synthesized de novo every time, shows the importance of DNA repair in cellular metabolism.

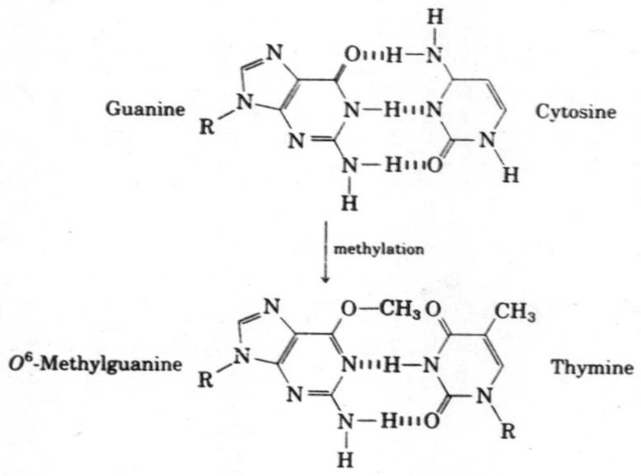

Direct repair of O^6-methylguanine is carried out by O^6-methylguanine-DNA methyltransferase, which catalyzes the transfer of the methyl group of O^6-methylguanine to a specific Cys residue on the same protein. This methyltransferase is not strictly an enzyme, because a single methyl transfer event inactivates the protein. The consumption of an entire protein molecule to correct a single damaged base is another vivid illustration of the central importance of maintaining the integrity of cellular DNA.

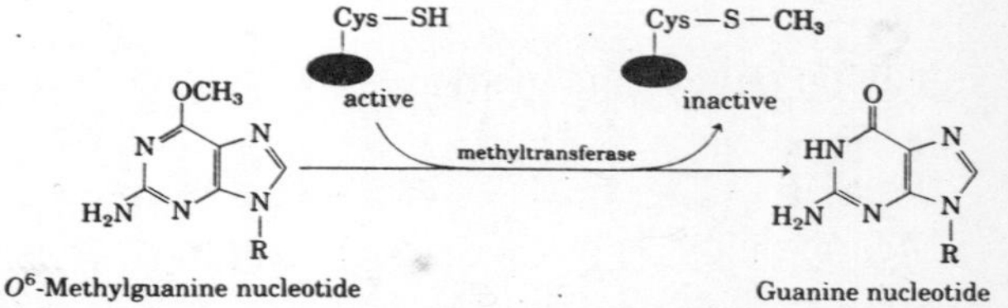

Fig. 11.10. Direct repair of O^6-methyl G by specific DNA methyl transferase. The methyl group from O^6-methyl G is transferred to Cys residue in the enzyme resulting in loss of biological activity of the enzyme.

B. Excision repair

In this type of repair, the damaged portion of the DNA is excised off and then this is replaced by fresh polynucleotide having correct bases. Based on the extend of damage, it could be either one of the following two types.

(a) *Base excision repair* : If only one base is damaged, then it is repaired by this method. The most common cause for a single base damage in the DNA is by spontaneous depurination or by deamination. To repair this damage, the damaged base is removed by a specific glycosilase which recognizes the altered base and removes it by hydrolysing the glycosidic bond between the base and the sugar. For example, uracil glycosilase removes an U from the DNA chain. As discussed, U is formed by spontaneous deamination of C. This is the most common one base damage and the enzyme uracil glycosilase is highly prevalent. It is highly specific for DNA only and does not act on RNA. Other glycosilases specifically remove the alkylated bases such as 3-methyl A or 7-methyl G. Still another glycosilase can remove a pyrimidine dimer. Once the base is removed, the DNA becomes abasic and this site in the DNA is referred as an AP site (AP is both for apurinated or apyrimidinated). Sometimes an AP site can also be produced by very slow hydrolysis of a glycosidic bond in a spontaneous manner. Once AP site is formed, then the abasic sugar is removed by specific endonuclease, the AP endonuclease, and a nick is created. The DNA polymerase I fills the gap. Finally, the DNA ligase seals the nick and the DNA is repaired (Fig. 11.11).

(b) *Nucleotide excision repair* : Whenever there is relatively large distortion and a large number of bases are damaged, a lesion is formed in the DNA. An enzyme, ABC excinuclease, recognizes the lesion and removes the damaged portion by making two simultaneous cuts at both the ends of the damage. The excinuclease thus differs from a common endonuclease as the excinuclease makes two simultaneous cuts in the DNA, therefore, removes a stretch of nucleotides and not a single cut as is made by endonuclease which would only form a nick. The ABC excinuclease is a three subunit enzyme of 246 KD, the subunits are coded by the genes urvA, urvB and urvC, respectively. The enzyme can recognize the damages such as the pyrimidine dimers formed by cyclobutane, the photoproducts of DNA bases and many other base adducts. Once the damaged region is removed, the polymerase I fills it and ligase seals it (Fig. 11.12).

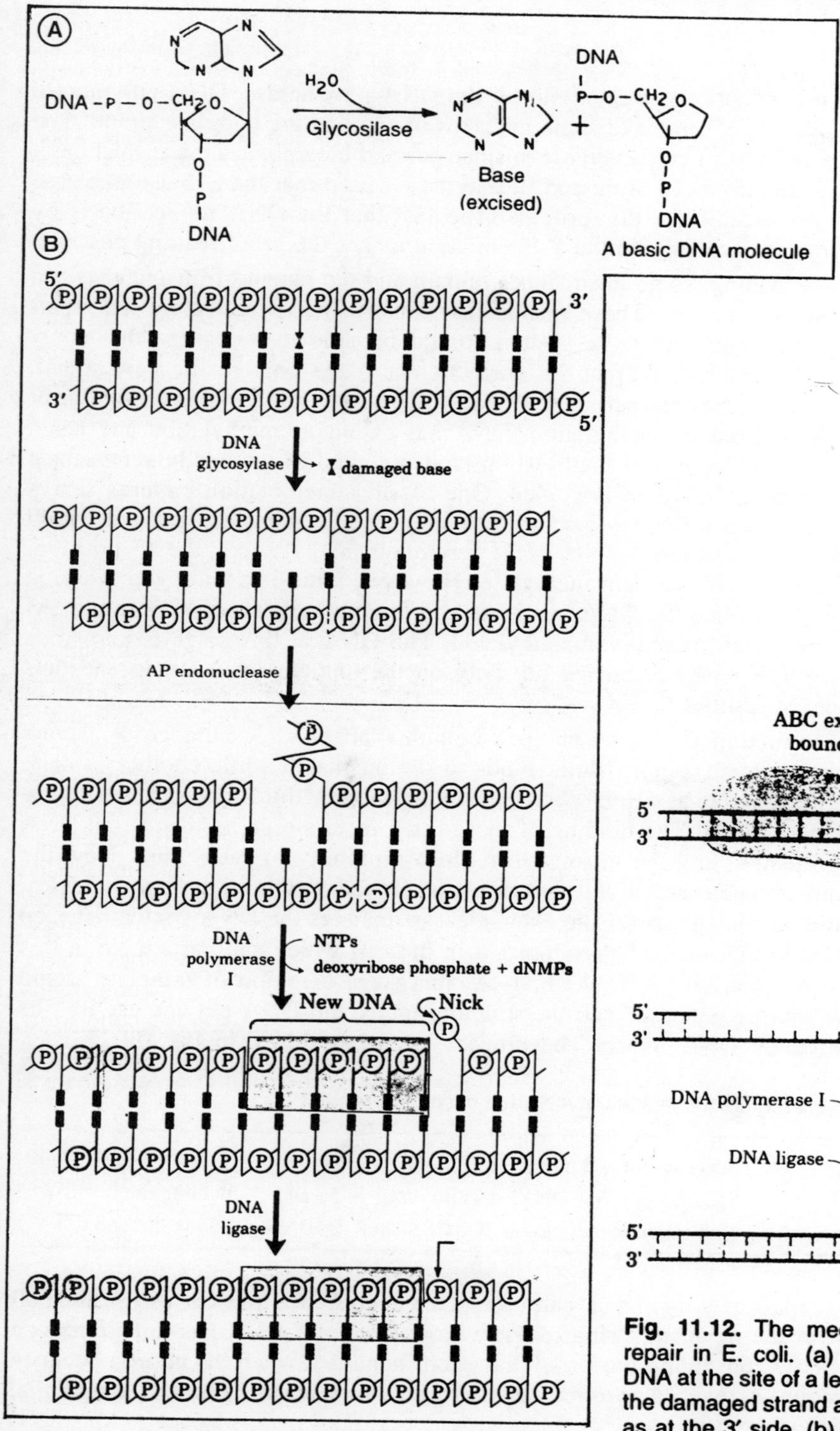

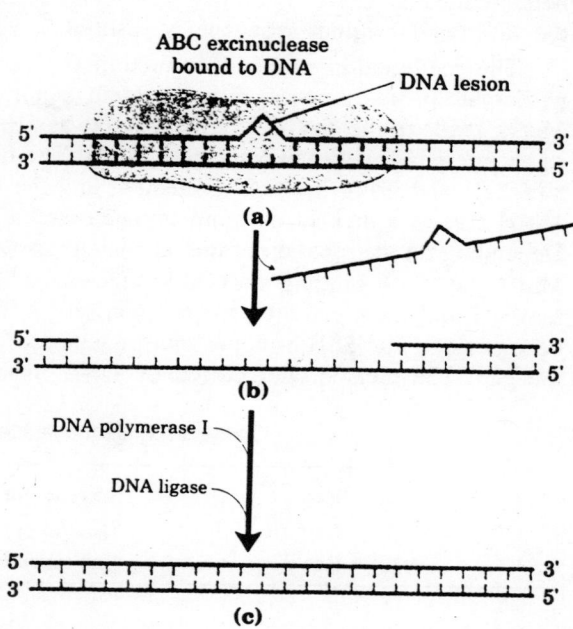

Fig. 11.12. The mechanism of nucleotide excision repair in E. coli. (a) The ABC excinuclease bind to DNA at the site of a lesion and simultaneously cleaves the damaged strand at the 5′ side of the lesion as well as at the 3′ side. (b) Excinuclease then removes the resulting oligonucleotide that spans the damaged base. (c) The resulting gap is filled in by DNA polymerase I and sealed by ligase.

Fig. 11.11. Base excision repair. (a) Formation of an AP site by specific glycosilase. (b) Repair of the damaged DNA by AP endonuclease.

C. Mismatch repair

As discussed earlier, the replication of DNA is carried out by the DNA polymerase. DNA polymerase faithfully copies the template, however, it can make some mistakes in copying the template strand. The proof reading function of DNA polymerase I corrects these mismatches and incorporates the correct base. The details of proof reading have already been discussed. It may be recalled that the 3'-5' exonuclease activity of DNA polymerase is responsible for this process. The fact that the DNA replication is by tail polymerization and the polymerase acts only in the 5'-3' direction makes the proof reading possible.

However, even after the proof reading, some mismatches remain and the extent of mismatches can still be too high to be acceptable by the cell. These mismatches have to be corrected by the repair enzymes. In order to repair, it is essential that the system should be able to recognize the newly synthesized strand from the template strand, so that the correction is made only in the new strand. Should the correction be made in the parent strand, it will lead to a mutation. This differentiation of new strand from old strand is carried out by methylation. DNA has extensive methylation and has a large number of methylated bases. The pattern of methylation is also copied in the newly synthesized strand in the same manner as the base sequence is copied. One of such methylation patterns serves as the 'tag' for the differentiation between the new and the old strands. The A residue present within a tetranucleotide, GATC, which is repeated many times in the genome is methylated at the N^6 position. The methylation is carried out by the enzyme dam methylase. However, there is a time gap (varying from few seconds to few minutes) between the DNA synthesis and the methylation of new strand. As a result, for a short time, the new strand remains unmethylated. The DNA at this stage is known as hemimethylated DNA. The mismatch repair is carried out only on the unmethylated strand and thus the fiditity of original sequence is ensured.

The methylation directed correction of mismatch is a complex process. A number of factors participate in this process. First a protein factor, MutS, binds to the mismatch while another protein, MutH, binds to the GATC site. MutH acts as a site specific endonuclease. A third factor, MutL serves as an interphase between MutS and MutH. The binding of these three factors together bends the DNA molecule and bring the GATC element and the mismatch in close proximity to each other. Now the MutH creates a nick in the unmethylated strand and makes a site for the action of the exonucleases. Depending on the location of the mismatch, one of the exonucleases removes the DNA stretch between MutH and MutL binding sites. Different exonucleases present in the cell which can participate in this removal and their activites are summarised in Table 11.1. At this stage a region of template strand becomes SS. The SSB proteins and the helicase keep the structure intact and DNA polymerase III fills the gap. The nick is later closed by DNA ligase. The process has been shown in Fig. 11.13.

Table 11.1. Exonucleases involved in mismatch repair

(a)	Exo I	Specific for SS DNA, acts in 3'-5' direction
(b)	Exo III	Specific for SS DNA, acts in both 3'-5' and 5'-3' direction
(c)	Rec J	Non-specific, acting on both SS and ds DNA in 5'-3' direction

It has been found that the repair of a mismatch can take place even if it is present as for as 1000 bp from the GATC site. Thus for the repair of a single base a large stretch of DNA has to be removed and re-synthesized. This is a energy consuming process. It has been found that when the genetic integrity of the cell is on stake, the amount of energy required for its repair is irrelevant. The DNA repair is, in general, very energy inefficient process.

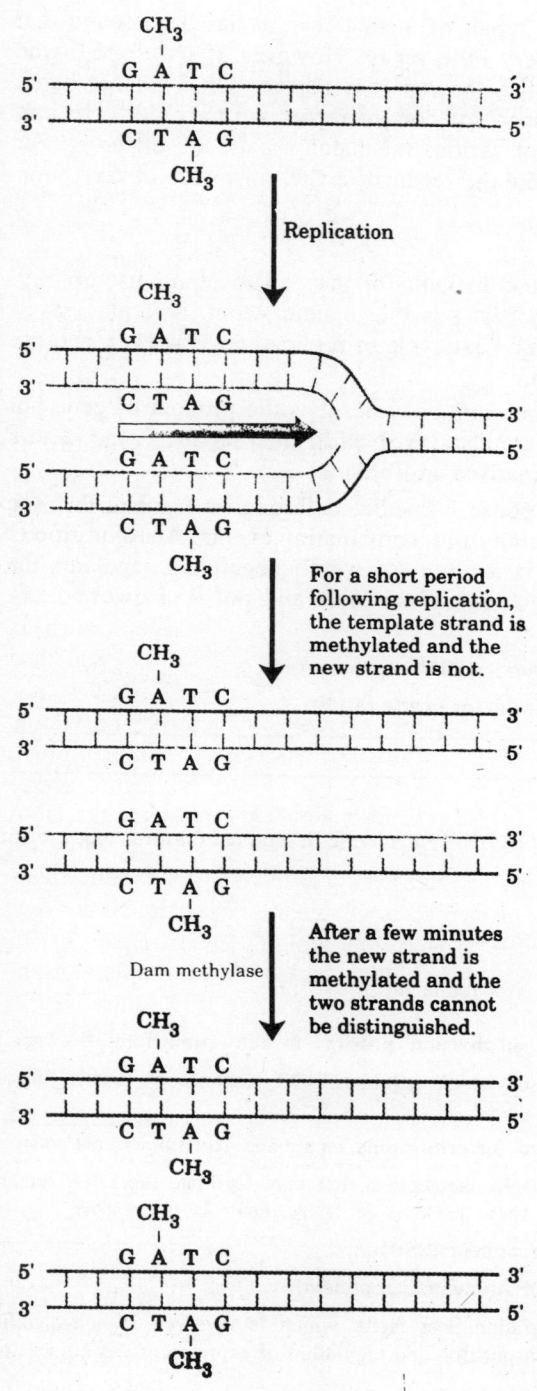

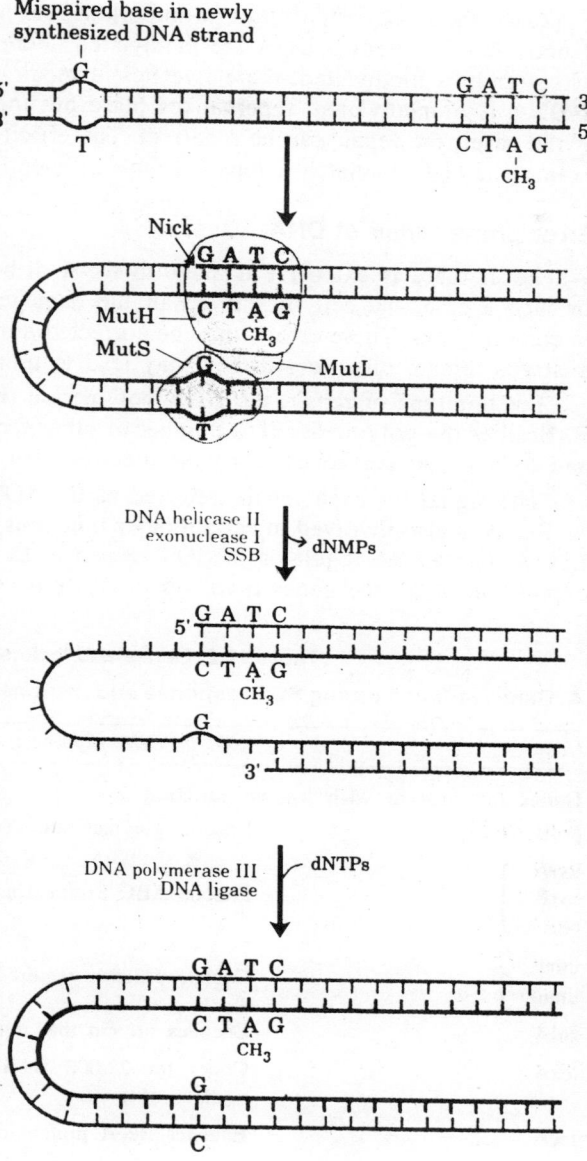

Fig. 11.13. Methylation of DNA strands can serve to distinguish the template strands from newly synthesized strands in E. coli DNA, which plays a critical role in mismatch repair. The methylation occurs at N6 of adenines in a palindrome GATC, which is repeated many times in the DNA. A number of protein factors and enzymes are involved in this repair process.

Thus, the methylation plays an important role in the repair of mismatches. It has been found that if both the strands of a DNA are methylated, there is very little repair. However, if only one of the two strands is methylated, there is efficient repair and also the repair is correct. On the other hand, if DNA is unmethylated, repair takes plase but the chances of correct repair are only 50%. In half of the cases, the repair can be incorrect. The efficiency of various mismatch repairs are different. For example, a G:T mismatch is repaired most efficiently while the repair of a C:C mismatch is very poor.

Error prone repair of DNA

Whenever there is extensive damage to DNA, it becomes difficult for the cell to repair it correctly. In such a case, the cell tries to repair the damage in a best possible manner, even if it may result in certain errors. These errors, may be corrected during the next cycle of replication. However, if these mistakes remain uncorrected they may lead to mutation.

For this type of repair, the DNA polymerase II is the main enzyme. It is the product of gene pol B. Besides the polymerase II, a number of other factors are also involved in such repair. These factors and their respective genes and their functions are summarised in Table 11.2.

The signal for such repair, referred as the SOS response is mediated through a protein, the Rec A. Rec A is also involved in certain other functions, specially in recombination events. Another protein Lex A acts as the regulator of SOS response. Lex A is a repressor which negatively regulates the expression of all the genes involved in this process, including the Rec A and pol B. However, Lex

Table 11.2. Genes and factors involved in DNA repair system

A. Genes induced during SOS response and responsible for error prone repair.

Gene	Role in DNA repair
Genes for protein with known function	
polB (dinA)	Encodes polymerization subunit of DNA polymerase II, required for error-prone repair
uvrA uvrB uvrC	Encode ABC excinuclease
umuC umuD	Encode proteins required for error-prone repair
sulA	Encodes protein that inhibits cell division, possibly to allow time for DNA repair
lexA	Codes for 22,000 Da repressor which regulates SOS response by controlling a number of genes
recA	Encodes RecA protein required for error-prone repair and recombinational repair
	Genes primarily involved in DNA metabolism, but may facilitate the DNA repair, however, the precise role of these proteins in DNA repair is not known
ssb	Encodes single-strand binding protein (SSB)
uvrD	Encodes DNA helicase II (DNA-unwinding protein)
himA	Encodes the subunit of integration host factor which is involved in site-specific recombination, replication, transposition and regulation of expression of a number of genes
recN	Involved in recombinational repair.

B. Genes involved in other repair mechanisms

recB	Codes for Exonuclease V (ATPase)	Needed for recombination and recombi
recC	Codes for Exonuclease V (DNA binding)	nation-repair
recD	Codes for Exonuclease V (58 K subunit)	
sbcB	Codes for Exonuclease I,	The precise role not known
recJ	Codes for single-strand DNA exonuclease	Precise function not known
recNOR	The product is not known	It is involved as part of recF pathway
recQ	Codes for DNA helicase; ATPase activity	
recE	Exonuclease VIII	Not known
dam	Methylase acts on GATC pattendrome	Identifies "old" DNA strand
mutH	Endonuclease	Components of repair
mutL	Not known	system, acting on newly
mutS	Recognizes mismatched pairs	synthesized DNA strand
uvrD	DNA helicase II	
mutY	Adenine glycosylase	Excises A from mismatches
ada	Guanine methyl transferase	Removes CH_3 from guanine
alkA	Methyl adenine glycosylase, it	Removes CH_3 from adenine/guanine
Ion	ATP-dependent protease that binds to DNA	May control genes for capsular polysaccharide

Genes with unknown function which may have role in DNA repair

dinB
dinD
dinE
recF

A, which is a 22.7 KD protein, can also undergo an autocleavage at a specific Ala-Gly site and is cleaved into two parts of roughly equal size. This cleavage takes place at high pH. At the normal pH, it requires Rec A protein for its cleavage. Rec A acts as a co-protease for this hydrolysis. It is not able to cleave the protein all by itself but can become a bioactive protease when only it is present along with Lex A. However, Rec A cannot carry out this co-protease function unless it is associated with SS:DNA also. While Rec A gene is under the influence of the repressor Lex A, a basal level of Rac A (about 1000 copies/cell) are always produced under the constitutive regulation.

The process of such repair is well understood in E. coli. The genes, dinF, uvrA, polB, dinB, urvB, sulA, umuC, umuD (often referred togather as umuCD) and recA, each has a operator which is repressed by Lex A. Thus under normal conditions none of these proteins are produced, except small amounts of RecA are produced in constitutive manner. Whenever there is extensive damage to DNA (such as the result of long exposure to UV), the regions of SS DNA are formed which remain uncorrected. The constitutively produced Rec A binds to these regions and the SSDNA:RecA complex, in association with LexA, breaks the LexA. The cleavage of Lex A results in derepression of all the repair genes and all these proteins, including the Rec A are synthesized. This triggers the SOS response and error prone repair of DNA takes place. DNA polymearse II tries to repair the DNA damage while the protein Sul A inhibits the cell division. Other factors essential for the repair are produced by the genes umu C and umu D. The process has been summariased in Fig. 11.13.

The RacA protein serves as the signal between the biological damage and the SOS response. During the SOS response, the cellular level of Rec A protein may increase by a factor of 50-100 fold.

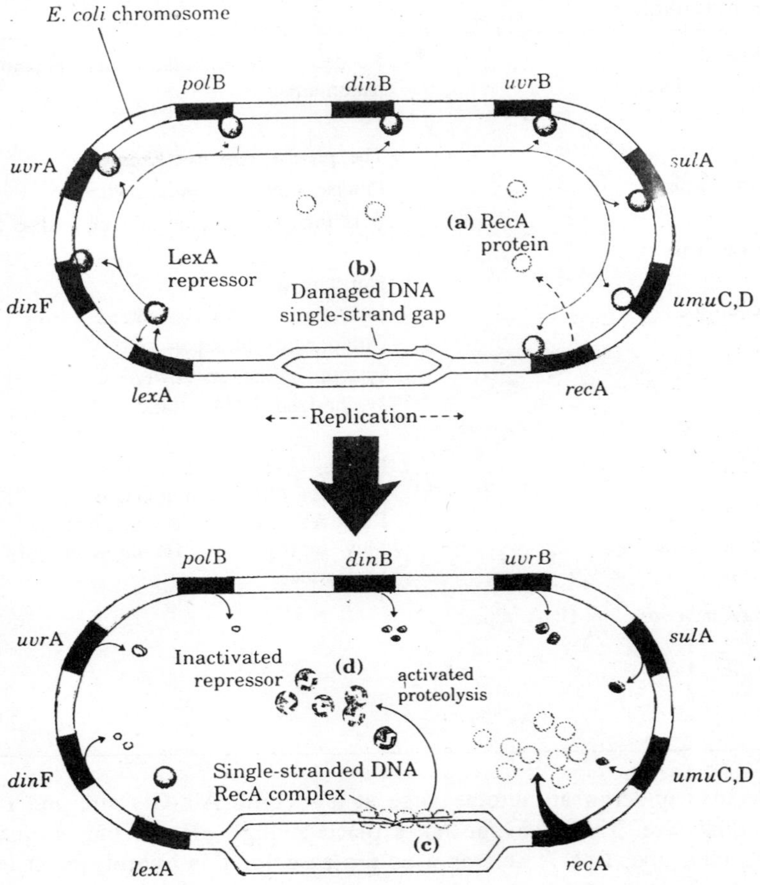

Fig. 11.14. The SOS response. The LexA protein is the repressor of entire system, and acts on an operator site present near each gene. The recA gene is not entirely repressed by the LexA repressor, and about 1,000 RecA protein monomers are normally found in the cell. When DNA is extensively damaged, the replication is halted and the number of single-strand gaps in the DNA are increased. RecA protein binds to this single-stranded region, activating the protein's coprotease activity. While bound to DNA the RecA protein facilitates the cleavage and inactivation of the LexA repressor. When the repressor is inactivated, the SOS genes, including recA, are induced. RecA protein levels increase 50- to 100-fold.

Other mechanisms of DNA repair

Other than the commonly used mechanisms of the DNA repair discussed so far, the cell sometimes uses extraordinary methods for the damage repair. These include the following.

Tolerance system

It enables the cell to overcome the problems which arise due to blockage of normal replication of the DNA as a result of the damage to DNA. In this system, the damaged template is copied. The regions of lesions in DNA can be copied with abnormally high frequency of error. Alternatively, the damaged region of the template is not copied but is later repaired by recombinational events between a fresh copy of the undamaged strand and the breakage in the damaged copy of the DNA strand. This type of system is more frequent in eukaryotes. For these recombinational events, the general rules of recombination are followed. The Holliday intermediates are formed between the two copies and there is either the horizontal cleavage or the vertical cleavage. In former, no recombination takes place while in later case the recombination takes place (Fig. 11.15). The type of damages which are generally repaired by the recombination events include the double stranded break in DNA, the ds crosslinking, the lesion in one strand and damage in other strand.

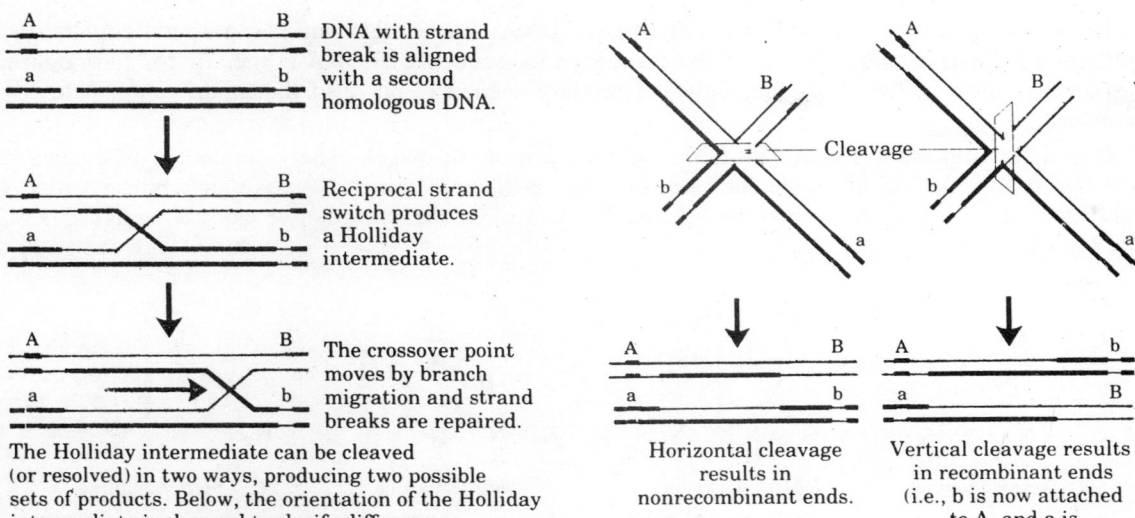

Fig. 11.15. The Holliday model for homologous genetic recombination. Two genes on the homologous chromosomes have different alleles, as indicated by uppercase and lowercase. Note which alleles are linked in the four final products. A Holliday intermediate is formed between two bacterial plasmids in vivo, which can be seen with electron microscope.

Occassionally this type of damage can be repaired by the formation of H DNA intermediate, which is triple stranded.

Retrieval System

If the damage is too extensive, the cell may prefer to abandon the damaged gene, provided another undamaged copy of the gene is present elsewhere in the genome. In such cases, the undamaged gene is later duplicated and the copy gets integrated in place of the damaged gene. This may involve the homologous recombination also.

The repair system in prokaryotes have been well understood, however, the mechanisms in eukaryotes are not very well understood. In certain cases the inefficient repair has been found. The genetic disease, Bloom Syndrome has been discussed earlier. Another disease Xeroderma Pigmentosum (XP), which is a recessive genetic disease has been very well characterized. It results in hypersensitivity to sunlight (specially to UV) resulting in a number of skin disorders.

In general, the DNA repair mechanisms try to repair the damage to DNA. In these processes, the cell does not care for energy conservation and repair processes are usually very energy inefficient. If correct repair is not possible due to extend of damage, the cell will try to minimise the effect of damage by making the error prone damage repairs.

DNA MODIFICATION

The basic structure of DNA is achieved by the polymerization of four different types of nucleotides, which have A, T, G and C as their nitrogeneous bases. However, these bases have a number of modified groups. These modifications serve a number of useful functions to the cell. One of these functions is to differentiate between the self and the foreign DNA. Each organism has a specific pattern of modification which is unique in the similar manner as the sequence of DNA is specific for an organism. During replication of the DNA, not only the primary sequence, but also the modification pattern is maintained.

The most important modification is the methylation of bases. The commonly used sites of methylation are adenine and cytosine. Adenine can be methylated at N^6 position while cytosine is methylated at C^5 position. Other methylated bases are N^2-methyl guanine and 7-methyl guanine (Fig. 11.16)

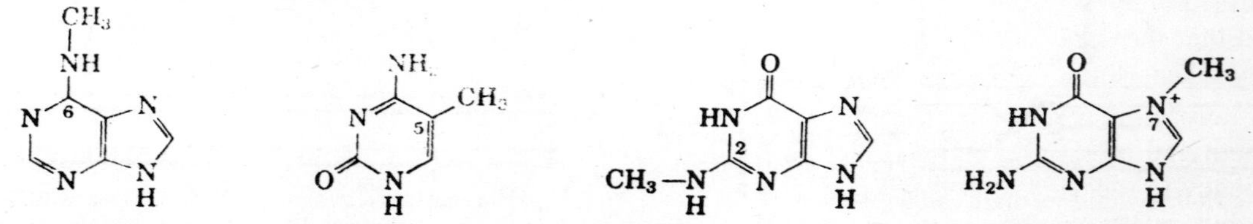

N^6-Methyladenine   5-Methylcytosine N^2-Methylguanine   7-Methylguanine

Fig. 11.16. Structure of methylated bases.

A number of different enzymes participate in methylation. The most commonly used enzymes for methylation are the product of following genes (Table 11.3).

Table 11.3. Enzyme involved in DNA methylation

Enzyme	Gene	Function
Adenosyl methylase	hsd	Methylation of adenosine at C_6 position
Cytosyl methylase	dcm	Methylation of cytosine residue at N_5 position
Dam methylase	dam	Methylation of adenosine in pallendromic sequence GATC, in the newly synthesized DNA stand
Maintenance methylase	—	Imprinting of methylation pattern in newly synthesized DNA
Establishment methylase	—	De novo methylation

(a) *hsd* : The product Hsd methylase causes the methylation of adenine residue.

(b) *dcm* : The product of this gene causes the methylation of cytosine.

(c) *dam* : The Dam methylase causes the methylation of newly synthesized DNA strand at A residue when it is present as a part of the tetranucleotide GATC. The details of this methylation have already been discussed.

In eukaryotes, about 2.7% of the total 'C' residues are methylated. Majority of the methylated 'C' (5-methyl cytosines) are present as the part of C:G duplex. The replication of genome results in the DNA, in which only one of the two strands (the parent strand) will be methylated. Such DNA is referred as the hemi-methylated DNA. The daughter cells contain this form of DNA. The hemi-methylated DNA is later fully methylated by an enzyme referred as maintenance methylase. Maintenance methylase will add methyl groups to the unmethylated strand and the pattern of methylation will be maintained precisely the same as the pattern in the parent strand. However, it cannot methylate an unmethylated DNA. It is possible that the methylation of an unmethylated DNA can take place in a *de novo* manner by another enzyme, the establishment methylase. However, the precise mechanism of establishment methylase action is not fully understood.

Role of methylation

The methylation of DNA plays many important functions. One of the roles is to differentiate between the self and the foreign DNA. In bacteria, there is a set of enzymes refered as the restriction endonucleases, which can break a foreign DNA and serve as the protection against the invading organisms. These enzymes recognize a specific DNA sequence and the pattern of methylation and do not break the self DNA in which this sequence is methylated. In fact, the restriction enzyme system is always present as coupled with the modifcation system.

Methylation also plays an important role in the regulation of gene expression. Many genes are expressed when these are not methylated and are not expressed if methylated. For example, it has been found that the addition of 5-aza cytidine which is an inhibitor of methylation, when added to a culture of myoblasts induces the myoblast cell for their differentiation into non-muscle cells.

Many other genes such as the actin gene, have different expression profile based on the degree of methylation. For example, the methylated and non-methylated genes are expressed with equal efficiency in the muscle cells. However, in the fibroblast cells there is no expression of non-methylated gene but relatively low level expression of the methylated gene takes place. The methylation, thus provides the tissue specificity for actin gene expression.

In the germ cells the methylation is parent specific. A certain pattern of methylation is present in the paternal cell while another methylation pattern may be present in the maternal genes. This specificity of methylation pattern between the two gametes is known as the imprinting. This imprinting may regulate the expression of certain genes and may account for the difference in behaviour between two alleles of a gene which have been inherited from different parents. For example, the genes for TGF II inherited from mother are not expressed, while the same gene inherited from the father is expressed.

Methylation plays a role in binding of regulatory proteins also. It has been found that some non-histone proteins bind specifically to the region of DNA which has a cluster of 5-methyl cytosine. This region is, thus, very rich in methylation. These proteins help in packaging of the DNA in a form which is hard to transcribe. Thus the gene expression is regulated.

Methylation may also result in switching a gene permanently off. For example, if a gene which has regulated expression has been switched off and then methylated, it is silenced permanantly and cannot be switched on again.

12

Transposable Elements

So far we have seen that the genome of an organism has a definite structure which is not variable. Its structure remains static throughout the life of an organism and also does not vary from individual to individual within the same species. It changes only on a leisurely time scale of evolution. However, it has been found that the conservation of structure in certain regions of the genome are not all that rigid. There are stretch of DNA which can move from one place to another place within the genome. These movable elements can not duplicate themselves and may be present in variable copy number in different cells of an individual. Such genes are often referred as the 'jumping genes' or the 'transposons'. The transposons or the transposable elements can be difined as the discrete sequences in the genome which are mobile. These are able to transport themselves from one location to another location within the genome. The presence of transposons has been shown in both the prokaryotes and the eukaryotes. For their movement, these elements donot use extrachromosomal elements (such as the plasmids) but move directly. These elements are of variable length varying from one to several thousand base pairs in length and usually code for a gene(s) which is flanked on both sides by a short direct or inverted repeats (DR or IR respectively, jointly called as the terminal repeats). Based on their structures, these can be divided into following classes.

A. Insertion sequences (IS)

These are the simplest transposition modules. These are the normal constituents of bacterial and plasmid genome. These are autonomous units which code for the proteins necessary for their own transposition. They donot code for any other protein which is beneficial to the the host. These are, therefore, also referred as the 'selfish DNA'. A bacteria such as E. coli may contain several copies of many of the common IS elements.

A number of IS elements have been isolated. These have been grouped in a number of classes each referred as IS-x, where x is a number alloted based on the history of its identification. All the IS elements are short DNA molecules (~ 1000 bp) which have short inverted repeats at their ends. During insertion a small sequence at the site of insertion is duplicated which generates short direct repeats in the target DNA (Fig. 12.1). The evidence for duplication can be obtained by comparing the sequence at the site of insertion before and after the insertion has taken place. The sequence of direct repeats varies from one transposition event to another event, suggesting that a particular IS element does not necessarily recoginize a specific sequence. However, the length of the repeat at the site of insertion is always the same for a particular IS element. A repeat of 9 bases seems to be most common for a number of IS elements. The inverted terminal repeats of an IS element is specific for each IS. Many times the two copies of a repeat may be very closely related rather than identical.

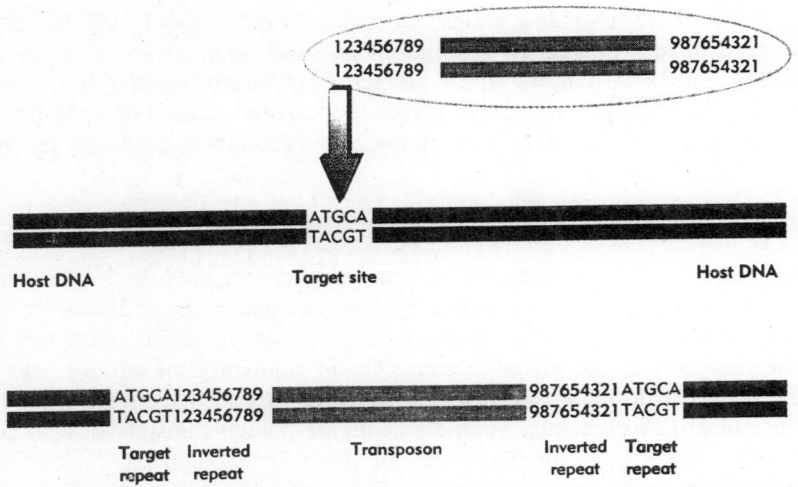

Fig. 12.1. Transposons have inverted terminal repeats and generate direct repeats of flanking DNA at the target site. The ends of the transposon consist of inverted repeats of 9 bp, where the numbers 1 through 9 indicate a sequence of base pairs.

Majority of the IS elements insert at the random sites in the genome. However, some of these show varying degree of preference for specific sites, usually within the 'hot spots'. The characteristics of some of the common IS elements are given in Table 12.1.

Table 12.1. Common IS elements of E. coli

Element	Size	No. of copies/genome
IS1	768 bp	8
IS2	1327 bp	5
IS3	1300 bp	1 or more
IS4	1426 bp	1 or more
IS10	1329 bp	Variable

The inverted repeats of IS-1 have been shown in Fig. 12.1. These repeats define the bounderies of an IS element. These are the recognition sites and any mutation in the ends can prevent the transposition. These ends are recognized by a protein, transposase which is responsible for the transposition. The main body of the IS element codes for the transposase. All the IS elements have only one ORF in this region. The ORF starts just inside the IR at one end and terminates just before or inside the IR on other end. Only known exception is the IS−1, which has two ORFs, both of which are used during the translation by virtue of making a frame shift.

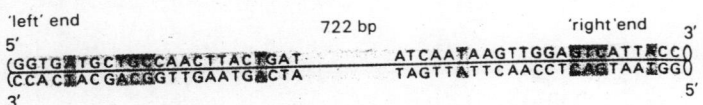

Fig. 12.2. The inverted teminral repeats of IS-1.

While the freguency of transposition varies, the overall rate is about 10^{-3} to 10^{-4} per elements/generation. The reversal of insertion or the removal of an IS element occurs at much lower frequency (about 10^{-6} to 10^{-10}). The insertion of an IS element will inactivate the target gene (insertional inactivation). Often it is associated with other types of mutations also. For example, it can increase or decrease the frequency of deletion and/or inversion of neighbouring genes (to the insertion site) by 100–1000 fold.

Transposons

These are independent transposable elements which are much larger than the IS elements. The function or the factor required for transpostion are coded by the transposon itself. However, it has a number of unrelated genes also. The unrelated genes usually code for certain useful characters such as the drug resistance. Thus the insertion of the element results in the aquisition of certain special characters at the target site. The ends of the elements have the inverted repeats which are relatively longer than the IR of many (but not all) IS elements. Such elements are named transposons and are designated as Tn followed by a number. For example Tn 3, has an IR of 38 nucleotides. It codes for three genes. Two of these genes are the transposition proteins, TnpA and TnpB and the third is the enzyme β-lactamase which provides ampicillin resistance to the target genome.

Composite transposons

These are relatively larger units which have a complex structure. In general, the structure is made of two modules, the transposon which is flanked by two copies of IS elements (Fig. 12.3) on both sides (the arms). These arms of IS elements may be present either as the direct repeat (eg Tn 9) or as the inverted repeats (eg Tn 903). Of course each IS module has its own inverted repeats. Thus the composite transposons are terminated in the same short inverted repeats in which its constituent IS elements were terminating.

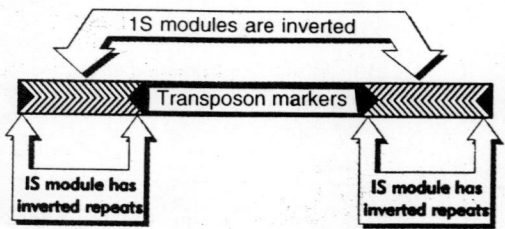

Fig. 12.3. A composite transposon has a central region carrying markers unconnected with transposition (such as drug resistance) flanked by 1S modules. The modules have short inverted terminal repeats. If the modules themselves are in inverted orientation (as shown in figure), the short inverted terminal repeats at the ends of the transposon are identical.

Sometimes the arms are not the true repeats of each other but may be closely related to one another. The example of such a case is Tn 10 and Tn 5. The structure of some of the composite transposons has been shown in Fig. 12.4.

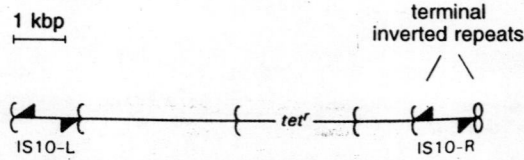

Fig. 12.4. The composite transposon Tn10 has two copies of IS10 flanking a central DNA segment. The central region codes for tetracyclin resistance.

If a composite transposon is inserted in a small circular molecule such as a plasmid, which has other markers also, then the IS elements within the transposon will border the original transposon in one orientation while these will also border the plasmid marker, but in other orientation. It is then possible to move either the original transposon or the plasmid marker gene as an 'in side out' of the original transposon (Fig. 12.5).

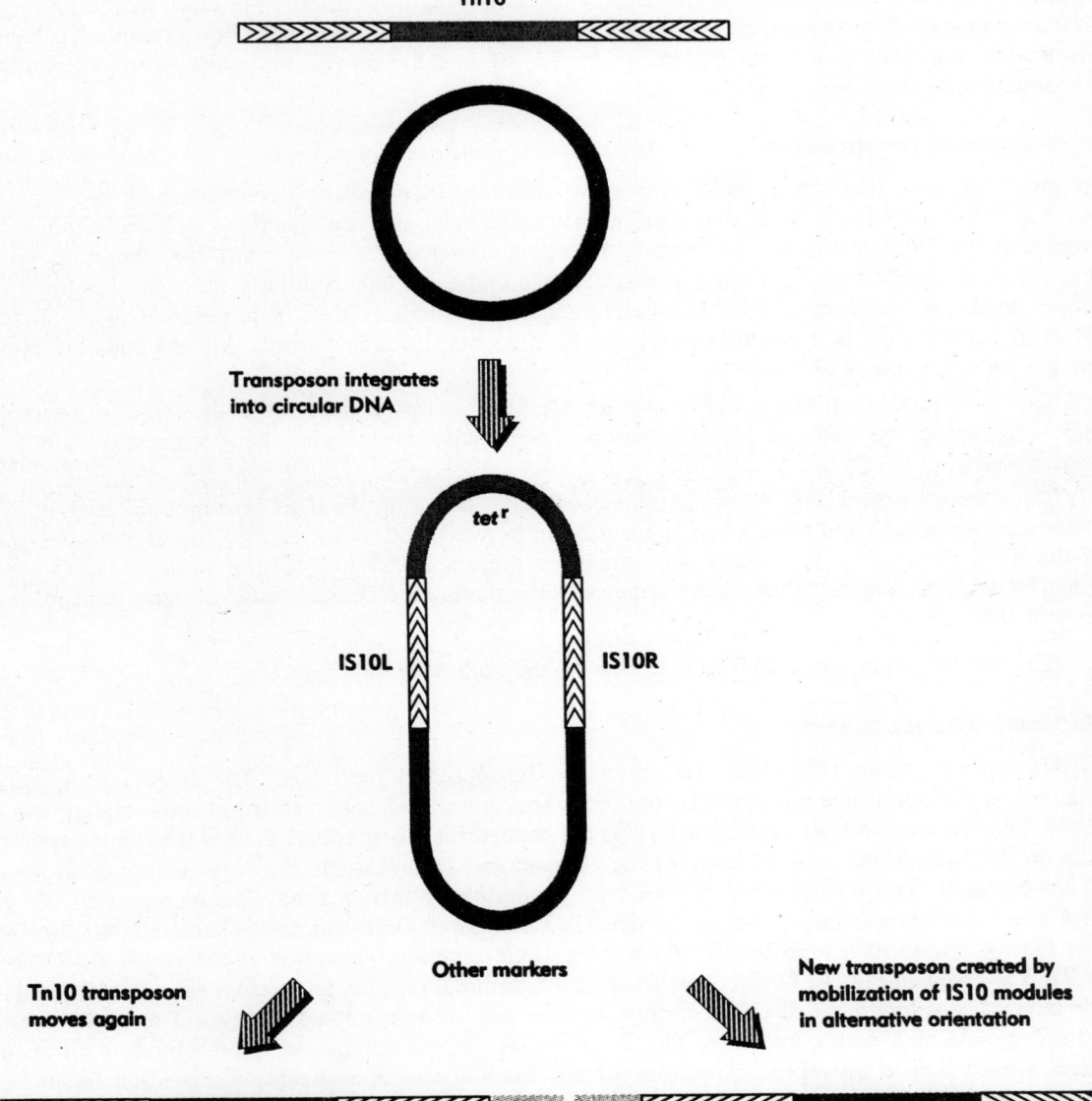

Fig. 12.5. Two IS10 modules create a composite transposon that can mobilize any region of DNA that lies between them. When Tn10 is part of a small circular molecule such as a plasmid, the IS10 repeats can transpose either side of the circle. Transposition of tetR corresponds to the movement of Tn10. Transposition of the markers on the other side creates a new "inside-out" transposon.

In a composite transposon, it is possible either to move the entire transposon or as an alternative, only the bordering IS sequences can move. However, if a selection pressure for the marker is present during the transposition, it fovours the movement of the entire gene.

As far as the target sites for the transposition are concerned, sometimes it has homology with the termini of the transposons. Sometimes, on the other hand, there may not be any homology and the insertion may be at random places. However, an A:T rich region is usually preferred over other regions. Certain elements have a tendancy to move along a palindromic sequence. For example Tn 5 inserts inself into the CTAG tetranucleotide while Tn 10 usually moves to a site with a palindromic septanucleotide sequence GCTNAGC.

Mechanism of transposition

As any composite transposon has a number of different independent elements which are capable of moving independently, it is valid to assume that these have evolved when two originally independent molecules (the IS elements) got associated with a central region (the transposon). It is, therefore, possible that the IS elements alone can move in place of the entire module. Similarly the central module could move alone too. As discussed in the above example of circuler DNA, it is possible to mobilize any DNA of correct size, if it is bordered by the IS elements. In other words, only the ends are required for the mobilization of the gene(s).

The transposase activity coded by the IS elements is responsible for both, creating a target site and recognizing the ends of the transposon. The precise events and their order is not very well understood.

The transposition occurs by a general procedure as following. First an asymmetrical nick is created at the target site and the transposon is inserted in between the nicks. Due to the assymetrical nature of the nick, there are a few bases which may be present as SS in both the strands. These are now filled by the polymerase. Thus at the target site the duplicated characteristic of each transposons are created (Fig. 12.6).

The transposition can take place in one of the following manners.

Replicative transposition

In this type of transposition, the element to be transposed is replicated. The original copy remains attached at the donor site while the second copy transposes and gets inserted at the recipient site (Fig. 12.7). Thus two separate enzymatic activities are needed for this purpose. First is the transposase which acts on the ends of the original copy of the element and second is the resolvase that acts on the copy of the element. The transposons of the group TnA family migrate by this method. The elements of the group TnA are large transposons of ~5 kb in size. Tn3 and Tn1000 are the best characterized elements of this family. These have ~38 bp IR and a 5 bp direct repeat is generated at the target site. The map of Tn 3 is given in Fig. 12.8. This has the inverted terminal repeats, an internal res site (for resolution, see later). It has a number of ORFs coding for two transposition related proteins, TnpA and TnpR and a third gene which codes for amp^r. The TnpA codes for the transposase which binds with about 25 bases within the 38 bp repeat. Adjacent to this binding site is a site for the binding of an E. coli protein, IHF. The transposase and the IHF bind co-operatively. However, IHF does not have a well defined role and is not essential for transposition. Protein TnpR acts as resolvase and also have a function as the regulator of gene expression. It is a repressor which inhibits TnpA as well as its own production. The two genes are present in opposite orientation to each other and are controlled from a common A:T rich region.

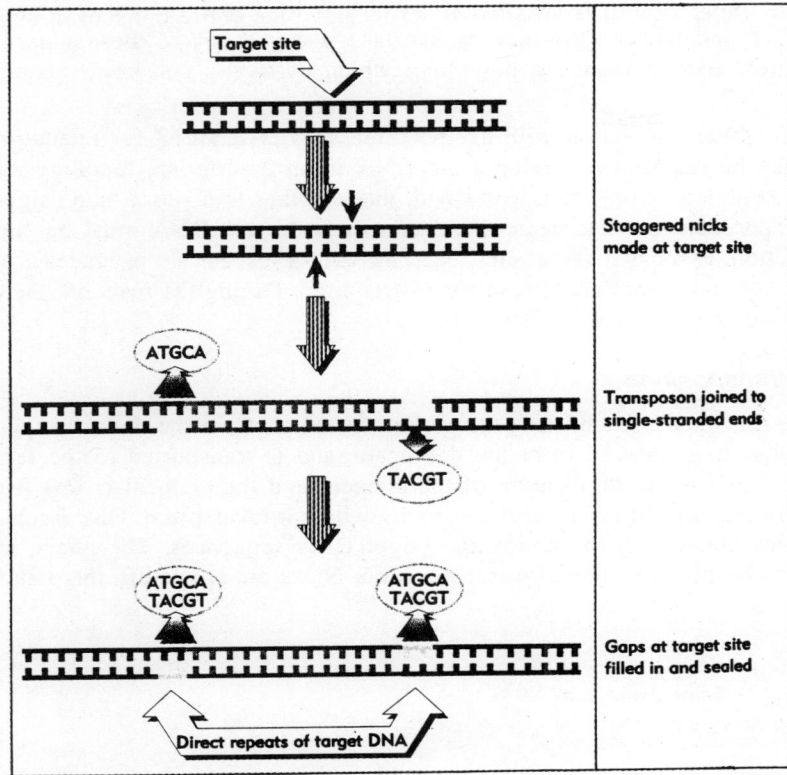

Fig. 12.6. The direct repeats of target DNA flanking a transposon are generated by the introduction of staggered cuts whose protruding ends are linked to the transposon.

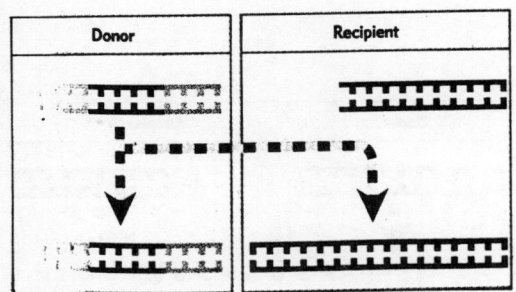

Fig. 12.7. Replicative transposition creates a copy of the transposon, which inserts at a recipient site. The donor site remains unchanged, so both donor and recipient have a copy of the transposon.

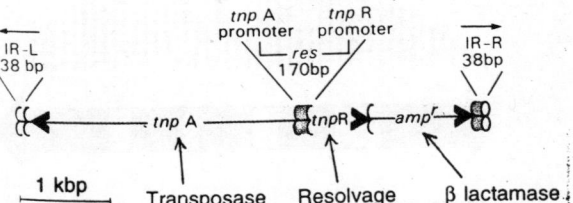

Fig. 12.8. The non-composite transposon Tn3. The direction of transcription of the three genes has been shown by arrows.

TnpR is involved in the recombination between the direct repeats of Tn3 for the formation of a co–integrate structure. It is then resolved by hemologous recombination at specific sites. The mechanism of resolution is shown in Fig. 12.9. The site of resolution is known as the res site. The resolution can take place in the absence of res by Rec A mediated general recombination. There are three sites, site I, II and III, and the binding can take place to any of these sites in an independent manner. These sites share a sequence homology which defines a consensus sequence with a dyad symmetry.

It is not clear if the interaction with all the three sites is required for resolution. Binding at all the three sites may be required for holding the DNA in an appropriate topology. The interaction of the protein-DNA complex of one transposon with that of other transposon may trigger the resolution. In the in vitro experiments, it has been found that the substrate DNA must be supercoiled. As the result of transposition, two catenated circles, each havaing a res site are produced. No host factors are needed but relatively large amounts of resolvase is required. During the reaction, the bonds are broken and rejoined without any demand of energy.

Non-replicative transposition

In non-replicative transposition the transposing element moves from the donor site to the recipient site as a physical entity. It is cleaved from the donor site and is transported to the recipient site where it gets integrated. There is no duplication of the element and the element is lost from the donor site (Fig. 12.10). There are two different mechanisms by which it takes place. One mechanism, as used by phage mu, involves connecting the donor and target DNA sequences. The phage integrates into the host genome by non-replicative mode of transposition. Nicks are created in the donor strand on either

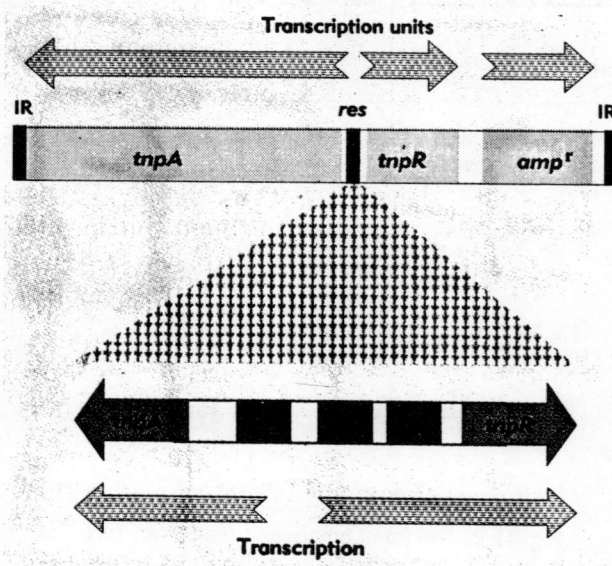

Fig. 12.9. Transposons of the TnA family have inverted terminal repeats, an internal res site, and three known genes coding for proteins $T_{np}A$, $T_{np}R$ and amp^r.

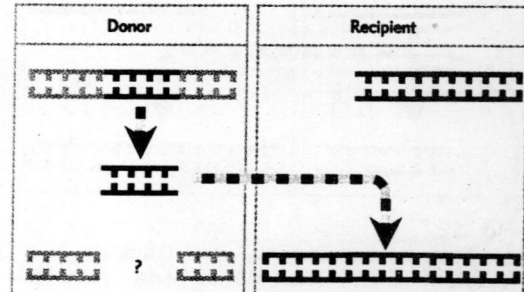

Fig. 12.10. Nonreplicative transposition allows a transposon to move as a physical entity from the donor site to a recipient site. This would leave a break at the donor site, which could be lethal to the genome unless it is repaired.

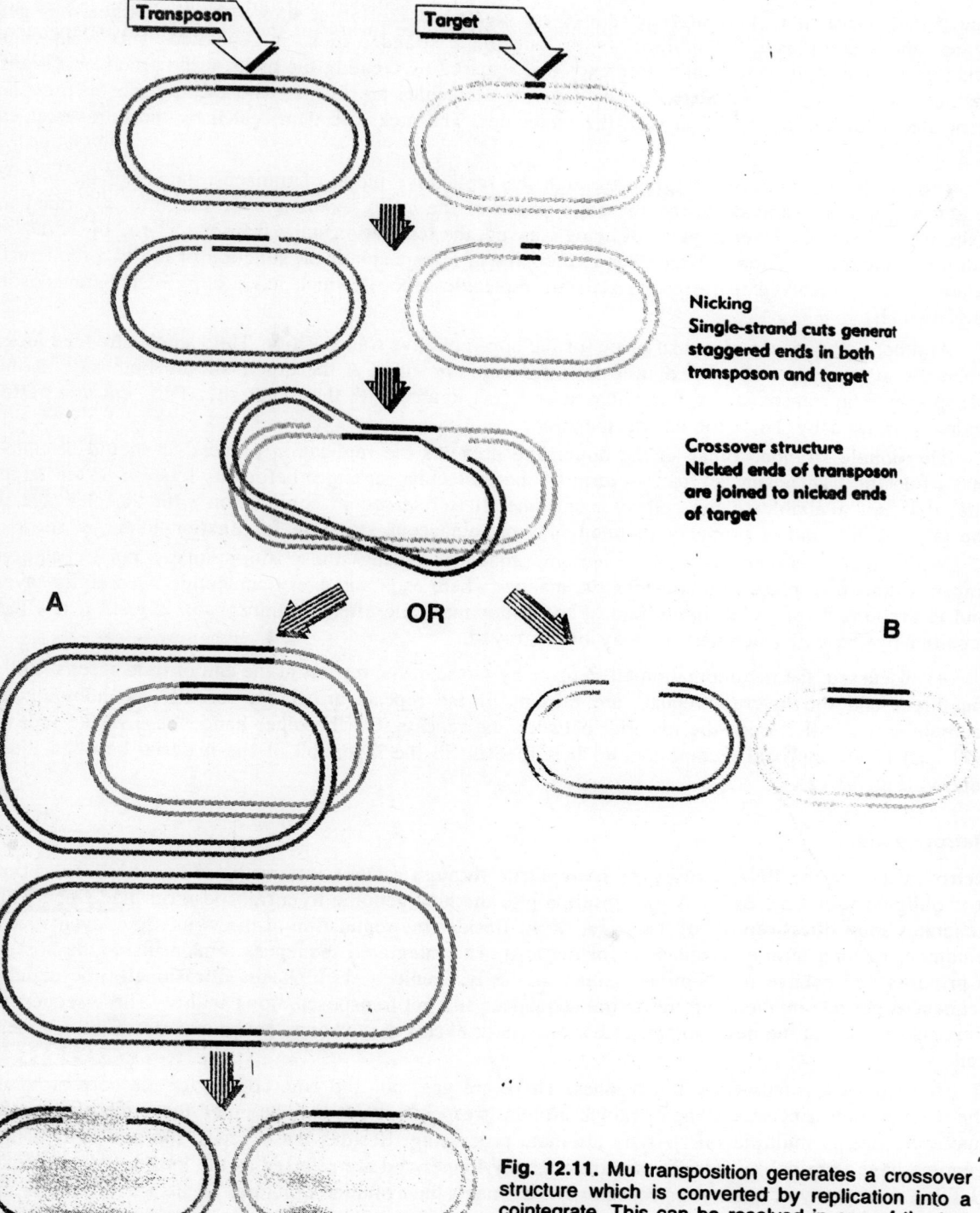

Nicking
Single-strand cuts generat
staggered ends in both
transposon and target

Crossover structure
Nicked ends of transposon
are joined to nicked ends
of target

Fig. 12.11. Mu transposition generates a crossover
structure which is converted by replication into a
cointegrate. This can be resolved in one of the two
ways; as shown in A & B.

side of the transposon. Similarly, the nicks are created at the target sites also. The target sites get ligated and a complex DNA molecule with four single stranded nicks is generated. This cross over structure is then replicated from 3' free ends and released by creating the nicks at the precise positions on the donor molecule. As a result, two separate molecules are formed and the transposon remains associated with the target site in both the molecules. The nicks are then sealed by the host enzymes (Fig. 12.11A).

The mu phage can also integrate through the replicative mode of transposition. Both the modes follow a common pathway during the early phase of the cycle. A cross over structure is formed in a similar manner. However in place of being cleaved, the replication starts from the 3'-end of the DNA and a co–integrate is formed which has two copies of transposon at the junction of the two replicons. These are then resolved to form two separate molecules one of which has a copy of the transposon (Fig. 12.11B).

Another pathway can also take place for the non-repliative transposition. Here single stranded nicks are made at the target site but double stranded cuts are made at the donor site on both side of the transposon. The transposon is thus released and gets ligated with the target site. This 'cut and paste' pathway is used by Tn10 for its transposition.

The double stranded break at the donor site prevents the replication process. It should be noted that while the transposon is 'free' in term of the molecular structure before its ligation to the target site, it is not available to the cell as a episome. It is released in conjunction with the cleavage in the target DNA and is probably retained in a proteinaceous structure for ligation to target site.

While there may be deletion of certain sequences during transposition, many non–repeatitive transpositions take place in a conservative manner where each and every nucleotide is carefully saved and is accounted for. What is the fate of the donor molecule after the transposon is lost? It is either repaired by the cell machinery or may be distroyed.

As discussed, the recombination takes place by virtue of the repeats at the end of transposons. Both, the direct and the inverted repeats are present. If the repeats are direct repeats, the homologous recombination will release the material between the repeats. On the other hand, the inverted repeats will lead to a reciprocal recombination. It will result in the inversion of the material between these repeats (Fig. 12.12).

Retroposons

Retroviruses are the RNA viruses which replicate through a DNA intermediate. For their replication it is obligatory that the ds DNA gets inserted into the host genome by a transposition like event. This generates short direct repeats of the target DNA. Besides the replication of the virus, these events have a number of long term consequences for the host. The integrated sequences remain inside the host as a provirus and behave in a similar manner as the lysogenic bacteriophage. Occasionally the cellular sequences get recombined with retroviral sequences and get transposed along with it. These sequences thus get inserted at the new genomic location. These events may change the properties of the recipient cell.

A retrovirus usually have three genes. These are gag, pol and env, coding for the core proteins, the reverse transcriptase and the envalope proteins, respectively. It may be noted that each of the gene may give rise to multiple mRNAs by alternate processing. Besides these genes, the two ends of the genome have terminal repeats. These are relatively longer and are referred as the long terminal repeats (LTRs). A majority of eukaryotic transposable elements have similar structure. These are referred as the

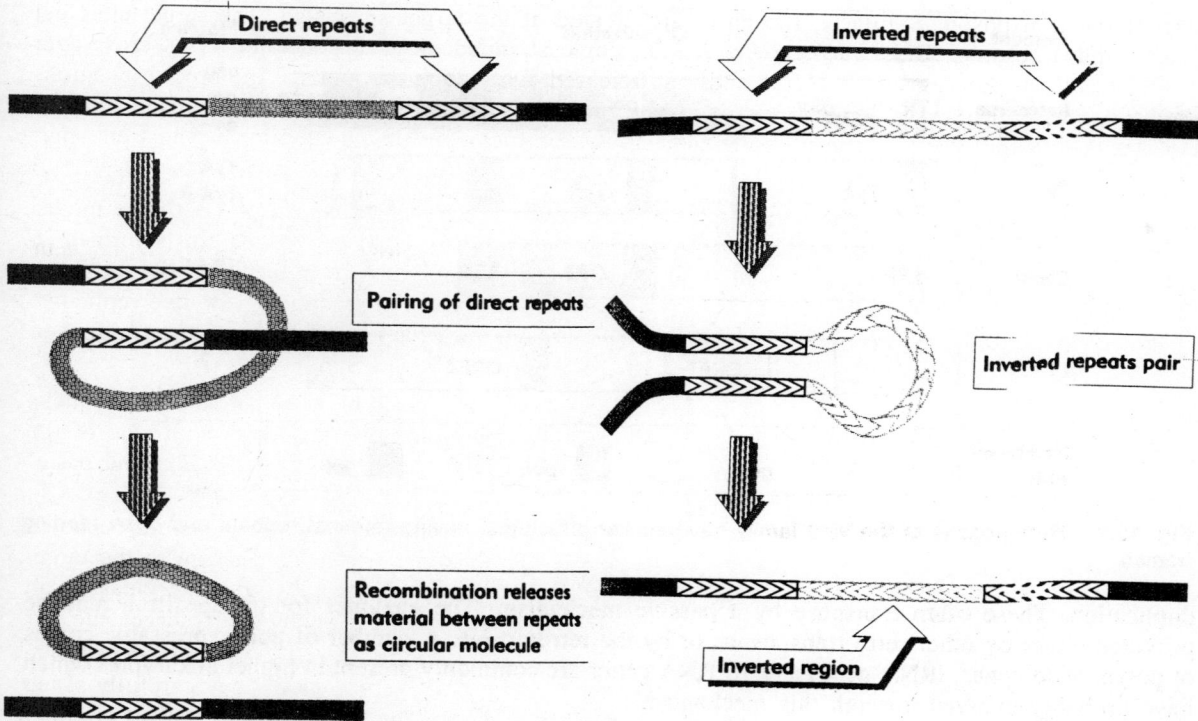

Fig. 12.12. Reciprocal recombination between direct repeats excises the sequences between them, producing two molecules each having one copy of the repeat. The recombination between inverted repeats on the other hand, inverts the region between them.

retroposons. The Ty elements of yeast, copia, FB and P elements of fruitfly and the L1 fragment of mammalian cells are the typical example of such elements. The structure of these elements is given in Fig. 12.13. The structure of a typical retrovirus has also been given along with it for comparision. In general, these fragments have a central fragment which is flanked by a direct repeat on both sides. The sequences in this direct repeat region may contain very short inverted repeats also, for example in copia. The P fragment on the other hand, has only short inverted repeats on both the ends.

Based on their structure, the retroposons can be of two types. These have been described below.

(a) Belonging to viral super family, these retroposons have LTRs. The target DNA has repeats of 4-6 bp and the reading frame has reverse transcriptase and/or integrase along with other genes. The genes may have introns which are removed at a later stage from the mRNA before its translation. Ty elements of yeast, copia of Drosophila and Lines 1 of mammals belong to this class.

(b) Belonging to non-viral super family, the retroposons of this class donot have the LTRs and use a relatively longer target repeats of 7-21 bp. The reading frames are either absent or donot code for any of the functions necessary for the transposition. The SINES and Alu repeats belong to this group of retroposons.

Many of the type 2 retroposons are often processed pseudogenes where there are no introns. These are also known as the retrogenes. The retrogenes often have an A-rich 3'-end and variable size target

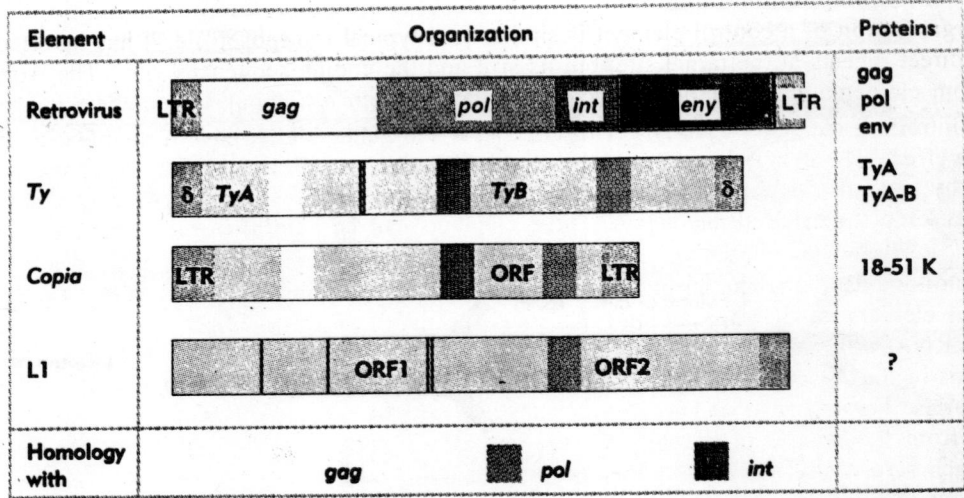

Fig. 12.13. Retroposons of the viral family have similar structures, having terminal repeats and open reading frames.

duplication. These often transpose by a passive mechanism. The enzymes for transposition may be provided either by other retro-transposons or by the retroviruses. A number of non-expressable copies of polypeptide genes, tRNA genes and 7S RNA genes are commonly present in higher eukaryotes which have probably evolved through this mechanism.

As discussed above, various types of transposons are present in both the eukaryotes and the prokaryotes. In higher eukaryotes, specially in the mammals, many copies of interspersed sequences are also present. These sequences, commonly known as the satellite DNA, move by transposon like mechanism. These are present in variable copy number between 20-50,000 copies/genome. If the repeats are of long repeat type, these are referred as the long interspersed sequences or LINES and if the repeats are short, then these are called SINES.

Some important transposons

Controling elements in maize

A number of controling transposable elements are known in maize. The number, types and the location of these elements is the characteristic of a particular strain of maize. These are either autonomous or non-autonomous elements. The autonomous elements can get excised from one location and move to another place by a transposition event. The insertion at a new location creates a unstable allele which is mutable. The loss of the element from an unstable allele renders it stable. The non-autonomous elements do not transpose spontaneously. However, the presence of another element of the same family (but autonomous type) in the same genome makes these elements unstable and causes their transposition. Thus when an autonomous element is provided in 'trans', the non-autonomous elements exhibit all the functions which are normally associated with the autonomous class.

A family of these elements usually includes one autonomous type of element and several non-autonomous elements. A non-autonomous element is included in a particular family if it can be 'activated' by the autonomous element of that family. In other words, all the elements of a single family can be activated by a single autonomous element.

The organization of a control element is similar to a typical transposon i.e. it has inverted repeats and short direct repeats at the target site, but its size and the coding sequences vary. The Ac elements and the Spm elements are the most characterized classes, each has about 10 members in the family.

The controlling elements usually get inserted near the genes which have a visible but non-lethal phenotypic effect. The genotypic effect of the transposition may result in an insertion, excision or break in the nearby gene also. It results in new phenotype in the affected descendents while the non-affected descendents keep the original characters. These elements can be helpful in providing the variegation by somatic development.

The autonomous elements can get converted to the non-autonomous group. In the Ac family, the autonomous element is 4563 bp, coding for a single primary transcript with 5 exons. It is spliced into a 3.3 kb mRNA with an ORF of 807 codons. It has an IR of 11 bp and 8 bp DR at the target site. By deletions in the Ac element, a related family of D5 elements have been generated. The extend of deletion varies. For example in Ds9 a small deletion of 152 bp has taken place while in Ds6, 2.5 kb region from the middle of the gene is lost. It has only 2 kb coding region, which represents 1 kb from each side of AC. The non-autonomous elements of each class are derived when the loss of internal sequences results in the activation of trans acting transposase but leaves the site of its action and the repeat termini intact. The loss of the enzyme activity may be due to minor mutation or large deletions and major rearrangements. The loss of certain cis acting factors may render a non-autonomous element stable for ever (i.e. it is no more a transposon in the true sense). There can be phase changes in these elements, which are the result of reversible changes and the element may be inactivited at one phase but gets activated in the other phase. Methylation of DNA may cause such changes. These changes may also be self regulating where an increase in the number of active elements converts these into inactive and thus regulates the number of transposition events.

The Ds elements transpose by a non–replicative mechanism. It has been found that Ds transposition almost always occurs after the replication of the chromosome. Usually the transposition is to another site on the same chromosome. It leaves a gap at the donor site, which may cause the chromosome breakage. In fact, the Ds element was originally recognized by its ability to provide a site for the chromosome breakage. If the Ds lies on one homologue of a heterologous zygote between the centromere and a series of dominant markers then this breakage will generate an acentric fragment with dominant markers which will get lost later during the mitosis. The descendants, thus have only the recessive markers present on the intact chromosome which results in the change of phenotype.

Similar arrangement of autonomous and non-autonomous elements is present in the supressor-mutator family (Spm). The non-autonomous elements of the Spm family are usually referred as dSpm (defective Spm) and are derived from Spm by various deletions.

Transposable elements in Drosophila

Drosophila has a number of transposable elements. One family of transposons is responsible for difficulty which is often encountered when one tries to interbreed certain strains of the fly. The progeny of such interbreeding results in a series of defects and mutations, chromosomal aberations and even sterility. The entire phenomenon is referred as the hybrid dysgenesis. The flies are divided into two types, I (inducer) and R (reactive). The crossing of an I male with a R female leads to the reduced fertility, however, no such effect is seen if a R male is crossed with an I female. In another system, the flies are grouped as the M (maternal contributing) and the P (paternal contributing). Cross of a P male with a M female leads to the sterile progeny which are normal otherwise. On the other hand, the crossing of M male and P female will give rise to a normal progeny. This phenomenon is due to the presence of a P factor in the P males. The P factor is distributed at various chromosomal locations. The M flies do not have the P factors. The P factor is due to the insertion of a transposon, the P element. The P element has the IR of 31 bp, generating a DR of 8 bp at the target site. The centre sequences vary in the length between different elements but are homologous. One of the elements has been mapped to contain 2.9 kb sequence with several ORFs. The shorter sequences arise by deletion, some of which donot produce transposase. However, these can be activated by certain 'trans' factors.

About 30-50 copies of P elements are present in a P strain which are inactive under normal conditions. However, by crossing of P male with a M female, these are activated and can transpose. The transposition is tissue specific, and takes place only in the germ line. No other cell types show this activity. This is achieved by a specific splicing pattern of the primary transcript (Fig. 12.14). It has four ORFs, the ORF O, ORF 1, ORF 2 and the ORF 3, present on a single primary transcript. The length of the transcript is either 2.5 kb (short RNA) or 3.0 kb (long RNA). The long RNA is formed due to a read through of a transcription terminator which is 'leaky'. The four ORFs are separated by three introns. In somatic cells, only 2 introns are removed and ORF O, ORF 1 and ORF 2 are joined together to form a translatable mRNA, which codes for a 66 KD protein. This protein acts as a repressor and the transposition is not possible. On the other hand in the germ cells, all the three introns are removed and a single mRNA from all the four ORFs is produced. This codes for a 87 KD protein which has transposase activity and causes the transposition of the sequences.

In a P line produced by the cross of homologous strain (P male and P female), only the 66 KD protein is formed in all the cells. Similarly the P female and M male cross also produces only the 66 KD protein. These crosses, thus, do not show any dysgenesis.

For the transposition of the P elements, the sequences at the termini (~ 150 bp) are needed. Ten bp region adjacent to the 31 bp IR acts as binding site for the transposase and transposition occurs by cut and paste type non-replicative mechanism.

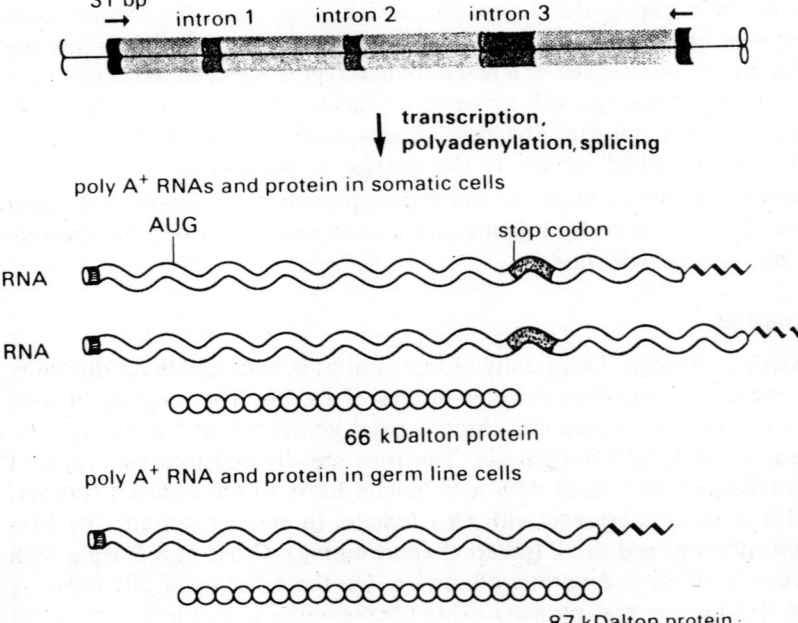

Fig. 12.14. Structure of a full length, active P element includes the 31 bp inverted terminal repeats, the four exons, and the three introns. The structures of two polyadenylated P RNAs found in somatic cells and the 66 kDalton protein they encode have been shown. Transcription initiates at base pair 87. The presumed structure of the polyadenylated RNA that occurs only in germ line cells and encodes an 87 kDalton transposase is shown at the bottom of the figure. In this RNA, all three introns have been removed by splicing.

Besides the P elements, Dosophila melano-gaster has a number of other transposable elements also. Some of these elements are the copia and the FB elements. The copia family includes a large number of closely related sequences and gets its name from the fact that these code for high abundant mRNAs. The copy number of copia elements is 20-60, depending on the strain. Each element has a 5 kb central fragment with a single large ORF of 4227 bp (coding for 1409 aa or approx 175 KD protein), flanked by a 276 bp DR. Each DR itself has a short IR on both its ends and a 5 bp DR is generated at the target site. It is a reteroposon and have high incidence of insertion in the cultured cells. The protein coded by the copia has homology with gag and pol proteins of retroviruses. However, no env like sequences are present, which means that it cannot generate virus like particles. The precise role for these sequences have not been assigned.

Another family of the transposable elements in fruit fly is the FB element (for fold back) which is an unknown family. It has IR repeats with variable length. Three common sizes of IRs are 10 bp, 20 bp and 31 bp, respectively. These have the sequences which have remained highly conserved (Table 12.2). Some of these have only the IRs and no central element may be present. The IRs resemble with the satellite DNA. The mechanism of transposition of the FB elements is not very clear.

The FB elements are capable of moving large stretches of unrelated elements. A region of DNA between two FB elements can transpose alongwith the FB elements. Several hundred kb of DNA has moved from X chromosome to chromosome 2 by this mechanism.

Table 12.2. Conserved sequences of FB elements

10 bp	C G T T T G C C C A	
20 bp	C G T T T G C C C A C C C T T T A A A A	
31 bp	C G T T T G C C C A C C C T T T A A A A T T A A A T T A T T T	

Ty elements of yeast

In yeast a family of dispersed repealitive sequences, known as the Ty elements (abbreviated form of transposon of yeast) are present. These are less frequently transposable elements of high divergence. Two major classes of the family, Ty 1 and Ty 917, are about 6.3 kb long with 330 bp DR on both the ends. These are transcribed into two overlapping RNAs, Ty A and Ty A-B. These mRNAs are highly abundant, constituting >5% of total cellular mRNA in a heploid yeast cell. The Ty A codes for a DNA binding protein, while Ty B proteins which expresses as the fused protein (the Ty A-B form) and is processed later to produce the mature Ty B, has homology with the enzymes such as RTase, protease and integrase of reterovirus. Belonging to retroposon class, Ty elements provide the region of homology. These are the targets for host mediated recombination events. Such recombination take place in bursts. If one recombination event is detected, chances are that other events will also be seen. The DR of Ty elements, referred as the delta sequences, help in the excision of the element by homologous recombination. The sequences are often present as independent elements without a centre region and are called as solo delta.

Ty elements transpose through the RNA intermediate. However, these donot form infectious particles. While present in high copy number, only some copies of the element are active. The inactive sequences provide a target for trans action of the protein produced by active element.

IAPs of mouse

These sequences are present in embryonic mouse cells and also in certain tumor cells. The elements give rise to a 80 nm reterovirus-like particle. Known as intra-cisternal A particles, these produce a 7.2 kb RNA which does not have resemblance with murine reteroviruses. The structural protein is 73 KD in size. IAPs move by retrotransposition and usually occupy previously empty genomic loci. Their insertion causes mutation in both germ line and in somatic cells.

Repeatitive sequences

It has been discussed that the eukaryotic genome contains a large number of repeatitive sequences. These sequences are usually interspersed with the single copy genes and are present at various locations within the genome. In Xenopus and the sea urchin, the middle repeatitive squences are about 300 bp long, in human these are between 8-1,200 bp while in Drosophilla these are upto 13,000 bp long. Depending on their size, these sequences are referred as LINEs (long interspersed nuclear elements) and SINEs (short interspersed nuclear elements), these sequences are capable of moving from one place to other. These have been speculated to have various regulatory roles. These are responsible for a number of mutations in the genome. Highly repeatitive sequences are usually present in genetically inactive heterochromatin region and may be important in organizational role, in involvement in chromosomal pairing, in crossing over and in protection of many important genes.

Transposable elements of Bacteria

In bacteria the genome is present in two forms; the chromosomal DNA and the extra-chromosomal DNA. The chromosomal DNA is packed in single chromosome. Relatively small amounts of extra-chromosomal DNA (also known as the episomal DNA)) is present in the form of plasmids. Some lower eukaryotes, such as yeast, and many plants also have plasmids. The plasmids can replicate in both ways; either as integrated part of the main genome of the host (stringent control) or as autonomous genetic material (relaxed control). The plasmids can be inherited and most of the plasmids are dispensable, even though these provide added characters to the bacteria. Based on the type of characters these provide to the cell, the plasmids can be of three type.

(i) F and F' plasmids which provide conjugation or fertility factor to the host.

(ii) R plasmids which provide the resistance to certain drug and are responsible for resistance transfer factor (RTF).

(iii) Col plasmids which produce a specific protein, namely colicin which will kill the sensitive bacteria. Some bacteriosins other than colicin such as vibriocin are also produced by Col plasmids.

Some of the plasmids are conjugative and are involved in transfer of DNA by conjugation.

As plasmids can move from one host to another, these are involved in the transfer of gene in a manner analogous to the movement of transposons. Besides, the bacteria also have a number of insertional sequences. For example, E. coli has 4 different IS elements. In fact, these were the first IS elements to be recognized. These elements referred as IS1, IS2, IS3, and IS4 are 768 bp, 1377 bp, 1300 bp and 1426 bp, respectively in length. E. coli K12 has 8 copies of IS1, 5 copies of IS2 and one or more copies of IS3 and IS4, respectively. The site of their integration depends on the presence of the F factor (a plasmid derived character) and their position in the chromosome. While these elements are movable themselves, these can also mediate the recombination between otherwise non–homologous elements and can mediate the integration of episome into the bacterial chromosome.

13

Principles of Genetic Engineering

It has been the dream of Molecular Biologists to be able to manipulate the genome of an organism in a desired manner. However, it was not possible to do so until the tools to cut the genome at precise locus and to join the pieces of different DNA molecules were available. Only after the discovery of the restriction endonucleases it became possible to digest any DNA molecule at a specific site and any two pieces of DNA could be joined together with the help of another modifying enzyme, the DNA ligase. Consequently, a new branch of molecular biology, namely genetic engineering, has been developed.

With the help of genetic engineering techniques, it is now possible to identify and isolate the gene(s) for a protein of interest and insert it into the genome of another organism with the help of a suitable vehicle. The foreign gene thus cloned, can be amplified to produce millions of its copies. The inserted gene can be expressed by the host to synthesize the gene product. The technique can also be used for understanding the regulation of expression of the cloned gene. The possibilities are endless and probably sky is the only limit. In this chapter we will briefly discuss the basic principles and the strategies involved in gene cloning.

Gene Cloning

The discovery of restriction endonucleases and the nucleic acid ligases (DNA ligase and the RNA ligase) has made it possible to cleave a DNA molecule at a desired place, isolate the gene fragments of interest and then put these at a desired locus. It can be compared with the work of a tailor, who cuts a cloth in desired manner and joins many pieces to design a dress. Using this technology, referred as the recombinant DNA (or rDNA) technology, it is possible to identify the pieces of DNA which code for the protein of interest, isolate these pieces and clone them into the genome of a totally unrelated organism. This has provided a very powerful tool in the hands of the molecular biologist which has enormous applications. The technique can be used to understand the regulation of expression of a particular gene in a non-ambiguous manner, to understand the structure-function relationship of a biomolecule, to see the mutual co-ordination between different genes as well as to produce a biomolecule by the cell of one's choice or by an organism which does not produce the molecule under normal physiological conditions. It is, atleast experimentally possible to cure a genetic disease or a disease which is produced as the result of a gene mutation by gene therapy. The DNA based diagnostic probes can detect many diseases at very early stage, even before the manifestation of the disease. The early detection as well as the time saved as the result of early detection can make a difference between the life and death of the patient in many cases, specially in the diseases such as the cancer. The entire gamut of molecular biology has undergone drammatic change during last 25 years. Today, using this technology, it is possible to get a number of studies done in a routine manner which one could not even imagine before the onset of gene cloning.

Enzymes used in gene cloning

Gene cloning is a complex and multistep process in which both, the gene to be cloned and the host genome are carefully manipulated in a calculated manner. These manipulations use a number of enzymes. Many of these enzymes are commonly used for all the gene cloning protocols, while certain others are used only for very specialized and specific experiments. Some of the commonly used enzymes have been very briefly described below.

Restriction endonucleases

Restriction endonucleases (commonly called as the restriction enzymes or RE) are one of the most important tool for the gene cloning. In fact the entire field of gene cloning could reach to its present form only after the discovery of REs. These are the specific endonucleases which digest a double stranded DNA molecule at specific sites. These are of bacterial origin and have evolved in the bacteria as a protection against the invading organisms. There are three types of REs; type I, type II and type III. The details of all these are beyond the scope of this chapter. The type II REs are the simplest of the three and are extensively used in gene cloning experiments. Type II REs recognize a specific DNA sequence and digest the DNA within this recognition sequence. If the target sequence is methylated, it is usually not recognized by the enzyme and the DNA is not digested. These require divalent cations, usually Mg^{++} but Mn^{++} can often replace Mg^{++}. Besides Mg^{++}, these also require a specific salt concentration. Majority of the enzymes use one of the three salt concentrations, the high salt (150 mM or more NaCl), the medium salt (50 mM NaCl) or the low salt (0-10 mM NaCl) for their activity. Except that SmaI is an enzyme which requires KCl for its activity. Most of the enzymes recognize either a six base pair sequence (6 base cutters) or a four base pair sequence (4 base cutters). The recognition sequence is almost always pallindromic in nature. The digestion of the DNA is within this sequence. The site of digestion may be either towards the 5'-end of the recognition sequence (usually after first base) in both the strands, or towards 3'-end of the target sequence. In both these cases it will produce a small region of single stranded DNA. This is referred as the sticky end or the overhang. Some enzymes cut at the centre of the recognition sequence, when these produce the blunt end. Thus a RE will produce either a 3' overhang, a 5' overhang or a blunt end (Fig. 13.1). It is possible that two enzymes which recognize different sequences can produce the same overhang sequence. Such overhangs are known as the compatible ends and can be ligated together. However, such ligations will result in the loss of cleavage sites for both the enzymes (Fig. 13.2). In certain other cases, two (or more) enzymes can recognize the same sequence yet digest at different place and produce different overhang. Sometimes, the recognition sequence of a 4 base cutter enzyme may lie within the sequence of a 6 base cutter. The examples of various types of enzymes are given in Fig. 13.3.

These enzymes are named after the host from which they are obtained. The first letter represent the genera and the last two letters represent the species of the bacteria from which it has been isolated. If only a specific strain of the bacteria synthesizes the enzyme then its name is added as 4th letter. If more than one enzymes have been isolated from a single organism, then a Roman numerical is added to represent the order of isolation. For example, EcoRI is the first enzyme isolated from the R starin of Escheria (E) coli (co). Table 13.1 lists a number of the commonly used REs.

Table 13.1. Common restriction endonucleases used in gene cloning.

Enzyme	Common isoschizomers	Optimum salt	Incubation temperature	Recognition sequence	Compatible cohesive ends
AccI		med	37ºC	GT↓(A/C) (T/G)AC	AcyI, AsuII, ClaI Hpall, Taq
AcyI			37ºC	G(A/G)↓CG(T/C)C	AccI, AsuII, ClaI, HpaII, TaqI
AluI		med	37ºC	AG↓CT	blunt
AosI			37ºC	TGC↓GCA	blunt
ApyI	AtuI, EcoRII		37ºC	CC↓(A/T)GG	
AsuI			37ºC	G↓GNCC	
AsuII			37ºC	TT↓CGAA	AccI, AcyI, ClaI, HpaII, TaqI
AtuII			37ºC	CC↓(A/T)GG	
AvaI		med	37ºC	G↓PyCGPuG	SalI, XhoI, XmaI
AvaII		med	37ºC	G↓G(A/T)CC	Sau96I
BalI			37ºC	TGG↓CCA	blunt
BamHI		med	37ºC	G↓GATCC	BclI, BglII, MboII, Sau3A, XhoII
BclI		med	60ºC	T↓GATCA	BamHI, BglII, MboI, Sau3A, XhoII
BglI		med	37ºC	GCCNNNN↓NGGC	
BglII		low	37ºC	AG↓ATCT	BamHI, BclI, MboI, Sau3A, XhoII
BpaI			37ºC	GT↓(C/A)(G/T)AC	
BstEII		med	60ºC	G↓GTNACC	
BstNI		low	60ºC	CC↓(A/T)GG	
ClaI			37ºC	AT↓CGAT	AccI, AcyI, AsyII, HpaII, TaqI
DdeI		med	37ºC	C↓TNAG	
DpnI	Sau3A	med	37ºC	G^{Me}A↓TC	blunt
EcoRI'		high	37ºC	G↓AATTC	
EcoB			37ºC	TGANNNNNNNTGCT	
EcoK			37ºC	AACNNNNNNGTGC	
EcoPI			37ºC	↓AGACC	
EcoRI			37ºC	(A/G)(A/G)A↓T(T/C)(T/C)	blunt
EcoRI*			37ºC	↓AATT	EcoRI
EcoRII	AtuI, ApyI	high	37ºC	↓CC(A/T)GG	
Fnu4HI		low	37ºC	GC↓NGC	
FnuDII	ThaI	low	37ºC	CG↓CG	blunt
HaeI		low	37ºC	(A/T)GG↓CG(T/A)	blunt
HaeII		low	37ºC	PuGCGC↓Py	
HaeIII		med	37ºC	GG↓CC	blunt
HgaI		med	37ºC	GACGCNNNNN↓	
				CTGCGNNNNNNNNNN↓	

(Contd.)

Enzyme	Common isoschizomers	Optimum salt	Incubation temperature	Recognition sequence	Compatible cohesive ends[2]
HgiAI		high	37°C	G(T/A)GC(A/T)↓C	
HhaI	CfoI	med	37°C	GCG↓C	
HincII		med	37°C	GTPy↓PuAC	blunt
HindIII		med	37-55°C	A↓AGCTT	
HinfI		med	37°C	G↓ANTC	
HpaI		low	37°C	GTT↓AAC	blunt
HpaII		low	37°C	C↓CGG	AccI, AcyI, AsuII, ClaI, TaqI
HphI		low	37°C	GGTGANNNNNNNN↓	
				CCACTNNNNNNN↓	
KpnI		low	37°C	GGTAC↓C	BamHI, BclI, BglII, XhoII
MboI	Sau3A	high	37°C	↓GATC	
MboII		low	37°C	GAAGANNNNNNNN↓	
				CTTCTNNNNNNN↓	
MspI		low	37°C	C↓CGG	
				C↓GMeGG	
MstI			37°C	T↓GCGCA	
PstI		med	21-37°C	CTGCA↓G	
PruI		high	37°C	C↓GATCG	
PruII		med	37°C	CAG↓CTG	blunt
RsaI		med	37°C	GT↓AC	blunt
SacI	SstI	low	37°C	GAGCT↓C	
SacII		low	37°C	CCGC↓GG	
SacIII		high	37°C	↓ACGT	
SalI		high	37°C	G↓TCGAC	AcaI[3], XhoI
Sau3A		med	37°C	↓GATC	BamHI, BclI, BglII, MboI, XhoII
				↓GMeATC	
Sau96I		med	37°C	G↓GNCC	
SmaI	XmaI		37°C	CCC↓GGG	blunt
SphI			37°C	GCATG↓C	
SstI	SacI	low	37°C	GAGCT↓C	
SstII		low	37°C	CCGC↓GG	
SstIII		high	37°C	↓ACGT	
TaqI		low	65°C	T↓CGA	AccI, AcyI, AsuII, ClaI, HpaII
ThaI	FnuDII	low	60°C	CG↓CG	blunt
XbaI		high	37°C	T↓CTAGA	
XhoI		high	37°C	C↓TCGAG	AraI, SalI
XhoII			37°C	(A/G)↓GATC(T/C)	BamHI, BclI, BglII, MboI, Sau3A
XmaI	SmaI	low	37°C	C↓CCGGG	AraI
XmaIII			37°C	C↓GGCCG	
XorII	PcuI, RshI	low	37°C	CGATC↓G	

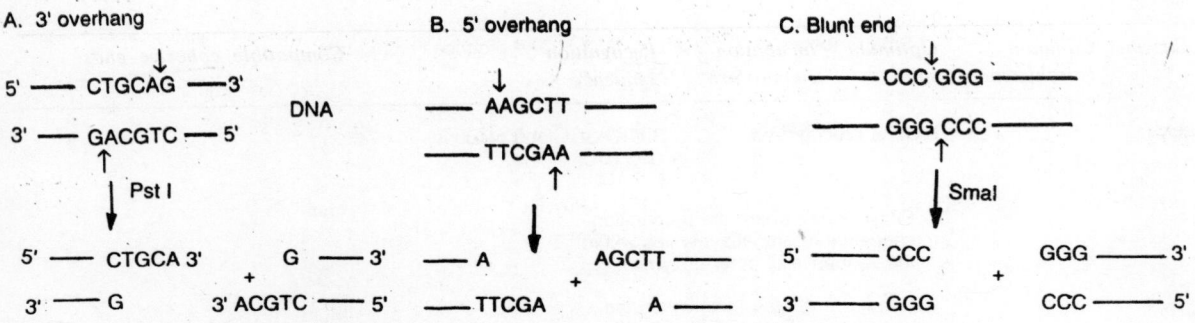

Fig. 13.1. Various restriction enzymes recognize and cleave the DNA at different sequences.

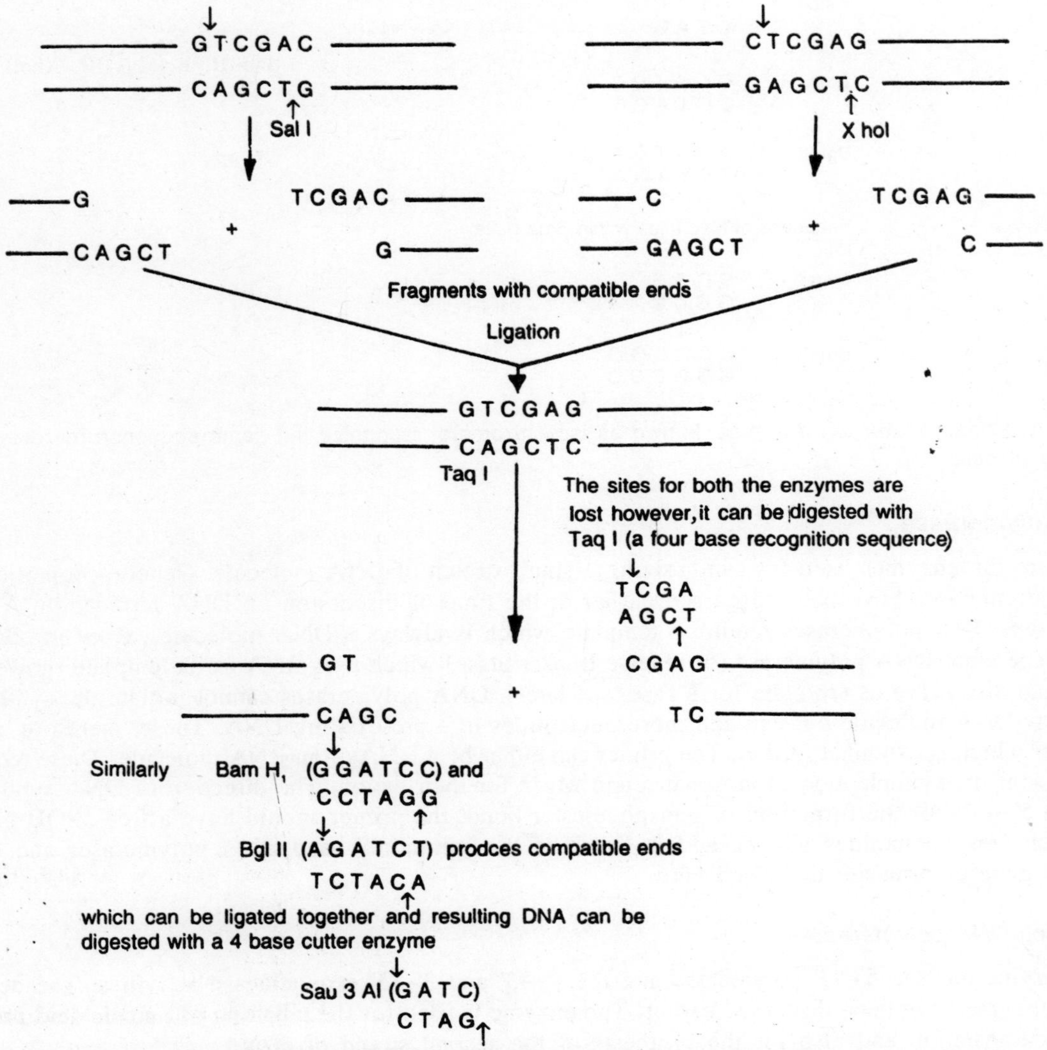

——————— G T C G A C ———————   ——————— C T C G A G ———————
——————— C A G C T G ———————   ——————— G A G C T C ———————
                    ↓ Sal I   ↓ X hol

——G   T C G A C ———   ——— C   T C G A G ——
——C A G C T   G ——   ——— G A G C T   C ——
            +   +

                        Fragments with compatible ends

                                Ligation

                    ——————— G T C G A G ———————
                    ——————— C A G C T C ———————
                    Taq I

The sites for both the enzymes are
lost however, it can be digested with
Taq I (a four base recognition sequence)
                                ↓
                            T C G A
                            A G C T
                                ↑

——————— G T   C G A G ———————
——————— C A G C   T C ———————
            +

Similarly   Bam H₁ (G G A T C C) and
                      C C T A G G
              ↓   ↑
            Bgl II (A G A T C T) prodces compatible ends
                    T C T A C A
                              ↑
which can be ligated together and resulting DNA can be
digested with a 4 base cutter enzyme
                                ↓
            Sau 3 AI (G A T C)
                      C T A G↑

Fig. 13.2. Sometimes two separate restriction enzymes can produce compatible ends which can be ligated.

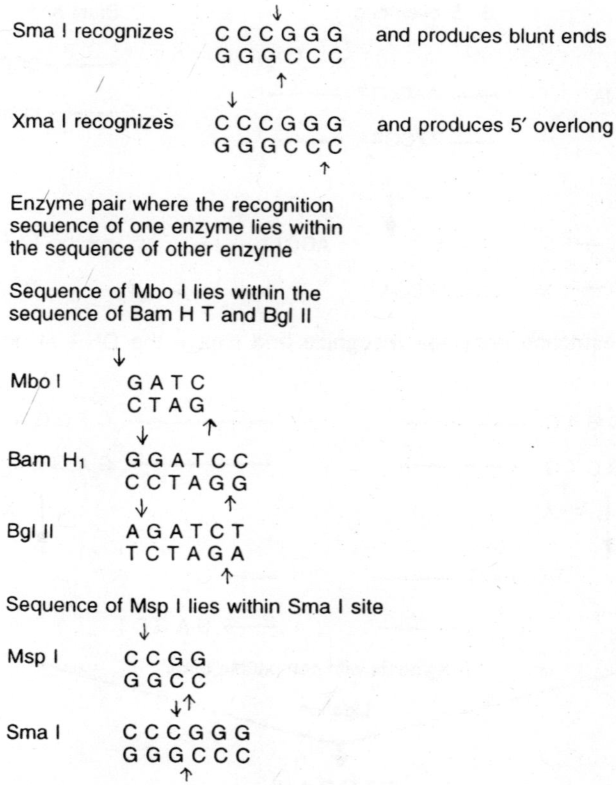

Sma I recognizes   C C C G G G   and produces blunt ends
                        G G G C C C

Xma I recognizes   C C C G G G   and produces 5′ overlong
                        G G G C C C

Enzyme pair where the recognition sequence of one enzyme lies within the sequence of other enzyme

Sequence of Mbo I lies within the sequence of Bam H T and Bgl II

Mbo I   G A T C
           C T A G

Bam H_1 G G A T C C
              C C T A G G

Bgl II   A G A T C T
          T C T A G A

Sequence of Msp I lies within Sma I site

Msp I   C C G G
          G G C C

Sma I   C C C G G G
         G G G C C C

Fig. 13.3. Certain restriction enzymes, known as isoschizomers, recognize the same sequence but digest at different places.

DNA polymerases

These are the enzymes used for synthesizing a small stretch of DNA molecule. General properties of DNA polymerases have been discussed earlier at the time of discussion on DNA replication. All of the known DNA polymerases require a template which is always a DNA molecule except in case of RNA dependent DNA polymerase (or reverse transcriptase) which uses RNA as its template (however, DNA can also serve as template for RTase, see later). DNA polymerases cannot initiate the synthesis of a new DNA molecule but can add more nucleotides to a pre-existing DNA. These, therefore, need a primer which is extended further. The primer can either be a DNA or an RNA molecule. These require all the four deoxynucleotide triphosphates and Mg^{++} for their action. The direction of DNA synthesis is from 5′→3′. For the formation of phosphodiester bond, the primer should have a free 3′-OH group to which new nucleotides will be added. Some of the commonly used DNA polymerases and their uses in gene cloning are described here.

1. E. coli DNA polymerase I

The enzyme has the 5′→3′ polymerase and the 5′→3′ and 3′→5′ exonuclaease activities. The details of the enzyme have been discussed earlier. The enzyme is used for the labelling of nucleic acid probes by nick-translation and also for the synthesis of the second strand of cDNA.

2. Klenow polymerase

It is the large subunit of DNA polymerase, has the 5'→3' polymerase and the 3'→5' exonuclease activity. It can degrade either ds or ss DNA in the absence of the nucleotide triphosphates. The details have been discussed earlier. It is used for filling the 5' over hangs created by RE digestion (Fig. 13.4), labelling the DNA by end filling, in 2nd strand cDNA synthesis and in DNA sequencing using Sanger's method. It can also be used for digesting the 3' over hang, but T_4 DNA polymerase is preferred for this purpose (see later).

(E. coli)

The enzyme consists of a single polypeptide chain (M_r = 76,000) produced by cleavage of DNA polymerase I. This peptide carries the 5' → 3' polymerase activity and the 3' →5' exonuclease activity but lacks the 5' →3' exonuclease activity.

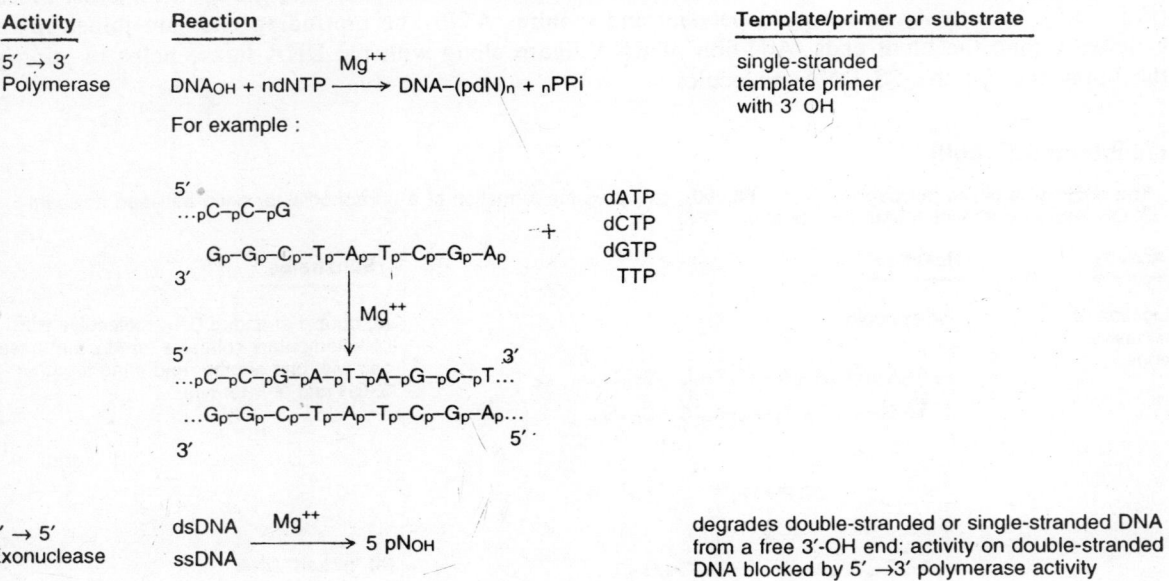

Activity	Reaction	Template/primer or substrate
5' → 3' Polymerase	$DNA_{OH} + ndNTP \xrightarrow{Mg^{++}} DNA-(pdN)_n + nPPi$	single-stranded template primer with 3' OH
3' → 5' Exonuclease	$\begin{array}{c} dsDNA \\ ssDNA \end{array} \xrightarrow{Mg^{++}} 5\ pN_{OH}$	degrades double-stranded or single-stranded DNA from a free 3'-OH end; activity on double-stranded DNA blocked by 5' →3' polymerase activity

Uses

1. Filling the 3' recessed termini created by digestion of DNA with restriction enzymes; for example :
2. Labeling the termini of DNA fragments (by using [32P] dNTPs in end-filling reactions).
3. Second-strand cDNA synthesis in cDNA cloning.
4. Sequencing DNA using the Sanger dideoxy system (Sanger et al. 1977).
5. At one time the 3' →5' exonuclease activity of the Klenow fragment was used to digest protruding 3' termini created by some restriction enzymes. Lately, T4 DNA polymerase has become the enzyme of choice for this purpose because of its more active 3' →5' exonuclease.

Fig. 13.4. Large fragment of DNA polymerase I (Klenow fragment), has three catalytic activities.

3. T_4 DNA polymerase

The enzyme has same activities as the Klenow enzyme except that the 3'→5' exonuclease activity is much higher. Further, this exonuclease activity is considerably higher on ss DNA than on ds DNA. It is the preferred enzyme for digesting the 3' protruding ends formed by RE digestion. Besides, the enzyme is also used to polish the ends of cDNA after it has been synthesized.

4. Reverse transcriptase

It is a specialised DNA polymerase which can use both the RNA as well as the DNA as template for DNA synthesis. Also it uses both the DNA as well as the RNA as the primer. Its activity is optimum at slightly alkaline pH (pH 8.3), other requirements are same as the DNA polymerase I. It is peimarily used for the synthesis of cDNA, specially the first strand, against an mRNA.

Other enzymes used in gene cloning

Besides the DNA polymerases, a number of other enzymes, specially the DNA modifying enzymes are used in gene cloming. Some of these are discussed below.

1. DNA ligase

This enzyme joins two fragments of DNA by forming a phosphodiester bond. The DNA pieces which are to be joined should have free 3'-OH group in one piece and a free 5'-PO_4 group in the other piece (Fig. 13.5). Its activity is energy dependent and requires ATP. The protruding ends are joined more efficiently than the blunt ends. Addition of RNA ligase along with the DNA ligase helps in joining the blunt ends or the SS DNA molecules.

(T_4-infected E. coli)

The enzyme, a single polypeptide (M r = 68,000), catalyzes the formation of a phosphodiester bond between adjacent 3'-OH and 5'- P termini in DNA (Weiss et al. 1968).

Activity	Reaction	Substrates
Ligation of cohesive ends	For example : 5' OH' ...pA–pC–pG pA–pA–pT–pT–pC–pG–pT... 3' ...Tp–Gp–Cp–Tp–Tp–Ap–Ap Gp–Cp–Ap... 3' OH 5' ATP | Mg++ ↓ ...pA–pC–pG–pA–pA–pT–pT–pC–pG–pT... Tp–Gp–Cp–Tp–Tp–Ap–Ap–Gp–Cp–Ap	(a) double-stranded DNA molecules with complementary cohesive termini that base pair with one another and bring together 3'-OH and 5'-P termini. (b) "nicked" DNA
Ligation of blunt ends	For example : 5' OH ...pC–pG–pA pC–pG–pT–pA... 3' ...Gp–Cp–Tp Gp–Cp–Ap–Tp... 3' OH, 5' ATP | Mg++ ↓ ...pC–pG–pA–pC–pG–pT–pA... ...Gp–Cp–Tp–Gp–Cp–Ap–Tp...	high concentrations of blunt-ended, double-stranded, DNA with 5'-P and 3'-OH termini.

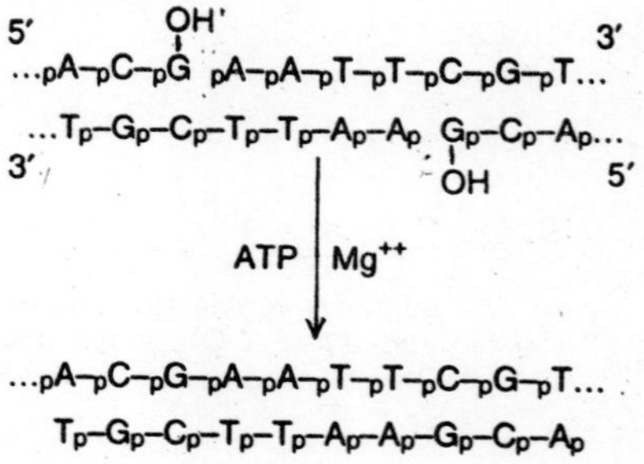

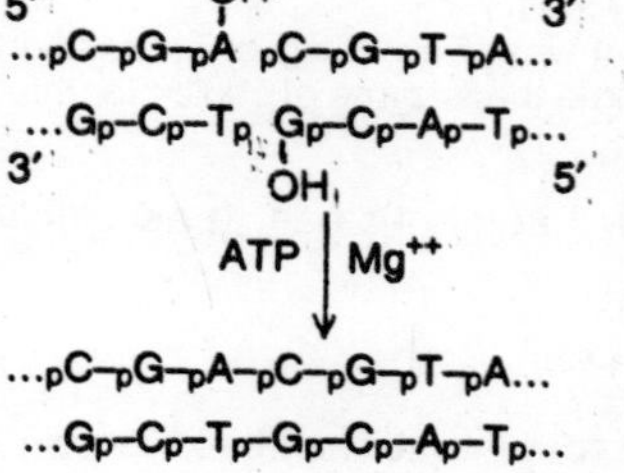

Uses

1. Joining together DNA molecules with compatible cohesive termini.
2. Joining blunt-ended, double-stranded DNA molecules to one another or to synthetic linkers. The activity of T4 ligase on blunt-ended DNA molecules can be stimulated approximately 20-fold by the addition of T4 RNA ligase (Sugino et al. 1977).

Fig. 13.5. Catalytic activity of T_4 DNA ligase.

DNA ligase can create a phosphodiester bond but cannot add any new nucleotides and cannot be used for filling a gap. The enzyme is extensively used for joining different DNA molecules for cloning an insert to the vector.

2. T_4 Polynucleotide kinase

The enzyme adds a phosphate group at the 5' end of a DNA molecule. The DNA molecule to be phosphorylated should have an OH group at the 5'-end. ATP serves as the phosphate group donor and its γ–PO_4 is added to the DNA (Fig. 13.6). No other nucleotide can replace ATP for this purpose. Under altered reaction conditions, it is possible to phosphorylate a DNA molecule with a 5'-PO_4 group. In such case, the 5'-PO_4 of the DNA can be exchanged with the γ–PO_4 of ATP (the exchange reaction). The enzyme is used for the purpose of end labelling a DNA molecule at the 5'-end with ^{32}P using γ-labelled ATP. The 5'-end labelling is done either for probe generation or during DNA sequencing by Maxam and Gilbert's method.

(T₄-infected E. coli)

The enzyme catalyzes the transfer of the γ-phosphate of ATP to a 5'-OH terminus in DNA or RNA.

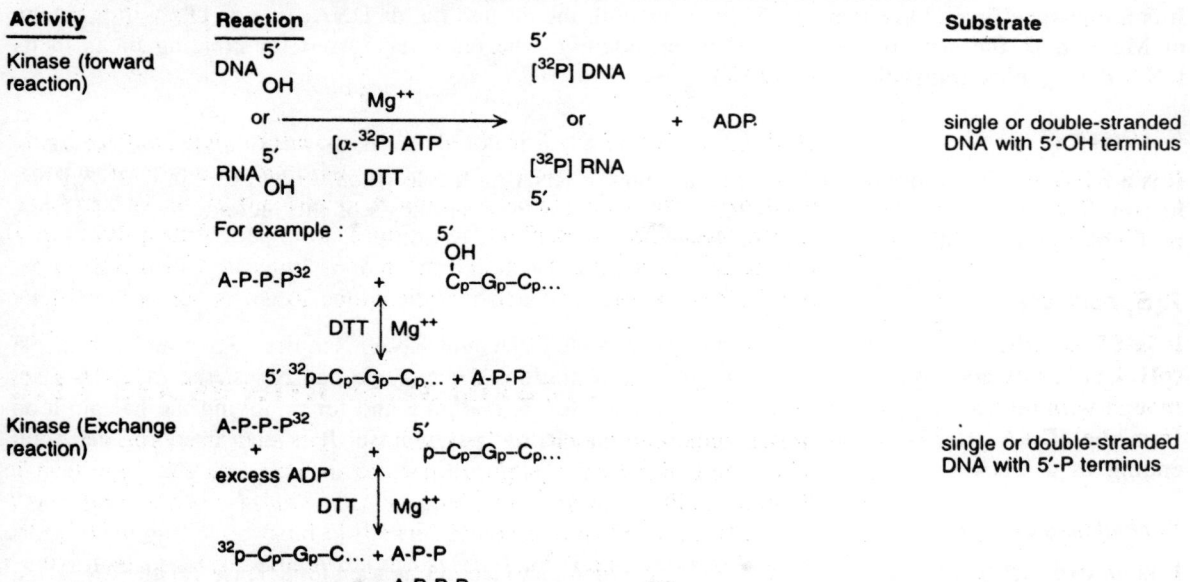

Activity	Reaction		Substrate

Kinase (forward reaction): DNA 5'-OH or RNA 5'-OH + [α-^{32}P] ATP, Mg^{++}, DTT → [^{32}P] DNA 5' or [^{32}P] RNA 5' + ADP.   single or double-stranded DNA with 5'-OH terminus

For example:

A-P-P-P^{32} + 5'-OH Cp–Gp–Cp... → (DTT, Mg^{++}) 5' ^{32}p–Cp–Gp–Cp... + A-P-P

Kinase (Exchange reaction): A-P-P-P^{32} + excess ADP + 5' p–Cp–Gp–Cp... → (DTT, Mg^{++}) ^{32}p–Cp–Gp–C... + A-P-P + A-P-P-P   single or double-stranded DNA with 5'-P terminus

The excess ADP drives the exchange reaction, causing polynucleotide kinase to transfer the terminal 5'-phosphate from DNA to ADP. The DNA is then rephosphorylated by transfer of the labeled γ-phosphate in the [α-^{32}P] ATP (Berkner and Folk 1977).

Uses

1. Labeling 5' termini in DNA for sequencing by the Maxam-Gilbert technique (Maxam and Gilbert 1977).
2. Phosphorylating synthetic linkers and other fragments of DNA lacking 5'-P termini prior to ligation.

Fig. 13.6. The properties and uses of T_4 polynucleotide kinase.

3. Alkaline phosphatase

The enzyme removes the PO_4 group from the 5'-end of a DNA molecule and converts it into the 5'-OH group. There are two commonly used alkaline phosphatases, one isolated from E. coli (the bacterial alkaline phosphatase or BAP) and other isolated from the calf intestine (CIP). BAP has higher activity than CIP. However, BAP cannot be fully inactivated by heat denaturation at 65°. As a result, the phenol extraction of the reaction mixture is essential after the BAP treatment, on the other hand, heating at 65° for 10 min is enough to inactivate CIP. The alkaline phosphatases are commonly used to dephosphorylate a DNA to generate the 5'-OH group either for labelling it later by kinase or to get dephosphorylated vector during cloning (see later).

4. Terminal deoxynucleotidyl transferase (TdT)

This enzyme can add a number of nucleotides at the 3'-end of a DNA molecule in a template independent manner. The dNTPs serve as the substrate for this purpose. The enzyme needs Co^{++} as cofactor for its activity. The length of the nucleotides added (the tail) can be upto 40 nucleotides, but the addit.. of a tail of about 20 nucleotides is very common. A 3' protruding or a blunt end is preferred but the tail can also be added to a 3' recessive end. The enzyme is used for adding a tail to the cDNA and the vector DNA for cloning by homopolymer tailing. It can also be used for labelling the 3'-end of a DNA molecule by tailing with radio-labelled nucleoside triphosphates.

5. DNase I

It is a non-specific endonuclease which cleaves both the SS and the ds DNA. In a ds DNA in presence of Mg^{++}, both the strands are digested independently. The enzyme is used for creating nicks in ds DNA during nick translation.

6. RNase H

It is a RNA specific endonuclease which can digest a RNA molecule when it is present in a DNA:RNA hybrid. The enzyme is used to digest the RNA strand during synthesis of the second strand of cDNA by Gubler and Hoffman's method (see later).

7. S₁ nuclease

It is SS specific endonuclease which can digest both DNA and RNA. Requires Zn^{++} and acidic pH (pH 4.5) for its activity. However, at higher concentrations the enzyme can digest the ds DNA also, though with reduced efficiency. The enzyme is used for S_1 mapping and for removing the hairpin loop from the cDNA after it has been synthesized with klenow polymerase. It is also used for the blunt ending of a DNA.

8. Nuclease Bal 31

It is an exonuclease for ds as well as SS DNA which can also act as a endonuclease for the SS DNA. The enzyme is used for the removal of nucleotides from the ends of a DNA molecule.

9. RNase A

The enzyme is specific for SS RNA. It is used for removal of unhybridized RNA from the hybridization reaction mixture during heteroduplex mapping. It is also used as a non-specific RNase for the removal of RNA from a DNA preparation, specially during the plasmid DNA isolation. It is also used to digest the cellular RNA during phage isolation.

RNase is heat stable enzyme and does not loose its activity even at 100°C. It is possible to remove the traces of DNase co-purified with the crude RNase preparation by boiling. RNase A is also one of the most widely present enzymes and can break a RNA preparation. It is therefore, essential that all the solutions are autoclaved if the aim of the experiment is to work with RNA.

10. Micrococcal nuclease

It is a Ca^{++} dependent RNase isolated from micrococcus. The enzyme can be inactivated by chelating the Ca^{++} with EGTA. This is used to digest endogeneous mRNA from the cell free translation system.

11. Methylases

These enzymes are present in association with the RE. Specific methylases for a number of REs have been isolated. These recognize a specific sequence in the same manner as a RE and add a $-CH_3$ group within the recognition sequence of the DNA. This specific methylation results in the protection of DNA by RE. The enzyme are used to protect the internal restriction sites during linker ligation for cloning of a DNA molecule.

12. RNA polymerase

The enzyme is used for transcription of a gene. A number of phage specific RNA polymerase are known which recognize the phage-specific promoters. A number of transcription vectors have been constructed, specially with SP64 and T_7 promoters which can be used to transcribe a cloned gene to get multiple RNA copies of a gene.

Construction of gene libraries

The first step in gene cloning is to collect all the genes of a genome present in a suitable way so that these can easily be studied. This is achived by making a gene library. In genetic engineering, the genes used are of two types, the natural genes and the cDNAs. The cDNA is an artificially made DNA copy of mRNA which has the entire coding sequence along with the translational regulatory elements but lacks all the transcriptional regulatory elements and also the introns. The cDNAs are synthesized with the help of reverse transcriptase (RTase), the enzyme present in many of the retroviruses. It may be worth mentioning that neither the enzyme nor a cDNA molecule occurs naturally in any of the known organism except the retroviruses, though there are some indirect evidences to suggest that a RTase like activity may have been present in eukaryotes also. Using the mRNA as the template and the RTase (usually obtained from AMV or from MMLV earlier, however, now the genes for RTase have been cloned and the enzyme is synthesized by r-DNA technology) in presence of a primer (an oligo-dT of 15-30 nucleotides can serve as an universal primer which anneals with the poly (A) tail present at the 3' end of the mRNA and initiates the DNA synthesis, as an alternate, the random hexamers can also be used), appropriate buffer and all the four dNTPs, a DNA molecule complementary to the mRNA is synthesized which forms a DNA : RNA hybrid. The RNA stand from this hybrid is later replaced by DNA, using one of the two routinely used (either the S_1 nuclease method or the Gubler and Hoffman's RNase H method) protocols. The practical details of the cDNA synthesis are beyond the scope of this book. However, these have been diagrammatically represented in Fig.s 13.7 and 13.8 respectively.

An obvious question arises here. Why should one take the trouble of synthesizing a cDNA molecule in the first place when one can clone a natural gene which is present in the genome of the organism. There are multiple reasons for this. Firstly, a cDNA is relatively smaller and simpler than the natural gene as it does not have many of the regulatory sequences or the introns. The complexiety of mRNAs of a cell is much simpler than the total genome. In any given cell, a very small percentage of the genome is transcribed at any given time. Further, in many cases specially if one is interested in a gene which is expressed in either tissue specific manner or in developmental stage related manner, then the use of cDNA makes a lot of sense. Some of the viruses have RNA genome (the retrovirus and reovirus, for example) and their genes can be cloned only in form of the cDNA. On the other hand, in many

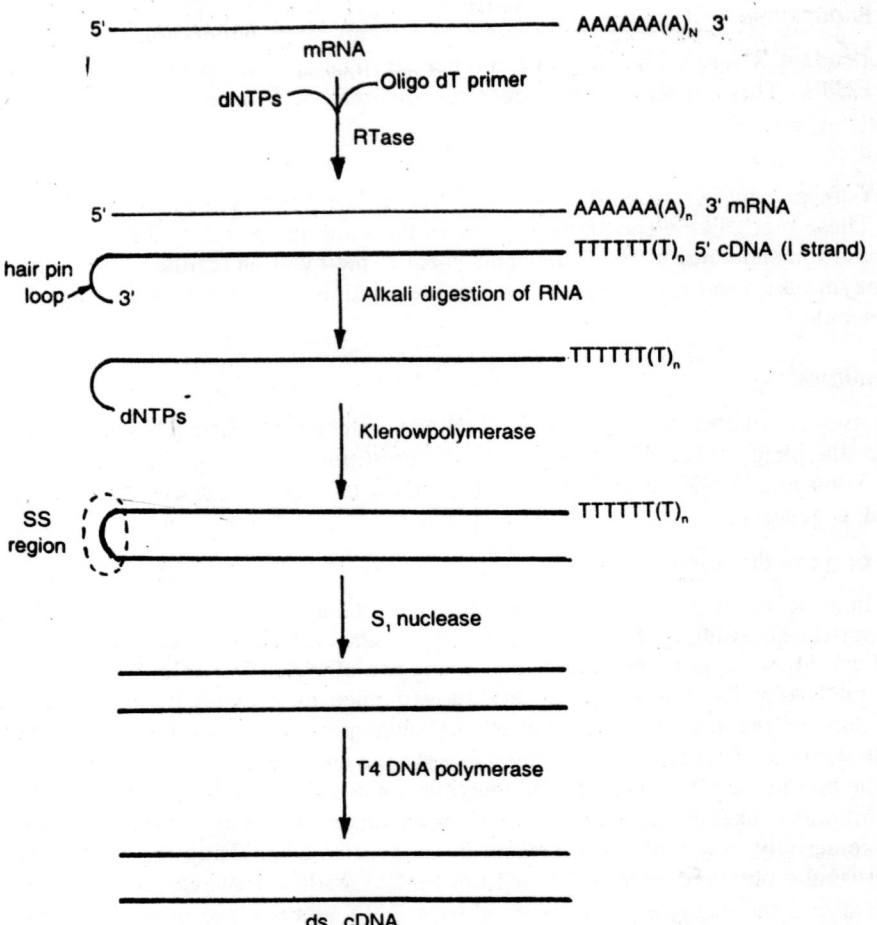

Fig. 13.7. cDNA synthesis by S_1 nuclease method using Klenow polymerase.

experiments one has no choice but to use natural gene. Some of the examples of such experiments are the study of the gene organization or the function of the regulatory elements of a gene. Similarly to express a gene in homologous system one will have to use a natural gene. Thus the choice of using either the cDNA or the natural gene primarily depends on the nature of the experiment.

When the natural gene is to be used, the size of the genome creates many problems. Being very large, the intact genome is difficult to handle experimentally and clone in any vector. It is therefore, fragmented into convenient size pieces by restriction enzyme digestions. Usually the fragments of 5-15 Kb size are used for the construction of a gene library. In a DNA with random sequences, on an average one site after every 4 kb is present for a restriction enzyme with a six base recognition sequence (4 different types of bases and a 6 base sequence; therefore, the size of an average fragment will be $4^6 = 4096$ bases). Similarly for a restriction enzyme with 4 base recognition sequence, the average length of a fragment will be $4^4 = 256$ or about 250 bp. It is therefore, essential that the DNA is only partially digested to get the fragments of right size. The fragmentation of genomic DNA can also be achieved

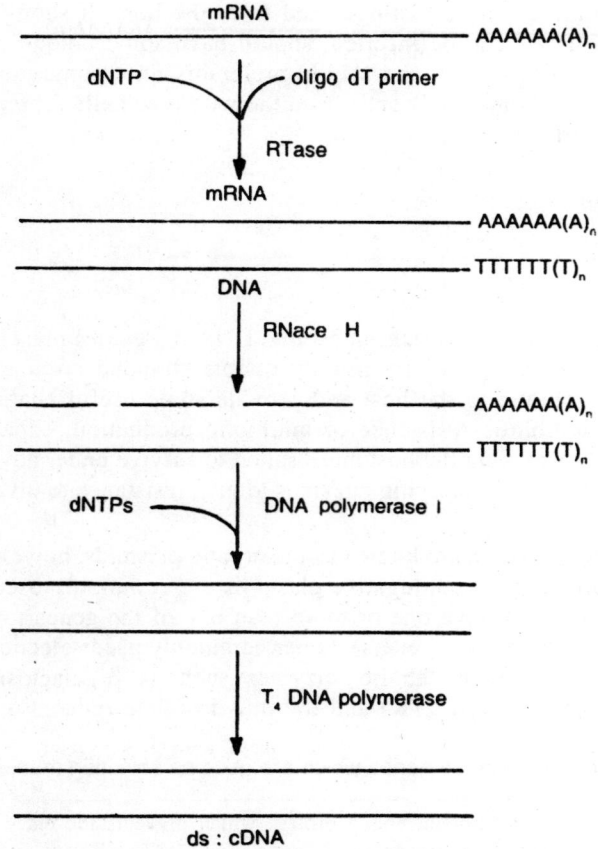

Fig. 13.8. cDNA synthesis by Gubler and Hoffman's method using RNase H and DNA polymerase I.

by physical shearing of DNA. It can be achieved either by limited sonication or by repeatedly passing the DNA through a low gauge hypodermic needle. However, in these cases the ends often get 'damaged' and have to be repaired by the enzymes such as Klenow and/or T4 DNA polymerase. It may be pertinent to point out that in gene cloning the term 'gene' is often used rather loosely. Both the cDNAs and the natural genes are generally referred as genes, even though the cDNAs are not the genes in true sense.

Cloning vectors

Once either the cDNA or the genomic DNA fragments of suitable size have been obtained, these are inserted in the specific vehicles which allows the transfer of the gene to desired place (the host). These vehicles are referred as the cloning vectors. The cloning vectors are defined as the vehicles which help in the transfer of a foreign DNA molecule into the host cell. The vectors are the DNA molecules of various size, shape and configuration. Some of the vectors are naturally occuring while others are the modified derivatives of the naturally occuring entities. To be suitable for this purpose, a vector should have autonomous replication, independent of the host cell. Its DNA should be characteristically different from the host DNA so that it can be distinguished from the host. It should have some non-essential region where the foreign DNA can be inserted, should have some unique restriction sites within this region for the cloning of foreign DNA and should preferably have some marker gene(s) which can be used to differentiate the transformed host cells from the wild type cells. Three different types of cloning vectors are commonly used. These are:

(a) Plasmids
(b) Bacteriophages and
(c) Cosmids.

Plasmids

Plasmids are the naturally occuring extrachromosomal DNA molecules present in many prokaryotes and also in some lower eukaryotes. These are usually double stranded circular molecules. The naturally occuring plasmids are symbiotic to the host and provide some useful characters to their hosts. Some of these characters are, antibiotic resistance or antibiotic production, capability to degrade complex organic compounds and thus making the host more suited to survive under adverse conditions, production of some enterotoxins and/or gene modifying enzymes to give resistance to invasion of the host by foreign DNA.

The naturally occuring plasmids are known as the cryptic plasmids, however, a number of derivatives of cryptic plasmids, referred as the conjugative plasmids are commonly used for cloning purpose. The commonly used plasmid vectors have one or more than one of the genes for antibiotic resistance (See Table 13.2) which serve as the marker gene(s). Other commonly used selection markers are the presence or the absence of some of the metabolic enzymes such as β-galactosidase, glutamine pyruvate transaminase (gpt), thymidine kinase (TK) and the dihydrofolate reductase (DHFR).

Table 13.2. Antibiotic resistance genes which are used as selection marker for cloning vectors

Tc^r	Codes for a 399 aa membrane bound protein which prevents the entry of tetracycline inside the cell and imparts tetracycline resistance
Amp^r	Codes for the enzyme β-lactamase which hydrolyses the β-lactom ring of ampicillin, thus detoxyfying it and providing ampicillin resistance
Cm^r	Cm^r or CAT codes for a 23 KD protein, chloramphenicol acetyl transferase which inactivates chloramphenicol by forming its hydroxyl acetoxyl derivatives
Kan^r/Nor^r	Codes for 25 KD amino-glycoside phosphotransferase which phosphorylates the antibiotic, preventing its transport to the cell. The neo^r gene, isolated from Tn 10 locus, provides resistance to G418 in mammalian cells

Based on the mode of replication, the plasmids are divided into two types, the relaxed and the stringent plasmids. The replication of stringent plasmids is coupled with the replication of host genome and as a result, these are present only in low copy number. On the other hand, the relaxed plasmids can continue replicating even in absence of the replication of host genome. These can, thus, be present in relatively high copy number. The precise number of the plasmid molecules which can be present in a single host cell is a property of the plasmid. Usually this property is vested in the replicon (see later) of the plasmid.

The replication of plasmids requires only a single trans element, the origin of replication. There is usually a single origin of replication. The only exceptions are certain derived plasmids which are generated by the fusion of more than one type of plasmids. These may have multiple origins of replication but only one of them is active. The host replicative machinery is used by the plasmid for its multiplication. The relaxed plasmids, which replicate independent of the host replication, also donot code for any function essential for plasmid replication. These rather use already existing enzymes within the host cell for their replication. The origin of replication of the plasmid alongwith all the necessary 'cis' factors is known as the replicon.

For a plasmid to be suitable for gene cloning, it should have following characteristics:

– It should be small in size which makes it easy to handle and manipulate.
– It should accept a relatively large foreign gene, sometimes many times larger than the plasmid genome itself.
– The plasmid should preferably be under the relaxed mode of control so that high copy number can be achieved. This results in relatively high percentage of plasmid DNA within the host and thus the abundance of foreign DNA is increased.
– The recombinants should be stable.
– It should have one or more of the marker genes so that differential selection (between recombinant and non-recombinants as well as between transfected and non- transfected cells) can be achieved.

Most of the commonly used cloning vectors have been derived from a natural plasmid ColE1. Plasmid pBR 322 is one of the most widely used cloning vector and has been extensively used during the early phase of the development of rDNA technology. Now a number of other plasmids such as pUC, pMBL etc. have been developed. The restriction maps of some of these plasmids are given in Fig. 13.9.

In a number of plasmids (and also in phages) a small synthetic oligonucleotide is often added at the cloning site. This oligonucleotide, which contains recognition sequence for a number of restriction enzymes in a continuous manner, next to each other is called the multiple cloning site (MCS) or a polylinker region. The pUC series of vectors are good example of such plasmids. the polylinker region of some of the pUC plasmids is shown in Fig. 13.10.

Bacteriophages

The bacteriophages are the bacterial viruses. Various phages have varying sizes. These are either single or double stranded DNA molecules. Bacteriophage λ is probably the most widely used phage in genetic engineering.

Bacteriophage λ is a double stranded DNA of 48.6 Kb. It is a linear molecule which circularizes inside the host and replicates as a circular molecule. There is a 12 nucleotide region present at the 5'–ends of both the strands which is single stranded and also complementary to each other. This region, known as the 'cos' site provides a cohesive site which allows the circularization of the genome. The DNA genome is encapsulated within a protein envalope and only the encapsulated DNA is infectious. The naked DNA is not infectious. The absorption of phage is mediated through the receptors present at the surface of the bacterial membrane. These receptors, which are the products of lamB gene of bacteria, are also involved in the transport of maltose. Their synthesis is enhanced by maltose and is inhibited by glucose. It is, therefore, essential that the bacteria which are to be transfected by bacteriophages are grown in presence of maltose. After infecting the bacteria the phage is internalised and the cohesive ends of the phage genome are annealed together. This results in the formation of a circular DNA which replicates by theta mode of DNA replication during the early stage of replication and by rolling circle mode during the late phase of infection. The envalope proteins are coded by the phage genome and the replicated genome is encapsulated to form the phage particles. Depending on the host phenotype and on the MOI, the phage selects either the lytic or the lysogenic mode of life cycle. In lytic cycle, the phage is maintained as an extrachromosomal entity, multiplies till a threshold

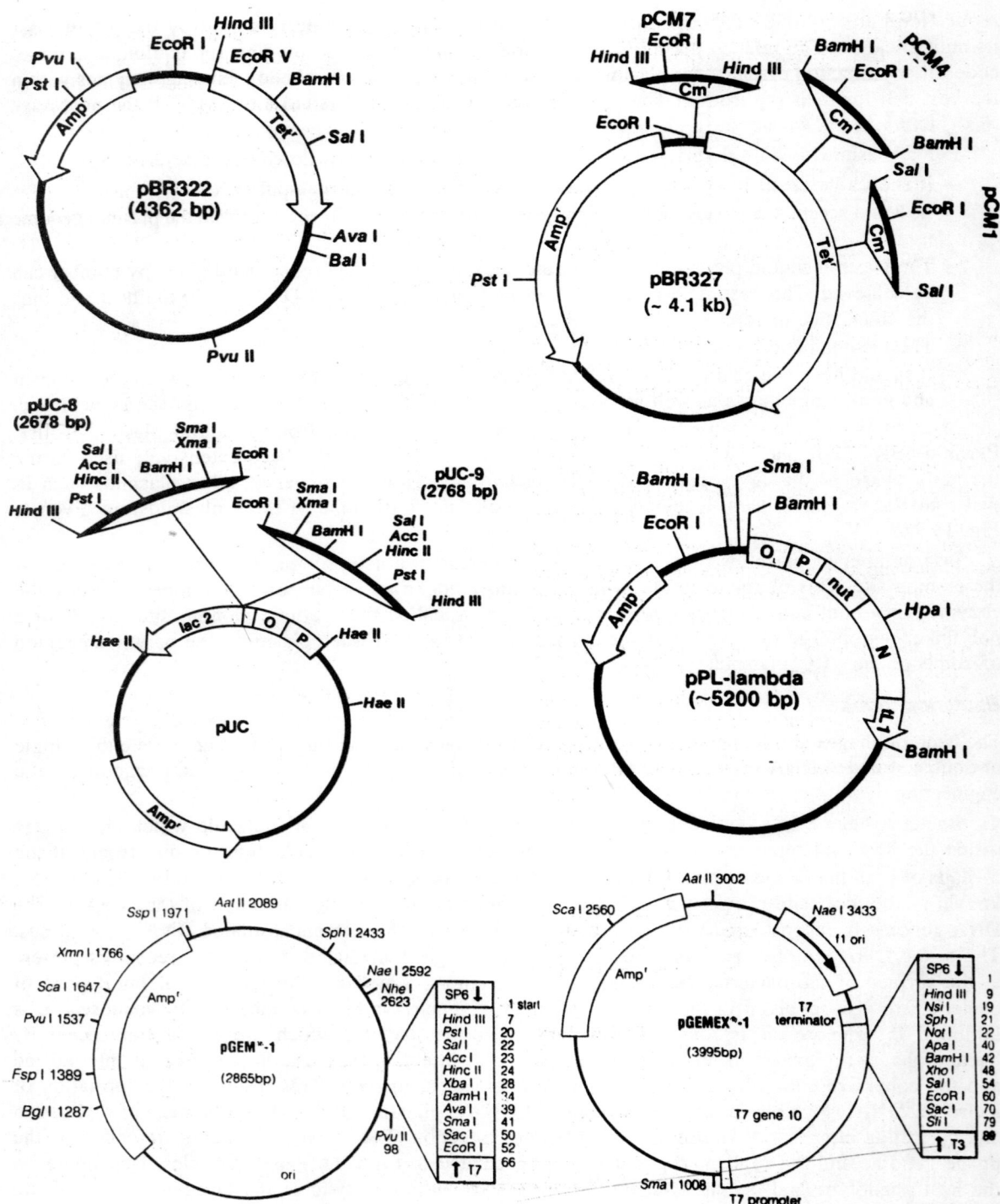

Fig. 13.9. Some of the commonly used cloning vectors.

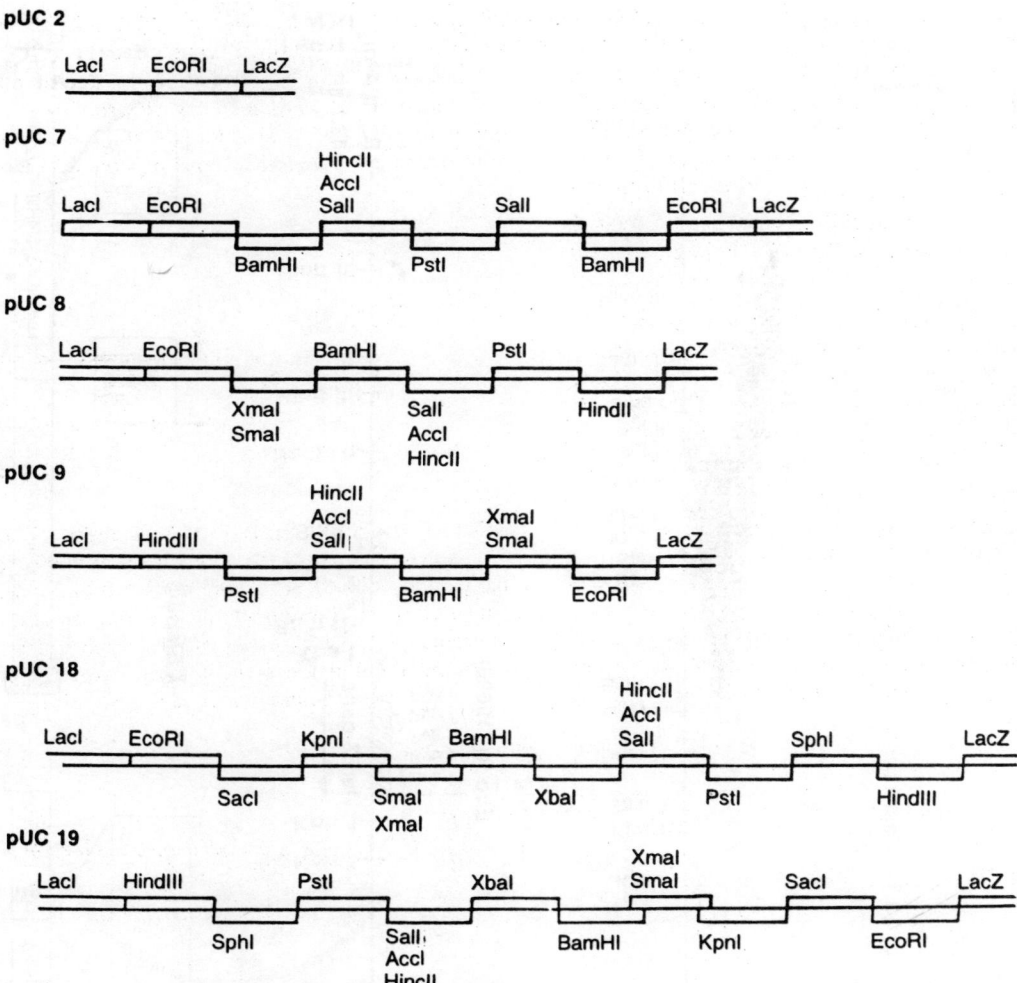

Fig. 13.10. The polylinker region of pUC plasmids.

copy number is achieved and then it kills the host. The particles are released into the culture medium and infect fresh cells. On the other hand, in the lysogenic cycle, the phage gets integrated into the bacterial genome and becomes its part. The phage genome continues to multiply alongwith the bacteria. The phage has the capability to switch over from one mode of life style to another mode. The mechanism of this switch has been discussed earlier.

About 18 Kb region at the center of the bacteriophase λ genome is non-essential. This portion can be used for the cloning of a foreign gene. The map of bacteriophage λ genome is shown in Fig. 13.11. However, the size of λ genome is relatively large and does not have convinient and unique restriction sites. This makes its use as a cloning vector relatively difficult. This problem has been overcome by making a number of derivatives which have convinient restriction sites.

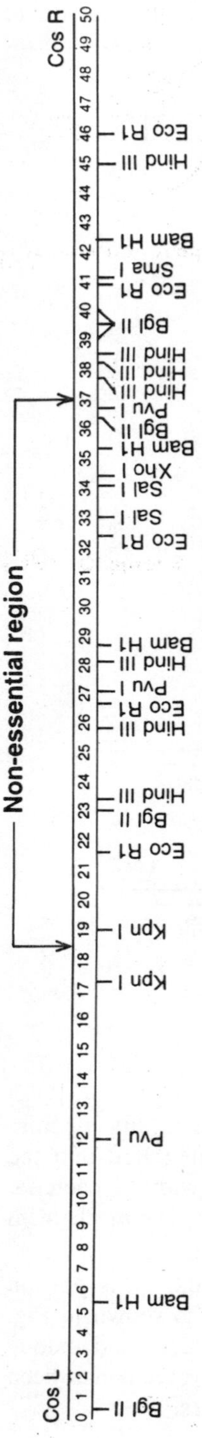

Fig. 13.11. Restriction map of bacteriophage λ.

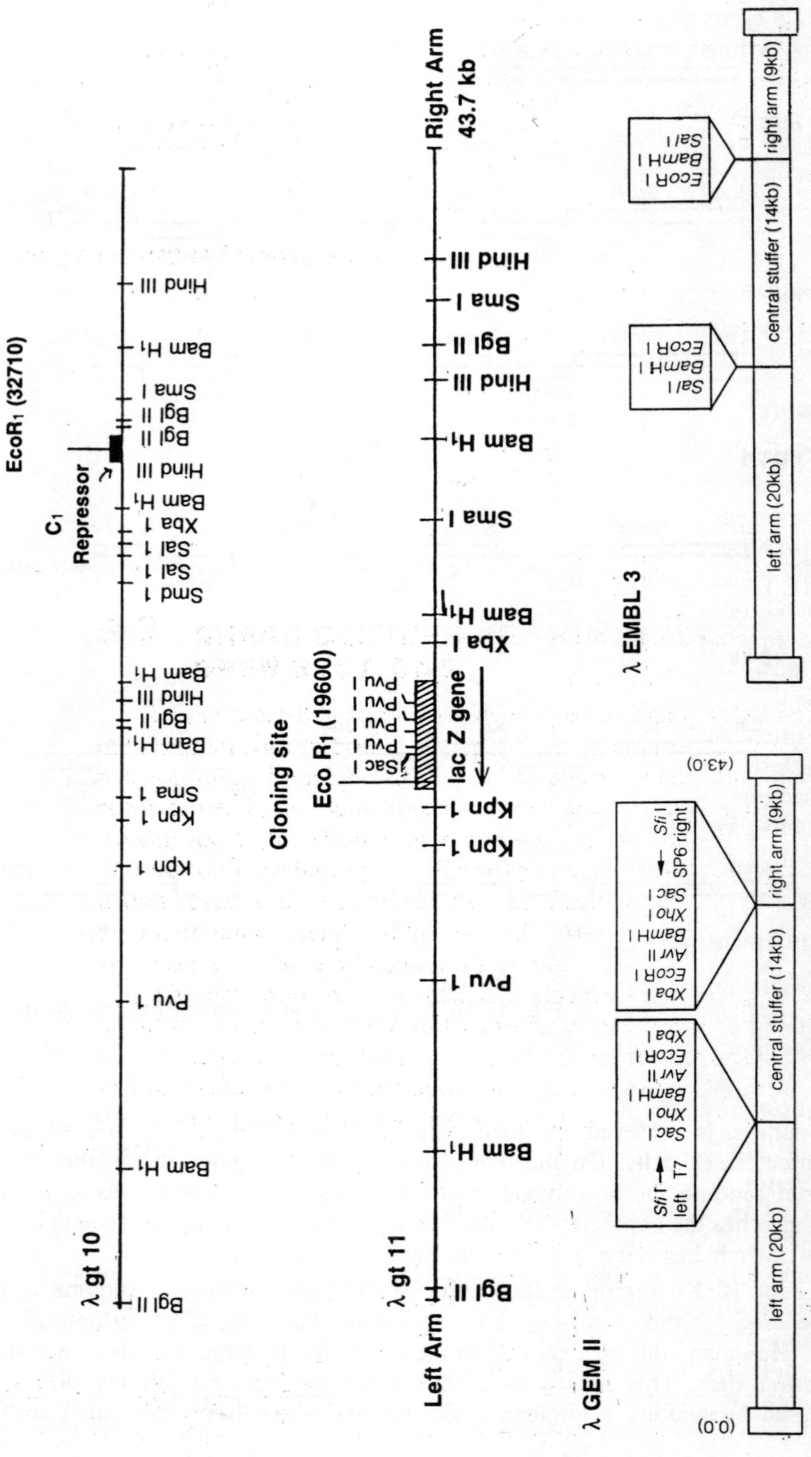

Fig. 13.12. Some of the λ phage-derived cloning vectors.

Two types of λ vectors have been constructed. In first type of vectors, referred as the insertional vectors, a foreign DNA is inserted in the non–essential region of the λ genome. However, it poses some size problems. It has been found that for the packaging of recombinant DNA into phage particles, the size of the genome cannot be more than 110% of the wild type genome. Larger DNAs donot get encapsulated. Thus a maximum of ~5 Kb of foreign DNA can be inserted. To overcome this limitation and making the vectors more versatile, a number of vectors have been designed in which a portion of the non–essential region has been excised off which can be replaced by a foreign DNA during cloning. This type of vectors, known as the replacement vectors, can accomodate much larger (upto 22 Kb) foreign DNA. In a number of vectors, many other useful features have also been added. Some of the commonly used vectors are λgt10, λgt11, λcharon vectors, EMBL series of vectors and the λZap vectors. The genomic maps and specific characteristics of some of these vectors are given in Fig. 13.12.

Cosmids

The cosmids are artificially made vectors. These have been constructed as a hybrid molecule between a plasmid and a phage and are also referred as the phagemids. These have the origin of replication from a plasmid (usually from pBR322) and the cos sites from a λ phage. This gives the name cosmid (cos from the cos sites and mid from plasmid). The cosmids infect the bacteria just like a phage. These require packging and the naked DNA is not infective. On the other hand, these replicate like a plasmid and the cosmid DNA can easily be obtained in the same manner as the plasmid DNA. These form colonies on an agar plate in a similar way as the colonies of the plasmid infected bacteria.

The cosmids are relatively small in size. However, these can accept the foreign DNA of very large size, often many times larger than the length of the cosmid DNA itself. If the size of foreign DNA is not large enough (a minimum and a maximum size is needed for efficient packaging of the DNA), a concatemer of the cosmid can be formed which can get packaged. The cosmids contain the antibiotic resistant genes within their genome and some of these also have a MCS. These vectors are very convinient for making genomic libraries with larege inserts. The structure of a typical cosmid and the mode of insertion of foreign gene is shown in Fig. 13.13.

Cloning strategies

Once suitable gene fragments (either the cDNA molecules or the genomic fragments) have been obtained, these are ligated with suitable vectors to form recombinants. A number of different strategies are used for this purpose. Some of these are described here very briefly.

Homopolymer Tailing

Here a 20-40 nucleotide long stretch of one of the four nucleotides is added at the 3'-end of both the strands of the insert. Similarly, the stretch of complementary nucleotides is added to the linearised vector. A template independent enzyme terminal deoxynucleotidyl transferase (TdT), is normally used for the addition of the 15-30 nucleotide long tails at 3'-ends (see earlier discussion). The tailed DNAs are then allowed to anneal with each other under appropriate buffer conditions which results in the formation of the open circular recombinant molecule. The hydrogen bonding between 20-40 nucleotides is strong enough to maintain the recombinant in a circular form, without the need for covalent bonding. This molecule is then used for the transformation of the host cells. This was the strategy used for most of the cloning experiments during the early periods of development of the techniques. A very common technique of cloning is by G : C tailing at Pst I site. This can be achieved by the digestion of pBR322

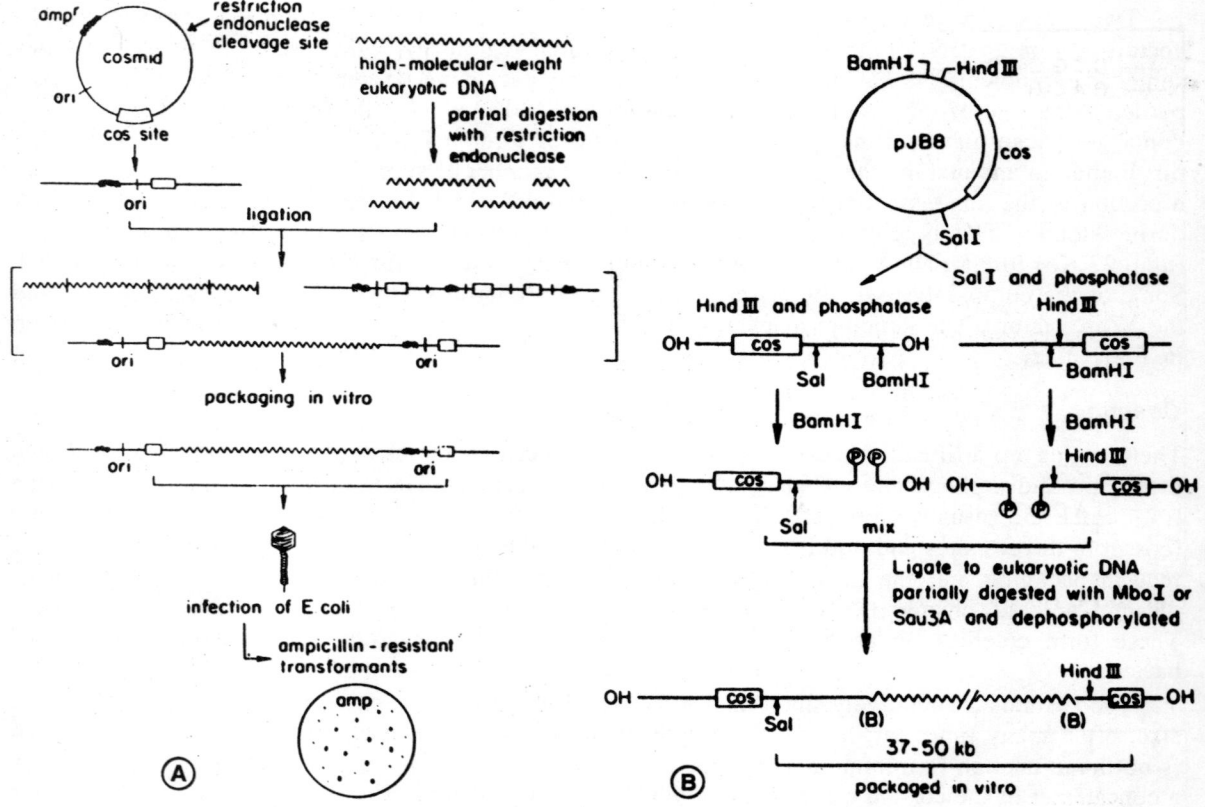

Fig. 13.13. Cloning in cosmids. Two different strategies have been shown.

with restriction endonuclease PstI (recgnition sequence 5'-CTGCA↓G-3') and adding a tail of poly(G) to it which also reconstitutes the PstI site (Fig. 13.14). The cDNA is tailed with poly(C) and two DNAs are allowed to anneal overnight in the presence of 150-500 mM NaCl. Similarly the A:T tailing can be used for cloning at HindIII site which could also reconstitute the restriction site (Fig. 13.15). As there are three hydrogen bonds between G and C and only two between A and T, a longer A:T tail is required than the G:C tail for the formation of open circular molecule. The deatiled strategy of cloning a cDNA by G:C tail at PstI site of pBR322 is shown in Fig. 13.16.

Cloning by Linker Ligation

The linkers are the synthetic oligonucleotides which have the recognition sequence for a particular restriction enzyme. These have one, two or three extra bases on both the sides of the sequence which help in maintaining a right reading frame when so desired. The linkers are ligated to both ends of the insert with the help of the enzyme T4 DNA ligase. The linkered molecule is then digested with the restriction enzyme to produce the cohessive ends. The internal sites present within the 'insert' molecule are protected by methylation of the insert DNA before the addition of the linkers. The vector DNA is also digested with the same enzyme which produces complementary ends. The two molecules (the vector and the insert) are mixed in appropriate molar ratio and are ligated togather. The resulting recombinants are then used for the transformation of the host cells. This is probably the most commonly used technique in most of the cloning experiments. This has been explained in Fig. 13.17.

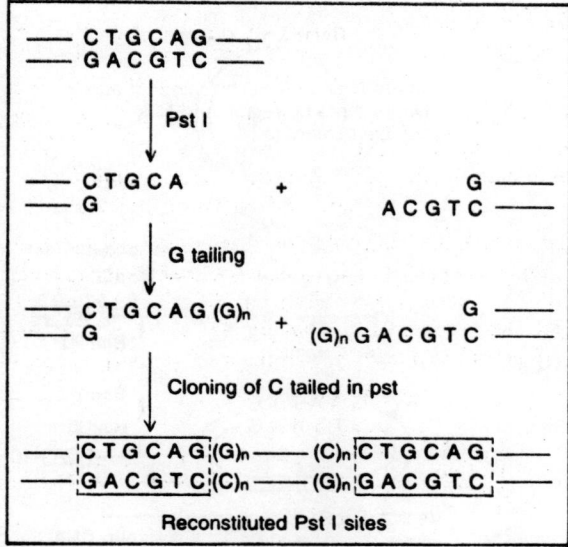

Fig. 13.14. Reconstitution of PstI site by G:C tailing.

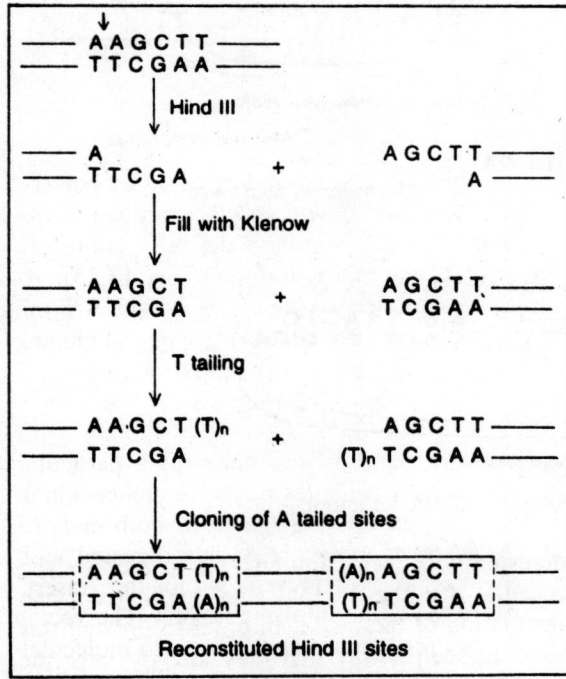

Fig. 13.15. Reconstitution of Hind III sites by A:T tailing.

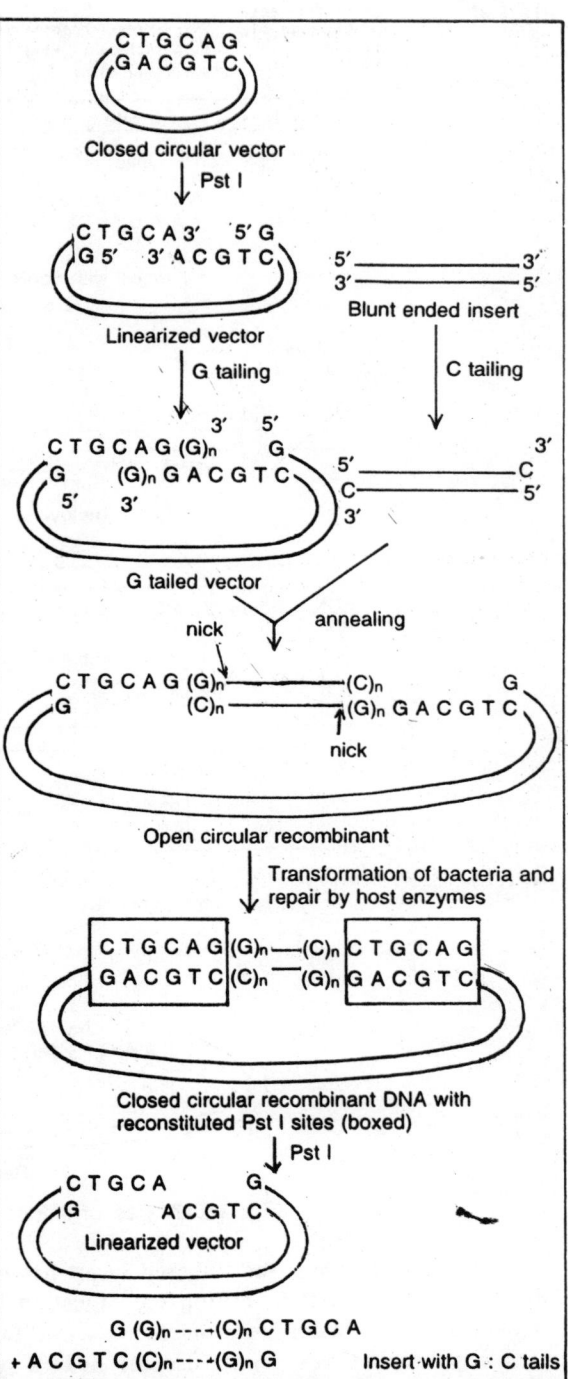

Fig. 13.16. Strategy for cloning of a cDNA in pBR322 by G:C tailing.

Use of linkers.

Linkers for RE

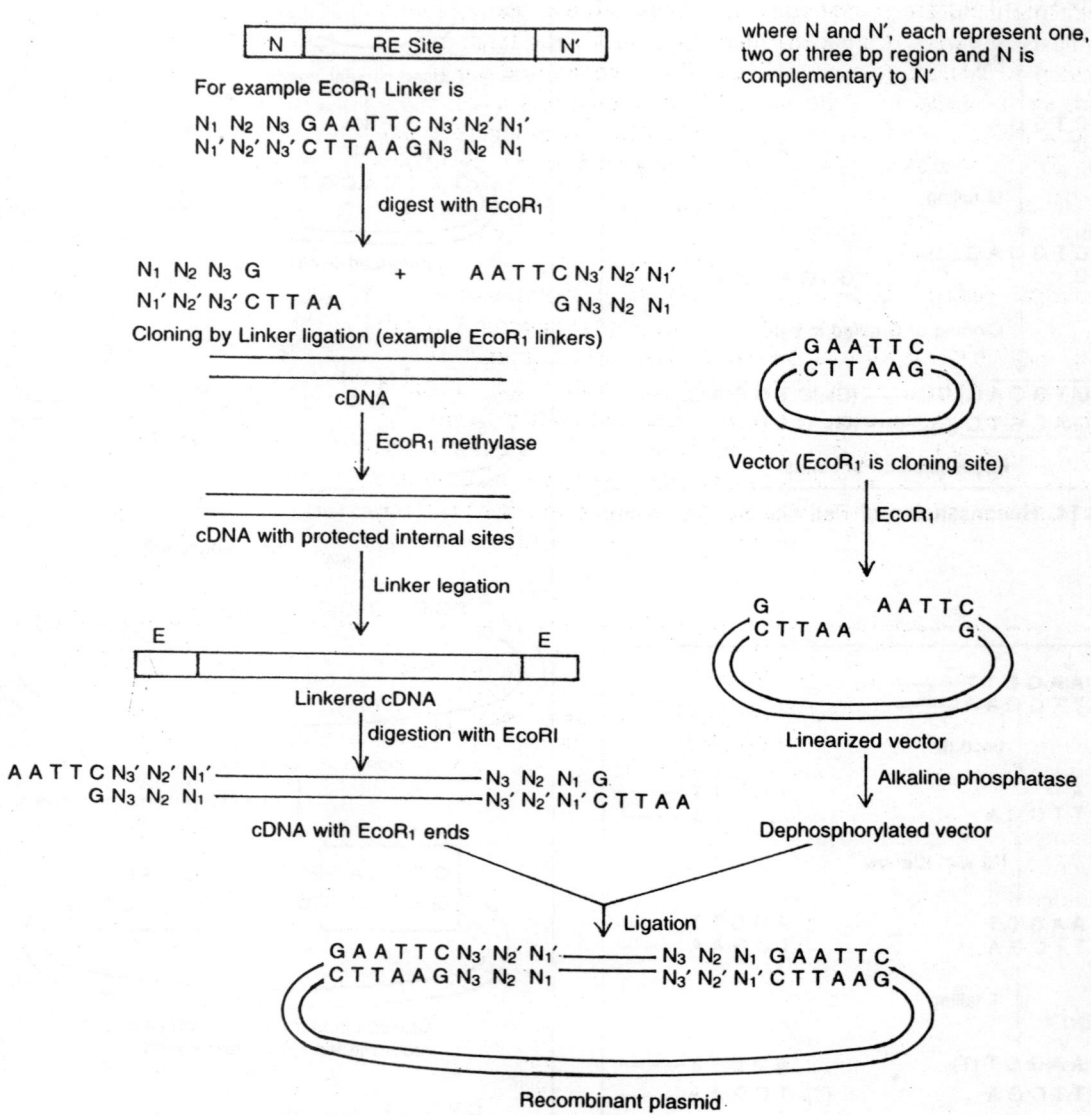

where N and N', each represent one, two or three bp region and N is complementary to N'

Fig. 13.17. Use of linkers for cloning a cDNA fragment.

As described above, the linkered insert has to be digested with restriction enzyme to produce the cohessive ends. However, during the digestion it is essential that the internal sites for that enzyme persent within the insert are protected to avoid the fragmentation of the insert. In order to prevent this possibility, many times people use the linkers synthesized in such a way that they already have the cohessive ends. These are often called as adopters. While these can help in avoiding the methylation as well as digestion steps, they require the use of very short single stranded oligonucleotide molecules which poses a lot of stability problems. Despite the convinience, the use of adopters is not very common.

Other strategies

While the two strategies discussed above are the most commonly used techniques, other strategies have also been occasionally used. These include the cloning of RNA:DNA hybrid which is formed during the synthesis of the first strand of the cDNA. This is useful as there is no need for the synthesis of second strand of DNA. Once inside the host cell, the repair enzyme digest the RNA strand and carry the synthesis of second strand. However, the efficiency of transformation of bacteria by the DNA:RNA hybrid is very low and this method is not used very often.

Other strategy is to clone the cDNA simultaneously as it is being synthesized. It is achieved by using a piece of DNA which is already linkered to the vector as the primer for the synthesis of cDNA. Paul Berg and his colleagues developed such a synthesis/cloning strategy which requires a number of complicated steps (Fig. 13.18). Even though it provided a very high cloning efficiency, it is not popular and is more of academic interest.

It may be pertinent to point out that when the genomic DNA fragments are produced by restriction digestion, these already have the cohessive ends and can be cloned into the vector directly without any modification of their ends. This is achieved by digesting the vector with the same enzyme which was used for fragmenting the genomic DNA.

During the ligation of the insert and the vector, some of the vector DNA molecules receive the insert molecule and form the recombinants. On the other hand, other vector molecules get recircularized without accepting the insert. Thus the efficiency of the cloning will be low. A number of modifications are used to increase the possibility of recombinant formation, these include the addition of insert DNA in several fold higher molar ratio and also the treatment of vector DNA with alkaline phosphate to remove the 5'–PO_4 group. The dephosphorylated DNA cannot get self ligated in absence of the 5'–PO_4. However, the 3'–end of the dephosphorylated vector can still ligate with 5'-end of the insert (having a phosphate group) to produce a open circular molecule. This can easily transform the cells and is repaired once it is inside the host cells (Fig. 13.19).

Once the cloning has been achievd, the ligation mixture is used to transform the host cells (usually one of the strains of E. coli) and the cells are plated on the agar containing the appropriate selection media where only the transformed cells will grow. The real number of colonies are counted and the actual number of independent clones in the mixture is calculated. This collection of the clones is known as the gene library or a gene bank. The library is now amplified so that multiple copies of each clone are obtained. To have a reasonable chance of obtaining a gene of choice, it is usually essential to screen about 100,000-250,000 clones if it is a cDNA library (which is less complex) and about 500,000-2,000,000 clones if it is a genomic library.

Isolation of the clone of interest

The gene library is like a stack of hay in which the gene of interest is hidden like a needle. In order to search the needle, one requires a specific tool which could be a magnet in this scenerio. Similarly in case of search for the gene of interest, the specific tool is required which is referred as the probe and the search is known as the screening of the library. The exact protocol for the screening will depend on the type of vector used and the type of probe being used for the screening. However, a plasmid library is usually screened by colony hybridization while the phage library is screened by plaque hybridization.

The most commonly used probes are the nucleic acid probes. If a gene of interest from another species has been cloned, it can be used as a probe. The chances are that it will have high degree of homology with the gene of interest which can easily be picked. Similarly if a clone for a closely related gene is known then it can be used to isolate a related gene. In certain cases, if the cDNA for a gene has been isolated then it can be used for the isolation of a genomic clone. Occasionly when only a small fragment of gene is available then it is used for isolation of the full length clone.

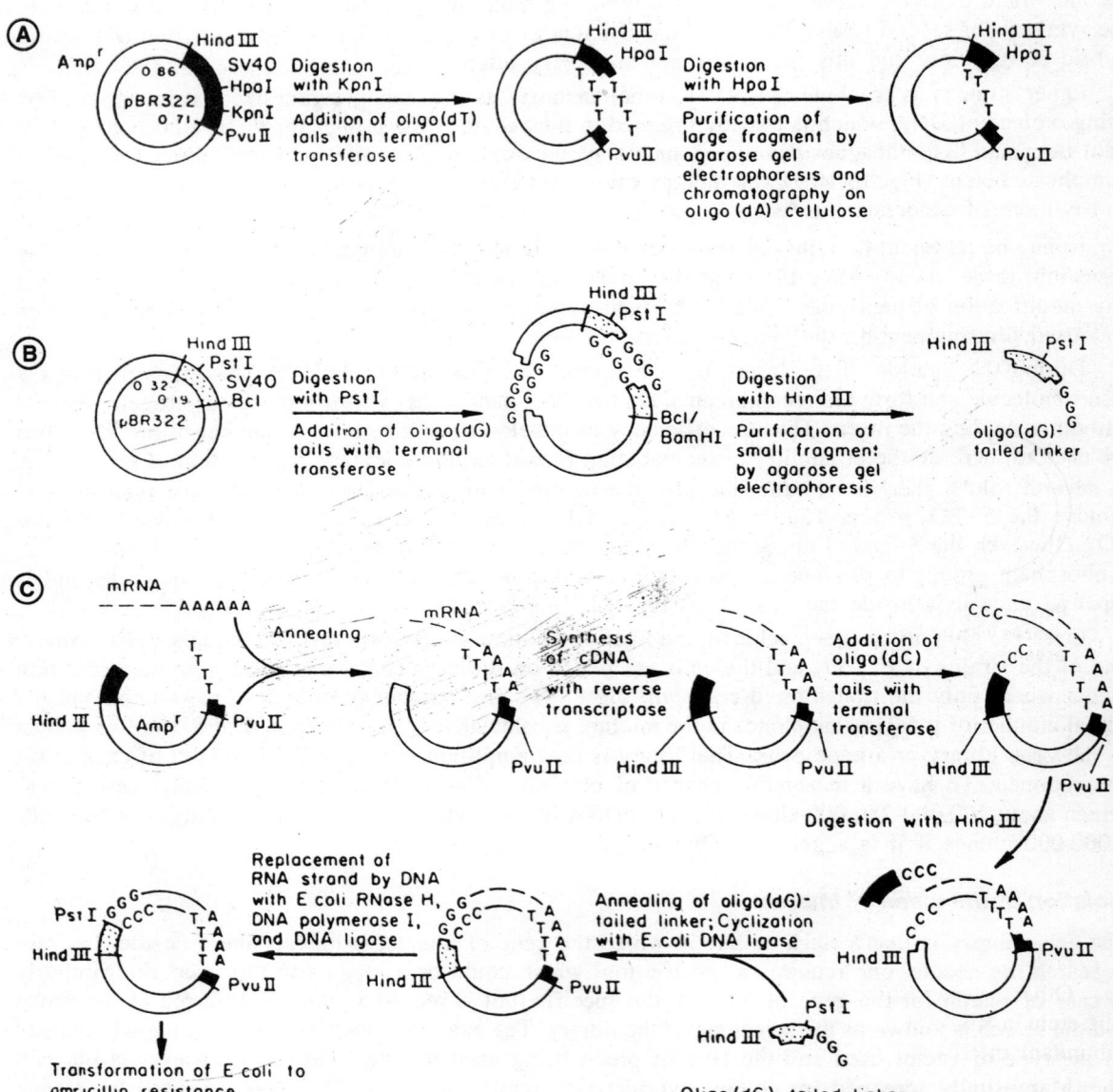

Fig. 13.18. Preparation of (A) plasmid primer and (B) oligo (dG)-tailed linked DNA. (C) Steps in the construction of plasmid-cDNA recombinants. pBR322 DNA is represented by the open sections of each ring; SV40 DNA is indicated by the darkened or stippled segments. The numbers next to the restriction site designations are the corresponding SV40 DNA map coordinates.

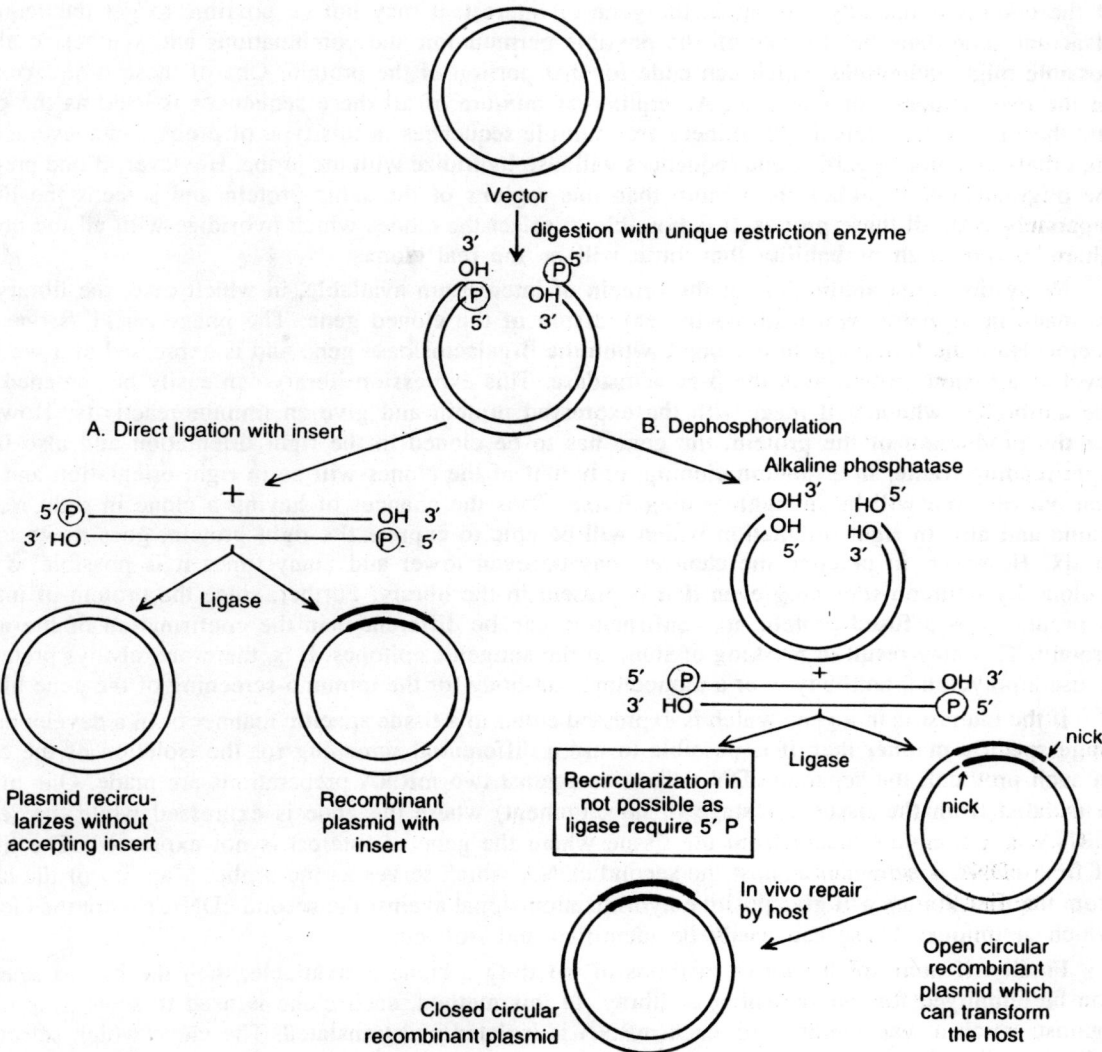

Fig. 13.19. Use of dephosphorylation to prevent self ligation of vector.

Other type of screening involves the use of mRNA against which the cDNA was made. Since different mRNAs are present in different abundance it is possible to isolate the clones for the most abundant mRNAs if hybridization studies are done under appropriate condition.

Many times none of the nucleic acid probes described above are available. However, if at least the partial sequence information about the sequence of the protein is known then it is possible to deduce the nuceic acid sequence for that portion of protein. An oligonucleotide for that portion can be chemically synthesized and can be used for the screening of the library. There is a point of caution here. As many aminoacids are coded by more than one codon and one can not be sure as to which of the codons is actually present in the gene of interest, it may not be possible to get the sequence of actual gene. One has to take all the possible permutation and combinations and synthesize all the possible oligonucleotides which can code for that portion of the protein. One of these sequences will be the real sequence of the gene. An equimolar mixture of all these sequences is used as the probe and the library is screened. Since there are multiple sequences in this type of probe, chances are quite high that some non-specific gene sequences will also hybridize with the probe. However, if one prepares the oligonucleotide probes from more than one regions of the same protein and screens the library separately with all these probes, it is possible to select the clones which hybridize with all the probes. There is very high probability that these will be the real clones.

Many times the antibodies for the protein of interest are available, in which case, the library can be made in a vector which allows the expression of the cloned gene. The phage λgt11 is one such vector. Here the foreign gene is cloned within the β-galactosidase gene and is expressed at a very low level as a fusion protein with the β-galactosidase. This expression library can easily be screened with the antibodies which will react with the expressed protein and give an immunoreactivity. However, for the production of the protein, the gene has to be cloned in the right orientation and also in the right reading frame. In a random cloning, only half of the clones will be in right orientation and only one out of three will be in right reading frame. Thus the chances of having a clone in right reading frame and also in right orientation which will be able to express the right protein, goes down to one in six. However, in practice the chances may be even lower and many times it is possible to miss a clone by immuno-screening even if it is present in the library. Further, since the protein of interest is produced as a fused protein, its confirmation can be different than the confirmation of the native protein. This may result in masking of some of the antigenic epitopes. It is, therefore, always preferable to use a polyclonal antibody over a monoclonal antibody for the immuno-screening of the gene library.

If the interest is in a gene which is expressed either in a tissue specific manner or in a developmental stage specific manner then it is possible to use a differential screening for the isolation of the clone. In such protocol, the separate cDNA libraries against two mRNA preparations are made. One mRNA is isolated from the tissue (or stage of development) where the gene is expressed while the second mRNA is a sample isolated from the tissue where the gene of interest is not expressed. The library of first cDNA is screened against the second cDNA which serves as the probe. Majority of the clones from the first library will give positive hybridization signal against the second cDNA except the clone(s) which ar unique. These can easily be identified and isolated.

Finally, if none of the above methods of isolating a clone is available, then the hybrid selection can be employed for the screening of library. In this method, each clone is used to select the mRNA against which it was synthesized, each mRNA is isolated and translated. The clone which selects the mRNA coding for desired protein is selected. In order to minimize the number of analyses, the clones are divided into a number of pools, each pool is analysed, one pool which hybridizes with the correct mRNA is selected and its clones are redistributed in many pools, each pool will have much less number of clones than the original pool and finally, by elimination a single clone is isolated. Cell free protein synthesis is used as the means to identify the mRNA. This is a very cumbersome process and is usually not preferred for the purpose of library screening. However, it is one of the final proofs for establishing the identity of the clones.

Characterization of gene clones

Once a clone has been obtained by screening of the library (it is still only a putative clone) it is essential that its identity should be established beyond any reasonable doubt. Following are some of he criterion which are used for this purpose.

1. Specific hybridization with related probes

The clone is digested with appropriate restriction enzyme(s) so that the insert is excised from the vector, it is then fractionated on agarose gels and Southern transferred to nitrocellulose filters. The blot is then hybridized with specific probe (see earlier section for the description of probes). Under high stringency conditions, the probe should specifically hybridize with the insert and should not give any signal with the vector band(s). As the experimental controls, some unrelated clones are also selected and digested in a similar manner. No hybridization with unrelated clones should take place.

2. Restriction analysis

The clone is digested with a number of restriction endonucleases, individually as well as in various combinations. A restriction map of the cloned gene is deduced by these analyses. If the restriction map of the same gene from another species is known or if the map of a related gene is known, the restriction map obtained for the isolated clone is compared with the map of the known gene. Very high degree of homology between the maps of two genes gives an indication that the clone may be right.

3. Hybrid selection, in vitro translation of selected mRNA and immuno-precipitation of the protein

The method of hybrid selection has been discussed earlier. The mRNA which hybridizes with the cloned gene is isolated and translated in vitro in a cell free system. The wheat germ S-30 or rabbit reticulocyte lysates are usually used for this purpose. The synthesized protein is characterized by SDS-PAGE to find out its molecular weight and is Western blotted and its reactivity with appropriate antibodies is checked. The entire protocol is described in Fig. 13.20. These analyses prove that the clone contains the correct gene.

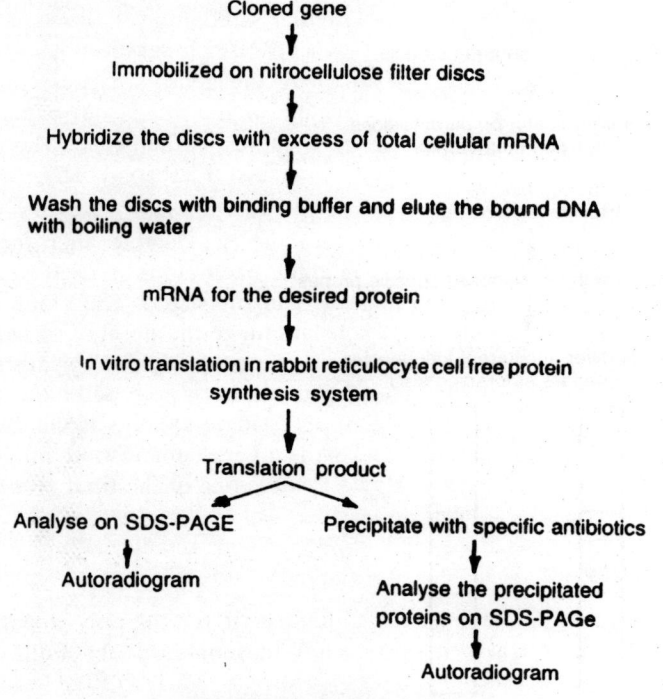

Fig. 13.20. Hybrid selection.

4. Nucleotide sequencing

The final identity of the gene is established by its nucleotide sequence. The clone should have a open reading frame coding for the correct protein. If the sequence of the protein is known then it establishes the identity of the clone beyond any doubt. If the sequence of the protein is not known then the sequencing data are used for deducing the amino acid sequence of the protein.

By a combination of all these analyses, the identity of the clone is established as well as it is characterized.

Genomic analysis

The purpose of carrying out the genomic analysis is to get an insight into the gene(s) which codes for the protein of interest. As discussed earlier, usually a cDNA clone is the first gene to be isolated, since it is much simpler in structure as well as in complexity. Using this clone as the probe, it is possible to identify and characterize the genes coding for the protein. The first step is to isolate the high molecular weight genomic DNA of the organism. In majority of the cases the blood is the most convinient tissue to obtain and is generally used for this purpose. The DNA is then digested with a number of different restriction enzymes and fractionated on agarose gels. The gels are Southern blotted to nitrocellulose membranes and hybridized with the cDNA probe. The bands obtained following the hybridization are analysed (Fig. 13.21).

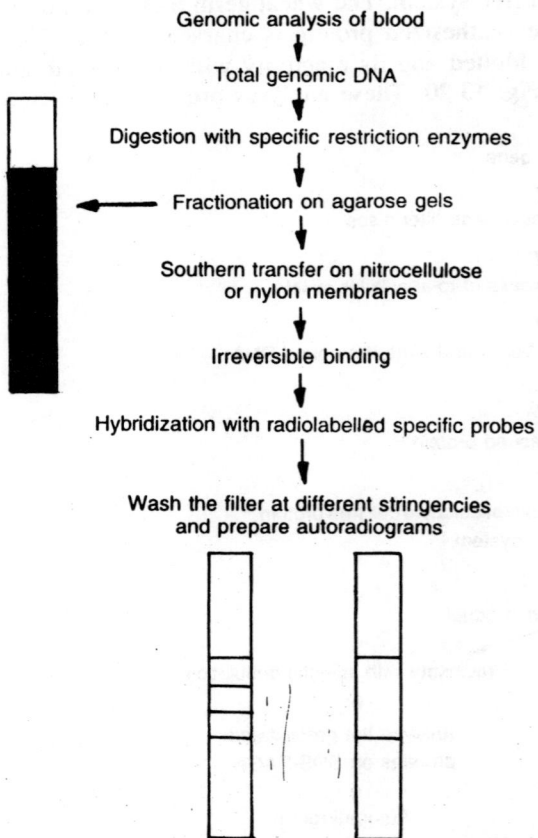

Fig. 13.21. Genomic analysis.

The restriction enzymes used in preliminary experiments are carefully selected. The enzymes should not have a site within the cDNA. Following the hybridization, if only one band is obtained in all the digests, it reflects that the protein is coded by a single gene. The size of the band will vary with each digestion. The band size doesnot reflect the actual size of the gene but only means that the gene is located within the restriction fragment of that size. However, if more than one bands are obtained then the scenerio becomes much more complex. it reflects that either there are multiple genes for the protein or the gene has site(s) for the specific restriction endonuclease (which give multiple bands) within the introns (as the enzymes used were such that no restriction sites were present in the cDNA, the exons will not have the site for the enzymes). In such case, it is possible to analyse the genes and find out which of the two possibilities exists. The subprobe analysis are done for this purpose.

Sub-probe analysis

The blot is first hybridized with the complete cDNA probe and hybridization pattern is analysed. Now the probe cDNA is fragmented by restriction digestion into 2-3 pieces. For the sake of simplicity, let us assume that the probe is cut into three pieces, the 5'-piece, the middle piece and the 3'-piece. Each of the three pieces is seperetely nick-translated and the blot is now hybridized with these probes individually (one probe at a time). It is possible to use a single blot for more than one hybridization by first obtaining a autoradiogram with one probe, stripping the blot and rehybridizing it with the second probe. The process can be repeated several times to get multiple analyses from the same blot. Should each of the bands obtained by hybridization with the complete probe represent a gene, this band would hybridize with each of the partial probes also. As a result, the number of bands will remain same irrespective of the probe used. However, if the multiple bands obtained in the first experiment were due to the presence of a restriction site within the intron, a band representing only part of a gene, will not hybridize with all the probe pieces (Fig. 13.22). By designing suitable probe pieces, it is possible to find out the exact number of genes which code for a specific protein.

Related genes

Many times, each of the multiple bands obtained during hybridization may represent a separate gene, however, each of these genes may not be the real gene. Some of the bands may represent the genes which have varying degree of homology with the real gene. This may be seen by doing a stringency analysis. After hybridization, the filter is washed at different stringencies, starting from low stringency (usually 6 X SSC, room temperature) and increasing the washing conditions in a stepwise manner to a high stringency. Higher the stringency, more homology is required for the probe to hybridize with the gene. At a stringency of 0.1 X SSC and 68°C temperature, almost 99% homology is required for hybridization. An autoradiogram is obtained for washing at each stringency. While the real gene will remain hybridized at each of the washings, the related genes will fade out at a stringencgy which exceeds its Tm. Thus it is possible to get a picture of related genes and also of the degree of homology of each of these genes with the gene of interest.

The exon-intron boundaries

By analysing the hybridization behaviour between an mRNA and its gene, it is possible to analyse the number of introns present in it and to find out their position within the gene. The analysis, referred as heteroduplex mapping or R-loop analysis is carried out by denaturing a gene and allowing it to hybridize with the mRNA. As the RNA:DNA hybrid is more stable than the DNA:DNA hybrid, the mRNA:gene duplex is formed. In such duplexes, the exons of the gene align with the

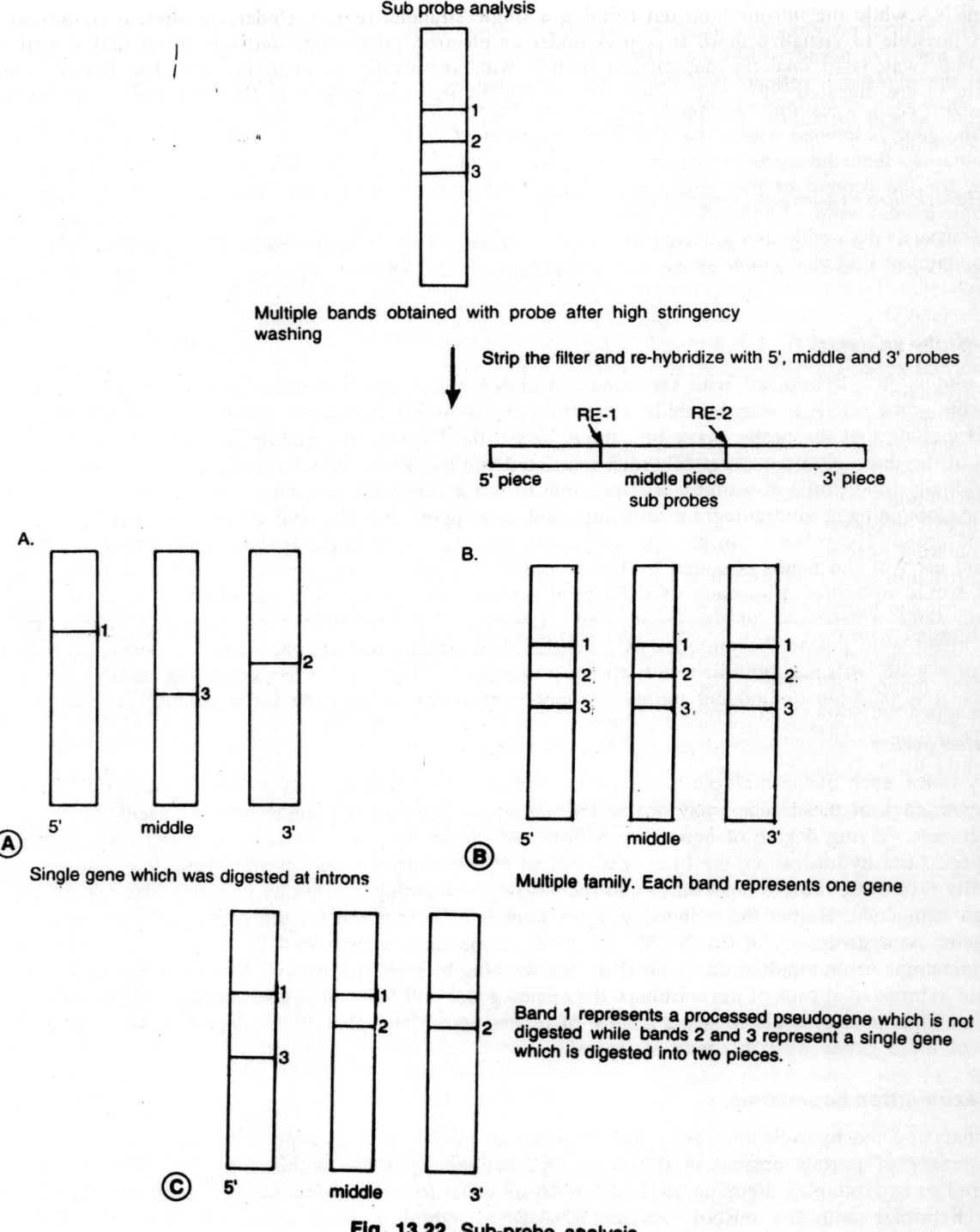

Sub probe analysis

Multiple bands obtained with probe after high stringency washing

Strip the filter and re-hybridize with 5', middle and 3' probes

A.

Single gene which was digested at introns

B.

Multiple family. Each band represents one gene

Band 1 represents a processed pseudogene which is not digested while bands 2 and 3 represent a single gene which is digested into two pieces.

Fig. 13.22. Sub-probe analysis.

mRNA while the introns loop out forming a single stranded region. Under appropriate conditions, it is possible to visualize these structures under an electron microscope and see the ds and ss regions. Other way is to take the duplex and treat it with ss specific S_1 endonuclease. The introns which are ss are digested while the exons are resistant as they are present in ds form due to the mRNA: gene hybrid formation. Resulting fragments are analysed on the gels and the sizes of the exons are determined.

Restriction Fragment Length Polymorphism

The analysis, commonly referred as RFLP, is used to determine a mutation in a gene when it (the mutation) is present within the site for a specific restriction enzyme. The genomic DNA from the normal as well as from the organism bearing the mutation of interest is isolated and digested with the restriction enzyme(s) which have site(s) within the gene of interest. Both the digests are fractionated on the gels and the gels are transferred to hybridization membranes. The blots are then hybridized with probe for normal gene. The DNA fragments containing the parts of gene will hybridize and give specific bands of certain size in the control DNA. The mutated gene on the other hand, will loose (or gain, as the case may be) some of the restriction sites. This will result in a different hybridization pattern than the pattern obtained with the DNA from the wild type organism. Any deviation from the pattern of the wild type DNA represents a mutation. When the site of mutation is not known, a number of different restriction enzymes are used for the fractionation of DNAs and hybridization pattern with each of these digests is obtained. By having a sufficiently high number of digests, the probability of detecting any mutation becomes reasonably high. However, if the mutation does not result in gain or loss of any restriction site, then it cannot be detected by the RFLP analysis.

If the purpose is to screen for a specific mutation which is well characterized then the DNA is digested with only the required enzyme and the presence or the absence of the band of the specific size is determined. For example, the mutations which result in a particular genetic disease have often been mapped. In such a case it is possible to detect the faulty gene by these analyses. Similarly the mapped mutation in a number of oncogenes can be detected much earlier than the onset of the disease. This type of analyses can also help in screening for a genetic diseases in the neonatal stage, if the child to be born is suspected of inheriting the disease because of the history of the parents.

Landmarks in Molecular Biology

1869 Friedrich Miescher discovered DNA.

1941 Beadle and Tatum demonstrated that a gene codes for a single protein.

1944 Avery proved that DNA is the genetic material.

1953 Watson and Crick proposed the double helical structure for DNA.

1958 Meselson and Stahl demonstrated that DNA replicates semiconservatively.

1961 The triplet nature of the genetic code was discovered.

1961 Messenger RNA was uncovered.

1961 Jacob and Monod proposed the operon model for gene regulation.

1970 Temin and Baltimore reported the discovery of reverse transcriptase in retroviruses.

1973 Type II restriction endonucleases were discovered.

1974 Eukaryotic genes were cloned in bacterial plasmids.

1976 Retroviral oncogenes were identified as the causative agents of cellular transformation.

1977 DNA sequencing became possible.

1977 Interrupted genes were discovered and splicing mechanism for their removal from the primary transcripts was deciphered.

1979 Cellular oncogenes were discovered by transfection.

1981 Catalytic activity of RNA was discovered.

1981 Transgenic mice and flies were obtained by introducing new DNA into the germline.

1997 A sheep was cloned from somatic cell genome, establishing the possible totipotency in animal cells.

Selected Readings

Biochemistry by L. Stryer, published by W.H. Freeman and Co. New York, USA

Principles of Bichemistry by A.L. Lehninger, D.L. Nelson and M.M. Cox, published by CBS Publishers and Distributor, New Delhi, India

Molecular Biology of Genes by, J.D. Watson, N.H. Hopkins, J.W. Roberts, J.A. Steitz and A.M. Weiner, published by Benzamin/ Cumminings Publishing Co. Inc. Reading USA

Molecular Biology of the Cell by B. Alberts, D. Bray, J. Lewis, M. Raff, K. Roberts and J.D. Watson, published by Garland Publishing, Inc. New York

Molecular Cell Biology by J. Darnell, H. Lodish and D. Baltimore, published by Scientific American Books, New York, USA.

Genes by B. Lewin published by Oxford University Press, Oxford, UK.

From Genes to Clone by E-L. Winnacker, published by VCH Verlagsgesellschaft, Weinheim, Germany.

Genetics by M.W. Strickberger, Published by Macmillan Publishing Company, New York, USA.

Recombinant DNA by J.D. Watson, M. Gilman, J. Witkowski and M. Zoller, publised by Scientific Americal Books, New York, USA.

Principals of Gene Manipulation by R.W. Old and S.B. Primrose, published by Blackwell Scientific Publications, Oxford, UK.

Microbial Genetics by S.R. Maloy, J.E. Cronan and D. Freifelder, published by Jones Bartlett Publishers, Boston, USA.

Glossary

α-helix (pl. α-helices): Common secondary structure of proteins in which the linear sequence of amino acids is folded into a right-handed spiral that is stabilized by hydrogen bonds between the carboxyl oxygen of each **peptide bond** and the amide group three residues away in the sequence.

Abundance of an mRNA: The average number of molecules per cell of a paritcular mRNA.

Abundant mRNAs: A small number of individual mRNA species, each of which are present in a large number of copies per cell.

Acceptor splicing site: Also referred as 3' splice site, it is the boundary between the 3' end of an intron and 5' end of the adjacent exon.

Acentric fragment: The piece of a chromosome which is generated by its breakage and lacks the centromere. It is lost during cell division.

Acrocentric chromosome: The chromosome which has the centromere located nearer to one of its end than to the other.

Activation energy: The input of energy required to overcome the barrier to initiate a chemical reaction.

Active transport: Movement of an ion or small molecule across a membrane against the concentration gradient or electrochemical gradient of the transported molecule by a process directly coupled to ATP hydrolysis.

Adenylate cyclase: Enzyme that catalyzes formation of **cyclic AMP** (cAMP), a second messenger. Building of ligands to certain **svenspanning** and other **receptors** leads to activation of membrane-bound adenylate cyclase and a rise in intracellular cAMP.

Allele: One of several alternative forms of a gene which occupy a given locus on a chromosome.

Allelic exclusion: The phenomenon of expression of only one allele coding for the expressed immuno-globulin.

Allosteric control: The regulatory mechanism where the interaction of a molecule at one site of a protein can influence the biological activity of another site of the same protein.

Alu family: A set of ~300 bp long dispersed and related sequences in human genome. Each of individual members have Alu cleavage sites at each end hence the name.

Alu-equivalent family: The sets of sequences in non-human mammalian genome that are related to human Alu family sequences.

α-Amanitin: A bicyclic octapeptide derived from the poisonous mushroom *Amanita phalloides* which can inhibit transcription process catalysed by certain eukaryotic RNA polymerases, especially the RNA polymerase II. Based on sensitivity to α-amanitin the RNA polymerases are classified as Pol I, Pol II and Pol III.

Amber codon: One of three stop codons with sequence UAG that causes termination of protein synthesis.

Amber mutation: Any change in genome that creates an amber codon at a site previously occupied by a codon representing an amino acid within a gene.

Amber suppressors: The mutant genes that code for tRNAs whose anticodons have been altered so that they can interact with amber codons in addition to or instead of their previous codons.

Ames test: A simple bacterial test for carcinogens, based on the assumption that carcinogens are mutagens.

Amino acids: A class of organic compounds in which an amino group and a carboxyl group are linked to a central carbon atom, called the α carbon, to which a variable side chain is bound. Twenty common amino acids are the monomers that polymerize to form proteins. Some of these amino acids can then become modified.

Aminoacyl-tRNA: The transfer RNA molecule carrying an amino acid; the covalent linkage is between the NH_2 group of the amino acid and either the 3′- or 2′-OH group of the terminal region (CCA) of the tRNA. Also referred as 'charged' tRNA.

Aminoacyl-tRNA synthetases: These are a group of enzymes which are responsible for covalently linking of an amino acid to the 2′- or 3′-OH position of its specific tRNA.

Amphipathic: The structures having two surfaces, one hydrophilic and one hydrophobic. Lipids are amphipathic; and some protein regions may form amphipathic helices, with one charged face and one neutral face.

Amplification: The production of additional copies of a DNA or gene sequence. These may be present as intrachromosomal or extrachromosomal DNA. It is possible to amplify a DNA *in vitro* using PCR.

Anaerobic: The term describes a cell, organism, or metabolic process that functions in the absence of air or, more precisely, in the absence of molecular oxygen.

Anchorage dependence: The need of normal eukaryotic cells for a surface for attachment in order to grow in culture.

Aneuploid: Chromosome constitution which differs from the usual diploid constitution by the loss or duplication of chromosomes or chromosomal segments.

Angstrom (Å): Unit of length used to measure atoms and molecules. Equal to 10^{-10} meter or 0.1 nanometer (nm).

Annealing: Pairing of complementary single strands of DNA or RNA to form double helix.

Antibody: A specialized group of proteins (immunoglobulins) produced by B lymphocyte cells that recognize a particular foreign "antigen," and thus triggers the humoral immune response.

Anticoding strand: The strand of duplex DNA which is used as a template to direct the synthesis of RNA that is complementary to it.

Anticodon: Sequence of three nucleotides in a transfer RNA (tRNA) that is complementary to a **codon** in a messenger RNA (**mRNA**). During protein synthesis, base pairing between a codon and anticodon aligns the tRNA carrying the corresponding amino acid for addition to the growing peptide chain.

Antigen: Any foreign molecule whose entry into an organism provokes the synthesis of an antibody.

Antiparallel strands: The two strands of the double helix of a nucleic acid which are organized in opposite orientation. The 5′ end of one strand is aligned with the 3′ end of the other strand and vice versa.

Antiport: Cotransport process in which the movement of a molecule or ion across a membrane against its concentration gradient is driven by the movement in the opposite direction of a second ion down its concentration gradient. Transport is mediated by specific membrane-bound proteins called antiporters.

Antitermination proteins: Also referred as antiterminators, these allow RNA polymerase to transcribe through certain terminator sites.

AP endonucleases: Special class of nucleases which makes incisions in DNA on the 5′ side of either an apurinic or an apyrimidinic site.

Apoinducer: A protein that binds to DNA and switches its transcription by RNA polymerase on.

Apoptosis: Programmed cell death; a specific suicide process in animal cells that includes fragmentation of nuclear DNA. Apoptosis occurs normally in development, as in the resorption of the tadpole tail during metamorphosis into a frog; or it can be induced, for example by DNA damage that exceeds the capacity of repair mechanisms.

Archebacteria: It is a minor group of prokaryotes which may have introns in their genome.

Asymmetric carbon atom: A carbon atom bonded to four differenct atoms; also called *chiral carbon atom*. The bonds can be arranged in two different ways producing **stereoisomers**, which are mirror images of each other.

ATP (adenosine 5′-triphosphate): Used as the currency of energy in the cell, it is an adenine **nucleotide** containing two high-energy phosphoanhydride bonds whose hydrolysis or transfer is accompanied by a large **free-energy change** ($\wedge G$) of ~7 kCal/mole each. It is the most important molecule for capturing and transferring free energy in all cells.

ATPase: One of a large group of enzymes that catalyzes hydrolysis of **ATP** to yield ADP and inorganic phosphate with release of free energy. The released energy is utilized in some coupled activity such as active transport, muscle contraction, unwiding of DNA, or movement of cilia and flagella.

ATP synthase, mitochondrial: Multimeric protein complex bound to inner mitochondrial membranes that catalyzes synthesis of ATP coupled to proton movement down its electrochemical gradient; also called $F_0 F_1$ *complex*. Similar enzymes are present in bacterial plasma membranes and the thylakoid membranes of chloroplasts ($CF_0 CF_1$ complex).

att **sites:** The loci on a phage as well as on bacterial chromosome upon recombination at which site the phage integrates into or excises from the bacterial chromosome during recombination.

Attenuation: A special mode of regulation of termination of transcription that is involved in controlling the expression of some bacterial operons. The coupled transcription and translation is essential for attenuation to work.

Attenuator: The terminator sequences at which attenuation occurs.

Autogenous control: The action of a gene product that either inhibits (negative autogenous control) or activates (positive autogenous control) the expression of the gene coding for it.

Autonomous controlling elements: Present in maize, these are the active transposons with the ability to transpose.

Autonomously replicating sequence (ARS): Sequence that permits a DNA molecule to replicate in yeast; an origin of yeast DNA replication.

Autoradiography: The process to detect radioactively labeled molecules by their ability of creating an image on photographic film.

Autosomes: All the chromosomes present in a cell except the sex chromosomes; a diploid cell has two copies of each autosome.

Autotroph: An organism that can synthesize its own complex molecules from very simple carbon and nitrogen sources, such as carbon dioxide and ammonia.

Auxotrophic mutant (auxotroph): A mutant organism defective in the synthesis of given bio-molecule, which must, therefore, be supplied for the organism's growth.

Axon: Process extending form the cell body of a neuron that is capable of conducting an electric impulse **(action potential)** generated at the junction with the cell body (called the axon hillock) toward its distal, branching end (called the axon terminal).

ß pleated sheet: A planar secondary structure element of proteins that is created by hydrogen bonding between the backbone atoms in two different polypeptide chains or segments of a single folded chain.

B lymphocytes (or B cells): These are the cells responsible for the synthesis of antibodies in response to antigen.

Back mutation or reverse mutation: A second mutation which reverses the effect of an earlier mutation that had inactivated a gene; thus it restores wild type phenotype of the cell.

Bacteriophages: The viruses that infect bacteria; often abbreviated as **phages**.

Balbiani ring: An extremely large puff at a band of a polytene chromosome.

Bands of polytene chromosomes: These are visible as dense regions that contain the majority of DNA.

Bands of normal chromosomes: These are relatively much larger and are generated in the form of regions that retain a stain on certain chemical treatments.

Base pair (bp): A partnership of complementary bases (A with T or of C with G) in a DNA double helix; other unusual pairs can be formed in RNA under certain circumstances. It is abbreviated as bp and the distance or length of DNA is usually measured in bp.

Bidirectional replication: Two replication forks moving away from the same origin in opposite directions.

Bivalent: The structure containing all four chromatids (two representing each homolog) at the start of meiosis.

Blocked reading frame: A set of codons that cannot be translated into protein because it is interrupted by termination codons. It is opposite of an open reading frame (ORF).

Blunt-end ligation: A reaction that joins two DNA duplex molecules directly at their ends.

Branch migration: The ability of a DNA strand partially paired with its complement in a duplex to extend its pairing by displacing the resident strand with which it is homologous.

Breakage and reunion: The mode of genetic recombination in which two DNA duplex molecules are broken at corresponding points and then rejoined crosswise. This involves the formation of hetero-duplex DNA around the site of joining.

Buoyant density: Measurement of the ability of a substance to float in some standard fluid, for example, the CsCI solution.

C banding: A technique for generating stained regions around centromeres.

C genes: The genes which code for the constant regions of immunoglobulin protein chains.

C value: Total amount of DNA present in the haploid genome of an organism.

CAAT box: Part of an eukaryotic promoter, these are the conserved sequences located upstream of the start points of eukaryotic transcription units; it is recognized by RNA polymerase and also by a number of transcription factors.

Cap: The structure at the 5′ end of eukaryotic mRNA; it is created post-transcriptionally by linking the terminal phosphate of 5′ GTP to the terminal base of the mRNA. The added G (and sometimes some other bases also) are methylated, giving a structure of the form $^{7Me}G^{5'}ppp^{5'}Np\ldots$

CAP (CRP): The catabolic gene activator protein or catabolic regulator protein; it is a positive regulator protein which is activated by cyclic AMP. It is needed for RNA polymerase to initiate transcription of certain (catabolite-sensitive) operons of *E. coli* (and other bacteria).

Capsid: The external protein coat of a virus particle.

Carbohydrate: Certain polyhdroxyaldehydes, polyhydroxyketones, or compounds derived from these with the formula $(CH_2O)_n$. They are classified as **monosaccharides, oligosaccharides,** and **polysaccharides.**

Catabolism: The physiological processes where complex biomolecules are enzymatically degraded to simpler ones and energy is released.

Catabolite repression: Decreased expression of many bacterial operons that results from addition of glucose. It is caused by a decrease in the level of cyclic AMP, which in turn inactivates the CAP regulator.

cDNA: A single-stranded DNA complementary to an RNA, synthesized from it by reverse transcription *in vitro.*

cDNA clone: A duplex DNA sequence representing an RNA, carried in a cloning vector.

Cell-adhesion molecules (CAMs): Integral membrane proteins that mediate cell-cell binding. These adhesive proteins primarily fall into three major classes: the Ca^2-dependent **cadherins** and selectins, and the Ca^2-independent **immunoglobulin superfamily** including N-CAM.

Cell cycle: The period from one cell division to the next cell division. The entire cell cycle can be divided into a number of phases.

Cell hybrid: A somatic cell containing chromosomes derived from parental cells of different species (e.g. a man-mouse somatic cell hybrid), generated by fusing the cells to form a heterokaryon in which the nuclei subsequently fused.

Centrifugation: Technique involving application of a large centrifugal force for collecting or separating macromolecules, particles, or cells from a suspension based on differences in mass, shape, or density.

Centrioles: Small hollow cylinders consisting of microtubules that become located near the poles during mitosis. They reside within the centrosomes.

Centromere: A constricted region of a chromosome that includes the site of attachment to the mitotic or meiotic spindle.

Centrosomes: The regions from which microtubules are organized at the poles of a mitotic cell. In animal cells, each centrosome contains a pair of centrioles surrounded by a dense amorphous region to which the microtubules attach.

Chaperones: The proteins that are needed for the assembly or proper folding of some other protein, but which is not itself a component of the target complex.

Chemical complexity: The amount of a DNA component measured by chemical assay.

Chi sequence: It is an octamer that provides a hotspot for RecA-mediated genetic recombination in *E. coli.*

Chi structure: A joint between two duplex molecules of DNA revealed by cleaving an intermediate of two joined circles to generate linear ends in each circle. It resembles the Greek letter, chi in outline, hence the name.

Chiasma: It is a site at which two homologous chromosomes appear to have exchanged material during meiosis.

Chimera: An animal or tissue composed of elements derived from genetically distinct individuals; also a protein molecule containing segments derived from different proteins.

Chiral compound: A compound that contains an asymmetric center (chiral atom or chiral center) and thus can occur in two nonsuperimposable mirror-image forms (enantiomers).

Chromatids: Two copies of a chromosome produced by replication. The name is usually used to describe these copies during the period before these are separated at the subsequent cell division.

Chromatin: The complex of DNA and protein in the nucleus of the cell at interphase, when individual chromosomes cannot be distinguished. It was originally recognized by its reaction with DNA specific stains.

Chromocenter: An aggregate of heterochromatin from different chromosomes.

Chromomeres: The densely staining granules visible in chromosomes under certain conditions, especially early in meiosis, when a chromosome may appear to consist of a series of chromomeres.

Chromosome: The discrete unit of the genome carrying a number of genes. Each chromosome consists of a very long molecule of duplex DNA and an approximately equal mass of proteins. It is visible as a morphological entity during the cell division only.

Chromosome walking: The technique of sequential isolation of clones carrying overlapping sequences of DNA, allowing large regions of the chromosome to be spanned. Walking is often performed in order to reach a particular locus of interest.

***cis*-acting locus:** A region of DNA which affects the activity only of DNA sequences present on its own molecule of DNA; this property usually implies that this locus does not code for protein.

***cis*-acting protein:** Such protein has the exceptional property of acting only on the molecule of DNA from which it was expressed.

***cis*-configuration:** This describes two sites on the same molecule of DNA.

***cis/trans* test:** An assay system for testing the effect of relative configuration on expression of two mutations. In a double heterozygote, two mutations in the same gene show mutant phenotype when both are present in *trans* configuration and wild-type phenotype when these are in *cis* configuration.

Cisterna (pl. cisternae): Flattened membrane-bounded compartment present in the **Golgi complex** and **endoplasmic reticulum** in various tissues.

Cistron: The genetic unit defined by the *cis/trans* test; equivalent to **gene** in comprising a unit of DNA representing a protein.

Class switching: A change in the expression of the C region of an immunoglobulin heavy chain during lymphocyte differentiation.

Clone: A large number of cells or molecules identical with a single ancestral cell or molecule.

Cloning vector: Extra chromosomal DNA molecule such as plasmid or phage that is used to "carry" inserted foreign DNA for the purposes of producing more copies of the genetic material or a protein product of the foreign DNA.

Closed reading frame: Same as blocked reading frame, it represents a DNA sequence which contains stop codon so that it can not be translated into a protein.

Coated vesicles: Transport vesicles whose membrane has a layer of specific protein coat such as clathrin on its surface.

Coding region: Sequences in DNA that encode the amino acid sequence of all or part of a protein, as distinct from regulatory sequences, which control transcription and translation, and other non-transcribed or non-translated regions of a gene such as **introns** and spacers.

Coding strand: The strand of DNA which has the same sequence as the mRNA represented by the gene. This strand does not serve as template during transcription.

Co-dominant alleles: Two alleles of a gene when both contribute to the phenotype; neither is dominant over the other.

Codon: A triplet of nucleotides that represents an amino acid or a termination signal.

Cognate: Describing two biomolecules that normally interact; for example, an enzyme and its normal substrate, or a receptor and its normal ligand.

Cognate tRNAs: A group of tRNAs specific for one amino acid which are recognized by a particular aminoacyl-tRNA synthetase.

Co-integrate structure: A structure which is produced by the fusion of two replicons, one originally possessing a transposon, the other lacking it; the cointegrate has copies of the transposon present at both junctions of the replicons, oriented as direct repeats.

Cold-sensitive mutants: A conditional mutant which is defective at low temperature but functional at normal temperature.

Colony hybridization: A technique which uses *in situ* hybridization to identify bacteria carrying chimeric vectors whose inserted DNA is homologous with some particular sequence (the probe).

Compatibility group: An element present on certain plasmids which renders the members unable to coexist in the same bacterial cell.

Complementary: Having a molecular surface with chemical groups arranged to interact specifically with chemical groups on another molecule.

Complementation: The ability of independent (nonallelic) genes to provide diffusible products that produce wild phenotype when two mutants are tested in *trans* configuration in a heterozygote.

Complementation assay (*in vitro*): A test for identifying a component of a wild-type cell that can confer activity on an extract prepared from a mutant cell. The assay identifies the component which is rendered inactive by the mutation.

Complementation group: A series of mutations unable to complement when tested in pairwise combinations in *trans*. These define a genetic unit (the cistron) that might better be called a *non-complementation* group.

Complex locus: A locus in *D. melanogaster* genome which has genetic properties inconsistent with the function of a gene representing a single protein. Complex loci are usually very large (100 kb or more) in terms of molecular size.

Complexity (Genomic): Total length of different sequences of DNA present in a given preparation of genomic DNA.

Composite transposons: Transposable elements which have a central region flanked on each side by insertion sequences. Either one or both of these sequences may be helpful for the transposition of entire element.

Concatemer: Form of DNA which is consisted of a series of unit genomes repeated in tandem.

Concatenated circles: Copies of circular DNA that are interlocked like rings on a chain.

Concerted evolution: The ability of two related genes to evolve together as though constituting a single locus.

Condensation reaction: A reaction in which a covalent bond is formed and a water molecule is given out, for example the addition of an amino acid to a polypeptide chain.

Conditional lethal mutations: The mutations which will kill a cell or virus under one set (non-permissive) of conditions, but allow it to survive under another (permissive) set of conditions.

Conjugation: The "mating" between two bacterial cells associated with the transfer of chromosome or its part from one cell to the other.

Consensus sequence: An idealized sequence in which each position represents the base most often found when many actual sequences are compared.

Conservative recombination: The breakage and reunion of pre-existing strands of DNA without any synthesis of new stretches of DNA.

Conservative transposition: The movement of large elements, originally classified as transposons, but now considered to be episomes. The mechanism of movement resembles that of phage lambda.

Constant regions of immunoglobulins: The part of antibody molecule which is coded by C genes and shows least degree of variation. The constant regions of heavy chains identify the type of immunoglobulin.

Constitutive genes: These genes are expressed as a function of the interaction of RNA polymerase with the promoter without additional regulation. Such genes are also called housekeeping genes in the context of describing their low level expression and function in all the cells.

Constitutive heterochromatin: The inert state of permanently nonexpressed sequences within the genome such as the satellite DNA.

Constitutive mutations: As a result of such mutations the genes that are normally expressed in regulated manner start expressing in constitutives manner without any regulation.

Contractile ring: A ring of actin filaments that forms around the equator at the end of mitosis and is responsible for separation of daughter cells.

Controlling elements of maize: The transposable units originally identified solely by their genetic properties. These may be autonomous (able to transpose independently) or non-autonomous (able to transpose only in the presence of an autonomous element).

Cooperativity: Property exhibited by some proteins with multiple ligand-binding sites whereby binding of one ligand molecule increases (positive cooperativity) or decreases (negative cooperativity) the binding affinity of successive ligand molecules.

Co-ordinate regulation: The term refers to a common control of a group of genes.

Cordycepin: It is 3' deoxyadenosine which is an inhibitor of polyadenylation of RNA.

Core DNA: The 146 bp segments of DNA that are present on a core particle of the nucleosome structure.

Core particle: A nuclease digestion product of the nucleosome that retains the histone octamer and has 146 bp of DNA. Its structure appears to be similar to that of the nucleosome itself.

Corepressor: A small molecule that triggers repression of transcription by binding to a regulator protein.

Cosmids: A artificially created hybrid vector, constructed by insertion of *Cos* sites of the bacteriophage lambda DNA into a plasmid. As a result, the plasmid DNA can be packaged *in vitro* in the phage coat. These particles infect like a phage but multiply like a plasmid.

Cot: The product of DNA concentration and time of incubation in a reassociation reaction.

Cot$\frac{1}{2}$: Cot required to proceed to half completion of the reaction; it is directly proportional to the unique length of reassociating DNA.

Co-transfection: Simultaneous transfection of a host with two plasmids, usually with separate markers.

Cotransport: The simultaneous transport, by a single transportor, of two solutes across a membrane.

Crossing-over: The reciprocal exchange of material between chromosomes that occurs during meiosis and is responsible for genetic recombination.

Crossover fixation: A possible consequence of unequal crossing-over that allows a mutation in one member of a tandem cluster to spread through the whole cluster (or to be eliminated).

Cruciform: The structure produced at inverted repeats of DNA if the repeated sequences pair with their complement on the same strand (instead of with its regular partner in the other strand of duplex).

Cryptic satellite: A satellite DNA sequence not identified as such by a separate peak on a density gradient, but, it remains present in the main-band DNA.

Cyclic AMP (cAMP): A monophosphate of adenosine in which the phosphate group is joined to two positions, the 3′ and the 5′, of the ribose; its binding activates the CAP (catabolic activator protein), which is a positive regulator of prokaryotic transcription. Cyclic AMP acts as second messenger in a number of cellular processes.

Cyclins: The proteins that accumulate continuously throughout the cell cycle and are later destroyed by proteolysis during mitosis.

Cytochrome: Any of a group of coloured, heme-containing proteins that transfer electrons during cellular respiration and photosynthesis.

Cytokine: A group of numerous secreted, small proteins (e.g., interferons, interleukins) that bind to cell-surface receptors on certain cells to trigger their differentiation or proliferation. Some cytokines, also called *lymphokines*, function to regulate the intensity and duration of the **immune response**.

Cytokinesis: The final process involved in separation and movement of daughter cells at the end of mitosis.

Cytoplasmic protein synthesis: The translation of mRNAs representing the nuclear genes to synthesize the proteins.

Cytoskeleton: A network of fibers in the cytoplasm of the eukaryotic cell. It provides the site for attachment of ribosomes and many other subcellular organelles.

Cytosol: The general volume of cytoplasm in which organelles (such as the mitochondria) are located.

D loop: A region within mitochondrial DNA in which a short stretch of RNA is paired with one strand of DNA, displacing the original partner DNA strand in this region. The same term is used also to describe the displacement of a region of one strand of duplex DNA by a single-stranded invader nucleic acid in the reaction catalyzed by RecA protein.

Dalton: Unit of molecular mass approximately equal to the mass of a hydrogen atom (1.66×10^{-24} g).

DNA (deoxyribonucleic acid): Long linear polymer, composed of four kinds of deoxyribose **nucleotides** linked by **phosphodiester bonds**, that is the carrier of genetic information. In its native state, DNA is a **double helix** of two antiparallel strands.

Degeneracy: A property of genetic code which refers to the lack of an effect of any change in the third base of the codon on the amino acid that is represented by this codon.

Deletions: These are generated by removal of a sequence of DNA, the regions on either side being joined together.

Denaturation of nucleic acid: The conversion of DNA (or double stranded RNA) from the double stranded to the single stranded state; the separation of the strands is most often accomplished by heating.

Denaturation of protein: The conversion of a protein from its physiological conformation to some other conformation, rendering it biologically inactive.

De novo pathway: Pathway for synthesis of a biomolecule, such as a nucleotide, from simple precursors; as distinct from a salvage pathway.

De-repressed state: A gene that has been turned on by a regulator molecule. It is synonymous with *induced* when describing the normal state of a gene; it has the same meaning as *constitutive* in describing the effect of mutation.

Dicentric chromosome: Formed by the fusion of two chromosome fragments, each of which has centromere, it is unstable and may break when both the centromeres are pulled to opposite poles during mitosis.

Differentiation: Process usually involving changes in gene expression by which a precursor cell becomes a distinct specialized cell type.

Diploid set of chromosomes: The set of chromosomes which have two copies of each autosome and two sex chromosomes.

Direct repeats: Identical or related sequences present in two or more copies in the same orientation in the same molecule of DNA. These may or may not be adjacent to each other.

Discontinuous replication: The synthesis of DNA in lagging strand in form of short (Okazaki) fragments that are later joined into a continuous strand.

Disjunction: The movement of members of a chromosome pair to opposite poles during cell division. During mitosis and the second meiotic division, disjunction applies to sister chromatids; at first mitosis division it applies to sister chromatid pairs.

Disulfide bridge: A common covalent cross link between two cysteine residues in different polypeptide chains or different part of the same polypeptide, resulting in the formation of a cystine residue. Formed by the oxidation of two sylfhydryl groups, these bridges (or bonds) are generally found only in extracellular proteins or protein domains.

Divergence: Percent difference in nucleotide sequence between two related DNA sequences or in amino acid sequences between two proteins.

Divergent transcription: The initiation of transcription starting from two promoters facing in the opposite direction, so that transcription proceeds away in both directions from a central region.

dna **mutants:** Temperature-sensitive mutants of bacteria which cannot synthesize DNA at 42°C, but can do so at 37°C.

DNAase or DNase: An enzyme that cleaves DNA by attacking the phosphodiester bonds.

DNA-driven hybridization: The hybridization reaction in presence of an excess of DNA with RNA to form DNA:RNA hybrid.

DNA polymerase: The primary enzyme that synthesizes a daughter strand(s) of DNA under direction from and complementary to a DNA template. It is involved in replication and/or repair.

DNA replicase: A specific DNA-synthesizing enzyme required for replication only.

Domain of a chromosome: *Either* a discrete structural entity within the chromosome which is defined as a region within which supercoiling is independent of other domains; *or* an extensive region including an expressed gene that has heightened sensitivity to degradation by the enzyme DNase I.

Domain of a protein: A distinct structural unit of a polypeptide chain representing the amino acid sequence that can be implicated with a particular function and can usually fold as an independent compact unit.

Dominant allele: The allele which determines the phenotype displayed in a heterozygote with another (recessive) allele.

Donor splicing site: Also referred as 5′ splicing site or left splicing junction, it is the boundary between the 3′ end of an exon with the 5′ end (begining) of adjacent intron.

Double helix: The natural coiled conformation of two complementary, antiparallel DNA chains.

Downstream: The term is used to identify sequences proceeding farther towards 3′ side in the direction of expression; for example, the coding region is downstream of the initiation codon.

Ectopic expression: The expression of a gene in a tissue in which it is not usually expressed; for example, expression of a foreign gene in a transgenic animal or its expression as the result of injection into an unusual location in an embryo.

Electorphoresis: Any of several techniques for separating **macromolecules** based on their migration in a gel or other medium subjected to a strong electric field.

Elongation factors: Abbreviated as an EF in prokaryotes and eEF in eukaryotes, these are proteins that associate with ribosomes during the addition of each amino acid to the growing polypeptide chain. Their functions include the regulation of binding of an aminoacyl-tRNA to a ribosome and release of tRNA after addition of an amino acid to the growing pepitede chain.

End labeling: The reaction which describes the addition of a radioactively labeled group to one end (5′ or 3′) of a DNA or RNA molecule.

End-product inhibition: The ability of a product of a metabolic pathway to inhibit the activity of an enzyme that catalyzes an early step in the pathway.

Endocytosis: The process by which proteins at the surface of the cell are internalized for transportation into the cell within membranous vesicles.

Endocytic vesicles: The membranous particles that transport proteins across the membrane through endocytosis; also known as clathrin-coated vesicles.

Endonucleases: The enzymes that cleave the phosphodiester bonds within a nucleic acid chain; they may be nonspecific or specific for RNA or for single-stranded or double-stranded DNA or for specific base or a short sequence within the nucleic acid.

Endoplasmic reticulum: A highly convoluted sheet of membranes, extending from the outer layer of the nuclear envelope into the cytoplasm.

Enhancer element: A *cis*-acting sequence that increases the efficiency of (some) eukaryotic promoters. These are position and orientation independent and can function in either orientation and in any location (upstream or downstream) relative to the promoter.

Envelope: The structure that surrounds some organelles (for example, nucleus or mitochondrion) and consists of concentric membranes, each membrane consisting of the usual lipid bilayer.

Epigenetic changes: The changes that influence the phenotype without altering the genotype. These consist of changes in the properties of a cell that are inherited but do not represent a change in genetic information.

Episome: A plasmid able to integrate into bacterial DNA.

Epistasis: A situation in which expression of one gene obscures the phenotypic effects of another gene.

Epitope: An antigenic determinant; the particular chemical group or groups within a macromolecule (antigen) to which a given anitbody binds.

Essential gene: a gene whose deletion or alteration is lethal to the organism.

Established cell lines: Eukaryotic cells that have been adopted to indefinite growth in culture (they are said to be immortalized).

Eubacteria: A class of unicellular organisms which is the major line of prokaryotes.

Euchromatin: The entire genome of the cell present in the interphase nucleus except for the heterochromatin. This is the active part of genome.

Eukaryotes: Class of organisms; including all plants, animals, fungi, yeast, protozoa, and most algae, that are composed of one or more cells containing a well-defined membrane-enclosed **nucleus** and **organelles**.

Evolutionary clock: It is defined by the rate at which mutations accumulate in a given gene.

Excision (of phage or episome or other sequences): The release of these sequences when present in integrated form with the host chromosome to produce an autonomous DNA molecule.

Excision-repair systems: DNA repair mechanism that removes a single-stranded sequence of DNA containing damaged or mispaired bases and replaces it with a correct sequence by synthesizing a sequence piece of DNA which is complementary to the remaining strand.

Exocytosis: the process of secreting proteins from a cell into the medium, by transport in membranous vesicles from the endoplasmic reticulum, through the Golgi, to storage vesicles, and finally (upon a regulatory signal) through the plasma membrane.

Exon: The segment of an interrupted gene that is represented in the mature RNA product.

Exonucleases: A nuclease that cleaves nucleotides, one base at a time, from the end of a polynucleotide. These may be specific for either the 5' or 3' end of DNA or RNA.

Expression: Production of an observable phenotype by a gene, usually by the synthesis of a protein.

Expression vector: A cloning vector so designed that a coding sequence inserted at a particular site will be transcribed and translated into protein.

Extranuclear genes: The DNA that resides outside the nucleus in organelles such as mitochondria and chloroplasts.

F factor: A bacterial sex or fertility plasmid.

F1 generation: The first generation produced by crossing two parental (homozygous) lines.

Facilitated diffusion: Diffusion of a polar substance across a biological membrane through a protein transproter; also called passive diffusion or passive transport.

Facultative cells: Cells that can live both in the presence as well as in absence of oxygen.

Facultative heterochromatin: The inert state of sequences that also exist in active copies; for example, one mammalian X chromosome in females.

Fibroblast: A type of connective-tissue cell, found in almost all vertebrate organs, that secretes collagen and other components of the extracellular matrix; it migrates and proliferates during wound healing and tissue culture.

Figure eight DNA: The term is used to describes two circles of DNA linked together by a recombination event that has not yet been completed.

Filter hybridization: The hybridization performed by incubating a denatured DNA preparation immobilized on a nitrocellulose filter with a solution of radioactively labeled RNA or DNA.

Fingerprint of DNA: A pattern of polymorphic restriction fragments that differ between individual genomes.

Fingerprint of a protein: The pattern of fragments (usually resolved on a two dimensional electrophoretic gel) generated by cleavage with an enzyme such as trypsin.

Flagellum (pl. flagella): Membrane-enclosed locomotory structure extending from the surface of eukaryotic cells and composed of a specific arrangement of microtubules, called an **axoneme**. Usually there is only one flagellum per cell (as in sperm cells), and its bending propels the cell forwards or backwards. Bacterial flagella are much simpler structures containing a single predominant type of protein.

Fluidity: A property of membranes; it indicates the ability of lipids to move laterally within their particular monolayer.

Focal contact (adhesion plaque): Small region on the surface of a fibroblast or other cell that is anchored to the extracellular matrix. The attachment is mediated by transmembrane proteins such as integrins, which are linked, through other proteins, to actin filaments in the cytoplasm.

Focus formation: The ability of transformed eukaryotic cells to grow in dense clusters, piled up on one another.

Focus forming unit (ffu): A quantitative measure of focus formation.

Foldback DNA: It consists of inverted repeats that have renatured by intra-strand reassociation of denatured DNA.

Footprinting: A technique for indentifying the site on DNA bound by some protein by virtue of the protection of bonds in this region against attack by nucleases.

Forward mutations: The mutations that inactivate a wild-type gene.

Founder effect: The presence of many individuals in a population, all with the same chromosome (or region of a chromosome) derived from a single ancestor.

Frameshift mutations: Such mutations arise by deletions or insertions that are not in multiple of 3 bp; they change the frame in which triplets (codons) are translated into protein. As a result, the polypeptide product has a garbled amino acid sequence begining at the mutated codon.

G banding: A technique that generates a striated pattern in metaphase chromosomes that distinguishes the members of a haploid set.

G1 phase: The period of the eukaryotic cell cycle between the last mitosis and the start of DNA replication (S-phase).

G2 phase: The period of the eukaryotic cell cycle between the end of DNA replication and the start of the next mitosis.

Gamete: The reproductive (germ) cell, either sperm or egg, which have haploid chromosome content.

Gap in DNA: The absence of one or more nucleotides in one strand of the duplex.

Gene: The segment of DNA responsible for producing a RNA molecule which may (i.e. mRNA) or may not (i.e. rRNA, tRNA and other small RNAs) lead to production of a polypeptide chain. It includes regions preceding and following the coding region (leader and trailer) as well as intervening sequences (introns) between individual coding segments (exons). A gene has the regulatory region and the transcription unit. Though there are many definitions, a gene may be defined as a sequence of DNA that codes for a product which defuses from the site of its synthesis and acts elsewhere, earlier the gene was defined as a segment of DNA that has necessary infomation for the production of a protein molecule.

Gene conversion: The alteration of one strand of a heteroduplex DNA to make it complementary with the other strand at any position(s) where there were mispaired bases.

Gene dosage: The number of copies of a particular gene in the genome.

Gene family: A set of genes whose exons are related; the members are derived by duplication and variation from some ancestral gene.

Gene cluster: A group of adjacent genes that are identical or related.

Gene expression: Overall process by which the information encoded by DNA in a gene is converted into an observable **phenotype** (most commonly the production of a protein).

Genetic code: The correspondence between triplets in DNA (or RNA) and amino acids in protein.

Genetic map: A diagram showing the relative sequence and position of specific genes along a chromosome.

Genetic marker: A DNA fragment representing an allele of interest coding for a known and well defined function which can be used in an experiment.

Genomic or chromosomal DNA clones: The sequence of genome carried by a cloning vector.

Genotype: It is the genetic constitution of an individual cell or organism.

Glycoprotein: A class of molecules in which one or more oligosaccharide chains are covalently linked to a protein; frequently found in the plasma membrane or secreted from the cell.

Glycosidic bond: The covalent linkage between two **monosaccharides** formed by a condensation reaction in which one carbon, usually carbon #1, of one sugar reacts with a hydroxyl group on a second sugar with the loss of a water molecule.

Glycosyl transferase: An enzyme that forms a **glycosidic bond** between a sugar residue (monosaccharide) and an amino acid side chain of a protein or a residue in an existing carbohydrate chain.

Golgi apparatus: It consists of individual stacks of membranes near the endoplasmic reticulum; involved in glycosylation of proteins and sorting them for transport to different cellular locations.

G proteins: These are guanine nucleotide-binding proteins which are involved in signal transduction. Usually trimeric in nature, these proteins reside in the plasma membrane. When bound with GDP, the trimer remains intact and is inert. When the GDP bound to the α-subunit is replaced by GTP, the α-subunit is released from the $\beta\gamma$ dimer. One of the separated units (either the α-monomer or the $\beta\gamma$ dimer) then activates or represses the activity of a target protein.

Gratuitous inducers: An inducer molcule which resembles authentic inducers of transcription but are not substrates for the induced enzymes.

Growth factor: An extracellular polypeptide molecule that binds to a cell-surface receptor triggering a **signal-transduction pathway** leading to cell proliferation or, in other cases, to specific differentiation responses. The receptors for many growth factors (e.g. epidermal growth factor, platelet-derived growth factor, insulin) are **receptor linked tyrosine kinases**.

GT-AG rule: This denotes the presence of these conserved dinucleotides as the first two and last two bases in the introns of almost all nuclear genes.

GTP (guanosine 5′-triphosphate): A **nucleotide** that is a precursor in RNA synthesis and also plays a special role in protein synthesis, signal-transduction pathways, and microtubule assembly.

GTPase superfamily: Group of guanine nucleotide-binding proteins that cycle between an inactive state with bound GDP and an active state with bound GTP. These proteins—including **G proteins, Ras proteins**, and certain polypeptide **elongation factors**—function as intracellular switch proteins.

Gyrase: A type II topoisomerase of *E. coli* with the ability to introduce negative supercoils into DNA.

Hairpin: A double-helical region formed by base pairing between adjacent (inverted) complementary sequences in a single strand of RNA or DNA.

Haploid set of chromosomes: The genome containing one copy of each of the autosomes and one sex chromosome; the haploid number *n* is characteristic of gametes of diploid organisms.

Haplotype: A specific combination of alleles in a defined region of some chromosomes, whose effect in the genotype is very little. Originally this term was used to describe combinations of MHC alleles, it is now used to describe particular combinations of RFLPs.

Hapten: A small molecule that acts as an antigen when conjugated to a protein or other large molecules.

Heat-shock response: Increased expression of a specific group of genes (*hsp* genes) in response to elevated temperature or other stressful treatment accompanied by decreased transcription of other genes and decreased translation of other mRNAs. This response is very widespread among both prokaryotic and eukaryotic organisms and helps the organism survive the stress.

HeLa cell: Cell of human epithelial cells, derived from a human cervical carcinoma, that grows readily in culture and is widely used in research.

Helicase: An enzyme that catalyzes the separation of strands in a DNA molecule before its replication.

Helix-loop-helix: A conserved protein dimerization **motif** present in DNA binding proteins such as **transcription factors**.

Helix-turn-helix: A DNA binding **motif** found in most bacterial DNA binding proteins.

Helper virus: A virus that provides functions absent in a defective virus, enabling the latter to complete the infective cycle during a mixed infection by both viruses.

Hemizygote: A diploid individual that has lost one of its copy of a particular gene (for example, because a chromosome has been lost) and which therefore has only a single copy.

Heterochromatin: The regions of the genome that are permanently in a highly condensed condition and are not genetically expressed. May be constitutive or facultative.

Heteroduplex DNA: Also known as hybrid DNA, it is generated by base pairing between complementary single strands derived from the different parental duplex molecules; it occurs during genetic recombination.

Heterogeneous nuclear RNA (hnRNA): Primary transcripts of nuclear genes made by RNA polymerase II; it has a wide range of size distribution and low stability, it is also referred as pre-mRNA.

Heteromultimeric proteins: A multimeric protein where the complex consist of nonidentical subunits (coded by different genes).

Heterokaryon: A cell containing two (or more) nuclei in a common cytoplasm, generated by the fusion of somatic cells.

Heterozygote: An individual with different alleles at some particular locus.

High-energy bond: Covalent bond that releases a large amount of energy when hydrolyzed under the usual intracellular conditions. Examples include the **phosphoanhydride bonds** in ATP, **thioester bond** in acetyl CoA, and various phosphate ester bonds.

Highly repetitive DNA: It is first component of DNA which reassociates and is generally equated with satellite DNA.

Histones: Highly conserved DNA-binding proteins of eukaryotes that associate tightly with the DNA to form the nucleosomes, the basic subunit of chromatin. These consist of a family of five basic proteins.

Holliday structure: Intermediate structure in DNA **recombination** whose resolution can result in **recombination** and/or **heteroduplex** formation.

Homeobox: Conserved sequence that is part of the coding region of *Drosophila melanogaster* homeotic genes; it is also found in amphibian and mammalian genes that are expressed in early embryonic development.

Homeostasis: The maintenance of a dynamic steady state by regulatory mechanisms that compensate for changes in external circumstances.

Homology: Similarity in the sequence of a protein or nucleic acid or in the structure of an organ that reflects a common evolutionary origin. In contrast, analogy is a similarity in structure or function that does not reflect a common evolutionary origin.

Homomultimeric protein: A multimeric protein which consists of identical subunits.

Homozygote: An individual with the same allele at corresponding loci on the homologous chromosomes.

Hormone: A chemical substance synthesized in small amounts by an endocrine tissue, and secreted directly in the blood which carries it to another tissue (target organ) where it acts as a messenger to regulate the function of the target tissue or organ.

Hormone receptor: A protein in, or on the surface of the membranes in target tissue which binds to hormone and initiates the cellular response.

Hotspot: A site in the genome at which the frequency of mutation (or recombination) is highly increased.

Hox genes: The clusters of mammalian genes containing homeoboxes; the individual members are related to the genes of the complex loci *ANT-C* and *BX-C* in *D. melanogaster*.

Housekeeping (constitutive) genes: The genes that are (theoretically) expressed in all cells because they provide basic functions needed for sustenance of all cell types.

Hybrid-arrested translation: A technique that identifies the cDNA corresponding to an mRNA by relying on the ability of DNA to base pair with the RNA *in vitro* to inhibit translation.

Hybrid dysgenesis: The inability of certain strains of *D. melanogaster* to interbreed, because the hybrids are sterile (although otherwise they may be phenotypically normal).

Hybridization: The pairing of complementary RNA and DNA strands to give an RNA-DNA, DNA-DNA or RNA-RNA (as the case may be) hybrid. These strands anneal together obeying the Watson-Crick base pairing.

Hybridoma: A cell line produced by fusing a myeloma wih a lymphocyte; it continues indefinitely to express the immunoglobulins of both the parents.

Hydrogen bond: A noncovalent association between an electronegative atom (often an oxygen or nitrogen) and a hydrogen atom covalently bonded to another electronegative atom. Although relatively weak, hydrogen bonds are numerous in macromolecules; they are particularly important in stabilizing the three-dimensional structure of proteins and are responsible for formation of **base pairs** in nucleic acids.

Hydrolysis: Reaction in which a covalent bond is cleaved with addition of an H from water to one product of the cleavage and of an OH from water to the other.

Hydropathy plot: A measure of the hydrophobicity of a protein region and therefore, of the likelihood that it will reside in a membrane.

Hydropathy groups: The reactive groups that interact with water, so that hydrophilic regions of protein or the faces of a lipid bilayer reside in an aqueous environment.

Hydrophobic groups: The reactive groups that repel water, so that they interact with one another to generate a nonaqueous environment.

Hyperchromicity: The increase in optical density (at 260 nm) that occurs when DNA is denatured.

hypersensitive site (DNAase I): A short region of chromatin detected by its extreme sensitivity to cleavage by DNAase I and other nucleases; probably comprises an area from which nucleosomes are excluded.

Hypervariable regions: The parts of the variable region of an immunoglobulin that show maximum alteration when different antibodies are compared.

Ideogram: A diagrammatic representation of the G-banding pattern of a chromosome.

Idling reaction: The production of ppGpp (sometimes pppGpp) by ribosomes when an uncharged tRNA is present at the A site. The formation of these molecules triggers the stringent response.

Immortalization: This term describes the acquisition of capability by a eukaryotic cell line to grow through an indefinite number of divisions in culture.

Immunity in phages: It refers to the ability of a prophage to prevent another phage of the same type from transfecting a cell which is already infected by the prophage. It usually results from interference with the ability to replicate.

Immunity in plasmids: It describes the ability of a plasmid to prevent another plasmid of the same type from becoming established in an already transformed cell. It usually results from interference with the ability to replicate.

Immunity in transposons: It refers to the ability of certain transposons to prevent other transposons of the same type from transposing to the same DNA molecule. It results from a variety of mechanisms.

Imprinting: A change in a gene that occurs during passage through the sperm or egg with the result that the paternal and maternal alleles have different properties in the very early embryo. May be caused by methylation of DNA.

in vitro: "In glass"; in the test tube. It denotes a reaction or a process taking place in an isolated cell free extract. The term is also used to distinguish the cells growing in culture from the cells in an organism.

in vivo: "In life"; that is, in the living cell or organism.

In situ hybridization: A specific type of hybridization that is performed by denaturing the DNA of cells squashed on a microscope slide so that reaction is possible with an added single-stranded RNA or DNA; the added preparation is radioactively labeled and its hybridization is followed by autoradiography.

Incompatibility: The inability of certain bacterial plasmids to coexist in the same cell. It is a cause of plasmid immunity.

Indirect end-labeling: a technique for examining the organization of DNA by making a cut at a specific site and isolating all fragments containing the sequence adjacent to one side of the cut; it reveals the distance from the cut to the next break(s) in DNA.

Induced mutations: These type of mutations are caused by specific chemicals known as mutagens.

Inducer: A small signal molecule that triggers the transcription of a gene by binding to a regulator protein.

Induction: The ability of bacteria (or yeast) to synthesize certain enzymes only when their substrates are present: when applied to gene expression, the term refers to switching on the transcription of the gene as a result of the interaction of the inducer with the regulator protein.

Induction of prophage: The excision of integrated phage from the host genome and its entry into the lytic (infective) cycle as a result the of destruction of the lysogenic repressor.

Initiation factors: Abbreviated as IF in prokaryotes and eIF in eukaryotes, these are proteins that specifically associate with the small subunit of the ribosome and are essential for the binding of ribosome to mRNA at the time of initiation of protein synthesis.

Initiator: An eukaryotic promoter sequence for RNA polymerase II that specifies transcription initiation within the sequence.

Insertion sequence (IS): Small bacterial transposons that carry only the genetic functions necessary for its own transposition.

Insertions: These identified events are result of incorporation of new sequnce at a locus and are identified by the presence of an additional stretch of base pairs in DNA.

Integral membrane protein: A protein (non-covalently) inserted into a membrane; it attains its membranous association by means of a stretch of ~25 amino acids that are uncharged and/or hydrophobic.

Integration of viral or another DNA sequence: The insertion of the foreign DNA into a host genome to become as its part. The inserted DNA gets covalently linked on either side of the host sequences.

Integrins: A large family of heterodimeric cell-surface receptors that promote adhesion of cells to the **extracellular matrix** by binding to **fibronectin, laminin**, and other matrix components, or to the surface of other cells by interacting with members of the Ig superfamily.

Interferon (IFN): A group of small proteins released from macrophages following stimulation or from many cells after virus infection that bind to **tyrosine kinase-linked receptors** on target cells inducing changes in gene expression leading to an antiviral state (IFNα, IFNβ, and IFNγ) or other cellular responses important in the immune response (IFNγ).

Interallelic complementation: The change in the properties of a heteromultimeric protein brought about by the interaction of subunits coded by two different mutant alleles; the mixed protein may be more or less active than the protein consisting of subunits only of one or the other type.

Inverted repeats: These comprise of two copies of the same sequence of DNA which are repeated in opposite orientation on the same molecule.

Interbands: Relatively dispersed regions of polytene chromosomes that lie between the bands.

Intercistronic region: The stretch of DNA forming the spacer region between the termination codon of one gene and the initiation codon of the next gene in a polycistronic transcription unit of a prokaryote.

Intermediate component(s): The DNA species which reassociate between the fast (satellite DNA) and slow (nonrepetitive DNA) component during a reassociation reaction. These contain moderately repetitive DNA.

Interphase: The period between two mitotic cell divisions; divided into G1, S, and G2 phases.

Intervening sequence: Commonly known as intron and present only in eukaryotic genes, it is a segment of DNA that is transcribed, but removed from the primary transcript by splicing. Absent in mature RNA, it does not code for biologically meaningful segment.

Inversion: A chromosomal change in which a segment has been rotated by 180° relative to the regions on either side and reinserted. Thus the sequence of this region becomes in opposite orientation.

Inverted terminal repeats: The short related or identical sequences present in reverse orientation at the ends of some transposons.

Isoacceptor tRNAs: Different tRNA molecules all of which accept the same amino acid, these may have different anticodons complementary to various codons for the same amino acid.

Isoforms: Multiple forms of the same protein whose amino acid sequences differ slightly but whose general activity is identical. They may be produced by alternative splicing of RNA transcripts from the same gene or be encoded by different genes.

Isotype: A group of closely related immunoglobulin chains.

Karyotype: The entire chromosomal complement of a cell or species (as visualized during mitosis).

kb (kilobase): An abbreviation for 1000 base pairs of DNA or 1000 bases of RNA.

Kinase: An enzyme that phophorylates (adds a phosphate group) to a substrate; ATP serves as the phosphate group donor. The substrates for **protein kinases** are amino acids present in other proteins. These are divided into those specific for tyrosine and those specific for threonine/serine.

Kinetic complexity: The complexity of a DNA component measured by the kinetics of DNA re-association.

Kinetochore: It is the structural feature of chromosome to which microtubules of the mitotic spindle attach.

Lagging strand: The strand of replicating DNA which seems to grow apparently in the 3'-5' direction. In fact it is synthesized discontinuously in the form of short fragments in 5'-3' direction and these fragments are later ligated covalently.

Laminin: A component of the **extracellular matrix** that is found in all basal laminae and has binding sites for cell-surface receptors, collagen, and heparan sulfate proteoglycans.

Lampbrush chromosomes: The large meiotic chromosomes found in amphibian oocytes.

Lariat: An intermediate in RNA splicing in which a circular structure with a tail is created by a 5'-2' bond.

Leader: The nontranslated sequence at the 5' end of mRNA that precedes the initiation codon.

Leader sequence of a protein: Also referred as signal sequence, it is a short sequence present at the N-terminal of a secretory protein. It is responsible for the passage of the protein into or through a membrane. Following the entry through the membrane, it is cleaved off by specific peptidase and is therefore, not present in mature protein.

Leading strand: The strand of DNA which is synthesized continuously in the 5'-3' direction.

Leaky mutations: The mutations that allow some residual but biologically detectable level of gene expression.

Lethal locus: An essential gene a mutions in which is lethal for the organism. The lethat mutation is usually obtained by deletion of the gene.

Leucine zipper: A coiled-coil of two helices that connect the polypeptide chains of one class of dimeric eukaryotic **transcription factors**.

Library or clone bank: This is a set of cloned fragments together representing the entire genome.

Ligand: Any molecule that binds to a specific site on a protein or other molecule. (From Latin *ligare*, to bind.)

Ligase: An enzyme that links together the *3′*-end of one nucleic acid strand with the *5′*-end of another, forming a continuous strand. Free *3′*-OH and *5′*-PO_4 groups are essential for the ligase to act.

Ligation: Formation of a phosphodiester bond to link two adjacent bases separated by a nick in one strand of a double helix of DNA. The term is also applied to blunt-end ligation and to joining of RNA. During genetic engineering technology, the joining of two DNA molecules is also referred as ligation. Specific enzymes, DNA ligase and RNA ligase, carry out this function which is ATP dependent.

LINES: The long interspersed nuclear elements are the long-period sequences found in mammalian genomes that are retroposons generated from RNA polymerase II transcripts.

Linkage: The tendency of genes to be inherited together as a result of their location on the same chromosome; measured by percent recombination between loci.

Linkage group: All the loci that can be connected (directly or indirectly) by linkage relationships; equivalent to a chromosome.

Linkage disequilibrium: A situation in which some combinations of genetic markers occur more or less frequently in the population than would be expected based on their distance. It implies that a group of markers has been inherited coordinately. It can result from reduced recombination in the region or from a founder effect, in which there has been insufficient time to reach equilibrium since the introduction of one of the markers into the population.

Linker DNA: All the DNA contained on a nucleosome in excess of the 146 bp core DNA.

Linker fragment: A short synthetic duplex oligonucleotide containing the target site for some restriction enzyme; may be added to ends of a DNA fragment prepared by cleavage with some other enzyme during reconstruction of recombinant DNA.

Linker scanner mutations: The mutations which can be introduced by recombining two DNA molecules *in vitro* at a restriction fragment added to the end of each; the result is to insert the linker sequence at the site of recombination.

Linking number: The number of times the two strands of a closed DNA duplex cross over each other.

Linking number paradox: The discrepancy between the existence of -2 supercoils in the path of DNA on the nucleosome compared with the measurement of -1 supercoil released when histones are removed.

Lipid bilayer: A specific form taken by concentration of lipids in which the hydrophobic fatty acids occupy the interior and the polar heads face the exterior. This form of lipid bilayer is present in the membrane structures.

Liquid (solution) hybridization: A hybridization reaction between complementary nucleic acid strands performed in solution.

Locus: The position on a chromosome at which the gene for a particular trait resides; locus may be occupied by any one of the alleles for the gene.

LOD score: A measure of genetic linkage, defined as the log_{10} ratio of the probability that the data would have arisen if the loci are linked to the probability that the data could have arisen from unlinked loci. The conventional threshold for declaring linkage is a LOD score of 3.0, that is, a 1000 : 1 ratio (which must be compared with the 50 : 1 probability that any random pair of loci will be unlinked).

Long-period interspersion: A pattern in the genome in which long stretches of moderately repetitive and nonrepetitive DNA alternate.

Loop: A single-stranded region at the end of a hairpin in RNA (or single-stranded DNA); corresponds to the sequence between inverted repeats in duplex DNA.

LTR: It is an abbreviation for **long-terminal repeat**, a sequence directly repeated at both ends of a retroviral DNA, sometimes these sequences may function as promoter.

Lumen: The interior of a compartment bounded by membranes, usually the endoplasmic reticulum or the mitochondrion.

Luxur genes: Those genes which code for specialized functions synthesized (usually) in large amounts in particular cell types.

Lysis: The death of bacteria at the end of a phage infective cycle when they burst open to release the progeny of an infecting phage. Also applies to eukaryotic cells, for example, infected cells that are attacked by the immune system.

Lysogen: A bacterium that possesses a repressed prophage as part of its genome.

Lysogenic immunity: The ability of a prophage to prevent another phage genome of the same type from becoming established in the bacterium.

Lysogenic repressor: The protein responsible for preventing a prophage from reentering the lytic cycle.

Lysogeny: The ability of a phage to survive in a bacterium as a stable prophage component of the bacterial genome.

Lysosomes: Small bodies present in cytoplasmic compartment of a cell, these are enclosed by membranes, and contain a number of hydrolytic enzymes.

Lytic infection: The infection of bacteria by a phage which ends in the destruction of bacteria and release of progeny phage proteins.

Main band of genomic DNA: A broad peak obtained on density gradient centrifugation of DNA excluding any visible satellite DNAs that form separate bands.

Major histocompatibility locus: A large chromosomal region containing a giant cluster of genes that code for transplantation antigens and other proteins found on the surfaces of lymphocytes.

Map distance: Measured as cM (centi-Morgans), it is the measurement of percent recombination (sometimes subject to adjustments).

MAR: The matrix attachment region; also known as SAR for scaffold attachment region, is a region of DNA that attaches to the nuclear matrix.

Maternal inheritance: The preferential survival in the progeny of genetic markers provided by one parent (the mother).

Mb (megabase): A abbreviation for 10^6 bp of DNA or 10^6 bases of RNA.

Melting of DNA: The denaturation of DNA resulting in opening of double stranded region to form two unpaired strands.

Melting temperature (Tm): The midpoint of the temperature range over which DNA gets denatured.

Membranes: The asymmetrical lipid bilayer that has lateral fluidity and contains proteins. These serve a number of important functions in the cell.

Membrane proteins: The integral part of membrane structure, these proteins have hydrophobic regions that allow part or all of the protein structure to reside within the membrane; the bonds involved in this association are usually non-covalent.

Metastasis: The ability of tumor cells to leave their site of origin and migrate to other locations in the body, where a new colony is established resulting in the spread of the tumor.

Microsomoes: The fragmented pieces of endoplasmic reticulum associated with ribosomes.

Minicell: An anucleated bacterial (*E. coli*) cell produced by a division that generates a cytoplasm without a nucleus.

Minichromosome: The nucleosomal form of circular DNA of viruses such as SV40 or polyoma.

Mitosis The division of a eukaryotic somatic cell where the number of chromosomes remains same.

Mobile DNA element: Any DNA sequence that is not present in the same chromosomal location in all individuals of a species. Examples include Tn elements in bacteria, *copia* and P elements in *Drosophila*, Ty elements in yeast. Ac and Ds in maize, and LINES and SINES in mammals.

Modification of DNA or RNA: This includes all changes made to the nucleotides after their initial incorporation into the polynucleotide chain.

Modified bases: These are all the bases except the usual four bases which are present in DNA (T, C, A, G) or RNA (U, C, A, G). They result from post-transcriptional changes in the nucleic acids.

Monocistronic mRNA: An mRNA that codes for one protein.

Monolayer: The growth of eukaryotic cells in culture as a layer only one cell deep.

Morphogen: A factor that induces development of particular cell types in a manner that depends on its concentration.

Motif: In proteins a unit exhibiting a particular three-dimensional architecture that is found in a variety of proteins and usually is associated with particular function. Many DNA-binding proteins contain one of a small number of DNA-binding motifs including the **helix-turn-helix, helix-loop-helix, homeodomain, leucine zipper**, and **zinc finger**.

MPF (maturation- or M phase- or mitosis promoting factor): A dimeric protein with kinase activity, containing the p34 catalytic subunit and a cyclin regulatory A or B type subunit, whose activation triggers the onset of mitosis.

mRNA (messenger RNA): Any **RNA** that specifies the order of amino acids in protein synthesis. It is produced by **transcription** of DNA by RNA polymerase and, in RNA viruses, by transcription of viral RNA. In eukaryotes, the initial RNA product (primary transcript) undergoes **RNA processing** to yield functional mRNA, which is transported to the cytoplasm.

Multiforked chromosomes: Present in bacterium, these have more than one replication fork, because a second initiation has occurred before the first cycle of replication has been completed.

Multimeric proteins: Proteins which consist of more than one subunit.

Mutagens: The substances that increase the rate of mutation by inducing changes in DNA structure.

Mutation: An inheritable change in the sequence of genomic DNA as well as the process by which such changes take place.

Mutation frequency: The frequency at which a particular mutant is found in the population.

Mutation rate: the rate at which a particular mutation occurs, usually given as the number of events per gene per generation.

Myeloma: A tumor cell line derived from a lymphocyte; usually produces a single type of immuno-globulin.

Negative complementation: Such processes occur when interallelic complementation allows a mutant subunit to suppress the activity of a wild-type subunit in a multimeric protein.

Negative regulators: The regulatory molecules that function by switching off the transcription or translation of a gene.

Negative supercoiling: The twisting of a duplex of DNA in space in the opposite direction to the turns of the strands in the double helix.

Neurotransmitter: Extracellular **signaling molecule** that is released by the presynaptic neuron at a chemical **synapse** and relays the signal to the postsynaptic cell. A neurotransmitter can elicit either an excitatory or inhibitory response, but the response is determined by the receptor activated by the neurotransmitter not by the chemical nature of the neurotransmitter. Examples include acetyl-choline, dopamine, GABA (γ-aminobutyric acid), and serotonin.

Neutral substitutions in a protein: Those changes of amino acids in the primary structure of a protein that do not affect its biological activity or function.

Nick translation: A process to prepare uniformly labelled DNA which uses the ability of *E. coli* DNA polymerase I to use a nick as a starting point from which one strand of a duplex DNA can be degraded and replaced by resynthesis of new material. Thus both strands act as template for each other. This process is used to introduce radioactively labeled nucleoticdes into DNA *in vitro*.

Nonautonomous controlling elements: The defective transposons that can transpose only when assisted by an autonomous controlling element of the same type.

Noncovalent bond: Any chemical bond between atoms that does not involve an intimate sharing of electrons. Although covalent bonds are relatively weak, large numbers of these bonds can stabilize the three-dimensional structure of biological molecules, particularly proteins and nucleic acids. The four main types of such bonds are the **hydrogen bond, hydrophobic interaction, ionic bond**, and **van der Waals interaction**.

Nondisjunction: The failure of chromatids (duplicate chromosomes) to move to opposite poles during mitosis or meiosis.

Non-permissive conditions: The growth conditions which do not allow conditional lethal mutants to survive.

Non-replicative transposition: The movement of a transposon that leaves a donor site (usually generating a double-strand break) and moves to a new site.

Nonsense codon: Any one of three triplets (UAG, UAA, UGA) that cause termination of protein synthesis, (UAG is known as amber; UAA as ochre and UGA as opal codon).

Nonsense mutation: Any change in DNA that result in generation of a termination codon to replace a codon representing an amino acid.

Nonsense suppressor: A gene coding for a mutant tRNA which can recognize and respond to one or more of the termination codons resulting in incorporation of an amino acid in place of termination of nascent polypeptide.

Non-transcribed spacer: The region between two transcription units in a tandem gene cluster.

Northern blotting: A technique for immobilization of RNA by transferring it from an agarose gel to a nitrocellulose filter (or nylon membrane) on which it can later be hybridized to a complementary DNA.

Nuclear envelope: A layer of double membranes surrounding the nucleus. It is penetrated by nuclear proes and bounded on the interior by the nuclear laminin.

Nuclear lamina: A proteinaceous layer on the inside of the nuclear envelope. It consists of (up to) three lamin proteins.

Nuclear matrix: A network of fibers surrounding and penetrating the nucleus.

Nuclear proes: The structure that extend across the nuclear envelope and are used for transport of macromolecules.

Nucleoid: The compact body that contains the genome in a bacterium.

Nucleolar organizer: The region of a chromosome carrying the genes coding for rRNA.

Nucleolus: A discrete region of the nucleus created by the transcription of rRNA genes. The processing of rRNA and assembly of ribosomes take place in this region.

Nucleosome: The basic structural subunit of chromatin, consisting of ~200 bp of DNA and an octamer of histone proteins.

Nucleus: Large membrane-bounded organelle that contains DNA organized into chromosomes; the synthesis and processing of RNA and ribosome assembly occur in the nucleus. Nearly all eukaryotic cells contain a nucleus, whereas prokaryotic cells do not.

Null mutation: A mutation that completely eliminates the function of a gene, usually becuase it has been physically deleted.

Ochre codon: Triplet UAA, one of three nonsense codons that cause termination of protein synthesis.

Ochre mutation: Any change in DNA that creates a UAA codon at a site previously occupied by another codon.

Ochre suppressor: A gene coding for a mutant tRNA able to respond to the UAA codon to allow continuation of protein synthesis; usually the ochre suppressors can also suppress amber codons.

Okazaki fragments: The short stretches of DNA, 1000-2000 bases in length, which are produced during discontinuous replication of the lagging strand; they are later joined covalently to form a continuous and intact strand.

Oncogenes: The genes whose products have the ability to transform eukaryotic cells so that they grow in a manner analogous to tumor cells. Oncogenes carried by retroviruses are known as *v-onc*.

Open reading frame (ORF): A series of triplets (codons) coding for amino acids without any termination codons. The sequence starts from an initiation codon and can be translated into a meaningful protein.

Operator: A regulatory site present on DNA at which a repressor protein can bind to regulate the transcription of the gene from initiating under the direction of the adjacent promoter.

Operon: A unit of bacterial gene involved in and regulation of its expression. It includes the structural genes and the control elements (operator) of the DNA which are recognized by regulator gene product(s).

Organelles: Specialized compartments located in the cytoplasm and surrounded by a membrane, each with specific structure and function.

Origin (*ori*): A sequence of DNA at which replication is initiated.

Orphan genes: These are isolated individual genes which are present in isolated locations, but are related to members of a gene cluster.

Overwinding of DNA: The winding of the DNA helices caused by positive supercoiling which applies further tension in the direction of winding of the two strands in the duplex.

Oxidative phosphorylation: The phosphorylation of ADP to form ATP driven by the transfer of electrons to oxygen (O_2) in bacteria and mitochondria. This process involves generation of a **protonmotive force** during electron transport, and use of the protonmotive force to power ATP synthesis.

Packing ratio: The ratio of the length of DNA to the unit length of the fiber containing it.

Palindrome: A sequence of DNA that is the same when one strand is read left to right or the other is read right to left; consists of adjacent inverted repeats.

Papovaviruses: A class of animal viruses with small genomes, including SV_{40} and polyoma.

Paranemic joint: A region of DNA in which two complementary sequences are associated side by side instead of being intertwined in a double helical structure.

Passive diffusion: Also called **simple diffusion**, it is the movement of the molecule across a membrane at a rate proportional to its concentration gradient across the membrane and the permeability of the membrane. Only water, gases (O_2, CO_2, N_2), small hydrophobic molecules, and small uncharged polar molecules such as urea and ethanol can move across biomembranes by simple diffusion.

pBR322: One of the most commonly used plasmid cloning vectors.

PCR (polymerase chain reaction): A technique in which sequential cycles of denaturation, annealing with primer, and extension with DNA polymerase are used to amplify the number of copies of DNA sequence of interest by millions of times.

Peptide: A small polymer usually containing fewer than 30 **amino acids** connected by peptide bonds.

Peptide bond: Covalent bond that links adjacent amino acid residues in proteins; formed by a condensation reaction between the amino group of one amino acid and the carboxyl group of another with release of a water molecule.

Peptide mapping: The characteristic two-dimensional pattern (on paper or gel) formed by the separation of a mixture of peptides resulting from partial hydrolysis of a protein; also known as peptide fingerprinting.

Perinuclear space: The space between the inner and outer membranes of the nuclear envelope.

Periodicity of DNA: The number of base pairs per turn of the double helix.

Peripheral proteins: Proteins that are loosely or reversibly bound to a membrane by hydrogen bonds or electrostatic forces; generally these proteins are water-soluble once released from the membrane.

Permissive conditions: The growth conditions that allow the conditional lethal mutants to survive.

Peroxisome: Small **organelle** in eukaryotic cells whose functions include degradation of fatty acids and amino acids by means of reactions that generate hydrogen peroxide, which is converted to water and oxygen by catalase.

Petite strains of yeast: A strain of yeast which lacks mitochondrial functions.

Phagocytosis: Process by which relatively large particles (e.g. bacterial cells) are internalized by certain eukaryotic cells. Phagocytosis of **pathogens** by macrophages and neutrophils is an important part of immune response in mammals.

Phase variation: An alternation in the type of flagella produced by a bacterium.

Phenotype: The appearance or other characteristics of an organism, resulting from the interaction of its genetic constitution with the environment.

Phosphatase: The enzyme that removes phosphate groups from the substrates.

Phosphodiester bond: A set of covalent bonds in which two hydroxyl groups form ester linkages to the same phosphate group. Adjacent nucleotides in DNA and RNA are joined by phosphodiester bonds.

Phosphorylation: Reaction in which a phosphate group becomes covalently linked to another molecule. The activity of many proteins is regulated by phosphorylation of hydroxyl-containing residues (serine, threonine, tyrosine) by various protein kinases.

Pinocytosis: The nonspecific uptake of small droplets of extracellular fluid into endocytic vesicles.

Plaque assay: Technique for determining the number of infectious viral particles in a sample by culturing a diluted sample on a layer of susceptible host cells and then counting the clear areas of lysed cells (plaques) that develop.

Plasma membrane: The continuous membrane defining the boundary of every cell.

Plasmid: An autonomous self-replicating extrachromosomal circular DNA. Present naturally in a number of prokaryotes and also in certain lower eukaryotes and plants.

Plastid: Cytoplasmic organelle present in plants, these are bounded by a double membrane that carries its own DNA and is often pigmented. Chloroplasts are one of the most abundant plastids.

Playback experiment: The retrieval of DNA that has hybridized with RNA to check whether or not it is nonrepetitive by a series of reassociation reactions.

Pleated sheet: The side-by-side, hydrogen-bonded arrangement of polypeptide chains in the extended ß conformation.

Plectonemic winding: The underwinding of the two strands in the classical double helix of DNA.

Pleiotropic gene: A gene that affects more than one (apparently unrelated) phenotypic characteristic set of an organism.

Ploidy: The number of copies of the chromosomes present in a cell; a haploid has one copy, a diploid has two copies, and so on.

Point mutations: The changes in DNA structure involving single base pairs.

Polar: Referring to a molecule or structure with a net electric charge or asymmetric distribution of positive and negative charges. Polar molecules are usually soluble in water.

Polarity: The effect of a mutation in one gene in influencing the expression (at the level of transcription or translation) of subsequent genes present in the same transcription unit.

Polyadenylation: The post-transcriptional addition of a sequence of polyadenylic acid to the 3′ end of an eukaryotic mRNA by a template independent enzyme, Poly(A) polymerase. A hexanucleotide sequence near the 3′ end of the transcript (AAUAAA) signals the Poly (A) addition.

Polyclonal antibodies: A heterogeneous pool of antibodies produced in an animal by a number of different B lymphocytes in response to an antigen. Different antibodies in the pool recognize different parts of the antigen.

Polycistronic mRNA: An mRNA that includes coding regions representing more than one gene. Majority of the prokaryotic mRNAs are polycistronic while eukaryotic mRNAs are generally monocistronic.

Polymorphism: The simultaneous occurrence in the population of genomes showing allelic variations as seen in alleles producing different phenotypes or in changes in DNA affecting the restriction pattern.

Polyploid cell: The cell having more than two sets of haploid genome.

Polyprotein: A gene product that is post-translationally cleaved into several independent proteins.

Polysome (polyribomosome): An mRNA associated with a series of ribosomes, each of which is actively engaged in translation and carries the growing polypeptide chain at different stage of elongation.

Polytene chromosomes: These are generated by successive replications of a chromosome set without separation of the replicas.

Position effect: A change in the level of expression of a gene caused by its translocation to a new site in the genome; for example, a previously active gene may become inactive if it is placed near heterochromatin.

Positive cooperativity: A phenomenon of some multisubunit enzymes or proteins in which binding of a ligand or substrate to one subunit facilitates binding to another subunit.

Positive regulator proteins: The proteins that are requried for the activation of a transcription unit or for switching the gene 'on'.

Positive supercoiling: The coiling of the double helix in space in the same direction as the winding of the two strands of the double helix itself.

Posttranscriptional processing: The enzymatic processing of the primary RNA transcript to produce functional mRNA, tRNA, and/or rRNA molecules.

Posttranslational modification: Enzymatic processing of a polypeptide chain after translation from its mRNA.

Primary structure: In proteins, the linear arrangement (sequence) of **amino acids** and the location of covalent (mostly disulfide) bonds within a polypeptide chain. In nucleic acids, the sequence of nucleotides.

Primary transcript: The original unmodified RNA product synthesized by the RNA polymerase corresponding to a transcription unit of a gene. The primary transcript is usually unstable in its original form and gets processed to produce the mature RNA.

Primase: A specialized RNA polymerase that synthesizes short stretches of RNA used as primer for DNA synthesis by the DNA polymerase.

Primer : A short sequence (often of RNA) that is paired with one strand of DNA and provides a free 3′-OH end at which a DNA polymerase can start the synthesis of a deoxyribonucleotide chain. The DNA polymerase always requires a primer.

Primosome: The complex of proteins involved in the priming action that initiates synthesis of each Okazaki fragment during discontinuous DNA replication; the primosome may move along DNA to engage in successive priming events.

Probe: Defined RNA or DNA fragment, radioactively or chemically labeled, that is used to locate specific nucleic acid sequences by **hybridization**.

Processed pseudogene: An inactive copy of a gene that lacks introns in contrast to the interrupted structure of the active gene. Such genes presumably originated by the reverse transcription of mRNA at some stage during evolution and insertion of this duplex copy of the DNA into the genome.

Prokaryote: The unicellular organisms including eubacteria and archaebacteria (bacteria) that lack a well defined nucleus and other organelles.

Promoter: An element of a gene, it is a region of DNA which directs the proper binding of RNA polymerase to DNA and its activation to a form which is capable of initiating the transcription of the gene.

-10 sequence: Also referred as Pribnow box, it is one of the regions of bacterial promoter with consensus sequence TATAATG centered about 10 bp before the transcription startpoint of the transcriptional unit of a bacterial gene. It is involved in the initial melting of DNA by RNA polymerase.

-35 sequence: The region of bacterial promoter with consensus sequence TTGACA centered about 35 bp before the transcription startpoint of a bacterial gene. It is involved in initial recognition of the promoter by RNA polymerase.

Promoter-proximal element: Any regulatory sequence in eukaryotic DNA that is located close to (within 200 base pairs of) a **promoter** and binds a specific protein thereby modulating transcription of the associated protein-coding gene. Many genes are controlled by multiple promoter-proximal elements.

Proof reading: A cellular mechanism for correcting the errors which may take place in protein or nucleic acid synthesis. It involves the scrutiny of individual units *after* they have been added to the chain.

Prophage: A phage genome covalently integrated as a linear part of the bacterial chromosome.

Protein: A linear polymer of **amino acids** linked together in a specific sequence and usually containing more than 50 residues. The most abundant macromolecules in cell, these serve as **enzymes**, structural elements, **antibodies, hormones, electron carriers**, etc. and are involved in nearly all cellular activities. X-ray crystallographic analysis of proteins has revealed four levels of structure: primary (the sequence of amino acids), secondary, tertiary, and quaternary.

Proton-motive force: The energy equivalent of the proton concentration gradient and electric potential gradient across membrane. In chloroplasts and mitochondria, these gradients are generated by **electron transport**, maintained by the thylakoid or inner mitochondrial membrane, and drive ATP synthesis by **ATP synthase**.

Proto-oncogenes: Present in eukaryotic genome, these are the normal counterparts of the oncogenes carried by certain retroviruses (V-onc). These are referred as *c-onc* and can become oncogenic by certain mutations.

Provirus: A duplex DNA sequence in the eukaryotic chromosome corresponding to the genome of an RNA retrovirus.

Pseudogenes: Inactive but stable components of the genome derived by mutation of an ancestral active gene.

Puff: An expansion of a band of a polytene chromosome associated with the synthesis of RNA at some locus in the band.

Quaternary structure of a protein: The multimeric constitution of a protein.

Quick-stop *dna* mutants: Diffective in DNA replication mechanism, these mutants of *E. coli* cease to replicate immediately when the temperature is increased to 42°C.

R loop: The structure formed when an RNA strand hybridizes with its complementary strand in a DNA duplex, thereby displacing the original strand of DNA in the form of a loop extending over the region of hybridization.

Rapid lysis (*r*) mutants: The mutants that display a change in the pattern of lysis of *E. coli* at the end of an infection by a T-even phage.

Ras protein: A monomeric guanine nucleotide-binding protein that occurs in **signal-transduction pathways** and is activated by binding of ligand to **receptor tyrosine kinases** and other receptors on the cell surface. Ligand binding leads to conversion of the inactive Ras.GDP form to the active Ras.GTP form. Constitutively active forms of Ras are **oncogenes**.

Reading frame: One of three possible ways of reading a nucleotide sequence as a series of codons (triplets).

Reassociation of DNA: It dercribes the pairing of complementary single strands of DNA to form a double stranded moleucle.

Rec A: It is a regulatory protein which is the product of the *recA* locus of *E. coli*. It has dual activities of activating proteases and also being able to exchange single strands of DNA molecules. The protease-activating activity controls the SOS response; the nucleic acid handling facility is involved in recombination-repair pathways.

Receptor: A transmembrane protein, located in the plasma membrane, that binds to a ligand through a specific domain present on the extracellular side. As the binding of ligand results in change in the activity of the cytoplasmic domain which causes the biological action of the ligand. (The same term is also used sometimes for the steroid receptors, which are transcription factors that are activated by binding of ligands that are steroids or other small molecules).

Recessive allele: The allele of a gene which is obscured in the phenotype of a heterozygote by the dominant allele, often due to inactivity or absence of the product of the recessive allele.

Reciprocal recombination: The production of new genotypes with the reverse arrangements of alleles according to maternal and paternal origin.

Reciprocal translocation: Such process exchanges part of one chromosome with the part of another chromosome.

Recombinant progeny: A daughter cell or organism which has a different genotype from that of either parent.

Recombinant joint: The point at which two recombining molecules of duplex DNA are connected (the edge of the heteroduplex region).

Recombinant nodules (nodes): The dense objects present on the synaptonemal complex; could be involved in crossing-over.

Recombination-repair: A mode of filling a gap in one strand of duplex DNA by retrieving a homologous single strand from another duplex.

Regulatory gene: The gene which codes for an RNA or a protein product whose function is to control the expression of other genes.

Regulon: A group of genes or operons that are coordinately regulated even though some or all, may be spatially distant within the chromosome or genome.

Relaxed mutants: Specialized mutants of *E. coli* that do not display the stringent response to starvation for amino acids or other nutritional deprivation.

Relaxed replication control: The ability of some plasmids to continue replicating even after the bacteria have ceased to divide.

Release (termination) factors: The protein factors that respond to termination codons and cause the release of the completed polypeptide chain and dissociation of ribosome from mRNA, thus causing the termination of translation.

Renaturation: The reassociation of denatured complementary single strands of a DNA double helix.

Repetition frequency: The (integral) number of copies of a given sequence present in the haploid genome; equals 1 for nonrepetitive DNA, 2 for repetitive DNA.

Repetitive DNA: The DNA species that behaves in a reassociation reaction as though many (related or identical) sequences are present in the component, allowing any pair of complementary sequences to reassociate.

Replacement sites: The loci in a gene at which the mutations alter the amino acid that was coded by original codon.

Replication-defective virus: A mutant virus that has lost one or more genes essential for completing the infective cycle.

Replication eye: A region of genome in which DNA has been replicated within a longer, unreplicated region.

Replication fork: The point at which the two strands of parental duplex DNA get separated so that the replication of DNA can proceed.

Replicative transposition: The movement of a transposon by a mechanism in which first it is replicated, and then one copy is transferred to a new site while one copy remains at the original locus.

Replicon: The unit of the genome in which DNA is replicated. It contains a single origin for the initiation of replication.

Replisome: The multiprotein structure that assembles at the bacterial replication fork to undertake synthesis of DNA. It contains DNA polymerase, other enzymes and factors needed for DNA replication.

Reporter gene: A gene which codes for a product which can be easily assayed and used as a marker, such as chloramphenicol transacetylase. The coding region of such genes may be connected to any promoter of interest so that expression of this gene can be used to assay the promoter function.

Repression: The ability of bacteria to prevent synthesis of certain enzymes when the final products of enzyme catalysed reactions are present in the cell; more generally, this term refers to inhibition of transcription (or translation) by the binding of repressor protein to a specific site on DNA (or mRNA).

Repressor protein: The regulatory proteins that bind to operator on DNA or RNA to prevent transcription or tanslation, respectively.

Residue: That part of a **monomer** (amino acid, sugar, nucleotide) that is retained as part of a **polymer** following chemical linkage of the monomers.

Resolvase: It is the enzyme activity involved in site-specific recombination between two transposons present as direct repeats in a cointegrate structure.

Restriction enzymes: Sequence specific endonucleases which recognize a specific short sequence of (usually) unmethylated DNA and cleave the duplex, sometimes at target site, sometimes elsewhere, depending on the type and nature of enzyme. Evolved as a protection against invading DNA molecules of foreign origin, these enzymes are very important in genetic engineering experiments and recombinant DNA technology.

Restriction fragment length polymorphism (RFLP): This term refers to inherited differences in sites for restriction enzymes (for example, caused by base changes in the target site) that result in differences in the lengths of the fragments produced by cleavage with the relevant restriction enzyme. RFLPs are used for genetic mapping to link the genome directly to a conventional genetic marker.

Restriction map: A linear array of sites on DNA which can be cleaved by various restriction enzymes.

Retroposon: A transposon that mobilizes via an RNA form; the DNA element is transcribed into RNA, and then reverse-transcribed into DNA, which is inserted at a new site in the genome.

Retro-regulation: It is the ability of a sequence present downstream of initiation codon to regulate the translation of an mRNA.

Retrovirus: A type of eukaryotic virus containing an RNA genome that replicates in cells by first making a DNA copy of the RNA, a process termed **reverse transcription**. This proviral DNA is inserted into cellular chromosomal DNA, and gives rise to further genomic RNA as well as the mRNAs for viral proteins.

Reverse translation: The synthesis of complementary DNA to an RNA using the RNA as template. It is accomplished *in vitro* by the enzyme reverse transcriptase, which is present only in retroviruses.

Reverse translation: A technique for isolating genes (or mRNAs) by their ability to hybridize with a short oligonucleotide sequence prepared by predicting the nucleic acid sequence from the known amino acid sequence of the protein.

Reversion of mutation: A change in DNA that either reverses the original alteration (true reversion) or compensates for it through a second mutation at another site in the same gene which nullifies the effect of first mutation and thus provides the original phenotype.

Revertants: The cells which are derived by reversion of a mutant cell or organism.

Rho factor: A protein involved in assisting bacterial RNA polymerase to terminate transcription at certain (rho-dependent) sites.

Rho-independent terminators: These are the sequences of DNA that cause *E. coli* RNA polymerase to terminate *in vitro* in the absence of rho factor. These sequences direct the RNA to attain a specific secondary structure which is unstable and results in its dissociation from the template DNA.

Ribozymes: Ribonucleic acid molecules with catalytic activities; RNA enzymes.

Rifamycins: A group of antibiotics that inhibit transcription in bacteria.

Right splicing junction: The boundary between the right end (3′ end) of an intron and the left end (5′ end) of the adjacent exon.

RNAase (RNase): An enzyme that cleaves the phosphodiester bond of an RNA molecule to break it. These may be specific or nonspecific in their action.

RNA-driven hybridization reactions: The hybridization reactions which use an excess of RNA to react with all the complementary sequences in a single-stranded preparation of DNA.

RNA polymerase: The main enzyme involved in transcription process that synthesizes RNA using a DNA template (formally described as DNA-dependent RNA polymerase). It is primer independent and can initiate a new RNA chain.

RNA replicase: An enzyme that synthesizes RNA using an RNA template (used for replication by certain RNA viruses such as reoviruses).

Rolling circle: A mode of DNA replication in which a replication fork proceeds around a circular template for an indefinite number of revolutions; the DNA strand newly synthesized in each revolution displaces the strand synthesized in the previous revolution, giving a tail containing a linear series of sequences complementary to the circular template strand. Specific nucleases later cleave and release individual copies of genome which form the provirus.

Rot: The product of RNA concentration and time of incubation in an RNA-driven hybridization reaction.

Rough ER: The region of endoplasmic reticulum which is associated with ribosomes. These ribosomes attach to ER in co-translational manner and give the characteristic rough texture to ER, hence the name.

S phase: The restricted part of the eukaryotic cell cycle during which the synthesis of DNA takes place.

S1 nuclease: An endonuclease enzyme that specifically degrades unpaired (single-stranded) sequences of DNA.

Salvage pathway: Synthesis of a biomolecule, such as a nucleotide, from intermediates in the degradative pathway for the biomolecule; a recycling pathway, as distinct from a de novo pathway.

Sarcoplasmic reticulum: Network of membranes, derived from the smooth endoplasmic reticulum, that surrounds each **myofibril** in a muscle cell and sequesters Ca^{+2} ions into the cytosol, triggering coordinated contraction along the length of the cell.

Satellite DNA: Highly repeated, nontranslated segments of a DNA in eukaryotic chromosomes; most often associated with the centromeric region. Its function is not clear.

Saturation hybridization: It refers to experiments which have a large excess of one component, causing all complementary sequences of the other component to get annealed and undergo duplex formation.

Scaffold of a chromosome: A proteinaceous structure in the shape of a sister chromatid pair, which is generated when the chromosomes are depleted of histones.

Scarce (complex) mRNA: Also referred as rare mRNA, this group of mRNAs consists of a large number of individual mRNA species (the majority), each of which is present in one or very few copies per cell.

scRNA: A group of several small cytoplasmic RNA molecules present in the cytoplasm and (sometimes) in nucleus also when these are known as snRNA.

scRNPs: Pronounced as 'scrups', these are small cytoplasmic ribonucleoproteins (scRNAs associated with a number of specific proteins).

Second messenger: An intracellular **signaling molecule** whose concentration increases (or decreases) in response to binding of an extracellular **ligand** to a cell-surface receptor and which participates in mediating the cellular response to the ligand. Examples include **cAMP**, Ca^{+2}, diacylglycerol, and inositol 1,4,5-triphosphate.

Secondary structure: In proteins, local folding of a polypeptide chain into regular structures including the α **helix**, β **pleated sheet**, and U-shaped turns and loops.

Segmentation genes: The genes that are concerned with controlling the number or the polarity of body segments in insects.

Selection: The use of particular conditions which allow the survival of only those cells which have a particular phenotype.

Semiconservative replication: This mode of replication is accomplished by the separation of the two strands of a parental duplex DNA, each strand then acts as a template for the synthesis of a complementary strand. The DNA replication takes place by this mode.

Semidiscontinuous replication: This is the mode of replication of DNA in which one new strand is synthesized continuously while the other is synthesized in a discontinuous manner. The cellular DNA replication is semidiscontinuous.

Septum: The structure that is formed at the center of a bacterial cell to divide it into two daughter cells at the end of a mitotic division cycle.

Sequence: The linear order of **monomers** in polymeric molecules, especially proteins and nucleic acids. Various techniques collectively termed sequencing, are used to determine the identity and position of each monomer in a polymer.

Serum dependence: The term describes the need of eukaryotic cells for factors contained in serum in order to grow in culture.

Sex chromosomes: These are the chromosomes whose contents are different in the two sexes; usually labeled X and Y (or W and Z), the females have XX (or WW), while the males have XY (or WZ).

Sex plasmid: Actually an episome; it is able to initiate the process of conjugation in bacteria, by which chromosomal material of one bacterium is transferred to another bacterium.

Shino-Dalgarno (SD) sequence: Also known as ribosome binding site (RBS), this sequence contains a part or all of the polypurine sequence AGGAGG and is located on bacterial mRNA just prior to an AUG initiation codon. It is complementary to the sequence at the 3′ end of 16S rRNA and is involved in binding of ribosome to mRNA and proper postioning of 30S subunit during the initiation of translation.

Short-period interspersion: A pattern in a genome where moderately repetitive DNA sequences of ~300 bp alternate with nonrepetitive sequences of ~1000 bp.

Shotgun experiment: The cloning of the entire genome in the form of randomly generated fragments.

Shuttle vector: A hybrid plasmid constructed to have origins of replication for two different hosts, such as, *E. coli* and *S. cerevisiae*, so that it can be used to carry a foreign gene or DNA sequence both in prokaryotes as well as eukaryotes.

Sickle-cell anemia: A human disease characterized by defective hemoglobin molecules; caused by a homozygous allele coding for the ß chain of hemoglobin.

Sigma factor: One of the subunits of bacterial RNA polymerase, it is essential for initiation of transcription. It causes the specific binding of RNA polymerase to promoter region of the genes.

Signal hypothesis: A theory that describes the role of about 15-30 amino acid long N-terminal sequence of a secretory protein in attaching the nascent polypeptide to membrane in a co-translational manner. It depicts that the mRNA and ribosome are attached to membrane via the N-terminal end of the protein at the time of its synthesis.

Signal sequence: The region of a protein (usually N-terminal) responsible for its co-translational insertion into membranes of the endoplasmic reticulum. It is about 15-30 amino acid long and is made up of a hydrophobic region followed by a negatively charged region. Following the entry of polypeptide into membrane, the signal sequence is cleaved by specific signal peptidase; the mature protein does not have this sequence.

Signal transduction: The process by which a receptor interacts with a ligand at the surface of the cell and then transmits a signal to trigger a pathway within the cell.

Silent mutations: A mutation that will not change the product of a gene.

Silent sites in a gene: Those positions within a gene at which mutations do not alter its expression product.

SINE: A class of retroposons that are found as short interspersed repeats in mammalian genome. These are derived from transcripts of RNA polymerase III.

Single-strand assimilation: The ability of RecA protein to cause a single strand of DNA to displace its homologous strand in a duplex; that is, the single strand is assimilated into the duplex.

Single-strand exchange: A reaction in which one of the strands of a duplex DNA leaves its former partner and instead pairs with the complementary strand in another molecule, displacing its homolog in the second duplex.

Sister chromatids: Two copies of a chromosome produced by its replication during cell division.

Site-specific mutagenesis: A set of methods used to create specific alterations in the sequence of a gene at desired location. This process is commonly used to modify genes during recombinant DNA experiments.

Site-specific recombination: A recombination that occurs between two specific (not necessarily homologous) sequences, as in phage integration/excision or resolution of cointegrate structures during transposition.

Slow-stop *dna* mutants: The mutant bacteria that complete the current round of bacterial replication but cannot initiate another round of replication at 42°C, thus inhibiting further growth when temperature is raised.

Smooth ER: A regions of endoplasmic reticulum devoid of ribosomes.

snRNA (small nuclear RNA): Many small RNA species present in the nucleus; several of the snRNAs are involved in splicing or other RNA processing reactions.

SnRNPs: Pronounced as 'snurps', these are small nuclear ribonucleoprotein practicles (SnRNAs associated with specific proteins).

Somatic cells: All the cells of an organism except those of the germ line. The somatic cells are diploid in nature.

Somatic mutation: A mutation occurring in a somatic cell, and therefore affecting only one generation of an organism, it is not inherited to next generation.

SOS box: The DNA sequence (operator) of ~20 bp recognized by LexA repressor protein which play an important role in SOS response.

SOS response: The coordinated induction of many enzymes, including repair activities, in response to irradiation or other major damage to DNA. It results from the activation of protease activity by RecA to cleave LexA repressor.

Southern blotting: The procedure for transferring denatured DNA from an agarose gel to a nitro-cellulose filter where it can be hybridized with a complementary nucleic acid.

Splicing: The removal of introns from the primary transcript and joining of exons during the maturation of RNA; thus introns are spliced out, while exons are spliced together.

Spontaneous mutations: The mutations that occur in the absence of any added reagent to increase the mutation rate.

Sporulation: Generation of a spore by bacterium by morphological conversion or by yeast as the product of meiosis.

SSB: The single-strand nucleic acid binding protein, that binds to single-stranded DNA (orRNA). These proteins stabilize the single-stranded form of DNA and play an important role in certain metabolic processes such as DNA replication.

Staggered cuts: Such cuts are made in duplex DNA when the two strands are cleaved at different points near each other.

Start point (start site): The position on DNA corresponding to the first base incorporated into RNA during transcription. It is the beginning of a transcription unit.

Stem: the base-paired segment of a hairpin.

Sticky ends: Complementary single stands of DNA that protrude from opposite ends of a duplex or from ends of different duplex molecules; can be generated by staggered cuts in duplex DNA.

Stop codons: Three triplets (UAA, UAG, UGA) which do not code for any amino acid and do not have corresponding tRNAs. These result in termination of protein synthesis.

Strand displacement: A mode of replication of some viruses in which a new DNA strand grows by displacing the previous (homologous) strand of the duplex.

Streptolydigins: A group of compounds that inhibit the elongation of transcription by bacterial RNA polymerase.

Stringent replication: The process describes the limitation of single-copy plasmids to replicate *pari passu* with the bacterial chromosome.

Stringent response: The ability of a bacterium to shut down synthesis of tRNAs and ribosomes in a nutritionally poor-growth medium.

Structural gene: The genes which code for any RNA or protein product other than a regulator molecule.

Supercoiling: The coiling of a closed duplex DNA in space so that it crosses over its own axis.

Super-repressed gene: A gene which is noninducible and has been permanently switched off.

Suppressor (extragenic) gene: A gene which usually codes for a mutant tRNA that reads the mutated codon either in the sense of the original codon or to give an acceptable substitute for the original meaning.

Suppressor (intragenic): A compensating mutation that restores the original reading frame after a frameshift.

Svedberg (S): A unit of measure of the rate at which a particle sediments in a centrifugal field.

Symbiosis: Intimate association between two organisms of different species from which both derive a long-term selective advantage.

Symport: Form of co-transport in which a membrane carrier protein transports two solute species across the membrane in the same direction.

Synopsis: The association of the two pairs of sister chromatids representing homologous chromosomes that occurs at the start of meiosis; the resulting structure is called a bivalent.

Synthase: Enzymes that catalyze condensation reactions in which no nucleoside triphosphate is required as an energy source.

Syntenic: The genetic loci that lie on the same chromosome.

Synthetases: Enzymes that catalyze condensation reactions using ATP or another nucleoside triphosphate as an energy source.

T cells: The mean lymphocytes of the T (thymic) lineage; may be subdivided into several functional types. They carry TcR (T-cell receptor) and are involved in the cell-mediated immune response.

T_m: The melting temperature of a double stranded DNA.

Tandem repeats: Multiple copies of the same sequence lying in a series.

TATA box: a conserved A.T-rich septamer found about 25 bp before the startpoint of each eukaryotic RNA polymerase II transcription unit; may be involved in positioning the enzyme for correct initiation. It has the same function as the Pribnow box in prokaryotes.

Temperature-sensitive mutation: Such mutations create a gene product that is functional at low temperature but inactive at higher temperature (the reverse relationship is usually called cold-sensitive).

Template: A molecular "mold" that dictates the structure of another molecule; most commonly, one strand of DNA that directs synthesis of a **complementary DNA** strand during DNA replication or of an RNA during **transcription**. An RNA molecule serves as template for RTase and RNA replicase.

Terminal redundancy: The repetition of the same sequence at both ends of (for example) a phage genome.

Termination codon: One of the three triplet sequences, UAG (amber), UAA (ochre), or UGA (opal) that cause termination of protein synthesis; not coding for any amino acid and not having a corresponding tRNA molecule, these are also called "nonsense" codons.

Terminal transferase: An enzyme that catalyzes the addition of a stretch of nucleotide residues of a single kind to the 3′ end of DNA chains.

Terminal factors: Protein factors of the cytosol required in releasing a completed polypeptide chain from a ribosome; also known as release factors.

Termination sequence: A DNA sequence that appears at the end of a transcriptional unit and signals the end of transcription.

Terminator: A sequence of DNA, represented at the end of the transcriptional unit that causes RNA polymerase to terminate transcription and release the primary transcript.

Tertiary structure of a protein: Three dimensional organization of the polypeptide chain in space.

Thalassemia: A disease of red blood cells resulting from lack of or defect in either the α or the β globin.

Thymine dimer: Chemically crosslinked pair of adjacent thymine residues in DNA, which are produced as a result of damage induced by ultraviolet irradiation.

Topoisomerase: The enzyme that can change the linking number of DNA (in steps of 1 by type I; in steps of 2 by type II).

Topological isomers: The molecules of DNA that are identical except for a difference in the linking number.

Tracer: A bio-molecule containing suitable **label** such as a radioactively labeled nucleic acid component included in a reassociation reaction in an amount too small to influence the progress of reaction or the radiolabeled hormone used in RIA reactions.

Trailer: The nontranslated sequence at the 3′ end of an mRNA down stream of the termination codon.

Trans **configuration:** It refers to the presence of two sites on two different molecules of DNA (chromosomes).

Transcribed spacer: The part of an rRNA transcription unit that is transcribed but discarded during maturation; it does not give rise to any part of mature rRNA.

Transcription: The synthesis of RNA corresponding to a DNA template. This is the first process in deciphering the genetic information from its stored form to functional form.

Transcription factor (TF): General term for any protein, other than RNA polymerase, required to initiate or regulate **transcription** in eukaryotic cells. A number of general factors, required for transcription of all genes, participate in formation of the transcription initiation complex near the start site. Specific factors stimulate (or repress) transcription of particular genes by binding to their regulatory sequences (e.g., **enhancers, promoter-proximal elements).**

Transcription unit: The region of the gene located between the sites of transcriptional initiation and transcriptional termination which is copied by RNA polymerase to produce RNA. In prokaryotes it may include more than one gene (polycistronic genes).

Transduction: The transfer of a bacterial gene from one bacterium to another by a phage; a phage carrying host as well as its own genes is called transducing phage. Also describes the acquisition and transfer of eukaryotic cellular sequences by retroviruses.

Transfection of eukaryotic cells: The acquisition of new genetic markers by incorporation of added DNA.

Transfection of bacteria: The acquisition of new genetic markers by incorporation of added DNA.

Transfection of eukaryotic cells: The conversion of an eukaryotic cell to a state of unrestrained growth in culture, resembling or identical with the tumorigenic condition.

Transgene: A cloned gene that is introduced and stably incorporated into a plant or animal and is passed on to successive generations.

Transgenic animals: The engineered animals created by introducing new DNA sequences into the germline, usually by its addition to the ovum.

Transit peptide: The short leader sequence cleaved from proteins that are imported into cellular organelles by post-translational passage through the membrane.

Transition: A mutation in which one pyrimidine is substituted by the other or in which one purine is substituted for the other.

Translation: The synthesis of protein corresponding to the mRNA template. This is the final step in deciphering the stored genetic information to its ultimate product, the proteins.

Translational control: The regulation of expression of a gene by controlling the rate of its translation on the ribosome, usually at the initiation of protein synthesis.

Translation repressor: The repressor that binds to an mRNA, blocking translation.

Translocation of a chromosome: A rearrangement of chromosomes in which part of a chromosome is detached by breakage and then it gets attached to some other chromosome.

Translocation of a gene: The appearance of a new copy of a gene at a location in the genome elsewhere than the location of the original copy.

Translocation of a protein: The movement of proteins across a membrane.

Translocation of the ribosome: The movement of ribosome along the mRNA, one codon at a time after the addition of each amino acid to the polypeptide chain during translation.

Transmembrane protein: These are the integral component of a membrane; the protein has a hydrophobic region or regions which resides in the membrane and hydrophilic regions which are exposed on one or both sides of the membrane.

Transposase: The enzyme activity involved in the insertion of transposon at a new site. This enzyme is coded by the corresponding transposon itself.

Transposition: The movement of a gene or set of genes from one site in the genome to another.

Transposition immunity: The ability of certain tansposons to prevent other transposons of the same type from transposing to the same DNA molecule.

Transposon: A DNA sequence able to insert itself at a new location in the genome (without any sequence relationship with the target locus). These are also referred as jumping genes.

Transposition: The movement of a transposon to a new site in the genome.

Transvection: The ability of a locus to influence activity of an allele on the other homolog only when two chromosomes are synapsed.

Transversion: A mutation in which a purine is replaced by a pyrimidine or vice versa.

Tropic hormone (tropin): A peptide hormone that stimulates a specific target gland to secrete its hormone; for example, thyrotropin produced by the pituitary stimulates secretion of thyroxine by the thyroid.

Twisting number of a DNA; The number of base pairs divided by the number of base pairs per turn of the double helix.

Underwinding of DNA: It is provided by the negative supercoiling (because the double helix is itself coiled in the opposite sense from the intertwining of the strands).

Unequal crossing-over: A recombination event in which the two recombining sites lie at nonidentical locations in the two parental DNA molecules.

Unidirectional replication: The movement of a single replication fork from a given origin, which is growing in only one direction.

Uninducible mutants: The mutants that cannot be induced by a molecule which is an inducer for a wild type organism.

Unipotent: Referring to a **stem cell** capable of giving rise to only a single type of differentiated cell. When a cell has the capacity to give rise to more than one type of cells it is referred as multipotent and if a cell can grow to become a fully differentiated organism, it is called a totipotent cell.

Unscheduled DNA synthesis: Any DNA synthesis occurring outside the S phase of the eukaryotic cell.

Up promoter mutations: The mutation that increases the activity of the promoter of a gene resulting in enhanced frequency of initiation of transcription.

Upstream: This term identifies sequences proceeding in the direction opposite to direction of expression i.e. towards 5′ direction, for example, the bacterial promoter is upstream from the transcription unit, the initiation codon is upstream of the coding region.

Upstream activating sequence (UAS): Any protein-binding regulatory sequence in the DNA of yeast and other simple eukaryotes that is necessary for maximal gene expression and is equivalent to an enhancer or **promoter-proximal element** in higher eukaryotes.

URF: It is an open (unidentified) reading frame, presumably coding for a protein, however, no product (protein) for this sequence is found in the cell.

V gene: The sequence coding for the major part of the variable (N-terminal) region of an immuno-globulin chain.

Variegation of phenotype: This is produced by a change in genotype during somatic development.

Vesicles: These are small bodies bounded by membrane, derived by budding from one membrane, often able to fuse with another membrane. A number of vesicles are involved in the transportation of proteins or other macromolecules from one subcellular location to other.

Virion: It is the physical form of a virus particle (irrespective of its ability to infect cells and reproduce).

Virulent phage mutants: The mutants that are unable to establish lysogeny.

Western blotting: The technique for detecting specific proteins in a mixture. After separation of the proteins by gel electrophoresis proteins are **blotted** to a filter paper and specific protein of interest are detected by labeled antibodies.

Wobble hypothesis: This hypothesis accounts for the ability of a tRNA to recognize more than one codon by unusual (non-G.G, A.T) pairing with the third base of a codon. Such a pairing is relatively loose. However, wobbling occurs only between two codons for the same amino acid and never between codons for different amino acids.

Writhing number: The number of times a duplex axis crosses over itself in space.

Zero time-binding DNA: The DNA that enters the duplex form at the start of a reassociation reaction; results from intramolecular reassociation of inverted repeats.

Zinc finger protein: These DNA binding protein motifs have a repeated motif of amino acids with characteristic spacing of cysteines that may be involved in binding zinc; is characteristic of some proteins that bind DNA and/or RNA.

Zoo blot: The use of Southern blotting to test the ability of a DNA probe from one species to hybridize with the DNA from the genomes of a variety of other species.

Zymogen: An inactive precursor of an enzyme; for example pepsinogen, the precursor of pepsin.

Index